Fourth Edition

Appleton & Lange's Review for the

USMLE STEP 1

D0206545

Michael W. King, PhD
Professor
Department of Biochemistry and Molecular Biology
Indiana University School of Medicine
Center for Regenerative Biology and Medicine
Terre Haute, Indiana

Appleton & Lange Reviews/McGraw-Hill
Medical Publishing Division

New York   Chicago   San Francisco   Lisbon   London   Madrid   Mexico City
New Delhi   San Juan   Seoul   Singapore   Sydney   Toronto

McGraw-Hill

A Division of The **McGraw·Hill** Companies

Appleton & Lange's Review for the USMLE Step 1, Fourth Edition

Copyright © 2003 by The **McGraw-Hill Companies**, Inc. All rights reserved. Printed in the United States of America. Except as permitted under the United States Copyright Act of 1976, no part of this publication may be reproduced or distributed in any form or by any means, or stored in a data base or retrieval system, without the prior written permission of the publisher.

Previous editions copyright © 2000, 1996, 1993, 1990 by Appleton & Lange; copyright © 1985 by Fleschner Publishing Co.

2 3 4 5 6 7 8 9 0   VFM/VFM   0 9 8 7 6 5 4

ISBN: 0-07-137742-5

This book was set in Palatino by Rainbow Graphics.
The editors were Catherine A. Johnson, Janene Matragrano, and Mary E. Bele.
The production supervisor was Catherine H. Saggese.
The cover designer was Aimee Nordin.
Von Hoffmann Graphics was printer and binder.

This book is printed on acid-free paper.

Library of Congress Cataloging-in-Publication Data

Appleton & Lange's review for the USMLE step 1 / [edited by] Michael W. King.–4th ed.
    p. ; cm.
  Includes bibliographical references.
  ISBN 0-07-137742-5 (alk. paper)
   1. Medicine–Examinations, questions, etc. 2. Medicine–Examinations, questions, etc.
I. Title: Appleton and Lange's review for the USMLE step 1. II. Title: Review for the USMLE step 1. III. King, Michael W. (Michael William)
  [DNLM: 1. Medicine–Examination Questions. 2. Medicine–Outlines. W 18.2 A649 2002]
R834.5 .A6634 2002
610'.76–dc21
                                      2002025495

International ISBN: 0-07-121216-7

Copyright © 2003. Exclusive rights by **The McGraw-Hill Companies,** Inc., for manufacturing and export. This book cannot be re-exported from the country to which it is consigned by McGraw-Hill. The International Edition is not available in North America.

Contents

Contributors

James F. P. Dixon, PhD
Professor
Department of Pathology and Laboratory Medicine
Keck School of Medicine
University of Southern California
Los Angeles, California

Taihung Duong, PhD
Associate Professor
Department of Anatomy and Cell Biology
Indiana University School of Medicine
Terre Haute Center for Medical Education
Terre Haute, Indiana

Bertram G. Katzung, MD, PhD
Professor Emeritus
Department of Cellular and Molecular
Pharmacology
University of California, San Francisco
San Francisco, California

Nicholas J. Legakis, MD
Professor and Chairman
Department of Microbiology and Immunology
University of Athens School of Medicine
Athens, Greece

Hoyle Leigh, MD
Professor
Department of Psychiatry
University of California, San Francisco
Fresno, California

Vishwanath R. Lingappa, MD, PhD
Professor of Physiology and Medicine
University of California, San Francisco
San Francisco, California

Clive R. Taylor, MD, DPhil
Professor and Chair of Pathology
Department of Pathology and Laboratory Medicine
Keck School of Medicine
University of Southern California
Los Angeles, California

Karen D. Tsoulas, MD
Instructor
Department of Family Medicine
Keck School of Medicine
University of Southern California
Los Angeles, California

William W. Yotis, PhD
Professor Emeritus of Microbiology and
Immunology
Loyola University
Stritch School of Medicine
Maywood, Illinois
Clinical Professor of Microbiology and
Immunology
University of South Florida
College of Medicine
Tampa, Florida

Preface

Success on the United States Medical Licensing Examination (USMLE) Step 1 requires a thorough understanding of the basic sciences covered in the first and second years of medical education. In order to offer the most complete and accurate review book, we assembled a team of authors and editors from around the country who are engaged in various specialties and involved in both academic and clinical settings. The author team was asked to research and write test questions using the parameters set forth by the National Board of Medical Examiners. All of the subjects, types of questions, and techniques that will be encountered on the USMLE Step 1 are presented in this book.

Appleton & Lange's Review for the USMLE Step 1 is designed to provide you with a comprehensive review of the basic sciences as well as a valuable self-assessment tool for exam preparation. A total of 1,200 questions are included in this edition.

Key Features and Use:

- Approximately 150 questions are covered in the basic sciences: Anatomy, Physiology, Biochemistry, Microbiology, Pathology, Pharmacology, and Behavioral Sciences.

- Questions are followed by a section with answers and detailed explanations referenced to the most current and popular resources available.

- A subspecialty list at the end of each chapter helps assess strengths and weaknesses, thus pinpointing areas for concentration during exam preparation.

- Three practice tests simulating the USMLE Step 1 are included at the end of this text.

We believe that you will find the questions, explanations, and format of *Appleton & Lange's Review for the USMLE Step 1* to be of great assistance to you during your review. We wish you luck on the USMLE Step 1.

The Editors and the Publisher
August 2002

Review Preparation Guide

If you are planning to prepare for the USMLE Step 1, then this book is designed for you. Here, in one package, is a comprehensive review resource with 1,200 examination-type basic science multiple-choice questions with referenced, paragraph-length explanations of each answer. In addition, the last section of the book offers three integrated practice tests for self-assessment purposes.

This introduction provides specific information on the USMLE Step 1, information on question types, question-answering strategies, and various ways to use this review.

THE USMLE STEP 1

The USMLE Step 1 has approximately 400 multiple-choice test items, divided into eight blocks of 50 questions, which are administered via computer. Students are allotted one hour to complete each question block. The exam is designed to test knowledge of Anatomy, Physiology, Biochemistry, Microbiology, Pathology, Pharmacology, and Behavioral Sciences. The questions have been proffered by senior academic faculty to test comprehension of basic science concepts that they feel are relevant to the future successful practice of medicine. In order to correctly answer these test questions, examinees may be required to recall memorized facts, to use deductive reasoning, or both. A minority of the questions will employ graphs, photographs, or line drawings that require interpretation.

The application materials you receive for the USMLE Step 1 will more fully discuss the exam procedure, rules of test administration, types of questions asked, and the scope of material you may be tested on.

ORGANIZATION OF THIS BOOK

This book is organized to cover sequentially each of the basic science areas specified by the National Board of Medical Examiners (NBME). There are seven sections, one for each of the basic sciences, plus three integrated practice tests at the end of the review. The sections are as follows:

1. **Anatomy** (including gross and microscopic anatomy; neuroanatomy; and development and control mechanisms).
2. **Physiology** (including general and cellular functions; major body system physiology; energy balance; and fluid and electrolyte balance).
3. **Biochemistry** (including energy metabolism; major metabolic pathways of small molecules; major tissue and cellular structures, properties, and functions; biochemical aspects of cellular and molecular biology; and special biochemistry of tissues).
4. **Microbiology** (including microbial structure and composition; cellular metabolism, physiology, and regulation; microbial and molecular genetics; immunology; bacterial pathogens; virology; and medical mycology and parasitology).
5. **Pathology** (including general and systemic pathology; and pathology of syndromes and complex reactions).

6. **Pharmacology** (including general principles; major body system agents; vitamins; chemotherapeutic agents; and poisoning and therapy of intoxication).

7. **Behavioral Sciences** (including behavioral biology; individual, interpersonal, and social behavior; and culture and society).

8. **Practice Tests** (each includes 100 questions from all seven basic sciences, presented in an integrated format).

Each of the ten chapters is organized in the following order:

1. Questions
2. Answers and Explanations
3. References
4. Subspecialty List

These sections and how you might use them are discussed below.

Question Formats

The style and presentation of the questions have been fully revised to conform with the USMLE Step 1. This will enable you to familiarize yourself with the types of questions to be expected, and provide practice in recalling your knowledge in each format. Following the answers in each chapter is a list of suggested references for additional consultation. Each of the seven basic science chapters contains multiple choice questions composed in the **Single Best Answer** query format (example question 1). This is the most frequently encountered format in the USMLE Step 1. It generally contains a brief statement, followed by five options of which only ONE is ENTIRELY correct. The answer options on the USMLE are lettered A, B, C, D, and E. Although the format for this question type is straightforward, the questions can be difficult because some of the distractors in the answer list are partially correct. An example of this question format follows.

DIRECTIONS (Question 1): Each of the numbered items or incomplete statements in this section is followed by answers or by completions of the statement. Select the ONE lettered answer or completion that is BEST in each case.

1. Liquefaction necrosis is the characteristic result of infarcts in the

(A) brain
(B) heart
(C) kidney
(D) spleen
(E) small intestine

The correct answer is A. There are two ways to attack this style of question. If after reading the query an answer immediately comes to mind, then look for it in the answer list. Alternatively, if no answer immediately comes to mind, or if the answer you thought was obvious is not a choice, then you will need to spend time examining all of the answer options to find the correct one. In this case anything you can do to eliminate an answer option will increase your odds of choosing the correct answer. With this in mind, scan all of the possible answers. Eliminate any that are clearly wrong and all that are only partially right. Even if you can eliminate one or two of the answer choices by this method you will have significantly increased your chance of guessing the right answer from the remaining choices. Always answer every question, even if you have to guess among all five answer choices, because there is no penalty for a wrong answer. Your test score is dependent only on the number of correct answers obtained.

STRATEGIES FOR ANSWERING SINGLE BEST ANSWER QUESTIONS

1. Remember that only one choice can be the correct answer.
2. Read the question carefully to be sure that you understand what is being asked.
3. If you immediately know the answer look for it in the answer choices.
4. If no answer is immediately obvious, quickly scan all the five answer choices for familiarity.
5. Eliminate any answer that is completely wrong or only partially correct. This increases your odds of picking the correct answer from a lesser number of remaining answer choices.
6. If two of the remaining choices are mutually exclusive, the correct answer is probably one of them.
7. Always answer every question even if you have to guess.
8. Don't spend too much time with any one question. In order to finish each 60-minute session you will need to answer a question about every 70 seconds.

Practice Tests

The three 100-question practice tests at the end of the book consist of questions from each of the seven basic sciences. This format mimics the actual exam and enables you to test your skill at answering questions in all of the basic sciences under simulated examination conditions.

The practice test section is organized in the same format as the seven earlier sections: questions; answers, explanations, and references.

HOW TO USE THIS BOOK

There are two logical ways to get the most value from this book. We will call them Plan A and Plan B.

In Plan A, you go straight to the Practice Tests and complete them according to the instructions. This will be a good indicator of your initial knowledge of the subject and will help you identify specific areas for preparation and review. You can now use the first seven chapters of the book to help you improve your relative weak points.

In Plan B, you go through chapters 1 through 7 checking off your answers, and then comparing your choices with the answers and discussions in the book. Once you have completed this process, you can take the Practice Tests and see how well prepared you are. If you still have a major weakness, it should be apparent in time for you to take remedial action.

In Plan A, by taking the Practice Tests first, you get quick feedback regarding your initial areas of strength and weakness. You may find that you have a good command of the material, indicating that perhaps only a cursory review of the seven chapters is necessary. This, of course, would be good to know early on in your exam preparation. On the other hand, you may find that you have many areas of weakness. In this case, you could then focus on these areas in your review—not just with this book, but also with the cited references and with your current textbooks.

It is, however, unlikely that you will not do some studying prior to taking the USMLE (especially since you have this book). Therefore, it may be more realistic to take the Practice Tests after you have reviewed the first seven chapters (as in Plan B). This will probably give you a more realistic type of testing situation since very few of us just sit down to a test without studying. In this case, you will have done some reviewing (from superficial to in-depth), and your Practice Tests will reflect this studying time. If, after reviewing the first seven chapters and taking the Practice Tests, you still have some weaknesses, you can then go back to the first seven chapters and supplement your review with your texts.

SPECIFIC INFORMATION ON THE STEP 1 EXAMINATION

The official source of all information with respect to the United States Medical Licensing Examination Step 1 is the National Board of Medical Examiners (NBME), 3930 Chestnut Street, Philadelphia, PA 19104 *(www.nbme.org)*. Established in 1915, the NBME is a voluntary, nonprofit, independent organization whose sole function is the design, implementation, distribution, and processing of a vast bank of question items, certifying examinations, and evaluative services in the professional medical field. You should contact the NBME directly for information regarding eligibility to sit for the USMLE, or visit the USMLE web site at *www.usmle.org*.

Scoring

Because there is no deduction for wrong answers, you should **answer every question.** Your test is scored in the following way:

1. The number of questions answered correctly is totaled. This is called the raw score.
2. The raw score is converted statistically to a "standard" score on a scale of 200 to 800, with the mean set at 500. Each 100 points away from 500 is one standard deviation.
3. Your score is compared statistically with the criteria set by the scores of the second-year medical school candidates for certification in the June administration during the prior four years. This is what is meant by the term, "criterion referenced test."
4. A score of 500 places you around the 50th percentile. A score of 380 is the minimum passing score for Step 1; this probably represents about the 12th to 15th percentile. If you answer 50 percent or so of the questions correctly, you will probably receive a passing score.

Remember: You do not have to pass all seven basic science components, although you will receive a standard score in each of them. A score of less than 400 (about the 15th percentile) on any particular area is a real cause for concern as it will certainly drag down your overall score. Likewise, a 600 or better (85th percentile) is an area of great relative strength. (You can use the practice test included in this book to help determine your areas of strength and weakness well in advance of the actual examination.)

Physical Conditions

The NBME is very concerned that all their exams be administered under uniform conditions in the numerous centers that are used. Since 1999, the USMLE examination has been administered electronically. Please visit *www.nmbe.org* for details, or contact your local Prometric center for scheduling and further information.

Standard Abbreviations

ACTH:	adrenocorticotropic hormone
ADH:	antidiuretic hormone
ADP:	adenosine diphosphate
AFP:	α-fetoprotein
AMP:	adenosine monophosphate
ATP:	adenosine triphosphate
ATPase:	adenosine triphosphatase
bid:	2 times a day
BP:	blood pressure
BUN:	blood urea nitrogen
CT:	computed tomography
CBC:	complete blood count
CCU:	coronary care unit
CNS:	central nervous system
CPK:	creatine phosphokinase
CSF:	cerebrospinal fluid
DNA:	deoxyribonucleic acid
DNAse:	deoxyribonuclease
ECG:	electrocardiogram
EDTA:	ethylenediaminetetraacetate
EEG:	electroencephalogram
ER:	emergency room
FAD:	flavin adenine dinucleotide
FSH:	follicle-stimulating hormone
GI:	gastrointestinal
GU:	genitourinary
Hb:	hemoglobin
HCG:	human chorionic gonadotropin
HDL:	high-density lipoprotein
Hct:	hematocrit
IgA, etc.:	immunoglobulin A, etc.
IM:	intramuscular(ly)
IQ:	intelligence quotient
IU:	international unit
IV:	intravenous(ly)
KUB:	kidney, ureter, and bladder
LDH:	lactic dehydrogenase
LDL:	low-density lipoprotein
LH:	luteinizing hormone
LSD:	lysergic acid diethylamide
mRNA:	messenger RNA
NAD:	nicotinamide adenine dinucleotide
NADP:	nicotinamide adenine dinucleotide phosphate
PO:	oral(ly)
prn:	as needed
RBC:	red blood cell
RNA:	ribonucleic acid
RNAse:	ribonuclease
rRNA:	ribosomal RNA
SC:	subcutaneous(ly)
SGOT:	serum glutamic oxaloacetic transaminase
SGPT:	serum glutamic pyruvic transaminase
TB:	tuberculosis
tRNA:	transfer RNA
TSH:	thyroid-stimulating hormone
WBC:	white blood cell

CHAPTER 1

Anatomy
Questions

Taihung Duong, PhD

155
75

48%

DIRECTIONS (Questions 1 through 155): Each of the numbered items or incomplete statements in this section is followed by answers or by completions of the statement. Select the ONE lettered answer or completion that is BEST in each case.

1. A patient returning from an extended backpacking trip complains of pain and paresthesia in the right upper limb. This patient also displays decrease in skin temperature, easy fatigability, and Raynaud's phenomenon in the right upper limb. She has edema in her right hand with distended superficial veins and cyanosis. As you palpate her radial artery, the nurse assistant draws the patient's shoulder inferiorly and posteriorly; this maneuver results in weakening of the pulse of the radial artery. Because she tested positive, you record a diagnosis of costoclavicular syndrome. The test was positive because the following artery was compressed:

   (A) axillary artery
   (B) brachial artery
   (C) radial artery
   (D) subclavian artery
   (E) ulnar artery

Questions 2 and 3

The following observations are noted while examining a patient in the emergency room: The pupil of the left eye is dilated and both direct and consensual pupillary light reflexes are absent in that eye. The left eye also appears to be deviated laterally and downward. The patient exhibits right hemiplegia with increased deep tendon reflexes and a positive Babinski sign on the right.

2. The deficits involving the left eye suggest involvement of the

   (A) left abducens nerve
   (B) left facial nerve
   (C) left oculomotor nerve
   (D) left trigeminal nerve
   (E) right trochlear nerve

3. The presence of unilateral ocular movement deficits, lateral strabismus, and mydriasis in combination with hemiplegia involving the contralateral extremities is referred to as

   (A) capsular hemiplegia
   (B) middle alternating hemiplegia
   (C) superior alternating hemiplegia
   (D) syringomyelia
   (E) Wallenberg syndrome

4. A pregnancy case is complicated by polyhydramnios due to esophageal atresia and tracheoesophageal fistula. The tracheal tube normally develops from the

   (A) first pharyngeal arch
   (B) foregut
   (C) fourth pharyngeal arch
   (D) second pharyngeal arch
   (E) third pharyngeal arch

5. Which of the following statements concerning the eye and photic stimulation is true?

   (A) Horizontal cells form direct synaptic connections with photoreceptors.
   (B) Light stimuli first pass through the lens and then penetrate all of the intervening layers of the retina before striking the photoreceptors.
   (C) The optic disc is located nasally (medially) with respect to the macula.
   (D) While in the dark, photoreceptors are depolarized due to dark current and are releasing neurotransmitter.
   (E) All of the above are true statements.

6. The structure indicated by arrow #1 in Figure 1–1 is the

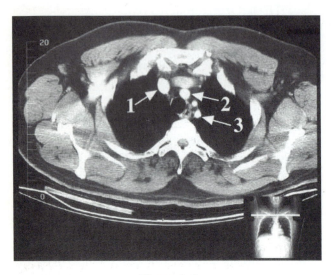

Figure 1–1

   (A) brachiocephalic artery
   (B) left brachiocephalic vein
   (C) left common carotid artery
   (D) right brachiocephalic vein
   (E) superior vena cava

7. In a case of appendicitis, the appendicular artery is thrombosed due to compression of the blood supply of the appendix by inflammatory edema. This artery arises directly from the

   (A) ileocolic artery
   (B) inferior mesenteric artery
   (C) middle colic artery
   (D) right colic artery
   (E) superior mesenteric artery

8. Which statement concerning the inverse myotatic reflex is correct?

   (A) A painful stimulus (i.e., pinprick) to the skin overlying a Golgi tendon organ is the typical mode of stimulation to elicit the reflex.
   (B) Sensory fibers originating in Golgi tendon organs synapse with interneurons that lead to inhibition of the muscle related to that tendon organ.
   (C) Type Ia sensory fibers synapse with interneurons that lead to inhibition of the muscle from which the sensory fibers originated.
   (D) Type Ib sensory fibers do not play a role in this reflex.
   (E) Type II sensory fibers are most active in this reflex and their input excites inhibitory interneurons that synapse with gamma motoneurons.

9. A newborn infant suffers from cyanotic heart disease caused by transposition of the great arteries (TGA). In this situation, the aorta arises from the

   (A) ductus arteriosus
   (B) left atrium
   (C) left ventricle
   (D) right atrium
   (E) right ventricle

10. Occlusion of the anterior spinal artery simultaneously damages the ipsilateral corticospinal fibers in the medullary pyramid and exiting fibers of the hypoglossal nerve. This clinical entity is known as

   (A) inferior alternating hemiplegia
   (B) middle alternating hemiplegia
   (C) spina bifida
   (D) superior alternating hemiplegia
   (E) syringomyelia

11. Internal hemorrhoids, also called piles, are painless and only sensitive to stretch. They are formed by folds of the mucous membrane and submucosa of the anal canal, which contain varicose branches of the

   (A) inferior rectal artery
   (B) inferior rectal vein
   (C) middle rectal artery
   (D) superior rectal artery
   (E) superior rectal vein

12. Which of the following structures in the medulla originates from the alar plate?

   (A) Cochlear nuclei
   (B) Dorsal motor nucleus of the vagus nerve
   (C) Hypoglossal nucleus
   (D) Nucleus ambiguus

13. Occlusion of which of the following vessels affects the entire dorsolateral part of the rostral medulla (level of the restiform body) and produce the lateral medullary (Wallenberg) syndrome?

   (A) Anterior inferior cerebellar artery
   (B) Anterior spinal artery
   (C) Posterior inferior cerebellar artery
   (D) Posterior spinal artery
   (E) Superior cerebellar artery

14. The structure indicated by arrow #5 in Figure 1–2 is the

   (A) abdominal aorta
   (B) inferior vena cava
   (C) left kidney
   (D) right kidney
   (E) small intestine

15. Which statement concerning the lateral medullary syndrome is MOST correct?

   (A) An infarct involving the anterior inferior cerebellar artery is typically the cause of this syndrome.
   (B) Due to involvement of fibers in the medullary pyramid, patients exhibit spastic paralysis involving the contralateral upper extremity.

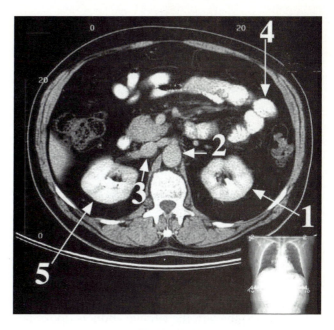

Figure 1–2

   (C) Pain and temperature sensibility is lost over the ipsilateral face and the contralateral trunk and extremities.
   (D) Patients typically exhibit loss of pain and temperature sensibility over the ipsilateral upper and contralateral lower extremities.
   (E) Patients usually exhibit a loss of pain and temperature sensibility on the side of the face contralateral to the lesion.

16. In addition to the inability to voluntarily adduct the right eye, which of the following would you expect to see in a patient with occlusion of paramedian branches of the basilar bifurcation on the right side (Weber syndrome)?

   (A) Complete paralysis of facial expression musculature on the left side
   (B) Deviation of the tongue to the right
   (C) Dilation of the right pupil
   (D) Ipsilateral hemiplegia
   (E) Paralysis of most movements of the left eye

17. While treating a patient with a ruptured eardrum, an attending physician quizzes a first-year resident on the microstructure of the tympanic membrane. The resident describes the inner surface of the eardrum as formed by a

    (A) pseudostratified epithelium
    (B) simple columnar epithelium
    (C) stratified columnar epithelium
    (D) stratified cuboidal epithelium
    (E) stratified squamous epithelium

18. You make the following observations during a neurologic examination of your patient. Both eyes can move conjugately to the right without difficulty. On attempted horizontal gaze to the left, the left eye abducts (looks laterally) but the right eye does not adduct. Based on this information, which of the following is the most likely site of the lesion?

    (A) Abducens nerve on the left
    (B) Abducens nerve on the right
    (C) Medial longitudinal fasciculus on the left
    (D) Medial longitudinal fasciculus on the right
    (E) Trochlear nerve on the right

19. In a medial medullary syndrome that involves a left-sided branch of the anterior spinal artery, which of the following deficits is seen?

    (A) Deviation of the tongue to the left, hemiplegia of arm and leg on left
    (B) Deviation of the tongue to the right, hemiplegia of arm and leg on right
    (C) Loss of conscious proprioception and precise tactile discrimination over the right side of the body exclusive of the face
    (D) Only deviation of the tongue to the left
    (E) Only hemiplegia on the right

20. A newborn infant presents with the Pierre Robin syndrome and displays hypoplasia of the mandible, a cleft palate, and defects of the ears, which render her deaf. During development, the malleus and incus in the middle ear develop from the

    (A) first pharyngeal arch
    (B) second pharyngeal arch
    (C) third pharyngeal arch
    (D) fourth pharyngeal arch
    (E) sixth pharyngeal arch

21. You are asked to evaluate a patient in the neurology clinic. Your neurologic examination reveals the following symptoms: (1) loss of pain and temperature sensation over the left side of the face, (2) loss of pain and temperature sensation in the right arm and leg, and (3) normal tactile and vibratory sensations on the face, body, and extremities. Identify this clinical entity.

    (A) Left capsular infarct
    (B) Left Wallenberg syndrome
    (C) Left Weber syndrome
    (D) Right lateral medullary syndrome
    (E) Syringomyelia

22. The structure indicated by arrow #2 in Figure 1–3 is the

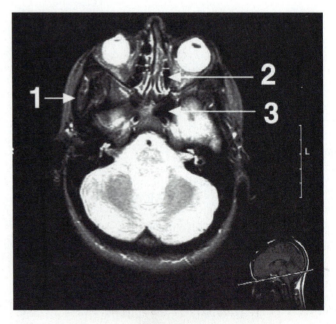

Figure 1–3

(A) ethmoidal sinus

(B) inferior nasal meatus

(C) infratemporal fossa

(D) maxillary sinus

(E) sphenoidal sinus

23. A patient comes to you in the ear, nose, and throat clinic complaining of dizziness. You have a vestibular caloric test done with the following results: Warm caloric irrigation of the right ear produces right beating horizontal nystagmus. Warm caloric irrigation of the left ear produces no response. You conclude which of the following?

(A) Receptors in the right ear have been damaged.

(B) The lateral vestibulospinal tract has been destroyed on the left side.

(C) The left labyrinth or VIIIth nerve has been affected either through trauma or possibly an acoustic neuroma.

(D) The right labyrinth or VIIIth nerve has been affected either through trauma or possibly an acoustic neuroma.

(E) There is no lesion in the vestibular system.

24. The structure indicated by arrow #2 in Figure 1–4 is the

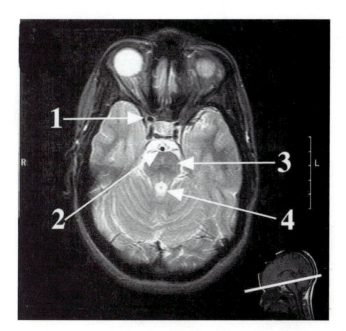

Figure 1–4

(A) basilar artery

(B) fourth ventricle

(C) great cerebral vein of Galen

(D) internal carotid artery

(E) vertebral artery

25. The structure indicated by arrow #2 in Figure 1–4 terminates by dividing into the

(A) anterior and middle cerebral arteries

(B) internal cerebral veins

(C) posterior cerebral arteries

(D) superior cerebellar arteries

(E) vertebral arteries

26. During development, the cerebellum arises from the following brain vesicle

(A) diencephalon

(B) mesencephalon

(C) metencephalon

(D) myelencephalon

(E) telencephalon

27. Which of the following are symptoms of cerebellar disease?

(A) Hyperreflexia

(B) Loss of pain and temperature sensation

(C) Resting tremor

(D) Spasticity

(E) Wide-based stance or staggering gait

28. A 12-year old soccer player suffers from tarsal tunnel syndrome with resulting pain on the heel. The structure involved in this condition is the

(A) anterior tibial artery

(B) deep peroneal (fibular) nerve

(C) peroneal artery

(D) superficial peroneal (fibular) nerve

(E) tibial nerve

Questions 29 and 30

In the emergency room, a 28-year-old male patient reports that he fell from a pine tree while attempting to install a satellite dish. In an effort to break his fall, he grabbed at a passing limb with his right arm but was unable to hold on. After a thorough examination, you suspect that he has damaged the brachial plexus on his right side at the point indicated in Figure 1–5.

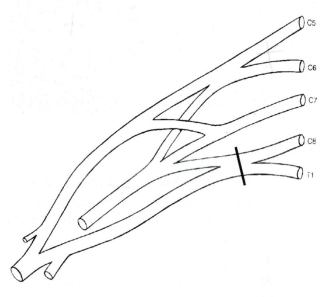

Figure 1–5

29. Which of the following muscles is likely to be the most adversely affected by this injury?

   (A) Biceps brachii
   (B) Deltoid
   (C) Opponens pollicis
   (D) Pronator teres
   (E) Supraspinatus

30. You would expect to observe a cutaneous sensory loss over the

   (A) deltoid muscle just above its insertion
   (B) dorsum of the wrist and the anatomic snuffbox
   (C) lateral side of the forearm
   (D) medial palm and small finger
   (E) web between the thumb and index finger

31. During surgery, the left middle suprarenal artery is ligated prior to resection of the left suprarenal gland. This artery arises from the

   (A) abdominal aorta
   (B) left inferior phrenic artery
   (C) left renal artery
   (D) splenic artery
   (E) thoracic aorta

32. Recanalization of the bile duct after the thirteenth week after fertilization allows for bile produced in the liver to reach the duodenum. However, if recanalization fails to occur and this cannot be corrected surgically, the affected infant will need a liver transplant. During development, the liver arises from the

   (A) foregut
   (B) hindgut
   (C) midgut
   (D) pleuroperitoneal membrane
   (E) septum transversum

Questions 33 and 34

Your patient presents with sensory loss over the areas indicated in Figure 1–6. He has no obvious motor difficulty.

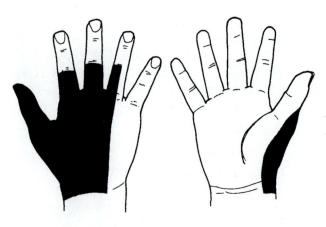

Figure 1–6

33. You suspect that he has damaged the

(A) dorsal cutaneous branch of the ulnar nerve
(B) posterior antebrachial cutaneous nerve
(C) radial nerve in the cubital fossa
(D) superficial branch of the radial nerve
(E) ulnar nerve at the elbow

34. The spinal cord segments supplying this area most likely include

(A) C5 and C6
(B) C6 and C7
(C) C7 and C8
(D) C8 and T1
(E) T1 only

35. A newborn infant, paralyzed from the waist down, suffers from a severe congenital anomaly of the spinal cord where the defect displays protrusion of an open, flattened spinal cord covered by a membrane. This type of congenital anomaly is called

(A) meroanencephaly
(B) spina bifida occulta
(C) spina bifida with meningocele
(D) spina bifida with meningomyelocele
(E) spina bifida with myeloschisis

36. A 27-year old male patient involved in a barroom brawl has suffered trauma to the right testis resulting in a hematocele. Surgical exploration reveals that branches of both the testicular artery and vein are ruptured. The right testicular vein normally drains to the

(A) hepatic vein
(B) inferior vena cava
(C) lumbar veins
(D) right renal vein
(E) superior mesenteric vein

37. The structure indicated by arrow #4 in Figure 1–7 is the

(A) abdominal aorta
(B) colon
(C) liver

(D) spleen
(E) stomach

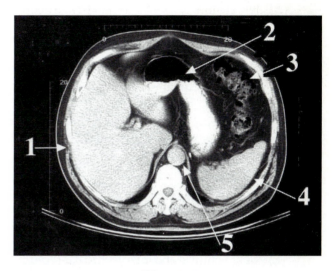

Figure 1–7

38. Which of the following is LEAST likely to be involved in a collateral anastomosis that bypasses an obstruction of the first part of the axillary artery?

(A) Dorsal scapular artery
(B) Posterior humeral circumflex artery
(C) Scapular circumflex artery
(D) Subscapular artery
(E) Suprascapular artery

39. In congenital coarctation of the aorta, aortic blood flow is usually obstructed past the left subclavian artery. Collateral circulation develops so that the superior epigastric arteries anastomosing with the inferior epigastric arteries carry the blood flow from the upper part to the lower part of the trunk. The superior epigastric artery arises from the

(A) anterior intercostals arteries
(B) internal thoracic artery
(C) lateral thoracic artery
(D) musculophrenic artery
(E) posterior intercostal arteries

40. A tumor in the posterior mediastinum most likely involves the

    (A) left atrium
    (B) phrenic nerves
    (C) recurrent laryngeal nerves
    (D) thoracic duct
    (E) tracheal bifurcation

41. Damaged heart muscle resulting from occlusion of the circumflex branch of the left coronary artery is most likely found in the

    (A) apex
    (B) left atrium and left ventricle
    (C) right and left ventricles
    (D) right atrium and right ventricle
    (E) right ventricle and interventricular septum

42. A 40-year old patient, who is a heavy smoker, complains of pain at the root of the neck and over the shoulder. Radiographic examination reveals an abnormal mass invading the mediastinal pleura and suggests that the pain is referred to the root of the neck and over the shoulder. The sensory innervation of the mediastinal pleura is mediated by the

    (A) celiac ganglia
    (B) intercostal nerves
    (C) phrenic nerve
    (D) T1–T4 paravertebral ganglia
    (E) vagus nerve

43. A surgeon's finger placed into the epiploic foramen (of Winslow) is related superiorly to the

    (A) caudate lobe of the liver
    (B) common bile duct
    (C) first part of the duodenum
    (D) head of the pancreas
    (E) hepatic veins

44. Cancer of the testis most likely metastasizes first to which set of nodes?

    (A) Aortic
    (B) Common iliac
    (C) Deep inguinal
    (D) Internal iliac
    (E) Superficial inguinal

45. Derivatives of the hindgut are typically supplied by the

    (A) celiac artery
    (B) ductus arteriosus
    (C) inferior mesenteric artery
    (D) superior mesenteric artery
    (E) umbilical artery

46. As you examine a newborn in the nursery, you notice an apparent oozing of fluid in the area of the umbilicus. You suspect that the leaking fluid is urine and is the result of

    (A) a persistent and patent vitelline duct
    (B) an incomplete obliteration of the lumen of the allantois
    (C) an omphalocele
    (D) an umbilical hernia
    (E) gastroschisis

47. During a surgical operation to repair a cleft palate, the surgeon locates the greater palatine foramen and injects the anesthetic agent. The greater palatine nerve is a branch of the

    (A) facial nerve (VII)
    (B) glossopharyngeal nerve (IX)
    (C) mandibular division of the trigeminal nerve (V)
    (D) maxillary division of the trigeminal nerve (V)
    (E) ophthalmic division of the trigeminal nerve (V)

48. A "claw hand" is usually associated with injury to which of the following nerves?

    (A) Axillary
    (B) Median
    (C) Musculocutaneous
    (D) Radial
    (E) Ulnar

49. Several days after your teenage male patient fell on his outstretched hand he reports increasing pain on movement of his wrist. Your examination reveals particular tenderness in the area of the anatomic snuffbox. Which of the carpal bones has most likely been injured?

(A) Capitate
(B) Hamate
(C) Lunate
(D) Pisiform
(E) Scaphoid

50. Your patient in the emergency room has an obvious fracture of the midshaft of the humerus. You support his extremity as you work and notice that with the forearm in a horizontal position his wrist drops and he is unable to extend his wrist or the metacarpophalangeal joints of the hand. Which nerve has been injured?

(A) Axillary
(B) Median
(C) Musculocutaneous
(D) Radial
(E) Ulnar

51. Cells in the pancreas that secrete glucagon and insulin are the

(A) A and B cells
(B) acinar cells
(C) D cells
(D) pancreatic D$_1$ cells
(E) pancreatic polypeptide cells

52. Damage to the coracobrachialis muscle and to the nerve passing through it could reasonably be expected to produce

(A) diminished cutaneous sensation over the medial forearm
(B) diminished cutaneous sensation over the medial palm
(C) weakened abduction at the shoulder
(D) weakened extension at the elbow
(E) weakened flexion at the shoulder

53. A 30-year-old patient displays ataxia of extremities and asynergy with decomposition of movement. He also has dysmetria (past-pointing phenomenon), dysdiadochokinesia (the inability to perform rapidly alternating movements), and intention tremor. These neurologic signs are characteristic of a lesion in the structure indicated by which arrow in Figure 1–8?

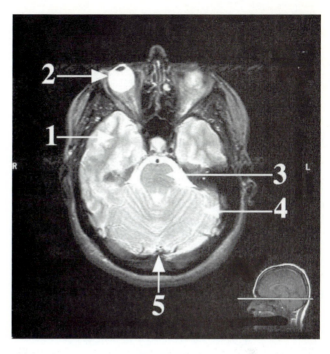

Figure 1–8

(A) #1
(B) #2
(C) #3
(D) #4
(E) #5

54. During cholecystectomy (surgical removal of the gallbladder), the cystic artery must be located and ligated. This arterial supply most commonly arises from the

(A) gastroduodenal artery
(B) hepatic artery proper
(C) left hepatic artery
(D) right hepatic artery
(E) superior pancreaticoduodenal artery

55. Premature infants may suffer from respiratory distress due an inadequate number of terminal air sacs and surfactant deficiency in the lungs. The number of terminal air sacs and the level of surfactant are sufficient for survival

(A) 5 to 17 weeks after fertilization
(B) 16 to 25 weeks after fertilization
(C) 20 weeks after fertilization
(D) 26 to 28 weeks after fertilization
(E) after birth only

56. Which label in Figure 1–9 indicates the typical plane of separation at which retinal detachment occurs?

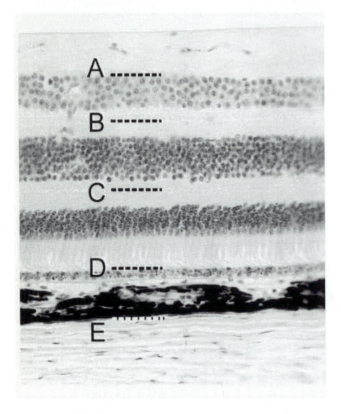

Figure 1–9

(A) A

(B) B

(C) C

(D) D

(E) E

57. The principal natural targets of cytotoxic T cells are

(A) allogenic tissue transplants

(B) bacteria

(C) bacterial toxins

(D) protozoans

(E) virus-infected cells

58. Which of the following is derived from neuroectoderm of the optic cup?

(A) Anterior iridal epithelium

(B) Choriocapillaris

(C) Ciliary muscle

(D) Lateral rectus muscle

(E) Lens epithelium

59. A patient has been admitted for hematemesis (vomiting of blood). Endoscopic examination reveals bleeding esophageal varices resulting from portal obstruction. These varices represent anastomoses between branches of the

(A) inferior vena cava with a patent ductus venosus

(B) left gastric, azygos, and hemiazygos veins

(C) right gastric vein and the inferior vena cava

(D) superior, middle, and inferior rectal veins

(E) veins running on the ligamentum teres and the epigastric veins

60. Which normal cell type is most severely affected by a chemotherapy regimen that includes an antimitotic drug such as vinblastine?

(A) Cardiac muscle cells

(B) Epithelial cells of the lens

(C) Intestinal epithelium

(D) Neurons in dorsal root ganglia

(E) Neurons of the cerebral cortex

61. Which structure most effectively prevents toxic molecules from penetrating an epithelium by passing between adjacent epithelial cells?

(A) Desmosome

(B) Gap junction

(C) Hemidesmosome

(D) Terminal bar

(E) Tight junction

62. Propagation of an action potential into the interior of a skeletal muscle fiber is a function of

(A) muscle spindles

(B) the endomysium

(C) the sarcoplasmic reticulum

(D) transverse (T) tubules

(E) Z lines

63. The macula densa, a component of the juxta-glomerular apparatus, is a specialization of

(A) Bowman's capsule
(B) mesangial cells
(C) the afferent arteriole
(D) the distal tubule
(E) the proximal tubule

64. During an epileptic attack, a patient accidentally bit his tongue resulting in profuse bleeding. Grasping the tongue between the finger and thumb posterior to the laceration stopped the bleeding. This action occluded the branches of the lingual artery. The lingual artery arises directly from the

(A) ascending pharyngeal artery
(B) external carotid artery
(C) facial artery
(D) internal carotid artery
(E) maxillary artery

65. Oxytocin is released from

(A) acidophils in the pars distalis
(B) basophils in the pars distalis
(C) nerve terminals in the hypothalamus
(D) nerve terminals in the pars nervosa
(E) pituicytes in the pars nervosa

66. Which of the following is characterized by an absence of lymphoid follicles and germinal centers?

(A) Axillary lymph node
(B) Peyer's patch
(C) Pharyngeal tonsil
(D) Spleen
(E) Thymus

67. The puborectalis muscle on one side of the pelvis joins with the one on the opposite side to form a U-shaped sling, which is responsible for the anorectal angle, an important structure in maintaining fecal continence. Relaxation of this muscle results in straightening of the anorectal angle and defecation. The puborectalis muscle is innervated by the

(A) nerve to coccygeus
(B) nerve to levator ani
(C) nerve to obturator internus
(D) pelvic splanchnic nerves
(E) pudendal nerve

Questions 68 and 69

A 19-year-old black female is brought to the emergency room complaining of severe abdominal pain that began immediately after eating dinner. The physical examination reveals extreme tenderness in the lower right abdominal quadrant, but no abdominal masses are noted. Her temperature is 100°F. Among other tests, a complete blood count is ordered, with the following findings (normal ranges in parentheses):

Hematocrit	39% (36–46%)
Hemoglobin	14.9 g/dL (12.0–16.0 g/dL)
Total leukocyte count	24,000/mm³
	(4500–11,000/mm³)

DIFFERENTIAL LEUKOCYTE COUNT

Segmented neutrophils	71% (54–62%)
Band form neutrophils	16% (3–5%)
Eosinophils	4% (1–3%)
Basophils	0.2% (0–0.75%)
Lymphocytes	3% (25–33%)
Monocytes	6% (3–7%)

68. For which leukocytes is there an elevation above the normal range in absolute numbers per microliter of blood?

(A) Only band form neutrophils
(B) Only monocytes and lymphocytes
(C) Only neutrophils
(D) Only neutrophils and eosinophils
(E) Only neutrophils, eosinophils, and monocytes

69. Which of the following conditions is most consistent with the laboratory findings?

(A) Acute inflammation in response to bacterial infection
(B) Chronic lymphocytic leukemia
(C) Parasitic worm infection
(D) Severe allergic condition
(E) Sickle cell disease

70. The space of Disse in the liver

    (A) constitutes the initial channel for the flow of bile
    (B) contains formed elements of blood
    (C) is a constituent of the portal triad
    (D) is bordered partly by microvilli of hepatocytes
    (E) is delimited entirely by hepatocytes

71. Production of specific granules occurs mainly during which stage of granulocyte development?

    (A) Granulocyte-colony–forming unit
    (B) Metamyelocyte
    (C) Myeloblast
    (D) Myelocyte
    (E) Promyelocyte

72. The acidophilic staining of the cytoplasm of gastric parietal (oxyntic) cells is most likely attributable to their high content of

    (A) hydrochloric acid
    (B) mitochondria
    (C) rough endoplasmic reticulum
    (D) secretory granules containing intrinsic factor
    (E) secretory granules containing pepsinogen

73. A resident is trying to perform an endotracheal intubation on a patient involved in a car accident. However, bleeding in the upper part of the larynx obscures her view. This region of the larynx is supplied by the superior laryngeal artery, which arises directly from the

    (A) ascending pharyngeal artery
    (B) inferior thyroid artery
    (C) lingual artery
    (D) superior thyroid artery
    (E) vertebral artery

74. In the placenta, maternal blood comes in direct contact with

    (A) connective tissue cells of secondary villi
    (B) endothelial cells of fetal capillaries
    (C) no fetally derived cells
    (D) the cytotrophoblast
    (E) the syncytiotrophoblast

75. Serous cells are glandular acinar cells that produce a watery, proteinaceous fluid. This cell type is most predominant in

    (A) esophageal glands
    (B) intestinal glands (of Lieberkün)
    (C) the parotid gland
    (D) the sublingual gland
    (E) the submandibular gland

76. A researcher wishes to examine the role of gastric cells in the absorption of vitamin B_{12}. A relevant initial experiment could be use of immunostaining to verify that

    (A) chief cells are stained using a primary antibody against pepsinogen
    (B) chief cells are stained using a primary antibody against lipase
    (C) enteroendocrine cells are stained using a primary antibody against gastrin
    (D) Paneth cells are stained using a primary antibody against lysozyme
    (E) parietal cells are stained using a primary antibody against intrinsic factor

77. Which of the following structures is located within the epidural space?

    (A) Anterior spinal artery
    (B) External vertebral venous plexus
    (C) Internal vertebral venous plexus
    (D) Middle cerebral artery
    (E) Posterior spinal arteries

78. The glossopharyngeal nerve provides the parasympathetic innervation of the

    (A) lacrimal gland
    (B) nasal mucus glands
    (C) parotid salivary gland
    (D) sublingual salivary gland
    (E) submandibular salivary gland

79. A blow to the side of the head can fracture the thin bones forming the pterion, rupturing the anterior branch of the middle meningeal artery, which lies deep to the pterion. If left untreated, this middle meningeal artery hemorrhage may be fatal in a few hours. The middle meningeal artery is a branch of the

(A) external carotid artery

(B) facial artery

(C) internal carotid artery

(D) maxillary artery

(E) superficial temporal artery

80. A 35-year-old male patient suffering from pulmonary hypertension has been diagnosed with ostium secundum atrial septal defect. Abnormal development of the following structure is responsible for this developmental defect:

(A) aorticopulmonary septum

(B) endocardial cushion

(C) interventricular septum

(D) septum primum

(E) sinus venosus

81. The photomicrograph in Figure 1–10 illustrates a section of

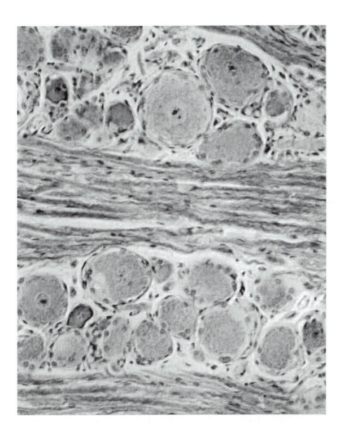

Figure 1–10

(A) cerebellar cortex

(B) dorsal root ganglion

(C) peripheral nerve

(D) pterygopalatine ganglion

(E) superior cervical ganglion

82. The dark spaces indicated by the arrows in Figure 1–11 are normally occupied by

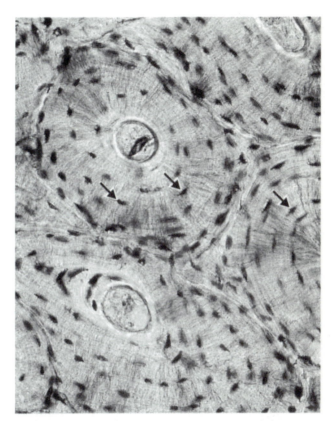

Figure 1–11

(A) blood vessels

(B) differentiating blood cell precursors

(C) osteoblasts

(D) osteoclasts

(E) osteocytes

83. As the body develops from embryo to fetus to newborn, the circulatory system changes at each stage. The portal vein in the infant derives from the embryonic

    (A) anterior cardinal vein
    (B) common cardinal vein
    (C) posterior cardinal vein
    (D) umbilical vein
    (E) vitelline vein

84. Which of the following statements concerning the control of reflexive ocular movements is correct?

    (A) Dilation of the pupil is the result of signals transmitted by postganglionic neurons in the ciliary ganglion.
    (B) Neurons in the left Edinger–Westphal nucleus receive input only from the right eye.
    (C) The blink reflex involves the oculomotor and trigeminal cranial nerves.
    (D) The near response or "near triad" involves activation of the ciliary, sphincter pupillae, and medial rectus muscles.
    (E) Signals originating in the right eye are directed only to the right pretectal region.

85. You are examining a 12-year-old male patient who has a slowly enlarging, painless swelling in the left inferior region of the neck. After careful palpation and consideration of the results of the radioimaging studies, you diagnose a branchial cyst in the left inferior parathyroid gland. This gland arose in development from the

    (A) fifth pharyngeal pouch
    (B) first pharyngeal pouch
    (C) fourth pharyngeal pouch
    (D) second pharyngeal pouch
    (E) third pharyngeal pouch

86. The axon of the second-order neuron in the pathway for conscious awareness of fine, discriminative touch and vibratory sensation from the upper limb

    (A) ascends the brainstem in the medial lemniscus

    (B) decussates in the ventral white commissure of the spinal cord
    (C) has its cell body in the nucleus gracilis
    (D) terminates in the nucleus cuneatus

87. Pathways for the conscious awareness of somatosensory signals

    (A) decussate at the level of the thalamus
    (B) pass through the ventral lateral nucleus of the thalamus
    (C) pass through the posterior limb of the internal capsule
    (D) terminate in the precentral gyrus
    (E) typically involve a two-neuron sequence from receptor to cortex

88. Choose the correct statement.

    (A) The ascending portion of the medial longitudinal fasciculus (MLF) gives off axons that terminate in the ipsilateral oculomotor nucleus.
    (B) The descending portion of the MLF (medial vestibulospinal tract) provides the vestibular system with control over extraocular musculature.
    (C) The medial vestibulospinal tract descends to lumbar levels of the spinal cord.
    (D) The lateral vestibulospinal tract primarily influences flexor musculature.
    (E) The lateral vestibulospinal tract originates from the medial vestibular nucleus.

89. Ocular movements termed nystagmus

    (A) are named for the direction of the slow phase of movement
    (B) are only observed in reference to horizontal eye movements
    (C) are unlikely to be induced in a patient with bilateral damage in the pontine and medullary levels of the brainstem
    (D) cannot be induced by caloric stimulation in a normal, conscious patient
    (E) indicate the presence of a lesion involving some portion of the vestibular system when observed following caloric stimulation

90. In performing a hysterectomy, care must be taken during ligation of the uterine artery because the following structure lies in close proximity and may be clamped or severed inadvertently:

    (A) the internal iliac artery
    (B) the ligament of the ovary
    (C) the ovarian artery
    (D) the ureter
    (E) the uterine tube

91. The accommodation–convergence reflex (near response) differs from the pupillary light reflex in that it (accommodation–convergence) involves

    (A) bilateral activation of lateral rectus motoneurons
    (B) conjugate eye movements
    (C) only the oculomotor nerve
    (D) only the optic nerve
    (E) the primary visual cortex

92. You are about to remove a small lesion from the mucosa of the laryngeal vestibule and want to anesthetize the nerve that supplies general sensation to the mucous membrane of that area. The nerve you are interested in is the

    (A) external laryngeal nerve
    (B) glossopharyngeal nerve
    (C) inferior laryngeal nerve
    (D) internal laryngeal nerve
    (E) pharyngeal plexus

93. The major support structure responsible for holding the liver in position in the right upper part of the abdominal cavity is the

    (A) attachment of the hepatic veins to the inferior vena cava
    (B) coronary ligament
    (C) falciform ligament
    (D) left triangular ligament
    (E) round ligament of the liver

94. A newborn infant suffers from a posterolateral defect on the left side of the body. His abdominal contents have herniated through the defect into the thoracic cavity, and as a result, the infant suffers from pulmonary hypoplasia. His breathing difficulty is life-threatening because the herniation has inhibited lung development and inflation. This congenital defect is due to a malformation of the

    (A) mesentery of the esophagus
    (B) muscular ingrowth of the body wall
    (C) pleuropericardial membrane
    (D) pleuroperitoneal membrane
    (E) septum transversum

95. In lingual carcinoma, malignant tumors in the posterior third of the tongue tend to metastasize most often to the

    (A) inferior deep cervical lymph nodes
    (B) retropharyngeal lymph nodes
    (C) submandibular lymph nodes
    (D) submental lymph nodes
    (E) superior deep cervical lymph nodes

96. The efferent limb of the pupillary light reflex is interrupted along with corticospinal and corticobulbar fibers in which of the following clinical entities?

    (A) Broca's aphasia
    (B) Inferior alternating hemiplegia
    (C) Middle alternating hemiplegia
    (D) Superior alternating hemiplegia
    (E) Wallenberg syndrome

97. Horner syndrome is sometimes seen in patients diagnosed with the lateral medullary syndrome. Which of the following is a characteristic feature of Horner syndrome?

    (A) Atrophy of tongue musculature
    (B) Mydriasis
    (C) Paralysis of muscles of facial expression
    (D) Profuse sweating
    (E) Red blushing of the skin in the affected area

98. A patient complains of heightened sensitivity to loud noises (hyperacusis) due to paralysis of the stapedius muscle. This patient also displays neurologic signs manifested by injury to the

    (A) Vth cranial nerve
    (B) VIIth cranial nerve
    (C) VIIIth cranial nerve
    (D) IXth cranial nerve
    (E) Xth cranial nerve

99. A large lesion involving the ventrolateral portion of the parietal lobe in the dominant hemisphere results in

    (A) Broca's aphasia
    (B) contralateral hemineglect
    (C) motor aprosodia
    (D) prosopagnosia
    (E) Wernicke's aphasia

100. The structure indicated by arrow #3 in Figure 1–12 is the

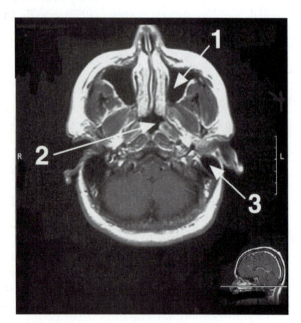

Figure 1–12

    (A) frontal sinus
    (B) mastoid sinus
    (C) maxillary sinus
    (D) pharynx
    (E) sphenoidal sinus

101. A large vascular infarct involving the posterior limb of the internal capsule on the right side is likely to produce which of the following deficits?

    (A) Deviation of the protruded tongue to the right
    (B) Hypertonia and hyperreflexia in the right upper limb
    (C) Paralysis of facial expression muscles on the lower left portion of face
    (D) Paraplegia involving the lower extremities
    (E) Spastic hemiplegia involving the right side of the body

102. Which of the following statements concerning the primary somatosensory (SI) cortex is correct?

    (A) A complete representation of the body surface is found only in cytoarchitectural subdivision 3b of SI cortex.
    (B) Areas 3a and 2 receive their major input from cutaneous receptors.
    (C) Areas 3b and 1 receive their major input from muscle spindle afferents and Golgi tendon organs.
    (D) Cytoarchitectural subdivisions of SI are numbered anterior to posterior as 3a, 3b, 1, and 2.
    (E) The somatotopic representation of the body surface in SI is arranged in a classic "tail-to-tongue" sequence from ventrolateral to dorsomedial.

103. Which of the following events is associated with vesicular release of neurotransmitter?

    (A) Activation of voltage-gated Ca^{++} channels allows calcium to enter the axon terminal.
    (B) Binding of neurotransmitter molecules to receptors on the presynaptic membrane follows vesicular release.
    (C) "Docking proteins" are present and attach vesicles to mitochondrial membranes.

(D) Fusion of vesicles with the presynaptic membrane allows 10 quanta of neurotransmitter to be released into the synaptic cleft.

(E) Movement of neurotransmitter occurs along actin "bridges," which structurally join the pre- and postsynaptic membranes.

104. Which of the following statements concerning muscle spindles is correct?

(A) Activation of type Ia sensory fibers from a given spindle leads to inhibition of the muscle in which that spindle is located.

(B) Alpha motoneurons synapse directly with intrafusal muscle fibers.

(C) Each intrafusal fiber is innervated by two different gamma motoneurons.

(D) Only one type of intrafusal muscle fiber (cell) is present in most muscle spindles.

(E) Type Ia sensory fibers from a spindle form direct synaptic contact with alpha motoneurons in the spinal cord.

105. Which of the following is characteristic of damage to the corticospinal (pyramidal) system?

(A) Babinski sign

(B) Flaccid paralysis and hypotonia

(C) Immediate muscle degeneration and atrophy

(D) Intention tremor

(E) Loss of deep tendon reflexes

106. Which of the following is a characteristic feature of spastic paralysis?

(A) It is observed as an increase in the resistance to passive movement.

(B) It usually involves paravertebral postural muscles most severely.

(C) The affected muscles are hypotonic.

(D) The affected muscles exhibit decreased (hypoactive) deep tendon reflexes.

(E) The affected muscles exhibit fibrillations and fasciculations.

107. The following artery in the adult forearm was derived from the primary axial artery in the embryo:

(A) anterior interosseous

(B) common interosseous

(C) posterior interosseous

(D) radial

(E) ulnar

108. Which of the following is directly involved with the descending modulation of pain transmission?

(A) Dopamine

(B) Medial longitudinal fasciculus

(C) Nucleus raphe magnus

(D) Rubrospinal fibers

(E) Ventral lateral thalamic nucleus

109. Which of the following statements concerning taste receptors is correct?

(A) Each receptor responds best to one stimulus quality (i.e., sweet, salty, sour, bitter) but also responds less vigorously to other stimulus qualities.

(B) Taste receptors are most numerous on the sides of the tongue.

(C) Taste receptors are stimulated when a food or fluid substance diffuses through the apical pore and hyperpolarizes the cell.

(D) Taste receptors have a life span of approximately 3 months.

(E) The receptors are arranged in a medial-to-lateral pattern on the tongue such that the most lateral respond best to sweet and salty stimuli.

110. Your patient is unable to dorsiflex and evert his right foot. The nerve most likely damaged is the

(A) common peroneal

(B) deep peroneal

(C) obturator

(D) superficial peroneal

(E) tibial

111. A 59-year old patient with a history of chronic alcoholism has developed bleeding esophageal varices. These varices represent a portal systemic shunt between the left gastric vein and the esophageal branch of the azygos vein. The azygos vein is indicated in the radiographic scan in Figure 1–13 by arrow

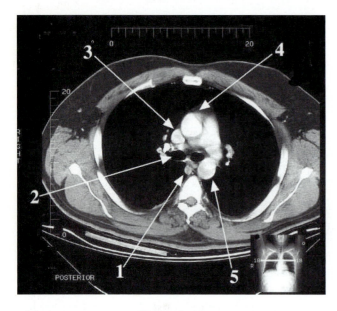

Figure 1–13

   (A) #1

   (B) #2

   (C) #3

   (D) #4

   (E) #5

112. An examination of your patient's injured knee reveals excessive posterior movement of the tibia on the femur. The chief ligament preventing posterior sliding of the tibia on the femur is the

   (A) anterior cruciate

   (B) fibular collateral

   (C) oblique popliteal

   (D) posterior cruciate

   (E) tibial collateral

113. A failure of the truncoconal septum to follow a spiral course results in

   (A) common atrium

   (B) persistent atrioventricular canal

   (C) persistent truncus arteriosus

   (D) tetralogy of Fallot

   (E) transposition of the great vessels

114. The azygos vein normally drains into the

   (A) inferior vena cava

   (B) right brachiocephalic vein

   (C) right jugular vein

   (D) right posterior intercostal veins

   (E) superior vena cava

115. The sensory innervation of the posterior one-third of the tongue is performed by cranial nerve IX (glossopharyngeal). During development, this region of the tongue develops from the

   (A) first pharyngeal arch

   (B) second pharyngeal arch

   (C) third pharyngeal arch

   (D) fourth pharyngeal arch

   (E) sixth pharyngeal arch

116. A male patient has suffered severe bilateral damage to the spinal cord in the thoracic region following a motorcycle accident. After the effects of spinal shock subside, he develops reflex erection of the penis. The nerve fibers that control erection of the penis are

   (A) branches of the genitofemoral nerve

   (B) parasympathetic branches from the vagus nerve

   (C) parasympathetic nerves from the middle sacral segments of the spinal cord

   (D) sympathetic nerves from the lumbar segments of the spinal cord

   (E) sympathetic nerves from the sacral segments of the spinal cord

117. In elderly patients (over 60 years of age), fractures of the neck of the femur following a fall are common. Arterial branches supplying the femoral head and neck are vulnerable to injury during these fractures and the resulting posttraumatic avascular necrosis affects the head of the femur. In the adult, the most important direct vascular source to the femoral head and neck is the

(A) artery to the head of the femur
(B) femoral artery
(C) lateral circumflex femoral artery
(D) medial circumflex femoral artery
(E) superior gluteal artery

118. Which of the following structures is located within the prevertebral layer of cervical fascia?

(A) Common carotid artery
(B) Esophagus
(C) Internal jugular vein
(D) Middle scalene muscle
(E) Vagus nerve

119. As an endocrine gland, the thyroid has a rich blood supply, receiving vessels derived directly or indirectly from the subclavian artery, the external carotid artery, and occasionally from the brachiocephalic trunk or the arch of the aorta. The superior thyroid artery is usually the first branch of the

(A) brachiocephalic trunk
(B) external carotid artery
(C) facial artery
(D) internal carotid artery
(E) thyrocervical trunk

120. A resident is about to perform a needle biopsy of the liver. She has marked the location for entry of the needle at the midaxillary line. To not penetrate the costodiaphragmatic recess, she asks the patient to breathe out forcefully and then to hold her breath before insertion of the needle. The resident remembered that, in the midaxillary line, the lower border of the pleura crosses the

(A) fourth rib
(B) sixth rib
(C) eighth rib
(D) tenth rib
(E) twelfth rib

Questions 121 and 122

Your patient presents in your office complaining of hoarseness. During your examination, you find that one vocal fold has deviated toward the midline and does not abduct during deep inspiration or vocalization. You also observe that touch sensation in the vestibule of the larynx appears to be intact.

121. Which laryngeal muscle is most important in abduction of the vocal folds?

(A) Cricothyroid
(B) Lateral cricoarytenoid
(C) Posterior cricoarytenoid
(D) Thyroarytenoid
(E) Transverse arytenoid

122. You suspect that a nerve has been damaged, but which nerve is most likely involved?

(A) External laryngeal
(B) Glossopharyngeal
(C) Inferior laryngeal
(D) Internal laryngeal
(E) Superior laryngeal

123. The rapid initial effect of parathyroid hormone is to increase the rate of release of calcium from bone to blood. Parathyroid hormone is secreted by

(A) chief or principal cells
(B) chromaffin cells
(C) follicular cells
(D) oxyphilic cells
(E) parafollicular cells

Questions 124 through 125

Your patient reports that several days earlier he "threw his back out" when he bent from the waist and picked up a very heavy package. The pain was immediate and extended from his hip, down the back of the thigh, and into his leg and foot. As he lies on the examining table, you raise his leg by the foot keeping the knee extended and elicit intense pain over the distribution of the sciatic nerve. A magnetic resonance imaging (MRI) scan confirms your conclusion that your patient has a herniated intervertebral disc between the fourth and fifth lumbar vertebrae.

124. Intervertebral discs may protrude or rupture in any direction, but they most commonly protrude in which direction?

(A) Anteriorly
(B) Anterolaterally
(C) Laterally
(D) Posteriorly
(E) Posterolaterally

125. Herniation of the intervertebral disc between the fourth and fifth lumbar vertebrae most likely impinges on the roots of which spinal nerve?

(A) L3
(B) L4
(C) L5
(D) S1
(E) S2

126. An opera singer, who has maintained a demanding work schedule, worries about the effect on her vocal cords. The epithelium covering the vocal cords is

(A) pseudostratified ciliated
(B) simple columnar
(C) simple cuboidal
(D) simple squamous
(E) stratified squamous

127. A patient suffers from Frey syndrome manifested by perspiration of the skin covering the left parotid gland whenever the patient eats. Upon inquiry, the patient reveals that he suffered deep injuries on that side of his face and neck in an automobile accident. You explain to him that his syndrome results from abnormal connections between the great auricular nerve and parasympathetic secretomotor fibers, which normally innervate only the parotid gland. This abnormal reinnervation occurred during the healing period after the accident. The parasympathetic secretomotor fibers to the parotid gland are carried by the

(A) auriculotemporal nerve
(B) buccal branch of the facial nerve
(C) buccal nerve

(D) greater petrosal nerve
(E) lesser petrosal nerve

128. Your young female patient has a large bulge on the anterior thigh below the inguinal ligament. You suspect an abdominal hernia that has passed through the femoral ring into the femoral sheath and then through the saphenous hiatus into the subcutaneous layer of the upper thigh. In addition to the hernial sac, you would expect the femoral canal to contain the

(A) connective tissue and lymph nodes
(B) femoral artery
(C) femoral nerve
(D) femoral vein
(E) great saphenous vein

129. The most anterior structure passing under the flexor retinaculum of the foot is the

(A) tendon of the flexor digitorum longus muscle
(B) tendon of the flexor hallucis longus muscle
(C) tendon of the peroneus longus muscle
(D) tendon of the tibialis posterior muscle
(E) tibial nerve

130. Corneal abrasions produce eye pain and excessive lacrimation. The cornea is innervated by cranial nerve

(A) II (optic)
(B) III (oculomotor)
(C) IV (trochlea)
(D) V (trigeminal)
(E) VI (abducens)

131. In examining radiographs of your patient's chest you notice that the contents of the middle mediastinum appear to be deviated to the right side. Which of the following structures is located within the middle mediastinum?

(A) Aortic arch
(B) Esophagus
(C) Heart
(D) Thymus
(E) Trachea

132. You are concerned that your patient may have compromised function of the mitral valve. The sound of the mitral valve is best heard

    (A) at the apex in the left fifth intercostal space in the midclavicular line
    (B) at the xiphisternal junction
    (C) in the fifth intercostal space to the right of the sternum
    (D) in the second intercostal space to the left of the sternum
    (E) in the second intercostal space to the right of the sternum

133. While performing surgery, you mobilize the duodenum and the head of the pancreas reflecting them to the left. Which of the following would you normally expect to find passing behind the first part of the duodenum?

    (A) Common hepatic artery
    (B) Common hepatic duct
    (C) Portal vein
    (D) Splenic artery
    (E) Superior mesenteric artery

134. A newborn infant displays wheezing respiration, which is aggravated when she feeds, flexes her neck, and/or cries. Radioimaging studies of her chest reveal a double aortic arch compressing her trachea and esophagus. This rare developmental defect results from persistence of the right dorsal aorta, which normally disappears. The arch of the aorta arises from the

    (A) second pair of aortic arches
    (B) third pair of aortic arches
    (C) fourth pair of aortic arches
    (D) fifth pair of aortic arches
    (E) sixth pair of aortic arches

135. After recovery from the surgical removal of the thyroid gland, the quality of the voice in a patient changed to a monotone. It was discovered that the cricothyroid muscle in this patient was paralyzed. The cricothyroid muscle is innervated by the

    (A) accessory nerve
    (B) ansa cervicalis
    (C) external laryngeal nerve
    (D) hypoglossal nerve
    (E) internal laryngeal nerve

136. Secretion of pulmonary surfactant is a function of

    (A) alveolar dust cells
    (B) endothelial cells of capillaries in the alveolar septum
    (C) small granule cells
    (D) type I pneumocytes (squamous alveolar cells)
    (E) type II pneumocytes (greater alveolar cells)

137. Which blood cell differentiates in a site other than the bone marrow?

    (A) B lymphocyte
    (B) Basophil
    (C) Eosinophil
    (D) Neutrophil
    (E) T lymphocyte

138. The cytoplasm of a typical acinar secretory cell in the pancreas contains

    (A) a poorly developed Golgi complex
    (B) abundant secretory granules at the cell apex
    (C) abundant smooth endoplasmic reticulum (sER)
    (D) mitochondria with tubular cristae
    (E) numerous lipid droplets

139. Which of the following is a mixed cranial nerve that includes axons with special visceral efferent, general visceral efferent, general visceral afferent, special visceral afferent, and general somatic afferent functions?

    (A) Abducens
    (B) Hypoglossal
    (C) Oculomotor
    (D) Trigeminal
    (E) Vagus

140. After removal of cancerous lymph nodes from the lateral pelvic wall, a patient develops painful spasms of the adductor muscles and sensory deficits in the medial thigh region. The adductor muscles are innervated by the

    (A) femoral nerve
    (B) inferior gluteal nerve
    (C) obturator nerve
    (D) pudendal nerve
    (E) sciatic nerve

141. A renal calculus (kidney stone) passing from the renal pelvis into the ureter causes excessive distension and severe ureteric colic. During development in the embryo, the ureter arose from the

    (A) mesonephric duct
    (B) metanephric diverticulum
    (C) metanephric mass of intermediate mesoderm
    (D) paramesonephric duct
    (E) pronephric duct

142. The presence in the plasmalemma of numerous receptors for the Fc portion of immunoglobulin E molecules is characteristic of

    (A) basophils and mast cells
    (B) B lymphocytes
    (C) monocytes and macrophages
    (D) neutrophils
    (E) platelets

143. Some fertility problems can be aided by procedures that require mixing of spermatozoa and ova *in vitro* to achieve fertilization. Strategies to optimize success in retrieving mature oocytes from the ovaries of a woman include the daily administration of both gonadotropins and gonadotropin-releasing hormone (GnRH) during the first half of the menstrual cycle. The daily doses of GnRH would be expected to

    (A) directly stimulate development of ovarian follicles
    (B) directly stimulate the proliferative phase of the endometrium
    (C) induce the second meiotic division by secondary oocytes
    (D) promote a luteinizing hormone (LH) surge
    (E) shut down the normal secretory activity of pituitary gonadotropic cells

144. During development, the permanent set of kidneys becomes functional around the ninth week. It originally developed from the

    (A) mesonephroi
    (B) metanephroi
    (C) paramesonephric ducts
    (D) pronephroi
    (E) ureteric bud

145. The root of a tooth is anchored in its bony socket by

    (A) dentinal tubules
    (B) fibers of the periodontal ligament
    (C) odontoblast processes
    (D) the stellate reticulum
    (E) the subodontoblastic plexus of Rashkow

146. Lymph nodes are populated by lymphocytes that exit the vascular compartment to gain access to the parenchyma of the node by passing through the walls of

    (A) afferent lymphatic vessels
    (B) arterioles
    (C) efferent lymphatic vessels
    (D) high endothelial postcapillary venules
    (E) medullary sinuses

147. Myelination of large-caliber axons in peripheral nerves is a function of

    (A) astrocytes
    (B) fibroblasts
    (C) oligodendroglial cells (oligodendrocytes)
    (D) perineurial cells
    (E) Schwann cells

148. In Figure 1–14, which labeled bracket spans a sarcomere?

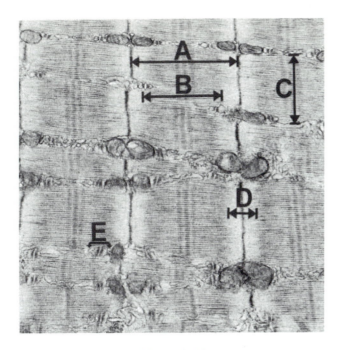

Figure 1–14

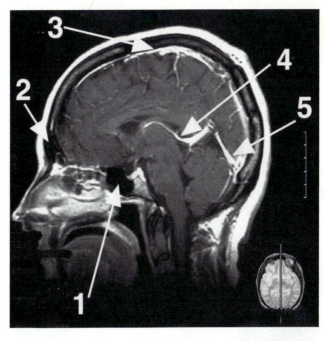

Figure 1–15

(A) A
(B) B
(C) C
(D) D
(E) E

149. The great cerebral vein of Galen (indicated by arrow #4 in Figure 1–15) is formed by the union of two internal cerebral veins and drains into the

(A) confluence of sinuses
(B) frontal sinus
(C) sphenoid sinus
(D) straight sinus
(E) superior sagittal sinus

150. A 42-year-old female patient has to undergo emergency cholecystectomy due to intense biliary colic. The structure to be removed during the surgery is indicated in Figure 1–16 by arrow

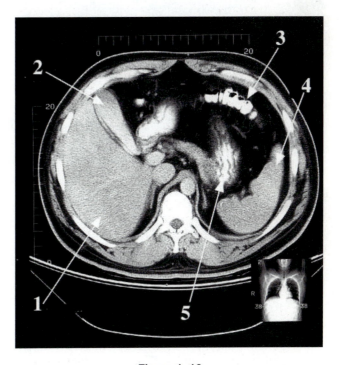

Figure 1–16

(A) #1
(B) #2
(C) #3
(D) #4
(E) #5

151. Inferiorly, the bile duct joins with the

    (A) ascending (fourth) part of the duodenum
    (B) descending (second) part of the duodenum
    (C) horizontal (third) part of the duodenum
    (D) pancreatic duct
    (E) superior (first) part of the duodenum

152. A 65-year-old male patient develops neuro-
    logic symptoms due to an embolus in the left
    common carotid artery. In the computerized
    tomographic (CT) scan in Figure 1–17, the in-
    volved vessel is indicated by arrow

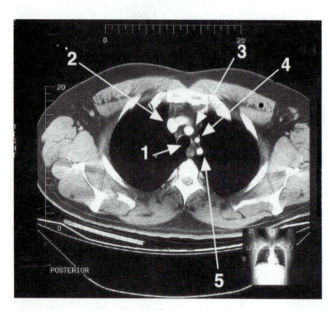

Figure 1–17

    (A) #1
    (B) #2
    (C) #3
    (D) #4
    (E) #5

153. A 22-year-old patient suffers from headaches
    due to pansinusitis. The inflammation and
    swelling of the mucosa are especially severe
    in the ethmoidal sinuses. The general sensory
    innervation of the ethmoidal sinuses is sup-
    plied by branches of the

    (A) facial nerve
    (B) infraorbital nerve
    (C) nasociliary nerve

    (D) olfactory nerve
    (E) optic nerve

154. A skydiver landing forcefully on his right
    lower limb suffered a central fracture of the
    acetabulum with dislocation of the femoral
    head into the pelvis. The acetabulum is
    formed by the joining of the ilium, ischium
    and pubis. These three bones are completely
    fused by

    (A) birth
    (B) 6 years
    (C) puberty
    (D) 16 years
    (E) 23 years

155. In the coronal section of the head shown in
    Figure 1–18, arrow #2 points to a structure
    that

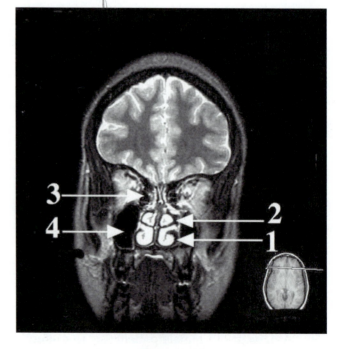

Figure 1–18

    (A) belongs to the ethmoid bone
    (B) belongs to the maxillary bone
    (C) belongs to the nasal septum
    (D) belongs to the vomer bone
    (E) is a separate bone

Answers and Explanations

1. **(D)** The right subclavian artery arises from the brachiocephalic artery and runs to the lateral border of rib 1. At that point, its name changes to the axillary artery. In costoclavicular syndrome, the divisions of the brachial plexus, the subclavian vein and artery, become compressed between the clavicle and the first rib. This is due to wearing a heavy backpack for prolonged periods of time. Compression of the divisions of the brachial plexus elicits pain and paresthesia. Compression of the subclavian vein results in edema of the hand with distended superficial veins and cyanosis. Compression of the subclavian artery gives rise to decreased skin temperature, easy fatigability and Raynaud's phenomenon (spasmodic constriction of the digital arteries). The test for the costoclavicular syndrome is positive because the maneuver depresses and retracts the pectoral girdle mimicking the condition that gives rise to the syndrome: this draws the clavicle closer to the first rib and compresses the subclavian artery, resulting in decreased pulsations in the radial artery distally.

2. **(C)** Traumatic lesions or compression of the left oculomotor nerve results in loss of parasympathetic innervation to the sphincter pupillae muscle and lead to mydriasis (dilation of pupil) along with lateral and downward deviation of the ipsilateral eye due to weakness in all ocular muscles innervated by the left third cranial nerve. Compression of the left abducens nerve (choice A) causes the left eye to be medially deviated and does not affect the sphincter pupillae muscle. Damage to the left facial nerve (choice B) or the left trigeminal nerve (choice D) has no effect on ocular motility or the sphincter pupillae of the left eye. Damage to the right trochlear nerve (choice E) denervates the right superior oblique muscle and has no effect on the left eye.

3. **(C)** These are the classic signs of uncal herniation, which involves compression of the third cranial nerve and the adjacent cerebral peduncle and its contingent of corticospinal fibers. This combination of symptoms is referred to as superior alternating hemiplegia and includes cranial nerve signs ipsilateral to the lesion and contralateral hemiplegia resulting from corticospinal tract involvement rostral to the pyramidal decussation. Capsular hemiplegia (choice A) results in contralateral hemiplegia and corticobulbar signs (upper motoneuron cranial nerve signs) and is not associated with lower motoneuron signs of cranial nerve dysfunction. The combination of corticospinal tract involvement and damage to the VIth cranial nerve is classified as middle alternating hemiplegia (choice B), and inferior alternating hemiplegia combines hypoglossal nerve (XII) damage with corticospinal tract involvement. Syringomyelia (choice D) and Wallenberg syndrome (choice E) are primarily sensory disorders that involve a loss of pain sensation.

4. **(B)** The tracheal tube arises from a diverticulum growing out of the foregut. The proximity of the esophagus and trachea during development may give rise to abnormal fistulas between these two structures. Normally, the embryo swallows the amniotic fluid, which is

absorbed by the digestive system. With atresia of the esophagus and/or abnormal fistulas between the trachea and esophagus, less amniotic fluid is absorbed by the fetus and polyhydramnios results. The fourth pharyngeal arch (choice C) develops into cartilages of the larynx. The second (choice D) and third pharyngeal arch (choice E) contribute to the formation of the hyoid bone. The first pharyngeal arch (choice A) plays no role in the development of structures of the neck.

5. **(E)** Horizontal cells in the retina do form synapses with the synaptic portion (rod spherules or cone pedicles) of the photoreceptor cells (choice A). Photons that pass through the lens eventually strike the photoreceptors after passing through all of the intervening layers of the retina (choice B). The optic disc is located nasally with respect to the macula (choice C). In the absence of photic stimulation (darkness), the photoreceptors are depolarized as a result of dark current and are therefore continuously releasing neurotransmitter in the dark (choice D).

6. **(D)** Remember that in viewing axial or transverse CT scans through the body, the right side of the patient is to your left and the left side to your right. In other words, the feet of the patient are toward you and the head away from you. The back of the patient is at the bottom of the image and the front of the patient toward the top. Directional terms are always in reference to the patient. The insert at the bottom right indicates the level of the section. Arrow #1 indicates the right brachiocephalic vein. The left brachiocephalic vein (choice B) is seen as the elongated structure immediately posterior to the manubrium of the sternum and to the left of the right brachiocephalic vein. Immediately posterior to the left brachiocephalic vein is the brachiocephalic artery (choice A, arrow #2). To the left of the latter are the left common carotid artery (choice C) and the left subclavian artery (arrow #3). The superior vena cava (choice E) is not seen at this level because the right and left brachiocephalic veins are still separate.

7. **(A)** The appendicular artery is a terminal branch of the ileocolic artery. The ileocolic, right colic (choice D) and middle colic (choice C) arteries are all terminal branches of the superior mesenteric artery (choice E). The ileocolic artery gives rise to jejunal and ileal branches, and also supplies the area of the ileoceal junction, including the appendix. The right colic supplies the ascending colon and the middle colic, the transverse colon. The inferior mesenteric artery (choice B) does not contribute to the blood supply of the appendix; it supplies the descending and sigmoid colon and the rectum.

8. **(B)** Sensory fibers that arise from Golgi tendon organs synapse with interneurons which inhibit those motoneurons that innervate the muscle to which the tendon organ is related. Stimulation of cutaneous pain endings (choice A) in the region of a Golgi tendon organ is not in itself sufficient to activate the reflex. Type Ib sensory fibers do play an important role in this reflex (choice D). Type Ia (choice C) and type II (choice E) sensory fibers originate from muscle spindles and are involved in the myotatic reflex but not the inverse myotatic reflex. An increase in the tension applied to the muscle tendon in which the tendon organ is located is the appropriate stimulus for this reflex.

9. **(E)** In TGA, the aorta arises from the right ventricle, and the pulmonary trunk arises from the left ventricle (choice C). This is the reverse of the normal situation and gives rise to the cyanotic condition in the newborn. The large arteries arise from the truncus arteriosus in the developing heart and thus could not develop from the atria (choices B and D), which are formed from the sinus venosus. The truncus arteriosus and the sinus venosus are at opposite ends of the heart. The ductus arteriosus (choice A) is the vessel that shunts oxygenated blood from the pulmonary trunk to the arch of the aorta in the fetus. It does not give rise to the aorta.

10. **(A)** In middle alternating hemiplegia (choice B), the involved structures are the corti-

cospinal tract and fibers of the abducens nerve. Superior alternating hemiplegia (choice D) involves corticospinal fibers and exiting fibers of the oculomotor nerve. Spina bifida (choice C) is a developmental defect involving failure of the neural tube to close. Syringomyelia (choice E) is due to the formation of a cyst-like cavity in the central portion of the spinal cord damaging the crossing pain fibers in the ventral white commissure, and resulting in a bilateral loss of pain and temperature sensation in the affected dermatomes.

11. **(E)** Internal hemorrhoids are formed by varicosities of the branches of the superior rectal vein. Varicosities of the branches of the inferior rectal vein (choice B) form external hemorrhoids. Hemorrhoids are thus varicose branches of the veins and not of the arteries of this region (choices A, C, and D).

12. **(A)** Sensory neurons such as those found in the cochlear, spinal trigeminal, solitary, and vestibular nuclei arise from the alar plate. The hypoglossal nucleus (choice C), dorsal vagal nucleus (choice B), and nucleus ambiguus (choice D) contain motoneurons that innervate either striated or smooth musculature, and such neurons arise from the basal plate.

13. **(C)** The posterior inferior cerebellar artery supplies the rostral, dorsolateral medulla. The posterior spinal (choice D) and anterior spinal (choice B) arteries supply dorsal and ventral portions, respectively, of the caudal medulla. The anterior inferior cerebellar (choice A) and superior cerebellar (choice E) arteries supply portions of the pons and mesencephalon.

14. **(D)** Arrow #5 indicates the right kidney. The abdominal aorta (choice A, arrow #2) lies anterior to the vertebra. The inferior vena cava (choice B, arrow #3) is located anterior and to the right of the abdominal aorta. At this level, the renal veins join with the inferior vena cava. The left kidney (choice C, arrow #1) is visible in the left side of the body and the small intestine filled with bright, contrast-

enhancing material lies anterior to the left kidney (arrow #4). The small intestine is recognizable by its regularly spaced constrictions.

15. **(C)** The characteristic feature of the lateral medullary syndrome is a loss of pain and temperature sensation that involves the ipsilateral face (the lesion side) and the contralateral side of the body. Pain and temperature sensation is lost in the ipsilateral and not the contralateral (choice E) face. The medullary pyramid (choice B) is typically not involved in this syndrome. Involvement of the ipsilateral upper and contralateral lower extremities (choice D) is not a feature of this syndrome. This syndrome is typically the result of a vascular lesion involving the posterior inferior (not anterior inferior) cerebellar artery (choice A).

16. **(C)** Patients with Weber syndrome exhibit involvement of the ipsilateral oculomotor nerve. Interruption of this nerve on the right eliminates parasympathetic outflow on that side, resulting in a dilated right pupil that does not react to light. Involvement of corticobulbar fibers coursing in the right crus cerebri might cause the protruded tongue to deviate to the left (not right, choice B), and cause paralysis of the facial expression musculature in the lower left portion (not complete paralysis on one side, choice A). Involvement of corticospinal fibers in the right crus (choice D) produces contralateral hemiplegia. Movements of the left eye (choice E) are not affected.

17. **(B)** The inner surface of the tympanic membrane is lined in patches with a ciliated simple columnar epithelium. Where this does not occur, the epithelium is simple squamous or cuboidal. The outer surface of the eardrum is covered with a stratified squamous epithelium (choice E). All the other epithelia (choices A, C, and D) are not found in association with the tympanic membrane.

18. **(D)** Failure of the right eye to adduct on attempted lateral gaze to the left, accompanied

by normal abduction of the left eye, suggests a lesion involving the right medial longitudinal fasciculus. Interruption of the left (choice A) or right abducens nerve (choice B) or the right trochlear nerve (choice E) alone does not result in defective conjugate horizontal eye movements, but unilaterally affects eye movements in the eye innervated by the injured nerve. Damage to the left medial longitudinal fasciculus (choice C) prevents adduction of the left eye on attempted right lateral gaze.

19. **(C)** A vascular lesion affecting the left caudal medulla involves the left medial lemniscus, left hypoglossal nerve fibers, and the left medullary pyramid. Involvement of the left medial lemniscus produces somatosensory deficits involving the right side of the body. Damage to the left hypoglossal nerve would result in deviation of the protruded tongue to the left (and other lower motoneuron signs), and damage to the left pyramid results in right hemiplegia (choices A and B involve incorrect combinations) along with other upper motoneuron signs. Choices D and E are incorrect because they fail to combine involvement of the tongue and contralateral hemiplegia.

20. **(A)** The malleus and incus arise from the first pharyngeal arch. The collection of congenital abnormalities displayed in this newborn infant is a manifestation of first arch syndrome, of which there are two: Pierre Robin syndrome and Treacher Collins syndrome (mandibulofacial dysostosis). The stapes of the middle ear is derived from the second pharyngeal arch (choice B). The third (choice C), fourth (choice D), and sixth (choice E) pharyngeal arches give rise to structures in the larynx and pharynx, and do not contribute to the ossicles of the middle ear.

21. **(B)** Lesions (usually vascular in nature) that involve the dorsolateral medulla produce the classic signs of the lateral medullary syndrome (Wallenberg syndrome), which include a loss of pain and temperature sensibility over the face ipsilateral to the lesion and

the contralateral side of the body. Unilateral lesions that involve somatosensory pathways coursing through the posterior limb of the internal capsule give rise to a loss of all or some somatosensation over the contralateral face (not choice A) and the contralateral body surface. Weber syndrome (choice C) does not typically produce somatosensory deficits. Because the left side of the face exhibits a loss of pain sensation, choice D is not correct. Syringomyelia (choice E) is a spinal cord lesion that typically does not affect the face.

22. **(A)** This axial scan is at the level of the orbits as indicated by the insert at the bottom right and the eyeballs in the orbits. Arrow #2 points to the ethmoidal sinus located medial to the orbits. The sinus is divided into compartments by the air cells. The maxillary sinus (choice D) and the inferior nasal meatus (choice B) are located inferior to the level of this scan and are not seen. The sphenoidal sinus (choice E) is indicated by arrow #3 and the infratemporal fossa (choice C) by arrow #1.

23. **(C)** The appearance of right beating horizontal nystagmus with warm caloric stimulation of the right ear, coupled with the absence of nystagmus following warm caloric stimulation of the left ear, suggests that the left labyrinth (and not the right, choice D) or the left VIIIth cranial nerve has been damaged. The absence of left beating nystagmus under these conditions does not indicate that only the left lateral vestibulospinal tract (choice B) has been affected. The presence of right beating nystagmus indicates that receptors in the right ear (choice A) have not been damaged. The absence of nystagmus upon warm water irrigation of the left ear suggests that there is a lesion (not choice E) in the vestibular system.

24. **(A)** Arrow #2 points to the basilar artery, which is located at the base of the pons (arrow #3). The basilar artery is formed by the union of the vertebral arteries (choice E), which cannot be seen at this level; they are located more inferiorly, at the junction of the

spinal cord with the medulla oblongata. The internal carotid artery (choice D) is located more anteriorly (arrow #1), and the cerebral vein of Galen (choice C) is located more superiorly and cannot be seen at this level. Arrow #4 indicates the fourth ventricle (choice B).

25. **(C)** The structure indicated by arrow #2 in Figure 1–4 is the basilar artery, which terminates by dividing into the posterior cerebral arteries. The anterior and middle cerebral arteries (choice A) are terminal branches of the internal carotid artery. The internal cerebral veins (choice B) drain into the great cerebral vein of Galen. The superior cerebellar arteries (choice D) are branches of the basilar artery. The vertebral arteries (choice E) unite to form the basilar artery.

26. **(C)** The cerebellum develops from the metencephalon. The telencephalon (choice E) gives rise to the cerebral hemispheres. The thalamus, hypothalamus, and epithalamnus arise from the diencephalon (choice A). The mesencephalon (choice B) eventually forms the midbrain and the myelencephalon (choice D), the medulla oblongata.

27. **(E)** The wide-based stance and staggering gait are two of the characteristic features of cerebellar disease. Hyperreflexia (choice A) and spasticity (choice D) are prominent signs of upper motoneuron dysfunction. Somatosensory deficits such as the loss of pain and temperature sensation (choice B) are not typically seen with cerebellar disease. Basal ganglia dysfunction, not cerebellar pathology, produces a resting-type tremor (choice C).

28. **(E)** Tarsal tunnel syndrome results from entrapment and compression of the tibial nerve as it passes deep to the flexor retinaculum between the medial malleolus and calcaneus. Compression of the anterior tibial artery (choice A) results in anterior compartment syndrome of the leg where structures distal to the compression are ischemic. A deep peroneal (fibular) nerve (choice B) entrapment results in this situation. Superficial peroneal (fibular) nerve (choice D) entrapment results

in pain along the lateral side of the leg and the dorsum of the ankle and foot. This may be due to chronic ankle sprains, which can lead to paralysis of the peroneal (fibular) muscles and inversion of the foot. Compression of the peroneal artery (choice C) does not result in tarsal tunnel syndrome because this artery supplies the inferior aspect of the lateral compartment of the leg.

29. **(C)** The intrinsic muscles of the hand are derived mostly from the T1 myotome and to a lesser degree from the C8 myotome and, consequently, derive their innervation from the corresponding segmental spinal nerves. The segmental innervation to the intrinsic muscles of the hand is overwhelmingly from the T1 segmental nerve with some input from the C8 nerve. The biceps brachii muscle (choice A) is innervated by the musculocutaneous nerve derived from the lateral cord of the brachial plexus. Although the lateral cord and musculocutaneous nerve contain fibers derived from the C5, C6, and C7 spinal nerves, the biceps muscle is mostly supplied by the C5 and C6 spinal nerves. The deltoid muscle (choice B) is an intrinsic muscle of the shoulder supplied by the axillary nerve. Although the posterior cord of the brachial plexus, which gives rise to the axillary nerve, contains fibers from the C5 to T1 spinal nerves, the axillary nerve largely consists of C5 and C6 fibers, which supply the deltoid and teres minor muscles. The pronator teres muscle (choice D) is supplied by the median nerve. Whereas the median nerve contains fibers derived from the C5 to T1 spinal nerves, the pronator teres muscle is mostly supplied by the C5 and C6 spinal nerves. The supraspinatus muscle (choice E) is supplied by the suprascapular nerve which is derived from the upper trunk of the brachial plexus. Consequently, it receives innervation from the C5 and C6 spinal nerves, as do the other intrinsic muscles of the shoulder.

30. **(D)** Injury to the lower trunk of the brachial plexus affects the C8 and T1 dermatomes. The C8 dermatome covers the little finger and the adjacent side of the ring finger and

the medial side of the hand, wrist, and lower forearm. The T1 dermatome extends up the medial side of the forearm across the elbow onto the medial side of the arm. The deltoid muscle just above its insertion (choice A) is covered by the C5 dermatome. The dorsum of the wrist and the anatomical snuffbox (choice B) are covered by the C6 dermatome. The lateral side of the forearm (choice C) is divided between the C5 and C6 dermatomes. The web between the thumb and index finger (choice E) is covered by the C6 dermatome.

31. **(A)** The middle suprarenal artery arises from the abdominal aorta. The left inferior phrenic artery (choice B) gives rise to the left superior suprarenal artery. The left renal artery (choice C) gives rise to the inferior suprarenal artery on the left side. The splenic artery (choice D) does not supply the suprarenal gland, nor does the thoracic aorta (choice E).

32. **(A)** The liver arises as a ventral outgrowth from the caudal portion of the foregut. The midgut (choice C) arises past the junction point between the bile duct and the duodenum, distal to the formative outgrowth of the liver. The midgut gives rise to the small intestine and part of the large intestine. The hindgut (choice B) arises further distally and gives rise to the rest of the large intestine, the superior part of the anal canal, the epithelium of the urinary bladder, and most of the urethra. The pleuroperitoneal membrane (choice D) and the septum transversum (choice E) are developmental components of the diaphragm.

33. **(D)** Figure 1–6 reflects the distribution of the superficial branch of the radial nerve over the dorsum of the hand. This nerve is entirely cutaneous and supplies no muscles. Damage to the dorsal cutaneous branch of the ulnar nerve (choice A) produces a sensory deficit over the dorsal surface of the medial one-third of the hand, little finger, and medial half of the ring finger. The posterior antebrachial cutaneous nerve (choice B) is a branch of the radial nerve in the posterior arm, and is distributed down the posterior forearm extending onto the dorsum of the wrist with distribution onto the hand. Damage to the radial nerve in the cubital fossa (choice C) produces the same cutaneous deficit as injury to the superficial radial nerve (the correct answer), but also affects the motor innervation to the muscles of the posterior compartment of the forearm. Damage to the ulnar nerve at the elbow (choice E) produces a sensory deficit over the dorsal and ventral surfaces of the medial one-third of the hand, all of the little finger, and the medial half of the ring finger.

34. **(B)** The blackened area in Figure 1–6 represents the C6 and C7 dermatomes. The C5 and C6 dermatomes (choice A) extend in a strip along the lateral surface of the upper extremity from the shoulder to the hand. The C6 dermatome extends onto the hand but the C5 dermatome does not. The C7 and C8 dermatomes (choice C) extend in a strip along the posterior and medial surfaces of the upper extremity from the shoulder to the hand. The C7 dermatome supplies the area indicated but the C8 dermatome covers the medial side of the hand rather than the lateral side. The C8 and T1 dermatomes (choice D) cover the little finger and the adjacent side of the ring finger and the medial side of the hand, wrist, and lower forearm (C8), and extend up the medial side of the forearm across the elbow onto the medial side of the arm (T1). The T1 dermatome (choice E) extends up the medial side of the forearm across the elbow onto the medial side of the arm. It has no representation on the hand.

35. **(E)** Spina bifida with myeloschisis is a severe form of spina bifida where the neural folds fail to fuse and the spinal cord is a flattened mass. The defect displays as a protrusion onto the skin covered by a membrane. Meroanencephaly (choice A) is the absence of part of the brain and is commonly seen with spina bifida with meningomyelocele (choice D). In the latter, the spinal cord is formed normally but is part of the protrusion onto the skin. Spina bifida with meningocele (choice C) involves a protrusion containing

only the meninges and cerebrospinal fluid. In spina bifida occulta (choice B), the arches of the vertebrae fail to fuse, but the anomaly usually does not involve the spinal cord.

36. **(B)** The right testicular vein drains directly to the inferior vena cava. The hepatic vein (choice A) is buried deep within the substance of the liver and has no relation to the testicular vein. The lumbar veins (choice C) drain the abdominal wall. The right renal vein (choice D) does not receive the right testicular vein. However, the left testicular vein does drain into the left renal vein. The superior mesenteric vein (choice E) drains peritoneal structures related to the digestive system and does not drain the testicular vein.

37. **(D)** The spleen (arrow #4) lies to the left of the abdominal cavity. It is in contact with the left side of the stomach (arrow #2) and lodges against the left paravertebral gutter. The abdominal aorta (choice A, arrow #5) is seen as the circular structure immediately anterior to the vertebra. The colon (choice B, arrow #3) is the convoluted structure to the left anterior aspect of the abdominal cavity. The large liver (choice C, arrow #1) occupies most of the right side of the abdominal cavity. The stomach (choice E, arrow #2) is located between the colon and the liver, and in this case, contains liquid contrast material.

38. **(B)** The posterior humeral circumflex artery arises from the third part of the axillary artery but has no anastomotic connections with branches of the subclavian artery. The dorsal scapular artery (choice A) arises from the subclavian artery and descends along the vertebral border of the scapula. It anastomoses deep to the infraspinatus muscle with branches of the scapular circumflex branch of the subscapular artery, from the third part of the axillary artery. The scapular circumflex artery (choice C) anastomoses around the scapula with the suprascapular artery, a branch of the thyrocervical trunk, and the dorsal scapular artery, a branch of the subclavian artery. The subscapular artery (choice D) is a branch from the third part of the axillary

artery and gives rise to the scapular circumflex artery. Through this branch, it makes anastomotic connections with the suprascapular artery in the infraspinous fossa. The suprascapular artery (choice E) is a branch of the thyrocervical trunk from the subclavian artery. As it descends in the infraspinous fossa deep to the infraspinatus muscle, it makes anastomotic connections with the scapular circumflex artery.

39. **(B)** The internal thoracic artery arises from the first part of the subclavian artery, and gives rise to the anterior intercostal arteries (choice A), the pericardiacophrenic artery, and the mediastinal arteries. It terminates by branching into the superior epigastric and the musculophrenic arteries (choice D). The superior epigastric artery enters the posterior aspect of the rectus sheath in the anterior abdominal wall, supplies the rectus muscle and anastomoses with the inferior epigastric artery arising from the external iliac artery. The lateral thoracic artery (choice C) arises from the second part of the axillary artery and supplies mainly the mammary gland. The posterior intercostal arteries (choice E) originate from the thoracic aorta and anastomose with the anterior intercostal arteries.

40. **(D)** The thoracic duct ascends in the posterior mediastinum between the azygous vein and the descending aorta. The left atrium (choice A) lies completely within the middle mediastinum, as does all of the heart. The phrenic nerves (choice B) descend through the superior and middle mediastina. The recurrent laryngeal nerves (choice C) have differing courses on the right and left sides: The left recurrent laryngeal nerve arises in the superior mediastinum adjacent to the aortic arch, and the right recurrent laryngeal nerve arises in the root of the neck, passing around the right subclavian artery to reenter the neck. The tracheal bifurcation (choice E) lies at the level of the sternal angle and lies largely in the middle mediastinum.

41. **(B)** The circumflex branch of the left coronary artery circles to the posterior surface of

the heart in the coronary sulcus (atrioventricular groove). It sends branches to the left atrium and left ventricle before anastomosing with the posterior interventricular branch of the right coronary artery. The apex of the heart (choice A) is supplied by the anterior interventricular branch of the left coronary artery as it descends in the anterior interventricular sulcus, and the posterior interventricular branch of the right coronary artery as it descends in the posterior interventricular sulcus. The right and left ventricles (choice C) are supplied by both the right and left coronary arteries, but the circumflex branch of the left coronary artery has little if any contribution to the right ventricle. The right atrium and right ventricle (choice D) are largely supplied by the right coronary artery as it descends in the coronary sulcus between them. The right ventricle and the interventricular septum (choice E) are supplied by both the right and left coronary arteries, but the circumflex branch of the left coronary artery has little if any contribution to the interventricular septum.

42. **(C)** The phrenic nerve (C3, C4, and C5) innervates the mediastinal pleura and central part of the diaphragmatic pleura. The pain is referred to the root of the neck and over the shoulder area because the supraclavicular nerves, which innervate this area, also originate from C3–C5. The celiac ganglia (choice A) are located in the abdomen and have no relation to the pleura. The intercostal nerves (choice B) innervate the costal pleura and peripheral parts of the diaphragmatic pleura. The paravertebral ganglia (T1–T4) (choice D) and the vagus nerve (choice E) form the pulmonary plexus and provide sympathetic and parasympathetic functions, respectively.

43. **(A)** The greater peritoneal sac communicates with the lesser sac, or omental bursa, through the epiploic foramen (of Winslow). The superior boundary is the caudate lobe of the liver. The common bile duct (choice B) lies in the free edge of the lesser omentum (the hepatoduodenal ligament) that forms the anterior boundary of the epiploic foramen. The first

part of the duodenum (choice C) is the inferior boundary of the epiploic foramen. The head of the pancreas (choice D) is separated from the epiploic foramen by the first part of the duodenum and does not form one of the boundaries of the opening. The hepatic veins (choice E) pass directly from the liver to join the inferior vena cava as it passes through the respiratory diaphragm. It is not related to the epiploic foramen.

44. **(A)** The lymphatic drainage of an organ is closely related to its blood supply. Lymphatic drainage from the testis travels along the testicular artery to reach lymph nodes along the aorta. The common iliac nodes (choice B) receive lymph from the inguinal, external iliac, and internal iliac nodes, none of which drain the testis. The deep inguinal nodes (choice C) lie alongside the femoral vein and drain the deep tissue of the thigh and leg. The internal iliac nodes (choice D) generally drain the structures supplied by branches of the internal iliac artery including the pelvic organs (but not the ovaries), the gluteal region, and the deep structures of the perineum. The superficial inguinal nodes (choice E) receive lymph from the superficial tissues of the thigh and leg, the buttock, the lower abdominal wall, and the external genitalia, but not from the testis.

45. **(C)** The artery to the hindgut and its derivatives is the inferior mesenteric artery. The celiac artery (choice A) supplies structures derived from the caudal foregut. In the fetus, the ductus arteriosus (choice B) shunts blood from the pulmonary trunk to the aorta to bypass the lungs. The superior mesenteric artery (choice D) supplies the structures derived from the midgut. In the fetus the umbilical artery (choice E) delivers blood to the placental circulation.

46. **(B)** Urine may leak from the umbilicus when the lumen of the allantois remains patent (a urachal fistula) allowing the urinary bladder to communicate with the umbilicus. A persistent and patent vitelline duct (choice A) may allow feces or mucus to leak from the umbili-

cus due to the communication between the terminal ileum and the umbilicus. An omphalocele (choice C) is a congenital hernia through the anterior abdominal wall at the umbilicus that is covered only by the amnion. An umbilical hernia (choice D) is a protrusion of the small intestine through the anterior abdominal wall at the umbilicus that is covered by peritoneum and skin. Gastroschisis (choice E) is a congenital defect in the anterior abdominal wall, not located at the umbilicus, that is accompanied by a herniation of the small intestine and part of the large intestine.

47. **(D)** The greater palatine nerve is a branch of the maxillary division of the trigeminal nerve. It comes from the pterygopalatine ganglion and emerges between the second and third molar teeth onto the hard palate. It supplies the glands, gingivae, and mucous membrane of the hard palate. The ophthalmic (choice E) and mandibular (choice C) divisions of the trigeminal nerve are, respectively, too far superior and too far inferior to contribute to the innervation of the hard palate. The facial (choice A) and glossopharyngeal (choice B) nerves do not supply branches to the hard palate.

48. **(E)** A "claw hand" is best associated with injury to the ulnar nerve at the wrist affecting the interosseus, lumbrical, and hypothenar muscles of the hand. It is characterized by a wasted palm and hypothenar eminence, hyperextended metacarpophalangeal joints, and flexed interphalangeal joints. Injury to the axillary nerve (choice A) affects the deltoid and teres minor muscles. The deltoid muscle is primarily an abductor of the upper limb, and the teres minor muscle is a lateral rotator of the shoulder. Injury to the median nerve (choice B) interferes with pronation of the forearm and flexion of the phalanges of the thumb and digits two and three. In addition, the thenar muscles waste with an accompanying inability to oppose the thumb and fingers. Injury to the musculocutaneous nerve (choice C) primarily involves the flexors of the arm and forearm. Injury to the radial nerve (choice D) may affect the extensor muscles of the arm and forearm depending on the point of injury. It is associated with "wrist drop" due to loss of the extensors of the wrist and fingers.

49. **(E)** The scaphoid bone lies in the floor of the anatomic snuffbox and acute tenderness over this area is indicative of a fracture of the scaphoid, even in the absence of radiographic verification. Approximately 70% of carpal fractures involve the scaphoid only. A fracture through its narrow middle part may deprive the scaphoid of its blood supply, causing its proximal part to undergo avascular necrosis. The capitate bone (choice A) is the largest of the carpal bones occupying a central position in the distal row of carpal bones. The hamate bone (choice B) lies in the distal row of carpal bones on the medial side of the wrist. It is not related to the anatomic snuffbox. The lunate bone (choice C) lies adjacent to the scaphoid in the proximal row of carpals and with the scaphoid articulates with the radius at the radiocarpal or wrist joint. It is not related to the anatomic snuffbox. The pisiform bone (choice D) is a sesamoid bone in the tendon of the flexor carpi ulnaris on the lateral wrist. It is not related to the anatomic snuffbox.

50. **(D)** Lesions of the radial nerve in the arm may paralyze all of the extensor muscles of the forearm, producing a "wrist drop" (flexion of the hand by gravity when the forearm is horizontal), as well as an inability to extend the digits at the metacarpophalangeal joints. Injury to the axillary nerve (choice A) affects the deltoid and teres minor muscles. The deltoid muscle is primarily an abductor of the upper limb and the teres minor muscle is a lateral rotator of the shoulder. Injury to the median nerve (choice B) in the arm interferes with pronation of the forearm and flexion of the phalanges of the thumb and digits two and three. In addition, the thenar muscles waste with an accompanying inability to oppose the thumb and fingers. Injury to the musculocutaneous nerve (choice C) primarily involves the flexors of the arm and forearm.

Injury to the ulnar nerve (choice E) in the arm affects the flexor digitorum profundus to the ring and little fingers and the interosseus, lumbrical, and hypothenar muscles of the hand. It is characterized by a wasted palm and hypothenar eminence, hyperextended metacarpophalangeal joints, and flexed interphalangeal joints.

51. **(A)** In the human pancreas, A and B cells of the islets of Langerhans secrete glucagon and insulin respectively. Pancreatic D_1 cells (choice D) release a product similar to vasoactive intestinal polypeptide. Pancreatic polypeptide cells (choice E) secrete pancreatic polypeptide and D cells (choice C) release somatostatin. All the aforementioned cells belong to the endocrine pancreas. Acinar cells (choice A) are part of the exocrine pancreas and do not secrete glucagon or insulin.

52. **(E)** The musculocutaneous nerve passes through the coracobrachialis muscle and continues distally between the biceps brachii and brachialis muscles. It supplies all three muscles. Injury to the nerve affects flexion at the shoulder (coracobrachialis and biceps brachii), flexion at the elbow (brachialis and biceps brachii), and supination of the forearm (biceps brachii). Diminished cutaneous sensation over the medial forearm (choice A) results from injury to the C8 or T1 spinal nerves, the medial cord of the brachial plexus, or the medial antebrachial cutaneous nerve arising from it. Diminished cutaneous sensation over the medial palm (choice B) results from injury to the C8 spinal nerve, the ulnar nerve, or the palmar cutaneous branch of the ulnar nerve. Weakened abduction at the shoulder (choice C) results from injury to the axillary nerve affecting the deltoid muscle or injury to the suprascapular nerve affecting the supraspinatus muscle. Weakened extension at the elbow (choice D) results from injury to the radial nerve affecting the triceps brachii muscle.

53. **(D)** The collective neurologic signs are characteristic of a lesion of the neocerebellum (cerebellar hemispheres). A lesion in the archicerebellum (cerebellar vermis; arrow #5, choice E) results in loss of equilibrium. None of the other choices apply to the collection of neurologic signs displayed by this patient: arrow #1 (choice A) points to the temporal lobe, arrow #2 (choice B) to the eyeball, and arrow #3 (choice C) to the pons.

54. **(D)** The cystic artery most commonly arises from the right hepatic artery. In decreasing order of occurrence, it can also arise from the left hepatic artery (choice C), gastroduodenal artery (choice A), or hepatic artery proper (choice B). The superior pancreaticoduodenal artery (choice E) is located too far inferiorly to contribute to the blood supply of the gallbladder.

55. **(D)** The number of terminal air sacs and the level of surfactant are sufficient by 26 to 28 weeks after fertilization to allow for survival of the premature infant. Before this time, the alveolar surface area is insufficient and the vascular system is underdeveloped. Choice A is the pseudoglandular period of lung development and choice B is the canalicular period. Choice C is the period when surfactant production begins, but the small amount present is insufficient for respiration. After birth (choice E), the lungs develop by a large increase in the number of pulmonary alveoli and capillaries. However, normal respiration by the premature infant is possible by 26 to 28 weeks.

56. **(D)** Retinal separation typically occurs at the interface between the retinal pigment epithelium and the outer limit of the sensory (neural) retina. The weakness of this plane is attributed to the manner in which the retina develops, a process that involves obliteration of the space between two of the layers of the optic cup—an inner layer from which the sensory retina arises, and an outer layer from which the retinal pigment epithelium arises. Other retinal layers are bridged by neuronal processes, and Müller cells (the retina's glial cells) span the entire thickness of the neural retina. Plane A (choice A) marks the boundary between the nerve fiber layer above and the ganglion cell layer below. The nerve fiber

layer is composed of axons of the retinal gan-glion cells. Plane B (choice B) is within the in-ner plexiform layer, the site of synaptic con-tacts between bipolar neurons, retinal ganglion cells, and amacrine cells. Plane C (choice C) is within the outer plexiform layer, the site of synapses between bipolar cells, rods and cones, and horizontal cells. The boundary between the choroid (of the middle vascular tunic or uvea) and the sclera (of the external, fibrous tunic) is marked by plane E (choice E).

57. **(E)** Virus-infected cells are the main natural targets of cytotoxic T cells (CD8$^+$). This class of lymphocyte recognizes antigens only when presented on the plasmalemmas of host (self) cells in association with class I MHC. Typically, these are viral antigens ex-pressed by infected cells. Cytotoxic cells are also activated by allogenic tissue grafts (choice A) via recognition of non-self-MHC molecules; however, this phenomenon (which is a result of the polymorphic nature of class I MHC genes) does not represent the typical natural function of these cells. Al-though regulatory T lymphocytes are impor-tant in defense against bacteria (choice B), bacterial toxins (choice C), and protozoan parasites (choice D), the direct destruction of these agents is brought about by other effec-tor mechanisms, such as the complement sys-tem, macrophages, and granulocytic leuko-cytes, that are triggered by immunoglobulins, which are produced by B lymphocytes.

58. **(A)** The neuroectoderm of the optic cup gives rise to the neural retina, pigmented retinal ep-ithelium, ciliary epithelium, posterior iridial epithelium, and anterior iridial epithelium. The lens epithelium (choice E) is derived from the lens placode, specialization of the surface ectoderm overlying the optic cup. The other structures (choices B, C, and D) are all mes-enchymal derivatives. The ciliary muscle (choice C) and choriocapillaris layer (choice B) are derived from the uvea (choroidal or vascular coat). The extraocular muscles, in-cluding the lateral rectus (choice D), are de-rived from mesenchyme, although there is some uncertainty about their precise origin.

59. **(B)** Obstruction of the portal vein results in an increase in the collateral circulation be-tween veins that normally drain to the portal vein and those that drain to the systemic veins. Choices A, B, D, and E all represent possible collateral venous circulation in case of portal obstruction. Choice A is rare be-cause the ductus venosus closes after birth. Choice B is correct because varicose veins in this region give rise to esophageal varices. Choice D results in varicose veins in the rec-tal region. Choice C is incorrect because there is no connection between the right gastric vein and the inferior vena cava. In choice E, enlargement of the epigastric veins results in varicose veins radiating from the umbilicus, the caput medusae.

60. **(C)** Antimitotic drugs disrupt microtubule assembly in the formation of the mitotic spin-dle. In addition to killing rapidly dividing tu-mor cells, this can deplete intestinal epithelial cells, blood cells, and other populations of normal cells that have a high rate of replace-ment. Because cardiac muscle cells (choice A), lens epithelial cells (choice B), and neu-rons (choices D and E) are all terminally dif-ferentiated, nondividing cells, they are not susceptible to spindle poisons.

61. **(E)** The space between plasmalemmas of ad-jacent epithelial cells is obliterated at the tight junction (zonula occludens), which forms by fusion of the membranes along narrow anas-tomosing bands. The tight junction is the api-cal-most part of the junctional complex, which is typical of epithelia lining tubular and hollow organs. The zonula adherens and desmosome (choice A) also contribute to the junctional complex, but they hold adjacent cells together. The gap junction (choice B) functions to electrically and chemically cou-ple adjacent cells. It consists of direct chan-nels (connexons) between cells, but there is a significant space (about 2 nm) separating the membranes between the channels. The hemidesmosome (choice C) is a specializa-tion for adhesion of a cell to its basement membrane. The terminal bar (choice D) is not a type of junction, but rather a manifestation

of the junctional complex seen with the light microscope.

62. **(D)** Action potentials (APs) are initiated at the myoneural junction on the surface of a muscle fiber. T tubules are narrow invaginations of the sarcolemma that channel the APs to the vicinity of the sarcoplasmic reticulum organized around myofibrils. Muscle spindles (choice A) are complex sensory structures that monitor changes in muscle length. The endomysium (choice B) is the thin connective tissue layer surrounding each muscle fiber. The sarcoplasmic reticulum (choice C) does not conduct APs; rather it responds to APs by releasing calcium. The Z line (choice E) is a component of the sarcomere that serves as an anchor for actin filaments.

63. **(D)** The macula densa is a modified segment of the distal tubule at the site of its passage adjacent to the vascular pole of the renal corpuscle. The name arises from the close spacing of nuclei of the epithelial cells forming this part of the distal tubule. These cells are thought to sense the chloride content in the passing filtrate and generate signals that regulate the caliber of the afferent arteriole. Bowman's capsule (choice A) encompasses the capillaries of the glomerulus in two layers of epithelium. The inner, closely applied, visceral layer of podocytes is continuous at the vascular pole with the outer, parietal layer of squamous cells. Between the two layers is the urinary space, which is continuous with the lumen of the proximal convoluted tubule (choice E), which is not a component of the juxtaglomerular apparatus. Mesangial cells (choice B) are incompletely understood cells found in the glomerulus and in the juxtaglomerular apparatus. The afferent arteriole (choice C) feeds blood to the glomerulus. As part of the juxtaglomerular apparatus, it is closely apposed to the macula densa.

64. **(B)** The lingual artery arises from the external carotid artery at the level of the tip of the greater horn of the hyoid bone. It courses medial to the posterior border of the hyoglossus muscle to supply the floor of the mouth and the tongue. The ascending pharyngeal, facial, and maxillary arteries (choices A, C, and E) are all branches of the external carotid artery, which do not supply the tongue. The internal carotid artery (choice D) does not have branches at this level and supplies mainly the brain along with the eye, forehead, and, partially, the nose.

65. **(D)** Oxytocin is synthesized by neurons that have their cell bodies in the hypothalamus. These cells project their axons to the pars nervosa, so this is where the hormone is secreted, not within the hypothalamus (choice C). Acidophils (choice A) secrete either growth hormone or prolactin. Basophils (choice B) of the adenohypophysis secrete corticotropin, thyrotropin, or gonadotropic hormones. Pituicytes (choice E) are not hormone-secreting cells, but are glial cells located in the pars nervosa.

66. **(E)** The thymus provides for development of new T lymphocytes in an environment shielded from foreign antigens. Like bone marrow, the thymus is a primary lymphoid organ, and not a site of reactions to foreign antigens. Lymphoid follicles are sites of B lymphocyte proliferation in response to antigen stimulation. These occur in the lymph nodes (choice A), Peyer's patches (choice B), tonsils (choice C), and white pulp of the spleen (choice D).

67. **(B)** The levator ani muscle forms part of the pelvic diaphragm and consists of the pubococcygeus, the puborectalis, and the iliococcygeus. The coccygeus is also part of the pelvic diaphragm, but its nerve (choice A) does not innervate the puborectalis, which is part of the levator ani. The nerve to obturator internus (choice C) innervates the muscle of the same name and the superior gemellus in the gluteal region. The pelvic splanchnic nerves (choice D) provide only the parasympathetic innervation of the pelvic structures. The pudendal nerve (choice E) is sensory to the genitalia and motor to the perineal muscles, the external urethral sphincter, and the external anal sphincter.

68. **(E)** The normal laboratory values can be used to calculate the upper limit of the normal range of absolute counts/mm³ for each leukocyte (maximum normal total leukocyte count times the maximum normal percentage for the cell type). The patient's differential percentages can each be multiplied by 24,000/mm³ to obtain total counts per mm³ for each leukocyte type. The following table shows the results of these calculations. Asterisks (*) indicate values that are elevated.

Leukocyte	Normal upper limit (per mm³)	Patient's count (per mm³)
Segmented neutrophils	6820	17,040*
Band form neutrophils	550	3840*
Eosinophils	330	960*
Basophils	82	48
Lymphocytes	3630	720
Monocytes	770	1440*

69. **(A)** Although numbers of eosinophils and monocytes are somewhat elevated, the most prominent change in circulating leukocyte numbers is a greatly elevated neutrophil count, with a "shift to the left" (increased numbers of immature forms). This is indicative of a bacterial infection. Chronic lymphocytic leukemia (choice B) results in lymphocytosis. Parasitic infections (choice C) and severe allergic reactions (choice D) are more likely to result specifically in an eosinophilia. Fragile, abnormally shaped erythrocytes are produced in sickle cell disease (choice E), resulting in chronic hemolytic anemia.

70. **(D)** The space of Disse separates hepatocytes from the endothelial cells that form the hepatic sinusoids. Thus, it is bordered partly by endothelium on one side and by microvilli of the hepatocytes on the other (choice E). The initial channel for flow of bile (choice A) is the bile canaliculus formed by junctions between adjacent hepatocytes. The endothelium of the sinusoids allows free passage of plasma, but not cells (choice B), into the space of Disse. The portal triad (choice C) is composed of an arteriolar branch of the hepatic artery, a venule conducting blood from the hepatic portal vein, and a bile duct. These are accompanied by one or more lymphatic vessels.

71. **(D)** Generation of specific granules occurs during the myelocyte stage. Development of all three types of granulocytes follows a similar sequence of stages. The granulocyte-colony–forming unit (choice A) is an undifferentiated progenitor cell of the granulocyte line. Buildup of the protein synthesis machinery occurs during the myeloblast (choice C) and promyelocyte (choice E) stages. The promyelocyte stage is also characterized by production of primary (nonspecific) granules. After the myelocyte stage, further condensation and reshaping of the nucleus occurs during the metamyelocyte stage (choice B).

72. **(B)** The term *acidophilic* describes the staining behavior of cellular components (e.g., proteins with a high content of basic amino acids) that attract acid dyes such as eosin. Concentrations of mitochondria, such as occur in parietal cells, confer cytoplasmic acidophilia. Parietal cells secrete hydrochloric acid (choice A), but they do not store it. Moreover, an acidic substance attracts basic dyes, such as hematoxylin. Rough endoplasmic reticulum (choice C), which occurs in only a small degree in parietal cells, is basophilic due to its high RNA content. Parietal cells are also the source of intrinsic factor (choice D), but they do not contain readily evident secretory granules. Chief cells, not parietal cells, synthesize pepsinogen (choice E) and store it in secretory granules.

73. **(D)** The superior thyroid artery gives rise to the superior laryngeal artery. The ascending pharyngeal artery (choice A), the lingual artery (choice C), and the superior thyroid artery (choice D) are all branches of the external carotid artery. However, both the ascending pharyngeal and the lingual arteries arise above the level of the larynx and do not contribute to its vascular supply. The inferior thyroid artery (choice B) gives rise to the inferior laryngeal artery. The vertebral artery (choice E) has no branches in the neck and gives a major vascular contribution to the brain.

74. **(E)** The syncytiotrophoblast forms the surface layer of the chorionic villi and is bathed by maternal blood flowing through the intervillus space. Fetal capillaries (choice B) course through the fetal connective tissue (choice A) that forms the core of all orders of villi and thus have no contact with maternal blood when placental structure is intact. Because the syncytiotrophoblast is a derivative of the embryonic trophoblast layer, it is incorrect to state that maternal blood has no contact with fetally derived cells (choice C). The syncytiotrophoblast is a product of division and fusion of cells in the underlying cytotrophoblast (choice D).

75. **(C)** The parotid gland is the only major salivary gland containing almost exclusively serous secretory cells. Esophageal (choice A) and intestinal glands (choice B) are small mucus-secreting glands. The sublingual glands (choice D) and submandibular (choice E) are mixed glands, with differing proportions of serous and mucous cells.

76. **(E)** The source of intrinsic factor in humans is parietal cells of gastric glands. Intrinsic factor is required for absorption of vitamin B_{12}. Pepsinogen (choice A) and lipase (choice B) are secreted by chief cells of gastric fundic glands, but pepsin and lipase are digestive enzymes unrelated to vitamin B_{12} absorption. Gastrin is a hormone that stimulates acid secretion by parietal cells. It is secreted by one type of enteroendocrine cell (choice C), type G, in the pyloric glands. Lysozyme is an enzyme found in Paneth cells (choice D) of the small intestine as well as in neutrophils. It hydrolyzes glycosides of the cell wall of some gram-positive bacteria, and may be involved in regulation of the intestinal flora.

77. **(C)** The spinal cord and its meninges do not entirely fill the vertebral canal. The space between the walls of this canal and the outer meninx of the cord, the dura mater, is the epidural space, which is filled with fat, connective tissue, and a plexus of veins. This is the internal vertebral venous plexus, which consists of anterior and posterior internal vertebral venous plexuses. The anterior spinal artery (choice A), posterior spinal arteries (choice E), and middle cerebral artery (choice D) are all located deep to the arachnoid mater. The external venous plexuses (choice B), which communicate with the internal venous plexus, are located anterior to the vertebral bodies and posterior to the vertebral arches.

78. **(C)** The glossopharyngeal nerve provides parasympathetic innervation for the parotid gland. The facial nerve provides the parasympathetic innervation of the lacrimal (choice A), nasal (choice B), sublingual (choice D), and submandibular (choice E) glands.

79. **(D)** The middle meningeal artery arises from the first or mandibular part of the maxillary artery. It runs superiorly through the foramen spinosum to reach the middle cranial fossa. From there, the artery divides into an anterior and a posterior branch supplying the meninges. The external carotid artery (choice A) supplies branches mainly to the neck, face (facial artery, choice B), and scalp (superficial temporal artery, choice E). The internal carotid artery (choice C) supplies branches mainly to the brain.

80. **(D)** Abnormal development of either the septum primum or septum secundum results in ostium secundum atrial septal defects in the area of the fossa ovalis. This common type of congenital heart defect is manifested by a patent foramen ovale between right and left atria. This is well tolerated during childhood but symptoms usually appear after 30 years of age. The aorticopulmonary septum (choice A) divides the truncus arteriosus of the developing heart and gives rise to the ascending aorta and pulmonary trunk. The endocardial cushions (choice B) give rise to the right and left atrioventricular canals. The interventricular septum (choice C) forms between the right and left ventricles. The sinus venosus (choice E) becomes incorporated into the atria as well as giving rise to the openings of the pulmonary veins and the venae cavae.

81. (B) Sensory ganglia are characterized histologically by the presence of clusters or columns of spherical neuronal cell bodies (somas or perikarya) interposed between bundles of nerve fibers. The micrograph illustrates some other features typical of somas of primary sensory (pseudounipolar) neurons: (1) centrally located nucleus, (2) a distinct covering of satellite cells (note the layer of small nuclei around each soma), and (3) a wide range of sizes. The cerebellar cortex (choice A) is composed of both cell bodies and nerve fibers, but these are organized in distinct layers. Moreover, the cell bodies (principally Purkinje cells and granule cells) have distinctive sizes and shapes. A peripheral nerve (choice C) is a bundle of nerve fibers; no cell bodies are seen. The pterygopalatine ganglion (choice D) and superior cervical ganglion (choice E) are autonomic ganglia, which are sites of synaptic contact between preganglionic nerve fibers and the multipolar postsynaptic neurons that project directly to effector organs. Like sensory ganglia, autonomic ganglia are composed of nerve fibers and neuronal cell bodies, but there are distinguishing features: (1) somas are scattered homogeneously among the nerve fibers rather than clustered, (2) somas have a narrow range of sizes, (3) nuclei tend to have an eccentric location within the soma, and (4) the satellite cells encompassing each soma are less prominent.

82. (E) The black areas in this section of dried, compact bone are empty spaces normally occupied by cells and soft tissues. The arrows indicate lacunae interspersed among lamellae of osteons (haversian systems). In life, these are occupied by osteocytes. The fine lines radiating from the lacunae are canaliculi, which contained processes of the osteocytes. Blood vessels (choice A) of compact bone course through Volkmann's canals (not shown) and haversian canals (seen here at the center of each osteon). Hematopoietic cells (choice B) occur in red marrow located within medullary canals of long bones and the cavities of cancellous bone. Osteoblasts (choice C) are restricted to surfaces of bone at sites of bone apposition.

When osteoblasts become entrapped in lacunae as a result of their synthetic activity, they become osteocytes. Osteoclasts (choice D) are large, multinucleated cells found at surfaces of bone at sites that are undergoing absorption.

83. (E) The portal system in the infant is derived from the vitelline vein, which drains the yolk sac in the embryo. The anterior (choice A) and posterior (choice C) cardinal veins respectively drain the cranial portion and caudal portions of the embryo. They join the common cardinal veins (choice B), which drain into the sinus venosus. The cardinal veins give rise to the caval system in the infant. The umbilical system (choice D), which carries oxygenated blood from the placenta to the embryonic heart, degenerates after birth.

84. (D) The ciliary, sphincter pupillae, and medial rectus muscles participate in the near response. Signals originating in the right eye are directed to both the right and left pretectal region, not only the right side (choice E). Dilation of the pupil is mediated via postganglionic neurons in the superior cervical ganglion, not the ciliary ganglion (choice A). Neurons in the left Edinger–Westphal nucleus receive input from both eyes, not only the the right eye (choice B). The blink reflex involves the trigeminal (sensory limb) and facial (motor limb), nerves but not the oculomotor nerve (choice C).

85. (E) The inferior parathyroid glands and the thymus arise from the third pharyngeal pouch. The superior parathyroid glands develop from the fourth pharyngeal pouch (choice C). The fifth pharyngeal pouch (choice A) in the human is rudimentary or absent. The first pharyngeal pouch (choice B) gives rise to the tympanic membrane, tympanic cavity, mastoid antrum, and pharyngotympanic tube. The palatine tonsil along with the tonsillar sinus and crypts develop from the second pharyngeal pouch (choice D).

86. (A) The sensations of discriminative touch and vibration are transmitted through the medial lemniscus. Pain and temperature pathways decussate in the ventral white commisssure (choice B). The nucleus gracilis (choice C) contains neurons that process sensory signals from the lower extremity. The second-order fibers carrying discriminative touch and vibration from the upper limb originate from neurons in the nucleus cuneatus (choice D).

87. **(C)** The principal somatosensory pathways course through the posterior limb of the internal capsule and terminate in the postcentral gyrus, not the precentral gyrus (choice D). The somatosensory pathways decussate in the spinal cord or brainstem, not in the thalamus (choice A). The ventral posterior nucleus of the thalamus is the principal processing station for somatosensation, not the ventral lateral nucleus (choice B). The somatosensory pathways typically involve a three-neuron chain, not a two-neuron sequence (choice E).

88. **(A)** The ascending MLF provides input to the oculomotor and abducens nuclei. The lateral vestibulospinal tract originates from the lateral vestibular nucleus, not the medial vestibular nucleus (choice E). The descending portion of the MLF courses into the spinal cord and has no influence over extraocular muscles (choice B). The medial vestibulospinal tract extends to cervical or upper thoracic levels but not to the lumbar spinal cord (choice C). The vestibulospinal tracts primarily influence extensor musculature, not flexors (choice D).

89. **(C)** A patient with extensive damage in the lower brainstem is likely to have some involvement of the vestibular nuclei or their connections, and this precludes nystagmus from being induced. In contrast, nystagmus can be induced (not choice D) with appropriate stimulation in a patient who has no involvement of the vestibular nuclei or their connections. The direction of nystagmus is defined as the direction of the fast component (not choice A) of the movement. Nystagmus is not limited to horizontal (choice B) eye movements. When observed following appropriate stimulation in a patient, the presence of nystagmus indicates that there is no damage to the vestibular system (not choice E).

90. **(D)** The uterine artery crosses anterior and superior to the ureter, near the lateral fornix of the vagina. The ureter is thus in danger of being clamped or severed by mistake during a hysterectomy. The internal iliac artery (choice A) is located lateral to and gives rise to the uterine artery. The ligament of the ovary (choice B), ovarian artery (choice C) and uterine tube (choice E) are located superior to the uterine artery. None of these structures (choices A, B, C, and E) are in close proximity to the uterine artery.

91. **(E)** The near response, but not the pupillary light reflex, involves the visual cortex. The near response includes bilateral activation of the medial rectus muscles, not the lateral rectus muscles (choice A). The near response includes disconjugate, not conjugate (choice B) eye movements. The near response involves both the oculomotor nerve (choice C) and the optic nerve (choice D).

92. **(D)** The internal laryngeal nerve supplies the laryngeal mucosa above the level of the vocal fold as well as the mucosa of the piriform recess and the epiglottic valleculae. The external laryngeal nerve (choice A) is motor to the cricothyroid muscle and the lowest part of the inferior pharyngeal constrictor muscle. The glossopharyngeal nerve (choice B) carries afferent fibers from the mucosa of the middle ear, auditory tube, pharynx, palatine tonsils, and posterior one-third of the tongue, but does not supply the laryngeal mucosa. The inferior laryngeal nerve (choice C) is motor to the intrinsic muscles of the larynx except the cricothyroid muscle, and is sensory to the mucosa of the larynx below the level of the vocal fold. The pharyngeal plexus (choice E) supplies most of the innervation to the pharynx, including general visceral afferent fibers from the pharyngeal mucosa that are carried in the glossopharyngeal nerve.

93. **(A)** The attachment of the hepatic veins to the inferior vena cava forms the major support of the liver. The peritoneal ligaments (choices B, C, and D) and the round ligament of the liver (choice E), a remnant of the fetal umbilical vein, play minor roles in supporting the liver.

94. **(D)** A congenital defect of the pleuroperitoneal membrane results in an abnormal opening in the posterolateral aspects of the diaphragm. This defect occurs more often on the left side of the body. It is due to the failure of the pleuroperitoneal membrane to form properly and/or to fuse with the other parts of the diaphragm: the mesentery of the esophagus (choice A), the muscular ingrowth of the body wall (choice B), and the septum transversum (choice E). The pleuropericardial membranes (choice C) participate in the formation of the mediastinum and do not contribute to the formation of the diaphragm.

95. **(E)** The lymph of the posterior one-third of the tongue drains to the superior deep cervical lymph nodes. The inferior deep cervical lymph nodes (choice A) drain the medial aspect of the anterior two-thirds of the tongue. The submandibular lymph nodes (choice C) drain the lateral portions of the anterior two thirds of the tongue. The apex of the tongue drains to the submental lymph nodes (choice D). The retropharyngeal lymph nodes (choice B) drain structures within and above the roof of the mouth.

96. **(D)** Compression of cranial nerve III, in combination with descending corticospinal and corticobulbar fibers occurs, as part of superior alternating hemiplegia. Patients with Broca's aphasia (choice A) typically do not exhibit involvement of the pupillary light reflexes. Inferior alternating hemiplegia (choice B) and middle alternating hemiplegia (choice C) involve cranial nerves XII and VI, respectively, in combination with corticospinal fibers. Wallenberg syndrome (lateral medullary syndrome) (choice E) typically does not include damage to the corticospinal tract.

97. **(E)** The skin in the affected area is red and dry (not moist as in choice D) due to diminished sympathetic activity. The pupil on the affected side is constricted (myosis) (not dilated as in choice B) due to unopposed activity of the sphincter pupillae muscle. Motor deficits such as atrophy of tongue musculature (choice A) or paralysis of facial expression muscles (choice C) are typically not part of Horner syndrome.

98. **(B)** The VIIth cranial nerve supplies the stapedius muscle, which dampens sounds by reducing the movements of the stapes in the oval window. A patient with injury to the facial nerve may also display paralysis of the facial musculature, loss of taste sensation, and loss of lacrimation on the affected side. The facial nerve provides motor innervation to the muscles of facial expression, taste sensation on the anterior two thirds of the tongue via the chorda tympani and parasympathetic innervation to the pterygopalatine ganglion via the greater petrosal nerve. Injury to the other cranial nerves (choices A, C, D, and E) does not affect the stapedius muscle.

99. **(E)** A lesion in the dominant hemisphere involving the ventrolateral parietal lobe is likely to include Wernicke's area. Damage to this cortical region produces a receptive (sensory) aphasia known as Wernicke's aphasia. Broca's (motor) aphasia (choice A) is the result of damage to the frontal operculum in the dominant hemisphere. Contralateral hemineglect (choice B) is typically caused by lesions in the nondominant parietal lobe, whereas motor aprosodia (choice C), the inability to impart proper emotional tone to speech, is due to damage to the frontal operculum in the nondominant hemisphere. Prosopagnosia (choice D), the inability to recognize familiar faces, most frequently results from bilateral damage to the ventral portion of the temporo-occipital association cortex.

100. **(B)** Arrow #3 indicates the mastoid sinus. The auricle can be seen as a flap of tissue lateral to the mastoid sinus. The scan, as indi-

cated by the insert at the bottom right, is at the level of the inferior nasal concha. The frontal (choice A) and sphenoidal (choice E) sinuses cannot be seen at this level. The maxillary sinus (choice C) is indicated by arrow #1, and the pharynx (choice D) by arrow #2.

101.   **(C)** Capsular lesions of the corticobulbar system produce the "central seven" symptoms. Loss of the descending cortical fibers to the contralateral facial nucleus (cranial nerve VII) primarily affects the muscles of facial expression in the lower portion of the face, particularly those around the angle of the mouth and the nasolabial fold. Deviation of the protruded tongue (choice A), hypertonia/hyperreflexia (choice B), and spastic hemiplegia (choice E) are symptoms that result from a capsular lesion, but they would be seen contralateral to the affected capsule, and in this case would involve the left side of the body. Paraplegia (choice D) is not typically seen following a unilateral capsular lesion.

102.   **(D)** The cytoarchitectural subdivisions of the SI cortex are numbered from anterior to posterior as 3a, 3b, 1, and 2. All four subdivisions of the SI cortex (not just 3b as in choice A) contain a complete representation of the entire body surface. Areas 3a and 2 (choice B) receive input from muscle spindle afferents and Golgi tendon organs, whereas areas 3b and 1 (choice C) receive mostly cutaneous inputs. The somatotopic representation of the body surface in the primary somatosensory cortex is arranged in a "tongue-to-tail" (not the reverse as indicated in choice E) sequence from ventrolateral to dorsomedial.

103.   **(A)** The entry of calcium into the axon terminal initiates the sequence of events leading to release of neurotransmitter. Following vesicular release, the neurotransmitter agent binds to receptors on the postsynaptic membrane, not the presynaptic membrane (choice B). Docking proteins (choice C) attach synaptic vesicles to the presynaptic membrane. Fusion of vesicles with the presynaptic membrane (choice D) results in the release of one quantum of the transmitter agent. There are no actin bridges (choice E) that join the pre- and postsynaptic membranes.

104.   **(E)** The type Ia sensory fibers from a spindle form direct excitatory synapses with alpha motoneurons. Activation of type Ia sensory fibers (choice A) leads to excitation of the muscle in which that spindle is located. Alpha motoneurons (choice B) synapse with extrafusal muscle fibers, whereas gamma motoneurons synapse with intrafusal muscle fibers. Each intrafusal muscle fiber (choice C) is innervated by only one gamma motoneuron. Each muscle spindle contains a mixture of both nuclear bag and nuclear chain intrafusal fibers, not just one type as indicated in choice D.

105.   **(A)** The Babinski sign—dorsiflexion of the great toe in response to stroking the plantar aspect of the foot—is a characteristic sign of pyramidal tract involvement. Signs and symptoms of corticospinal tract injury that are nearly always apparent to some degree include spastic paralysis, hypertonia, loss of deep tendon reflexes, and hyperactive abdominal and cremasteric reflexes. Flaccid paralysis and hypotonia (choice B) are commonly seen following lower motoneuron injury, as is loss of deep tendon reflexes (choice E). Muscle degeneration and atrophy (choice C) are not characteristic symptoms of corticospinal tract damage. The presence of an intention tremor (choice D) is a sign of cerebellar damage, and is not seen with corticospinal tract lesions.

106.   **(A)** Spastic muscles exhibit an increase in the resistance to passive manipulation by the examiner. The muscles typically affected by spasticity are physiologic limb extensors and not postural muscles as indicated in choice B. Muscles that exhibit spastic paralysis are hypertonic, not hypotonic (choice C). Muscles that exhibit fibrillations (choice E) or decreased deep tendon reflexes (choice D) are demonstrating signs of lower motoneuron damage, not involvement of upper motoneurons that form the corticospinal tract.

107. (B) The primary axial artery in the embryo gives rise to the common interosseous artery in the adult. The anterior interosseous (choice A) and posterior interosseous (choice C) arteries are branches of the common interosseous artery. The radial (choice D) and ulnar (choice E) arteries are branches of the brachial artery (the primary axial artery in the arm).

108. (C) The nucleus raphe magnus receives input from the periaqueductal gray and gives rise to descending serotonergic fibers of the raphespinal projection. The latter fibers activate enkephalinergic spinal cord interneurons that presynaptically inhibit incoming pain fibers at their initial synapse in the spinal cord dorsal horn. The neurotransmitter dopamine (choice A) has not been shown to be involved in the descending systems that modulate pain transmission. The medial longitudinal fasciculus (choice B) is an ascending fiber system in the brainstem that is primarily involved in the control of eye movements. The rubrospinal system (choice D) is a descending fiber tract involved with the control of limb musculature. The ventral lateral nucleus of the thalamus (choice E) is primarily involved with motor function and does not contribute to descending pathways that influence pain transmission.

109. (A) Each taste receptor responds best to a specific type of stimulus quality, but may respond with less vigor to the other stimuli. The taste receptors are arranged in a rostro-caudal pattern (not medial to lateral as indicated in choice E), such that the most anterior respond best to sweet and salty stimuli, whereas sour and bitter sensations are represented posteriorly. Taste receptors are not typically found on the lateral surfaces (choice B) of the tongue. Taste receptors are stimulated when a solid or fluid substance diffuses through its apical pore and depolarizes the cell. The only receptors that hyperpolarize (choice C) in response to their preferred stimulus are retinal photoreceptors. Taste receptors generally have a relatively short life span of 7 to 10 days (not 3 months as indicated in choice D).

110. (A) The muscles that dorsiflex the ankle joint are located in the anterior compartment of the leg and are innervated by the deep peroneal nerve. The evertors of the foot occupy the lateral compartment of the leg and are supplied by the superficial peroneal nerve. Thus, the common peroneal nerve innervates both the dorsiflexors and evertors of the foot. The deep peroneal nerve (choice B) supplies the dorsiflexors of the foot located in the anterior compartment of the leg, but not the evertors of the foot located in the lateral compartment. The obturator nerve (choice C) supplies the adductor muscle group of the medial thigh. The superficial peroneal nerve (choice D) supplies the evertors of the foot located in the lateral compartment of the leg, but not the dorsiflexors of the foot located in the anterior compartment. The tibial nerve (choice E) supplies the muscles of the posterior leg which are plantar flexors and invertors of the foot.

111. (A) Arrow #1 points out the azygos vein, which is seen at this level posterior to the carina of the trachea (arrow #2, choice B). Arrow #3 (choice C) indicates the superior vena cava, and arrows 4 (choice D) and 5 (choice E) respectively show the ascending aorta and descending aorta.

112. (D) The posterior cruciate ligament prevents backward sliding of the tibia on the femur. Abnormal anteroposterior movement when the knee is flexed is a "drawer" sign. The anterior cruciate ligament (choice A) prevents forward sliding of the tibia on the femur, but not backward movement. The fibular collateral ligament (choice B) extends from the lateral femoral epicondyle to the head of the fibula. It does not significantly restrict anterior or posterior sliding movements between the tibia and femur. The oblique popliteal ligament (choice C) is an upward and lateral extension of the semimembranosus tendon, which reinforces the capsule of the knee joint posteriorly. It helps to resist hyperextension of the knee, but does not significantly restrict anterior or posterior sliding movements between the tibia and femur. The tibial collateral ligament (choice E) extends from the medial femoral condyle to the medial tibial condyle, blending with and reinforcing the medial part of the fibrous capsule. It does not significantly restrict anterior or posterior sliding movements between the tibia and femur.

113. **(E)** Transposition of the great vessels occurs when the truncoconal ridges fail to spiral as they divide the outflow tract into two channels. This produces two totally independent circulatory loops with the right ventricle feeding into the aorta and the left ventricle feeding into the pulmonary artery. Common atrium (choice A) results from a complete failure of the septum primum and septum secundum to form. Persistent atrioventricular canal (choice B) results from a failure of the endocardial cushions to fuse and partition the atrioventricular canal into a right and left component. It is accompanied by defects of the atrial and ventricular septa. Persistent truncus arteriosus (choice C) results from a total failure of the truncoconal ridges to develop and partition the outflow tract of the developing heart. Tetralogy of Fallot (choice D) is a related group of defects with the primary malformation being an unequal division of the outflow tract resulting in pulmonary stenosis. The other features of tetralogy are an interventricular septal defect, an overriding aorta, and right ventricular hypertrophy. Survival of the infant depends on the maintenance of a patent ductus arteriosus.

114. **(E)** The azygos vein normally drains into the superior vena cava. The inferior vena cava (choice A) mainly drains venous blood from the hepatic veins from the liver. The right posterior intercostal veins (choice D) drain into the azygos vein, and not the reverse. The right brachiocephalic vein (choice B) and the right jugular vein (choice C) unite to form the superior vena cava.

115. **(C)** The posterior one-third of the tongue is derived from the third pharyngeal arch and is thus innervated by cranial nerve IX (glossopharyngeal). The first pharyngeal arch (choice A) and second pharyngeal arch (choice B) give rise to the anterior two-thirds of the tongue. The mandibular division of cranial nerve V (trigeminal) provides general sensation to the anterior two thirds of the tongue, and cranial nerve VII via the chorda tympani provides special sensation (taste). The fourth pharyngeal arch (choice D) gives rise to the epiglottis and, along with the sixth pharyngeal arch (choice E), to the laryngeal cartilages. The nerve to the fourth pharyngeal arch is cranial nerve X (vagus).

116. **(C)** Parasympathetic nerves originating from the second, third, and fourth sacral segments of the spinal cord control erection of the penis. The genitofemoral nerve (choice A) is a branch of the lumbar plexus, which is motor to the cremaster muscle and sensory to the inner aspect of the thigh. Parasympathetic branches of the vagus nerve (choice B) terminate at the level of the splenic flexure of the transverse colon and do not reach the penis. Sympathetic nerves from the lumbar segments of the spinal cord (choice D) control ejaculation, but not erection of the penis. The sympathetic system is also called the thoracolumbar system because its preganglionic fibers arise only from these segments of the spinal cord, and not from the sacral segments (choice E).

117. **(D)** The medial circumflex femoral artery supplies the most important source of blood to the femoral head and neck. This artery anastomoses with the artery to the head of the femur (choice A), which arises from the obturator artery. However, if the medial circumflex femoral artery is injured, the blood flow in the small artery to the head of the femur may not be sufficient to prevent posttraumatic avascular necrosis of the femoral head. Normally, the medial and lateral circumflex femoral arteries arise from the deep artery of the thigh, but occasionally they arise from the femoral artery (choice B). However, the femoral artery is not a direct vascular source to the head of the femur. The lateral circumflex femoral artery (choice C) and superior gluteal artery (choice E) also supply

the hip joint but their contribution to the head and neck of the femur is less than that of the medial femoral circumflex artery.

118. **(D)** The prevertebral fascia crosses the midline anterior to the prevertebral muscles and continues laterally, covering the scalene muscles and forming the floor of the posterior triangle. The common carotid artery (choice A) lies within the carotid sheath. The esophagus (choice B) is surrounded by the pretracheal (visceral) fascia. The internal jugular vein (choice C) lies within the carotid sheath. The vagus nerve (choice E) lies within the carotid sheath.

119. **(B)** The superior thyroid artery is usually the first branch of the external carotid artery. The brachiocephalic artery (choice A) gives rise to the right subclavian artery, the right common carotid artery, and occasionally a single thyroidea ima (lowest thyroid) artery. The facial artery (choice C) and the lingual artery arise as independent branches of the external carotid artery. The internal carotid artery (choice D) gives off no major branches in the neck. The thyrocervical trunk (choice E) arises from the subclavian artery and gives rise to the inferior thyroid artery.

120. **(D)** The lower border of the pleura crosses the tenth rib at the midaxillary line. It crosses the eighth rib (choice C) at the midclavicular line and the twelfth rib (choice E) at the sides of the vertebral column. The lower border of the lungs cross the sixth rib (choice B) at the midclavicular line, the eighth rib at the midaxillary line and the tenth rib at the sides of the vertebral column. The space between the lower borders of the lungs and the pleura forms the costodiaphragmatic recess. Rib 4 (choice A) is superior to the nipple and thus to the lower border of the pleura.

121. **(C)** The vocal folds are abducted and the rima glottidis is widened by the posterior cricoarytenoid muscles that rotate the arytenoid cartilages laterally. The cricothyroid muscles (choice A) tense and lengthen the vocal ligament by tilting the thyroid cartilage

forward. The lateral cricoarytenoid muscles (choice B) adduct the vocal folds by medially rotating the arytenoid cartilages. The thyroarytenoid muscles (choice D) decrease the tension and length of the vocal ligaments by tilting the thyroid cartilages posteriorly. The transverse arytenoid muscle (choice E) adducts the vocal folds by pulling the arytenoid cartilages together.

122. **(C)** The inferior laryngeal nerve is motor to the intrinsic muscles of the larynx except the cricothyroid muscle, and is sensory to the larynx below the level of the vocal fold. The external laryngeal nerve (choice A) is the branch of the superior laryngeal nerve that contains the motor fibers to the cricothyroid muscle and to the cricopharyngeus muscle. The glossopharyngeal nerve (choice B) does not supply either motor or sensory fibers to the larynx. The internal laryngeal nerve (choice D) is the branch of the superior laryngeal nerve that contains the sensory fibers to the laryngeal mucosa above the vocal fold. The superior laryngeal nerve (choice E) is sensory to the laryngeal mucosa above the vocal fold and also includes motor fibers to the cricothyroid muscle.

123. **(A)** Chief or principal cells of the parathyroid gland secrete parathyroid hormone in response to the level of calcium in the blood. The other type of cells in the parathyroid gland is the oxyphilic cell (choice D), which does not appear to be involved in hormone synthesis or secretion. Follicular (choice C) and parafollicular (choice E) cells belong to the thyroid gland. They release thyroid hormones and thyrocalcitonin, respectively. Chromaffin cells (choice B) are catecholamine-secreting cells. They are not distributed to the parathyroid gland and are not involved in parathyroid hormone secretion.

124. **(E)** Intervertebral discs may protrude or rupture in any direction but do so most commonly in a posterolateral direction, just lateral to the strong central portion of the posterior longitudinal ligament. This is usually the weakest part of the disc, because the

annulus is thinner here and is not supported by other ligaments. Anteriorly (choice A) the intervertebral discs are supported by the broad and strong anterior ligament. Herniation is less common in this direction. Anterolaterally (choice B) the intervertebral disc is supported by the broad anterior longitudinal ligament. The nucleus pulposus is also situated posteriorly in the disc, making herniation here less likely. Herniation of the intervertebral disc laterally (choice C) is not particularly common. Posteriorly (choice D) the intervertebral discs are supported by the posterior longitudinal ligament. Herniation is less common in this direction.

125. **(C)** A bulging or protruded disc typically affects the traversing nerve root; that is, the nerve affected is one number greater than the number of the disc. The L3 spinal nerve (choice A) would be affected by protrusion of the L2 intervertebral disc. The L4 spinal nerve (choice B) would be affected by protrusion of the L3 intervertebral disc. The S1 spinal nerve (choice D) would be affected by protrusion of the L5 intervertebral disc. The S2 spinal nerve (choice E) exits through the foramina of the fused sacrum and therefore is not subject to compression by herniated intervertebral discs.

126. **(E)** A stratified squamous epithelium covers the vocal cords or folds. This epithelium protects the underlying tissue from the mechanical stress acting on the surface of the vocal cords. A simple squamous epithelium (choice D) is not suitable for protection. The rest of the larynx is covered with a pseudostratified ciliated epithelium (i.e., a respiratory epithelium [choice A]). Simple columnar (choice B) and simple cuboidal (choice C) epithelia are found more commonly in organs with secretory or absorptive functions.

127. **(A)** The auriculotemporal nerve is a branch of the mandibular division of the trigeminal nerve. It carries postganglionic parasympathetic fibers from the otic ganglion to the parotid gland. The buccal nerve (choice C) is a sensory branch of the mandibular division of the trigeminal nerve. It innervates the gingiva adjacent to the two posterior molar teeth, the mucosa and skin of the cheek. The buccal branch of the facial nerve (choice B) provides motor innervation to the muscles around the mouth. The greater petrosal nerve (choice D) is a branch of the facial nerve from the geniculate ganglion. It carries preganglionic parasympathetic fibers to the pterygopalatine ganglion. The lesser petrosal nerve (choice E) is a continuation of the tympanic branch of the glossopharyngeal nerve and carries preganglionic parasympathetic fibers to the otic ganglion.

128. **(A)** The femoral canal, the medial compartment of the femoral sheath, contains only a slight amount of loose connective tissue and one or two lymphatic vessels and nodes. The femoral artery (choice B) is found in the lateral compartment of the femoral sheath with the genital branch of the genitofemoral nerve. The femoral nerve (choice C) is the most lateral structure in the femoral triangle, but it does not lie within the femoral sheath. The femoral vein (choice D) occupies the intermediate compartment of the femoral sheath. The saphenous vein (choice E) is a superficial vein that passes through the saphenous hiatus to end in the femoral vein. It does not lie within the femoral canal.

129. **(D)** The flexor retinaculum of the foot runs between the medial malleolus and the calcaneus. The tendon of the tibialis posterior muscle passes under the flexor retinaculum immediately posterior to the medial malleolus. The tendon of the flexor digitorum longus muscle (choice A) passes beneath the flexor retinaculum immediately posterior to the tendon of the tibialis posterior. The tendon of the flexor hallucis longus muscle (choice B) passes beneath the flexor retinaculum posterior to the tendons of the tibialis posterior and flexor digitorum longus muscles. The tendon of the peroneus longus muscle (choice C) and the tendon of the peroneus brevis muscle pass beneath the superior and inferior peroneal retinacula on the lateral side of the foot. The tibial nerve (choice E) and the

posterior tibial vessels pass beneath the flexor retinaculum between the tendons of the flexor digitorum longus and the flexor hallucis longus muscles.

130. **(D)** The ophthalmic division of cranial nerve V (trigeminal) provides general sensory innervation to the eyeball, including the cornea. Cranial nerve II (optic, choice A) carries the visual function of the retina of the eye. Cranial nerves IV (trochlea, choice C) and VI (abducens, choice E) innervate the superior oblique and lateral rectus muscles, respectively. The innervation of all other extraocular muscles is performed by cranial nerve III (oculomotor, choice B).

131. **(C)** The pericardial sac, the heart, and the roots of the great vessels occupy the middle mediastinum. The aortic arch (choice A) lies completely in the superior mediastinum, beginning and ending at the level of the sternal angle. The esophagus (choice B), vagus nerves, descending thoracic aorta, azygos veins, and thoracic duct are all located in the posterior mediastinum. The thymus (choice D) or its remnant lies in the superior mediastinum and the anterior mediastinum. The trachea (choice E) descends from the neck through the superior mediastinum and divides into the primary bronchi at the level of the sternal angle.

132. **(A)** There is only one point of the heart that can be directly identified on the precordium: the apex. A cardiac impulse may be visible at the apex, and palpation over it confirms the presence of the apex beat. The apex is located in the left fifth intercostal space just medial to the midclavicular line, and is the point where the mitral valve is best heard. None of the heart sounds are best heard at the xiphisternal junction (choice B). The tricuspid valve is best heard in the fifth intercostal space to the right of the sternum (choice C). The pulmonary valve is best heard in the second intercostal space to the left of the sternum (choice D). The aortic valve is best heard in the second intercostal space to the right of the sternum (choice E).

133. **(C)** The portal vein forms posterior to the neck of the pancreas and ascends behind the first part of the duodenum to pass to the liver through the hepatoduodenal ligament. The common hepatic artery (choice A) arises from the celiac trunk in the bed of the stomach and passes to the right to enter the hepatoduodenal ligament. It passes above, not behind, the first part of the duodenum. The common hepatic duct (choice B) forms from the right and left hepatic ducts in the porta hepatis and becomes the common bile duct when it is joined by the cystic duct. The common bile duct descends behind the first part of the duodenum to join the main pancreatic duct. The splenic artery (choice D) arises from the celiac trunk in the bed of the stomach and passes to the left along the upper border of the pancreas. The superior mesenteric artery (choice E) arises from the abdominal aorta and enters the root of the mesentery where it passes anterior to the third part of the duodenum.

134. **(C)** The arch of the aorta is formed from the left fourth aortic arch. Part of the right fourth aortic arch becomes the proximal portion of the right subclavian artery whereas the rest of the fourth arch disappears. However, if it persists, a right aortic arch is formed passing posterior to the trachea and esophagus. With the formation of the normally occurring left aortic arch, which runs anterior to the trachea and esophagus, a double aortic arch is created. This defect clamps the trachea and esophagus resulting in the respiratory symptoms. The second pair of aortic arches (choice A) partially forms the stapedial arteries in the middle ear of the embryo. The third pair of aortic arches (choice B) forms the common carotid arteries and contributes to the internal carotid arteries. The fifth pair of aortic arches (choice D) either does not develop or forms primitive vessels, which disappear eventually. The sixth pair of aortic arches (choice E) contributes to the formation of the pulmonary arteries and ductus arteriosus.

135. **(C)** The external laryngeal nerve, a branch of the superior laryngeal nerve from the vagus,

innervates the cricothyroid muscle. Normally, the cricothyroid muscle varies the length and tension of the vocal cord, and in its absence, the voice acquires a monotonous quality. The accessory nerve (XI, choice A) only innervates the sternocleidomastoid and the trapezius muscles in the neck. The ansa cervicalis (choice B) supplies motor branches to the infrahyoid muscles. The hypoglossal nerve (XII, choice D) innervates intrinsic and extrinsic muscle fibers of the tongue. The internal laryngeal nerve (choice E) provides sensory innervation to the interior of the larynx.

136. **(E)** All the listed cell types are components of the respiratory system. Type II pneumocytes are the source of pulmonary surfactant. Alveolar dust cells (choice A) are macrophages. Endothelial cells (choice B) and type I pneumocytes (choice D) are components of the blood–air barrier. Small granule cells (choice C), which are members of the diffuse neuroendocrine system, function in paracrine and endocrine signaling.

137. **(E)** Although it is likely that T lymphocyte progenitor cells arise in bone marrow, differentiation and programming of new T lymphocytes occurs in the thymus. Bone marrow provides the environment for development of stem and precursor cells into B lymphocytes (choice A), granulocytes (choices B, C, and D), erythrocytes, platelets, and monocytes.

138. **(B)** Cells that secrete proteinaceous substances in response to endocrine signals characteristically store these products (or their precursors) in membrane-delimited granules in the apical (toward the lumen of the acinus) region of the cytoplasm. Steroid hormones have several stereotypical ultrastructural features related to their function. Although a Golgi complex is a ubiquitous feature of metabolically active cells, it is particularly well developed in cells that synthesize and package proteins for secretion (choice A). Synthesis of steroid hormones is a cooperative activity of the well-developed sER (choice C) and mitochondria with specializations that include tubular rather than shelf-like cristae (choice D). None of these features typify protein-secreting cells. Lipid precursor molecules are stored in lipid droplets (choice E), but there is no storage of the end product in secretory granules.

139. **(E)** The vagus nerve is a mixed nerve with functions including special visceral efferent (innervation of laryngeal muscles), general visceral efferent (parasympathetic innervation of thoracic and abdominal viscera), general visceral afferent (sensory innervation of thoracic and abdominal viscera), special visceral afferent (sensory innervation of pharyngeal taste buds), and general somatic afferent (cutaneous innervation of a portion of the external ear), but not general somatic efferent. The abducens nerve (choice A) provides motor innervation of the lateral rectus extraocular muscle, and the hypoglossal nerve (choice B) provides motor innervation of the intrinsic and extrinsic skeletal muscles of the tongue. Thus, both nerves are classified as having somatic efferent as their sole functional component. The oculomotor nerve (choice C) contains nerve fibers that serve either a somatic efferent (motor innervation of extraocular muscles) or general visceral efferent (parasympathetic innervation of pupillary constrictor and ciliary body) function. The trigeminal nerve (choice D) consists of axons that are either general somatic afferent (sensory innervation of face and anterior oral and nasal cavities or special visceral efferent (motor innervation of mastication muscles).

140. **(C)** The obturator nerve innervates the adductor muscles and the medial region of the thigh. The nerve originates from the lumbar plexus, runs on the lateral aspect of the pelvic wall, and exits through the obturator canal to reach the medial aspect of the thigh. Lying on the lateral pelvic wall, it may be injured by surgical mishap. The femoral nerve (choice A) innervates the anterior aspect of the thigh and the muscles contained within: the sartorius and the quadriceps femoris. The inferior gluteal nerve (choice B) innervates the gluteus

maximus muscle and is confined to the gluteal region. The pudendal nerve (choice D) is sensory to the genitalia, motor to the perineal muscles, the external urethral sphincter and the external anal sphincter. The sciatic nerve (choice E) innervates the hamstring muscles in the posterior aspect of the thigh.

141. **(B)** The metanephric diverticulum or ureteric bud gives rise to the ureter, renal pelvis, calices, and collecting tubules. The metanephric mass of intermediate mesoderm (choice C) gives rise to the nephrons in the kidney. The mesonephric and paramesonephric ducts (choices A and D) play essential roles in the development of the male and female reproductive system, respectively. The pronephric duct (choice E) is derived from the transitory, nonfunctional first set of kidneys or pronephroi and does not contribute to the development of the ureter.

142. **(A)** The source of IgE molecules is a subpopulation of antigen-stimulated B lymphocytes (choice B) and their immunoglobulin-secreting plasma cell progeny. The IgE that is secreted by plasma cells into tissue fluid and blood is sequestered by the IgE receptors of mast cells and basophils. Mast cells and basophils are triggered to degranulate when antigen (typically allergens) binds to the IgE molecules that occupy their IgE receptors. This is the basis of allergic reactions. Macrophages (choice C) and neutrophils (choice D) have Fc receptors for immunoglobulins of the IgG class. Binding of IgG molecules to bacteria promotes their phagocytosis and destruction by neutrophils and macrophages. Platelets (choice E), which function primarily in hemostasis, are not directly involved in immune responses.

143. **(E)** GnRH normally acts on pituitary gonadotropic cells, those cells in the pars distalis that secrete follicle stimulating hormone (FSH) and LH. For the gonadotropes to function normally, hypothalamic neurons must intermittently secrete GnRH into the hypothalamohypophyseal portal system in brief pulses at an interval of about 90 minutes. Paradoxically, if the gonadotropic cells are

exposed to a prolonged high level of GnRH signal, as when a pharmacologic dose of an agonist is administered, gonadotropic cells cease secretion of FSH and LH (choice D) and become desensitized; that is, they no longer respond to the normal estrogens and progestins in the normal feedback mechanisms. When the objective is to retrieve mature (fertilizable) oocytes, it is important to know the exact timing of the LH surge. This is a necessary event because it brings about the final maturation of the oocyte; however, ovulation occurs about 40 hours after the LH surge and the oocytes can be harvested effectively only before they are released from the ovary. Thus, the reason for disabling the normal hormonal signaling by gonadotropic cells is to avoid a natural LH surge and substitute a controlled surge by administering an LH analog when numerous large follicles have emerged as a result of gonadotropic hormone therapy. The midcycle LH surge is normally brought about by the response of gonadotropes to elevated levels of estrogens (mainly estradiol) secreted by the ovarian follicle that has established dominance. The primary extra-ovarian signals that regulate development of ovarian follicles are FSH and LH. GnRH (choice A) is only indirectly involved. Immediately before ovulation, the primary oocyte of the (usually single) dominant follicle resumes meiosis, completing the first division to produce a polar body and a secondary oocyte, which begins the second division (choice C), but becomes arrested in metaphase. This is one of many preovulatory changes that are brought about by the LH surge. The proliferative phase of the endometrium (choice B) is induced by estrogens released by developing ovarian follicles.

144. **(B)** The permanent set of kidneys develops from the metanephroi. During development, three sets of kidneys are formed in the embryo. The first set or pronephroi (choice D) are transitional, nonfunctional structures that appear around the 4th week of development. The second set or mesonephroi (choice A) appear late in the 4th week and are functional until the permanent kidneys or metanephroi

are fully developed. The paramesonephric ducts (choice C) are structures developing lateral to the gonads and mesonephric ducts. They play an essential role in the female reproductive system, but are not involved in the formation of the kidneys. The ureteric bud (choice E) is an outgrowth from the mesonephric duct that gives rise to the ureter, renal pelvis, calices, and collecting tubules.

145. **(B)** Collagenous fibers of the periodontal ligament function to form a resilient suspension system for the tooth. These fibers are attached to the cementum covering of the root and to the alveolar bone of the tooth socket. Dentinal tubules (choice A) are minute canals that extend through the thickness of the dentin in both the crown and root. Each dentinal tubule contains processes of an odontoblast (choice C). Odontoblasts are the cells that produce dentin. The stellate reticulum (choice D) is a component of the enamel organ, a temporary epithelial structure that produces the enamel of the crown before the tooth erupts. The subodontoblastic plexus of Rashkow (choice E) is a network of nerve fibers in the dental pulp.

146. **(D)** High endothelial venules (HEV), located primarily in the deep cortex, are specialized to recruit circulating lymphocytes from the blood. Lymphocytes in the circulating blood adhere to the lining endothelial cells of HEV by way of an integrin-based recognition. Lymphocytes then gain access to the lymph node tissue by actively migrating (a process called *diapedesis*) between or through endothelial cells. Afferent lymphatic vessels (choice A) conduct lymph, not blood, into the lymph node. The source of the lymph is either upstream lymph nodes or tissue fluid from the region supplied by the node. This component of the system serves as a filter and as a mechanism for antigen-presenting cells to enter the node. Arterioles (choice B) are a component of the circulation of the lymph node, but they are not permeable to cell traffic. Efferent lymphatic vessels (choice C) conduct lymph and cells from the lymph node to either the blood circulation or down-stream lymph nodes. Lymph in efferent lymphatic vessels conveys immunoglobulins and recirculating lymphocytes to the bloodstream. Medullary sinuses (choice E) are part of a system of passages that filter lymph and direct it from the afferent lymphatic vessels to the efferent lymphatic vessels. Medullary sinuses occupy spaces between medullary cords, which are occupied by large numbers of plasma cells, the cells that secrete immunoglobulins.

147. **(E)** Schwann cells are neural crest derivatives that form the myelin sheaths of large axons in peripheral nerves. The myelin is composed of multiple, tightly packed layers of Schwann cell membrane. Astrocytes (choice A) are restricted to the central nervous system where they have multiple functions in support of neurons. These functions include mechanical support, scavenging of neurotransmitters, metabolic support, and contributions to the isolation of brain tissue from blood and cerebrospinal fluid. Fibroblasts (choice B) contribute to the formation of the perineurium, which is a sleeve covering bundles (fascicles) of nerve fibers, and to formation of the epineurium, a connective tissue sleeve that covers the entire nerve. Oligodendrocytes (choice C) also form myelin, but they are restricted to the central nervous system. Cells of the perineurium (choice D) are flattened, epithelium-like cells that contribute to the blood–nerve barrier.

148. **(A)** An individual sarcomere, the unit of contraction in striated muscle, spans the interval between successive Z lines. Each sarcomere encompasses an A-band (choice B) and half of each of two I bands (choice D). Each myofibril (choice C) of a striated muscle fiber is composed of a tandem series of sarcomeres. Coupling of excitation and contraction is a critical function of the triad (choice E), which is composed of a T tubule interposed between two cisternae of the sarcoplasmic reticulum.

149. **(D)** The great cerebral vein of Galen (arrow #4) drains posteriorly into the straight sinus

(arrow #5). The union of the superior sagittal sinus (choice E; arrow #3) and the straight sinus forms the confluence of sinuses (choice A). The straight sinus and superior sagittal sinus are dural venous sinuses: they contain venous blood draining from the brain, skull and scalp. The frontal sinus (choice B) and the sphenoid sinus (choice C) are bony sinuses: they are hollow, air-filled structures and do not drain venous blood.

150. **(B)** Arrow #2 points to the gallbladder, which will be removed during the cholecystectomy (surgical removal of the gallbladder). Biliary colic may be due to impaction of a gallstone in the cystic duct, resulting in cholecystitis (inflammation of the gallbladder). Arrow #1 (choice A) points to the liver. Arrow #3 (choice C) points to the transverse colon. Arrow #4 (choice D) points to the spleen and arrow #5 (choice E) indicates the stomach, recognizable by its internal rugae.

151. **(D)** The bile duct joins with the pancreatic duct and they form the hepatopancreatic ampulla (of Vater). The distal end of the hepatopancreatic ampulla opens into the descending (second) part of the duodenum (choice B). The ascending (choice A), horizontal (choice C), and superior (choice E) parts of the duodenum are not related to the opening of the bile duct.

152. **(D)** Arrow #4 points to the left common carotid artery. The three arteries arising from the arch of the aorta are lined anteriorly to posteriorly on a slanted line: arrow #3 (choice C) shows the brachiocephalic artery, arrow #4 (choice D) points to the left common carotid artery and arrow #5 (choice E) indicates the left subclavian artery. Arrow #2 (choice B) points to the right brachiocephalic vein, which is joined here by the left brachiocephalic vein. Arrow #1 (choice A) points to the trachea, which is filled with air and thus is not radiopaque.

153. **(C)** The anterior and posterior ethmoidal branches of the nasociliary nerve (from the ophthalmic division of the trigeminal nerve) innervate the ethmoidal sinuses. The facial nerve (choice A) does not provide general sensory innervation. The infraorbital nerve (choice B) supplies the cheek area of the face. The olfactory nerve (choice D) provides for the special sensation of smell and the optic nerve (choice E) provides for vision.

154. **(E)** Fusion of the ilium, ischium and pubis at the acetabulum is usually complete by age 23. From birth to the early 20s (choices A to D), the three bones are held together by a Y-shaped cartilage.

155. **(A)** Arrow #2 points to the middle nasal concha, which is part of the ethmoid bone. Arrow #3 points to the ethmoid sinus, which also belongs to the ethmoid bone. The inferior nasal concha (arrow #1) is a separate bone (choice E). The maxillary bone (choice B) is located more laterally and does not contribute to the nasal conchae. The maxillary sinus, a part of the maxillary bone, is indicated by arrow #4. The vomer bone (choice D) forms part of the nasal septum (choice C), which can be seen here as the thin line between the nasal conchae. The nasal conchae have no attachment to the septum.

REFERENCES

Moore KL, Dalley AF. *Clinically Oriented Anatomy,* 4th ed. Philadelphia: Lippincott Williams & Wilkins; 1999.

Moore KL, Persaud TVN. *The Developing Human. Clinically Oriented Embryology,* 6th ed. Philadelphia: Saunders; 1998.

Slaby FJ, McCune SK, Summers RW. *Gross Anatomy in the Practice of Medicine.* Philadelphia: Lea & Febiger; 1994.

Snell RS. *Clinical Anatomy for Medical Students,* 6th ed. Philadelphia: Lippincott Williams & Wilkins; 2000.

Waxman SG. *Correlative Neuroanatomy,* 24th ed. New York: Lange Medical Books/McGraw-Hill; 2000.

Williams PL (ed). *Gray's Anatomy. The Anatomical Basis of Medicine and Surgery.* New York: Churchill Livingstone; 1995.

Subspecialty List: Anatomy

Question Number and Subspecialty

1. Trunk and upper extremity
2. Nervous system
3. Nervous system
4. Respiratory system
5. Eye
6. Thorax
7. Abdomen
8. Nervous system
9. Heart
10. Nervous system
11. Perineum
12. Nervous system
13. Nervous system
14. Abdomen
15. Nervous system
16. Nervous system
17. Auditory system
18. Nervous system
19. Nervous system
20. Head and neck
21. Nervous system
22. Head and neck
23. Vestibular system
24. Head and neck
25. Vascular system
26. Nervous system
27. Nervous system
28. Lower limb
29. Trunk and upper extremity
30. Trunk and upper extremity
31. Abdomen
32. Digestive system
33. Trunk and upper extremity
34. Trunk and upper extremity
35. Spine
36. Vascular system
37. Abdomen
38. Trunk and upper extremity
39. Thorax
40. Thorax
41. Heart
42. Thorax
43. Abdomen
44. Reproductive system
45. Vascular system
46. Abdomen
47. Head and neck
48. Trunk and upper extremity
49. Trunk and upper extremity
50. Trunk and upper extremity
51. Pancreas
52. Trunk and upper extremity
53. Nervous system
54. Digestive system
55. Respiratory system
56. Eye
57. Hematopoietic system
58. Eye
59. Abdomen
60. Cellular biology
61. Cellular biology
62. Muscular system
63. Urinary system
64. Head and neck
65. Endocrine system
66. Lymphoid system
67. Pelvis
68. Hematopoietic system
69. Hematopoietic system
70. Liver
71. Hematopoietic system
72. Digestive system
73. Larynx
74. Placenta

75. Digestive system
76. Digestive system
77. Nervous system
78. Nervous system
79. Head and neck
80. Heart
81. Nervous system
82. Skeletal system
83. Vascular system
84. Eye
85. Parathyroid gland
86. Nervous system
87. Nervous system
88. Nervous system
89. Eye
90. Pelvis
91. Eye
92. Larynx
93. Liver
94. Diaphragm
95. Tongue
96. Nervous system
97. Nervous system
98. Auditory system
99. Nervous system
100. Head and neck
101. Nervous system
102. Nervous system
103. Cellular biology
104. Muscular system
105. Nervous system
106. Nervous system
107. Vascular system
108. Nervous system
109. Taste
110. Lower extremity
111. Thorax
112. Lower extremity
113. Heart
114. Thorax
115. Tongue

116. Perineum
117. Lower extremity
118. Head and neck
119. Thyroid
120. Thorax
121. Larynx
122. Larynx
123. Parathyroid gland
124. Spine
125. Spine
126. Larynx
127. Head and neck
128. Lower extremity
129. Lower extremity
130. Eye
131. Thorax
132. Heart
133. Abdomen
134. Vascular system
135. Head and neck
136. Respiratory system
137. Hematopoietic system
138. Digestive system
139. Nervous system
140. Pelvis
141. Urinary system
142. Hematopoietic system
143. Endocrine system
144. Urinary system
145. Head and neck
146. Lymphoid system
147. Nervous system
148. Muscular system
149. Head and neck
150. Abdomen
151. Abdomen
152. Thorax
153. Head and neck
154. Lower extremity
155. Head and neck

CHAPTER 2

Physiology
Questions

Vishwanath Lingappa, MD, PhD

74%

94   127

DIRECTIONS (Questions 156 through 282): Each of the numbered items or incomplete statements in this section is followed by answers or by completions of the statement. Select the ONE lettered answer or completion that is BEST in each case.

156. A 17-year-old primigravida asks you what to expect during her pregnancy. You tell her that normally during pregnancy

    (A) blood volume increases
    (B) GI muscle tone and motility increase
    (C) hematocrit increases
    (D) pulmonary functional residual capacity increases
    (E) respiratory tidal volume decreases

157. Tremor caused by a cerebellar lesion is most readily differentiated from that caused by loss of the dopaminergic nigrostriatal tracts in that

    (A) it is decreased during activity
    (B) it is present at rest
    (C) it only occurs during voluntary movements
    (D) its amplitude remains constant during voluntary movements
    (E) its frequency is very regular

158. Antidiuretic hormone (ADH) secretion is stimulated by which of the following?

    (A) Angiotensinogen
    (B) Extracellular fluid osmolality increase
    (C) Temperature decrease
    (D) Thyroid hormone
    (E) Volume increase

159. Elderly patients often lose control over their bladder function. Which of the following statements about micturition is correct?

    (A) Higher centers in the brainstem primarily serve to enhance the micturition reflex.
    (B) Patients with damage to the lumbar spinal cord lose their micturition reflex (atonic bladder).
    (C) Patients with damage to the sacral spinal cord have an intact micturition reflex, but lose almost all voluntary control over micturition (automatic bladder).
    (D) Sympathetic fibers originating in L1 and L2 provide continuous tone to the external sphincter, thereby preventing micturition unless desired.
    (E) Urination occurs if inhibition of the external sphincter, through spinal reflex pathways, is stronger than the voluntary constrictor signals to the external sphincter from the brain.

Questions 160 and 161

Figure 2–1 illustrates histologic changes in the endometrium during the menstrual cycle.

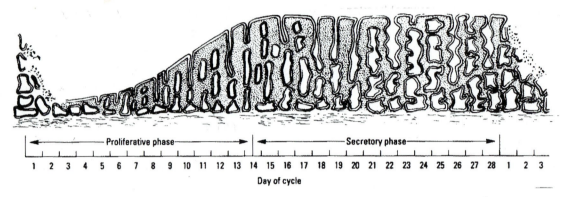

Figure 2–1

160. Progesterone levels are highest around day

  (A) 7
  (B) 12
  (C) 14
  (D) 21
  (E) 28

161. Estrogen levels are highest around day

  (A) 7
  (B) 12
  (C) 14
  (D) 21
  (E) 28

162. Pupil size is an important indicator of brainstem function. Which of the following statements about pupil diameter is correct?

  (A) Atropine causes pupil constriction.
  (B) Decreased parasympathetic activity in fibers innervating the inner eye muscles during darkness results in pupil constriction.
  (C) General increase in sympathetic tone during emotional excitement results in pupil constriction.
  (D) Increase in sympathetic activity in fibers innervating the inner eye muscles during darkness results in pupil constriction.
  (E) Phentolamine causes pupil constriction.

163. The introduction of cold water into one ear may cause vertigo and nausea. The primary cause of this effect of temperature is

  (A) convection currents in endolymph
  (B) decreased discharge rate in vestibular afferents
  (C) decreased movement of ampullar cristae
  (D) increased discharge rate in vestibular afferents
  (E) temporary immobilization of otoliths

164. Reliable, quick, and cost-effective laboratory tests are often needed to determine what is specifically wrong before treating a patient. Radioimmunoassays are commonly used for this purpose, as a quantitative and fast, albeit indirect, way to measure hormone levels (e.g., in blood). To set up a radioimmunoassay, you need

  (A) a biological assay for the hormone to be measured
  (B) a cell culture system in which the hormone has activity
  (C) an antibody to the hormone to be measured and a sample of purified hormone
  (D) an antibody to the hormone to be measured but not a sample of purified hormone
  (E) column chromatography conditions to separate hormone isoforms

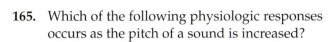

165. Which of the following physiologic responses occurs as the pitch of a sound is increased?

(A) A greater number of hair cells become activated.
(B) The amplitude of maximal basilar membrane displacement increases.
(C) The frequency of action potentials in auditory nerve fibers increases.
(D) The location of maximal basilar membrane displacement moves toward the base of the cochlea.
(E) Units in the auditory nerve become responsive to a wider range of sound frequencies.

166. Drug detoxification by the liver occurs in two phases. Phase I results in activation of drugs, making them more reactive. Phase II results in conjugation of drugs to bulky hydrophilic groups that facilitates their excretion. What is/are the most dangerous condition(s) of dysregulation of the phases of drug detoxification, as commonly occurs, for example, in acetaminophen (Tylenol) toxicity?

(A) Diminished phase I activity
(B) Diminished phase II activity
(C) Increased phase I activity and decreased phase II activity
(D) Increases in both phase I and II activity
(E) When the drug bypasses both phase I and II activity

167. A 54-year-old insulin-dependent diabetic notes that her insulin requirements have gone up dramatically in the past year (from 50 U to nearly 200 U of recombinant human insulin) and her blood glucose is still poorly controlled. Possible explanations for worsening of her diabetes include which of the following?

(A) A high titer of anti-insulin antibodies
(B) An improved diet
(C) An improved exercise program
(D) Progression of macrovascular disease
(E) Weight loss

168. The stimulation of nerve endings in the Golgi tendon organs leads directly to

(A) contraction of extrafusal muscle fibers
(B) contraction of intrafusal muscle fibers
(C) increased activity in group II afferent fibers
(D) increased gamma-efferent discharge
(E) reflex inhibition of motor neurons

169. Lipids are the precursors for synthesis of numerous classes of hormones, including

(A) adrenocorticotrophin (ACTH)
(B) catecholamines
(C) leukotrienes
(D) nitric oxide
(E) thyrotropin releasing hormone (TRH)

170. A large body of evidence implicates dietary fiber as being protective against various diseases. The physiologic basis for the benefits of dietary fiber are numerous, and include

(A) promotion of GI blood flow
(B) promotion of pancreatic bicarbonate secretion
(C) promotion of satiety
(D) slowing of GI transit time
(E) stimulation of acid secretion

171. Two patients are admitted to the intensive care unit after acute episodes of GI bleeding that has lowered each of their hematocrit levels from 45% to 30%. Neither patient is currently actively bleeding. The first patient has no heart disease, the second has significant aortic stenosis. What normal protective response would be impaired in the second patient that could increase the risk of death in the event of another episode of bleeding?

(A) Ability to augment cardiac output by increasing heart rate and contractility
(B) Ability to augment venous return and maintain preload
(C) Aortic stenosis is associated with an impaired cardiac conduction system
(D) Increased sympathetic tone in the patient with aortic stenosis
(E) The patient with aortic stenosis should be anticoagulated, increasing risk of bleeding

172. Distinguishing sinus tachycardia from ventricular tachycardia can be particularly difficult when a patient has what electrocardiographic feature due to a conduction system defect?

    (A) Bundle branch block
    (B) Heart rate > 100
    (C) Inverted T waves
    (D) Prolonged QT interval
    (E) P waves in fixed relationship to QRS complexes

173. Responses to starvation include which of the following?

    (A) Decreased corticotrophin releasing hormone (CRH)
    (B) Decreased gonadotrophin releasing hormone (GnRH)
    (C) Decreased parasympathetic tone
    (D) Increased energy expenditure
    (E) Increased sympathetic tone

174. One of the most feared acute complications of insulin-dependent diabetes mellitus is severe ketoacidosis. The classic metabolic derangements distinctive of this disorder can be traced in large measure to excessive activity of which metabolic pathway?

    (A) Fatty acid oxidation
    (B) Fatty acid synthesis
    (C) Glycogen synthesis
    (D) Protein catabolism
    (E) Protein synthesis

Questions 175 through 177

A 52-year-old man has a history of anginal pain that until recently was responsive to nitrates. He is now evaluated for possible angioplasty.

175. The graph in Figure 2–2 shows the ECG of this patient. Blood flow across the mitral valve is largest around

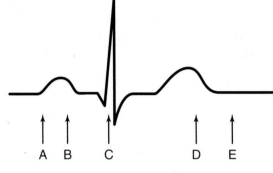

A   B   C   D   E

Figure 2–2

    (A) point A
    (B) point B
    (C) point C
    (D) point D
    (E) point E

176. The graph in Figure 2–3 shows the pressure–volume curve of the left ventricle of this patient (shaded area). The pressure–volume curve of a normal subject is shown for comparison (broken lines). Compared to normal this patient most likely has a (an)

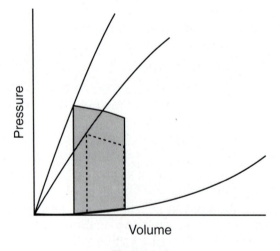

Figure 2–3

    (A) decreased afterload
    (B) decreased preload
    (C) decreased stroke volume
    (D) increased force of contraction
    (E) increased preload

177. The graph in Figure 2–4 shows the jugular vein pressure curve of this patient. Which part of the curve represents the atrial contraction?

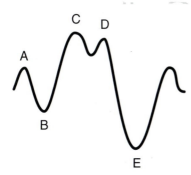

Figure 2–4

(A) Peak A
(B) Peak B
(C) Peak C
(D) Peak D
(E) Peak E

178. Reticuloendothelial cells of the liver are important in both physiologic function and liver disease. A key cell type in pathophysiology of cirrhosis is the Stellate cell, which transforms into an overproducer of collagen upon loss of its' normal characteristics, including

(A) an intracellular vitamin A droplet
(B) association with Kupffer cells
(C) bile synthesis
(D) insulin receptors
(E) periportal location

179. Hormones known to increase glomerular filtration rate (GFR) include

(A) endothelin
(B) epinephrine
(C) norepinephrine
(D) prostaglandins
(E) renin

180. Which of the following hormones is produced by the kidney?

(A) Aldosterone
(B) Angiotensinogen
(C) Erythropoietin
(D) Insulin
(E) Parathyroid hormone

181. Ascites formation in patients with protein calorie malnutrition is due to

(A) decreased plasma oncotic pressure
(B) elevated intravascular hydrostatic pressure
(C) insufficient energy to drive Na^+/K^+ ATPase
(D) opportunistic parasitic infections due to immunosuppression
(E) portal hypertension

182. Complications of high-dose glucocorticoid therapy include which one of the following?

(A) Excessive growth in children and acromegaly in adults
(B) Hyperkalemia
(C) Hyponatremia
(D) Suppression of the hypothalamic–pituitary–adrenal axis
(E) Volume depletion

183. Which of the following statements correctly describes effects of autonomic nerve activity on the cardiovascular system in a healthy subject?

(A) Inhibition of parasympathetic nerves decreases total peripheral resistance.
(B) Inhibition of parasympathetic nerves increases heart rate.
(C) Inhibition of parasympathetic nerves increases total peripheral resistance.
(D) Stimulation of parasympathetic nerves decreases the strength of cardiac ventricular contractions.
(E) Stimulation of sympathetic nerves decreases the strength of cardiac ventricular contractions.

184. Collapse of alveoli, termed atelectasis, is a common finding in various forms of acute lung injury and can greatly increase the work of breathing, sometimes to the extent of causing respiratory failure. The mechanism that normally prevents atelectasis involves which of the following?

(A) A phospholipid–protein complex termed surfactant that lowers surface tension

(B) Antioxidants that prevent damage due to cigarette smoke

(C) Neutrophil proteases that maintain lung compliance

(D) Smooth muscle relaxation to decrease airway resistance to airflow

(E) The role of prostaglandins in distribution of pulmonary blood flow

185. A patient with acute glomerulonephritis has a total plasma Ca^{2+} of 2.5 mM/L and a glomerular filtration rate of 160 L/day. What is the estimated daily filtered load of calcium?

(A) 64 mM/day

(B) 120 mM/day

(C) 240 mM/day

(D) 400 mM/day

(E) 800 mM/day

186. The work of breathing is determined by elastic forces and compliance, and airway resistance to airflow. Mechanisms by which airway resistance to airflow can be increased include

(A) diminished neutrophil infiltration of the lung mucosa

(B) excessive smooth muscle relaxation in medium-sized bronchioles

(C) increased pulmonary blood flow

(D) mucus gland hypertrophy and mucus oversecretion

(E) overproduction of anti-oxidants in response to lung irritants

187. Normally, O_2 transfer is perfusion limited; that is, the amount of O_2 taken up is a function of pulmonary blood flow. Which of the following conditions would favor a diffusion limitation of O_2 transfer from alveolar to pulmonary capillary blood?

(A) Breathing hyperbaric gas mixture

(B) Chronic obstructive lung disease

(C) Increased ventilatory rate

(D) Lung edema

(E) Mild exercise

188. Obesity in humans is generally associated with which of the following?

(A) Increased estrogen level

(B) Decreased low-density lipoproteins

(C) Increased high-density lipoproteins

(D) Increased insulin resistance

(E) Leptin sensitivity

189. The action potentials shown in Figure 2–5 represent those of

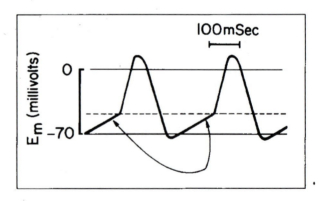

Figure 2–5

(A) cardiac nodal cells

(B) myelinated motor axons

(C) skeletal muscle fibers

(D) vascular smooth muscle cells

(E) ventricular Purkinje cells

Questions 190 and 191

Refer to Figure 2–6, which displays the relationship of ventricular performance to ventricular end diastolic volume (stretching of the myocardium) normally at rest and under other conditions.

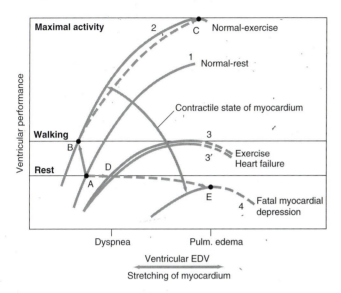

Figure 2–6. *(Modified from E. Braunwald et al:* Mechanisms of Contraction of the Normal and Failing Heart. *Boston, Little, Brown, 1976.)*

190. Factors that shift this curve upward and to the left include which of the following?

   (A) Changes in the number of myocardial cells induced to contract

   (B) Decrease in ATP levels that affects the function of the sarcoplasmic reticulum

   (C) Development of systemic acidosis

   (D) The parasympathetic nervous system operating via acetylcholine

   (E) The sympathetic nervous system operating via norepinephrine

191. Factors capable of shifting the curve downward and to the right include

   (A) calcium ions

   (B) cardiac glycosides

   (C) circulating catecholamines

   (D) inotropic agents such as isoproterenol, dopamine, and dobutamine

   (E) myocardial apoptosis

Questions 192 and 193

A middle-aged man with smaller-than-normal-sized kidneys on ultrasound and a history of chronic glomerulonephritis has the following laboratory values.

Arterial blood	Urine
pH = 7.33	pH = 6.0
Pao_2 = 95 mm Hg	protein = positive
$Paco_2$ = 35 mm Hg	glucose = negative
HCO_3^- = 18 mEq/L	

192. This patient most likely has

   (A) diabetic ketoacidosis

   (B) metabolic acidosis with some respiratory compensation

   (C) metabolic acidosis without respiratory compensation

   (D) respiratory acidosis with some renal compensation

   (E) respiratory acidosis without renal compensation

193. The most likely cause of his acid–base imbalance is

   (A) decreased ability to produce adequate urinary NH_4^+ excretion

   (B) decreased catabolism of sulfur-containing amino acids (e.g., methionine, cysteine)

   (C) excess β-hydroxybutyric and acetoacetic acids in his blood

   (D) hyperventilation

   (E) hypoventilation

194. Edema occurs when intravascular hydrostatic pressure exceeds plasma oncotic pressure

   (A) by an amount greater than the capacity of the lymphatic drainage

   (B) by any amount

   (C) in the presence of excess antidiuretic hormone (ADH)

   (D) only when portal venous pressure is also elevated

   (E) when total body sodium is depleted

195. The adverse consequences on the body of severe acidemia include

    (A) arteriolar constriction
    (B) decreased catabolism
    (C) hyperkalemia
    (D) hypoventilation
    (E) insulin sensitivity

196. During a routine preschool examination, a 5-year-old boy is found to have difficulty focusing on distant objects. Which of the following is true during far accommodation of the eyes?

    (A) The ciliary muscles are relaxed
    (B) The focal length of the lens is short
    (C) The lens is rounded
    (D) The pupils are constricted (accommodation response)
    (E) The zonula fibers are relaxed

197. Although most cases of hypertension are "essential," meaning the underlying disorder is unknown, about 10% of cases are "secondary hypertension" due to a specific, usually treatable cause, including

    (A) adrenal insufficiency
    (B) estrogen deficiency
    (C) hyperparathyroidism
    (D) renal artery stenosis
    (E) volume depletion

198. A 47-year-old woman presents for elective cholecystectomy. Shortly after induction of anesthesia with halothane, the patient develops circulatory instability, tachypnea, and a sharp rise in body temperature (malignant hyperthermia). What is the cause of fever in this patient?

    (A) Decreased convectional heat loss
    (B) Increased blood levels of interleukin-1
    (C) Increased heat production by skeletal muscle
    (D) Increased hypothalamic temperature set point
    (E) Increased sweat production

199. Hypoxia can be due to many different causes. The alveolar to arterial (A–a) oxygen gradient is useful for discriminating between the possible causes of hypoxia in a patient. In which of the following conditions would a patient with hypoxia demonstrate an elevated A–a oxygen gradient?

    (A) A patient with neuromuscular disease impairing ventilatory effort
    (B) Hypoventilation in a patient with a narcotic overdose
    (C) Inspiration of air lacking sufficient oxygen (e.g., at high altitude)
    (D) Shunting of venous blood bypassing the lungs

200. Sensory input from a variety of receptors contributes to control over-respiration. Receptors whose activity modify the frequency, depth, and timing of spontaneous breathing include

    (A) chemoreceptors in the peripheral vasculature and brainstem
    (B) histamine receptors in bronchial smooth muscle
    (C) monitors of inflammation in the airway epithelium
    (D) pH receptors in the diaphragm
    (E) stretch receptors in the left atrium

201. A patient with chronic renal insufficiency due to renal vascular disease has a net functional loss of nephrons. If we assume that production of urea and creatinine is constant and that the patient is in a steady state, a 50% decrease in the normal GFR will

    (A) decrease plasma urea concentration
    (B) greatly increase plasma Na⁺
    (C) increase the percent of filtered Na⁺ excreted
    (D) not affect plasma creatinine
    (E) significantly decrease plasma K⁺

202. Which of the following events typically occurs during REM sleep?

    (A) Enuresis
    (B) Night terrors

(C) Penile erections

(D) Sleep spindles

(E) Somnambulism

203. A patient with multiple trauma in the ICU is on artificial respiration. If alveolar ventilation is halved (and if CO_2 production remains unchanged), then

(A) alveolar CO_2 pressure ($PACO_2$) will be halved

(B) alveolar O_2 pressure (PAO_2) will double

(C) arterial CO_2 pressure ($PaCO_2$) will double

(D) arterial O_2 pressure (PaO_2) will double

(E) arterial O_2 pressure (PaO_2) will not change

204. A 4-year-old child with signs of precocious puberty is brought to clinic for evaluation and found to have a congenital deficiency of 21 β-hydroxylase. As a result of this genetic defect, feedback inhibition of the pituitary gland is lost, excess ACTH is secreted, and which one of the following happens?

(A) Adrenal cortical atrophy occurs.

(B) Adrenal medullary hypertrophy occurs.

(C) Excess cortisol is released.

(D) Precursors to cortisol back up and spillover into the adrenal androgen synthesis pathway.

(E) There is a dramatic fall in serum cholesterol.

205. Pulmonary embolism is a devastating complication of venous thrombosis. Risk factors for thrombosis include venous stasis caused by which of the following?

(A) Anemia

(B) Bed rest and immobilization

(C) High-output cardiac failure

(D) Oral anticoagulant therapy

(E) Strenuous activity

206. A 35-year-old weightlifter who has been injecting testosterone for muscle mass augmentation is evaluated for infertility and found to have an extremely low sperm count. The likely explanation is that injected testosterone serves to effectively feedback inhibit gonadotropin secretion centrally, but fails to

(A) feedback inhibit hepatic testosterone-binding protein synthesis

(B) feedback inhibit gonadotropin-releasing hormone (GnRH) secretion by the hypothalamus

(C) saturate androgen binding protein in the seminiferous tubules

(D) stimulate leydig cell proliferation

(E) stimulate sertoli cell maturation

207. Findings that suggest a metabolic cause in a comatose patient include

(A) failure to withdraw from painful stimuli

(B) gross blood in the cerebrospinal fluid

(C) impaired pupillary light responses

(D) posturing of limbs

(E) serum sodium of 115 mEq/L

208. Peripherally injected insulin differs physiologically from endogenously secreted insulin in a number of respects, including which of the following?

(A) Endogenous insulin achieves a higher concentration in the liver than in the periphery.

(B) Exogenous insulin is able to bypass insulin resistance observed with endogenous insulin.

(C) Exogenous insulin is always extracted from animal sources and therefore is less effective due to sequence differences and anti-insulin antibodies.

(D) Injected insulin contains C peptide, which is missing from endogenous insulin because it is degraded in the pancreatic β-cell prior to secretion.

(E) Injected insulin is in the form of proinsulin, whereas endogenous insulin has had C peptide removed.

209. A routine ECG on a patient reveals a prolonged PQ interval. Which of the following cardiac systems is most likely damaged and responsible for this patient's prolonged PQ interval?

(A) AV node

(B) Between the sinoatrial (SA) and the atrioventricular (AV) nodes

(C) Bundle of His

(D) Purkinje fibers

(E) Ventricular muscle

210. In excess, glucocorticoids have which of the following effects?

(A) Increased renal reabsorption of calcium

(B) Increased synthesis of bone matrix proteins

(C) Partial block of intestinal calcium absorption

(D) Stimulation of osteoblast activity

(E) Suppression of osteoclast activity

211. Restrictive lung disease is often associated with

(A) bronchial wall thickening due to mucous gland hypertrophy

(B) increased or normal diffusing capacity

(C) increased pulmonary fibrosis

(D) increased total lung capacity (TLC)

(E) reduced forced expiratory volume in 1 second/forced vital capacity (FEV_1/FVC) ratio

212. Hepatocytes in the liver carry out a remarkable array of functions that are specialized with regard to both location of the cell and level of activity as a function of location of the cell along the zones of the liver acinus. An example of a liver function that is limited to the apical plasma membrane is

(A) bile acid conjugation

(B) bile acid export out of the hepatocyte

(C) bile acid synthesis

(D) carbohydrate metabolism

(E) protein synthesis

213. Inappropriate transient relaxation of the lower esophageal sphincter (LES) is responsible for common clinical symptoms and findings ranging from "heartburn" to more severe cases of esophageal injury. Which of the following causes diminished LES tone?

(A) β-adrenergic receptor antagonists

(B) Antacids

(C) Chocolate

(D) Gastrin

(E) High-protein meals

214. Effects of angiotensin II include which of the following?

(A) Enhanced GFR

(B) Enhanced renin secretion

(C) Inhibition of aldosterone secretion

(D) Thirst, through a central action on the hypothalamus

(E) Vascular smooth muscle relaxation

215. Regulation of one particular anterior pituitary hormone is distinctive in that its primary control is by inhibition rather than stimulation of secretion. Thus, with pituitary stalk transection (e.g., after a motor vehicle accident) that separates the pituitary gland from the hypothalamic hormones by which their secretion is regulated, secretion of all pituitary hormones is lost except one, whose blood level actually increases. The hormone in question is

(A) gonadotropin releasing hormone (GnRH)

(B) growth hormone (GH)

(C) prolactin

(D) proopiomelanacortin (POMC)

(E) thyroid stimulating hormone (TSH)

216. Typical symptoms in hypothyroidism include which of the following?

(A) Abdominal pain

(B) Constipation

(C) Heart palpitations

(D) Heat intolerance

(E) Weight loss

217. Endocrine disease can occur due to hormone excess, hormone lack, or dysregulation of hormone action including hormone resistance, where hormone is present—often at elevated levels—but is not as effective as it normally is (e.g., due to downregulation or desensitization of receptors). An example of such a resistance state to a hormone is

    (A) ACTH resistance in Cushing syndrome in patients with pituitary adenomas

    (B) glucocorticoid resistance in Addison disease in patients with adrenal tuberculosis

    (C) hypoparathyroidism following parathyroid surgery

    (D) leptin resistance in most human obesity

    (E) thyroid hormone resistance in Graves disease in patients with thyroid hormone excess

218. Which of the following statements regarding fetal circulation is correct?

    (A) PO_2 of fetal blood leaving the placenta is slightly greater than maternal mixed venous PO_2.

    (B) The foramen ovale closes during the third trimester unless the fetus has an atrial septal defect.

    (C) The liver and heart of the fetus receive blood with very high O_2 saturation.

    (D) The major portion of right ventricular output passes through the lungs.

    (E) The presence of fetal hemoglobin shifts the oxyhemoglobin dissociation to the right.

219. Resistance to blood flow in the cerebral circulation of humans increases when

    (A) an individual inhales a gas mixture enriched with CO_2

    (B) an individual suffers an epileptic seizure

    (C) an individual's hematocrit is decreased to < 0.30 by isovolemic exchange transfusion

    (D) PaO_2 decreases to < 50 mm Hg

    (E) systemic arterial pressure increases from 100 to 130 mm Hg

220. A 68-year-old coal miner with decades of work-related exposure to dust is examined for pulmonary fibrosis. His FEV_1 is 75% (normal > 65%) and his arterial oxygen saturation is 92%. His alveolar ventilation is 6000 mL/min at a tidal volume of 600 mL and a breathing rate of 12 breaths/min. Pathologic changes in lung compliance and residual volume are also documented in this patient. Which of the following describes this patient's lung compliance measured under static conditions?

    (A) Change in distending pressure ($P_{alv} - P_{pl}$) divided by change in lung volume

    (B) Change in distending pressure ($P_{alv} - P_{pl}$) minus the change in lung volume

    (C) Change in elastic recoil pressure ($P_{alv} - P_{pl}$)

    (D) Change in lung volume divided by change in distending pressure ($P_{alv} - P_{pl}$)

    (E) Lung volume divided by recoil pressure ($P_{alv} - P_{pl}$)

221. Typical physical and laboratory findings in hyperthyroidism include which of the following?

    (A) Bradycardia
    (B) Delayed reflexes
    (C) High serum cholesterol
    (D) Thick, rough skin
    (E) Tremor

222. Effects of long-term ACTH treatment on the adrenal cortex include which of the following?

    (A) Adrenal hyperplasia
    (B) Decreased blood flow to the adrenal gland
    (C) Decreased conversion of cholesterol to pregnenolone
    (D) Decreased glucocorticoid production
    (E) Increased insulin sensitivity

223. A patient's arterial blood analysis shows a pH of 7.56, bicarbonate 21 mEq/L, P_{O_2} of 50 mm Hg, and P_{CO_2} of 25 mm Hg. This patient probably

    (A) has severe chronic lung disease
    (B) is a lowlander who has been vacationing at high altitude for 2 weeks
    (C) is a subject in a clinical research experiment who has been breathing a gas mixture of 10% oxygen and 90% nitrogen for a few minutes
    (D) is an adult psychiatric patient who swallowed an overdose of aspirin
    (E) is an emergency room patient with severely depressed respiration as a result of a heroin overdose

224. A patient with newly diagnosed schizophrenia is given chlorpromazine. Which of the following is an expected side effect of this medication?

    (A) Bradycardia
    (B) Decreased GI sphincter tone
    (C) Dry mouth
    (D) Emptying of urinary bladder and rectum
    (E) Increased GI motility

225. Which of the following conditions is associated with a decrease in skeletal muscle tone?

    (A) Activation of γ-fibers
    (B) Anxiety
    (C) Lower motoneuron lesions
    (D) Parkinson disease
    (E) Upper motoneuron lesions

226. Risk factors for developing osteoporosis include

    (A) complete abstinence from alcohol
    (B) excessively vigorous physical activity
    (C) late menopause
    (D) low calcium intake
    (E) obesity

227. On routine examination a patient has an arterial oxygen (P_{aO_2}) slightly below the alveolar oxygen (P_{AO_2}). This finding is

    (A) due to reaction time of O_2 with hemoglobin
    (B) due to significant diffusion gradient
    (C) due to unloading of CO_2
    (D) normal and due to shunted blood
    (E) the result of a major cardiac right-to-left shunt (ventricular septal defect)

228. Which of the following statements about cystic fibrosis is correct?

    (A) Cystic fibrosis is caused by a defective Na^+ transporter across airway epithelial cells, resulting in thick airway mucus.
    (B) Cystic fibrosis is more common in African-Americans than in Caucasians.
    (C) The gene that is abnormal in cystic fibrosis encodes a cAMP-regulated Cl^- channel.
    (D) The gene that is abnormal in cystic fibrosis is located on the X chromosome.
    (E) The sweat of cystic fibrosis patients has elevated Na^+ and low Cl^- content.

229. Cutting sympathetic nerve fibers that supply blood vessels in the arms or legs usually results in acute vasodilatation due to

    (A) compensatory increase of epinephrine release from the adrenal medulla
    (B) compensatory increase of norepinephrine release from the adrenal medulla
    (C) development of hypersensitivity to circulating catecholamines
    (D) loss of sympathetic tone
    (E) parasympathetic fibers dilating blood vessels

230. Figure 2–7 shows an EEG recording of a 12-year-old child with suspected attention deficit hyperactivity disorder (ADHD). Which of the following events most likely causes the change at the time marked by the arrow?

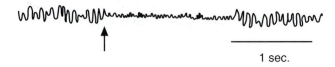

1 sec.

Figure 2–7

(A) Patient closes eyes

(B) Patient falling asleep

(C) Patient opens eyes

(D) Patient's mind "wandering off"

(E) Petit mal attack

231. Prostaglandins are important mediators of inflammation. Which of the following statements about the role of prostaglandins during inflammatory processes is correct?

(A) PGE_2 contracts bronchial smooth muscle.

(B) PGE_2 sensitizes nociceptive nerve endings, causing pain.

(C) $PGF_{2\alpha}$ and PGE_2 relax uterine smooth muscle.

(D) $PGF_{2\alpha}$ relaxes bronchial smooth muscle.

(E) Thromboxane A_2 inhibits platelet aggregation.

232. Patients with cardiomyopathy who develop new-onset atrial fibrillation often have a clinically significant fall in cardiac output due to

(A) hyperthyroidism

(B) hypotension

(C) left atrial clot formation

(D) loss of the augmentation of left ventricular filling by atrial contraction

(E) poor conduction through the AV node

233. Figure 2–8 shows four flow-volume curves. Which one is consistent with asthma?

(A) Curve A

(B) Curve B

(C) Curve C

(D) Curves B and C

234. A 28-year-old woman with chronic fatigue is admitted to the sleep laboratory for 24-hour monitoring of her sleep and breathing patterns. Her sleep latency is 90 minutes (normal 20 to 30 minutes). An hour later she appears asleep but her EEG pattern reverts to beta waves. Most likely, this patient

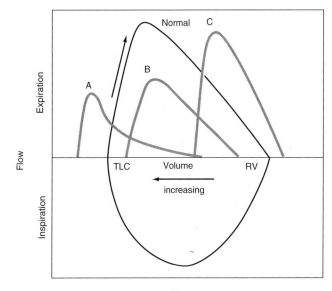

Figure 2–8. *(Reproduced with permission from Braunwald et al: Harrison's Principles of Internal Medicine, 15th ed., McGraw-Hill, 2000.)*

(A) has entered REM sleep

(B) has just entered deep sleep (stage 4)

(C) has just entered light sleep (stage 1)

(D) just woke up

(E) suffers from central sleep apnea

235. A patient with acute myocardial infarction is treated with streptokinase to reduce a blood clot in his left coronary artery. Fibrinolysis in this patient is

(A) due to activation of tissue plasminogen activator by streptokenase

(B) due to hydrolysis of fibrin by plasmin

(C) due to hydrolysis of fibrin by streptokinase

(D) inhibited by plasmin

(E) inhibited by streptokinase

Questions 236 and 237

236. The graph in Figure 2–9 shows the static expiratory pressure–volume curve of a patient's lung and thorax (solid line). The broken line indicates the pressure–volume curve of a normal person for comparison. The lung compliance (at point x) of this patient is approximately

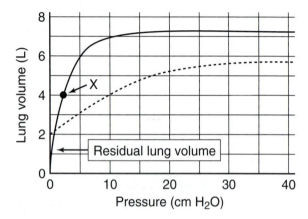

Figure 2–9

(A) 0.5 cm H_2O/L
(B) 1 cm H_2O/L
(C) 1 L/cm H_2O
(D) 2 L/cm H_2O
(E) 4 L/cm H_2O

237. This patient most likely suffers from

(A) acute obstruction of the glottis
(B) α_1-antitrypsin deficiency
(C) asbestosis
(D) sarcoidosis
(E) tuberculosis

238. Gout results from the initiation of acute inflammation by monosodium urate crystals deposited in typically distal joints. These crystals serve directly and indirectly to

(A) activate endothelial cells to attract neutrophils
(B) downregulate neutrophil effector functions

(C) downregulate prostaglandin production
(D) suppress complement activation
(E) suppress kinin activation

239. A newlywed 23-year-old woman and her 28-year-old husband are evaluated for infertility. They have been unable to conceive a child despite regular intercourse for the past 12 months. The first step of this couple's infertility workup is to determine whether ovulation occurs regularly. Which of the following hormones is primarily responsible for ovulation?

(A) Estradiol
(B) Estriol
(C) Follicle-stimulating hormone (FSH)
(D) Inhibin
(E) Luteinizing hormone (LH)

240. Neuronal function is critically dependent on oxygen supply. Blood flow through the brain is most increased by

(A) barbiturates
(B) decreased arterial oxygen to 75 mm Hg
(C) increased arterial carbon dioxide to 45 mm Hg
(D) increased arterial pressure to 160/90 mm Hg
(E) intensive thinking

241. The solid line in Figure 2–10 represents a normal hemoglobin oxygen-binding curve. Strenuous physical exercise will shift this oxygen binding curve to

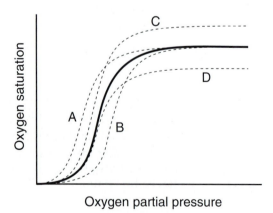

Figure 2–10

(A) line A
(B) line B
(C) line C
(D) line D
(E) no change

242. One way of appreciating the complex and myriad functions of the GI tract is to consider the location and direction of secretion. Molecules secreted into the GI tract lumen by cells in the stomach include

(A) gastrin
(B) histamine
(C) hydrogen ions (H^+)
(D) intrinsic factor
(E) transferrin

243. In type IV renal tubular acidosis (RTA), which is often seen in patients with diabetes mellitus, the capacity of the distal tubule to transport which of the following ions is affected?

(A) Hydrogen and potassium in exchange for sodium
(B) Hydrogen only
(C) Potassium only
(D) Sodium and bicarbonate
(E) Sodium only

244. During a marathon attempt a runner collapses and is admitted with severe acute dehydration. This patient most likely has

(A) decreased baroreceptor firing rate
(B) decreased plasma osmolarity
(C) high renal water excretion
(D) low plasma ADH levels
(E) low water permeability of collecting duct tubular cells

245. An important long-term measure of the "tightness" of blood glucose control in patients with diabetes mellitus is the level of a particular nonenzymatic modification. The most commonly measured example of this modification is

(A) hemoglobin A_{1c} (also known as glycohemoglobin)
(B) lipoprotein (a)
(C) modified albumin
(D) myoinositol
(E) sorbitol

246. A patient on intensive care is ventilated with a frequency of 12 per minute and a tidal volume of 0.6 L. His arterial pH increases to > 7.6. To correct this respiratory alkalosis, you should

(A) decrease dead space
(B) decrease tidal volume
(C) increase minute ventilation
(D) increase oxygen fraction
(E) use positive end-expiratory pressure (PEEP)

247. Figure 2–11 illustrates the extracellular and intracellular volume–osmolarity status of a patient (broken lines) and that of a normal subject (solid lines) for comparison. This patient most likely suffers from

(A) adrenal insufficiency
(B) chronic vomiting
(C) iatrogenic fluid overload with 0.9% NaCl
(D) iatrogenic fluid overload with hypertonic solution
(E) syndrome of inappropriate hypersecretion of antidiuretic hormone (SIADH)

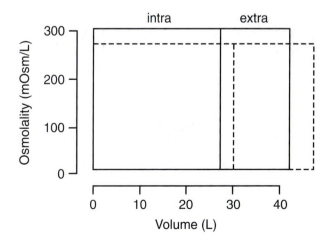

Figure 2–11

248. A series of oxygen-binding curves is shown in Figure 2–12. Which of these curves represents the binding of oxygen to myoglobin?

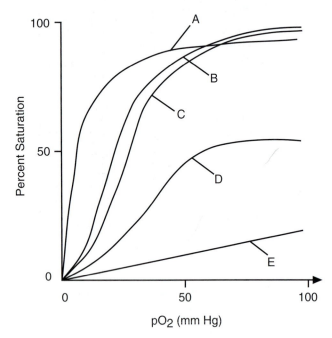

Figure 2–12

(A) Curve A
(B) Curve B
(C) Curve C
(D) Curve D
(E) Curve E

249. The "dark current" of retinal photoreceptors is generated by

(A) Cl^- channels
(B) nonselective anion channels
(C) nonselective cation channels
(D) the Na^+/K^+ pump
(E) the ryanodine receptor

250. Creatinine clearance is often used to evaluate glomerular function. Which of the graphs in Figure 2–13 best represents the relationship between plasma creatinine concentration and creatinine clearance in a normal healthy person?

(A) Curve A
(B) Curve B
(C) Curve C

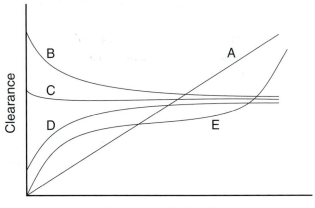

Concentration in plasma

Figure 2–13

(D) Curve D
(E) Curve E

251. Which of the following cytokines is produced by T cells and induces major histocompatibility (MHC-II) proteins?

(A) α-Interferon (INF-α)
(B) β-Interferon (INF-β)
(C) γ-Interferon (INF-γ)
(D) Interleukin-1 (IL-1)
(E) Tumor necrosis factor (TNF)

252. Under resting conditions athletes (compared to untrained persons) have a higher

(A) cardiac output
(B) cardiac stroke volume
(C) heart frequency
(D) oxygen consumption
(E) respiratory frequency

253. A 56-year-old man presents with headache, nausea, left-sided ocular pain, and blurred vision. On examination his cornea appears cloudy and the pupils are fixed in a mid-dilated position. Ocular pressure is 48 mm Hg (normally < 20 mm Hg). Which of the following statements about intraocular pressure is correct?

(A) Anti-inflammatory corticosteroids are the drug of choice for this patient.
(B) Decreased pupil size reduces flow out of ocular chamber.

(C) Glaucoma is a rare cause of blindness in the United States.

(D) Intraocular pressure is mainly determined by the rate of production of the aqueous humor.

(E) Intraocular pressure varies by as much as 50% from day to day.

254. Which of the following hormones is produced in the duodenum and stimulates the pancreas to produce an enzyme-rich secretion?

(A) Cholecystokinin (CCK)

(B) Gastric inhibitory peptide (GIP)

(C) Gastrin

(D) Secretin

(E) Vasointestinal inhibitory peptide (VIP)

255. Chronic nonerosive gastritis is often associated with decreased gastric acid secretion. Which of the following best describes the main ion transport at the apical membrane of gastric parietal cells?

(A) Active H^+ and Cl^- cotransport

(B) Active secretion of H^+ in exchange for K^+

(C) Cl^-/HCO_3^- exchange

(D) Na^+/K^+ pump

(E) Passive diffusion of H^+

256. Plasma renin levels are decreased in patients with

(A) heart failure

(B) primary aldosteronism

(C) renal artery stenosis

(D) salt restriction

(E) upright posture

257. A 19-year-old patient has a 5-year history of moderate to severe asthma and comes in for his yearly pulmonary function test. Illustrated in Figure 2–14 are four different patterns of forced expiratory volume in one second (FEV$_1$) and forced vital capacity (FVC). Which of these patterns do you expect to see in this patient?

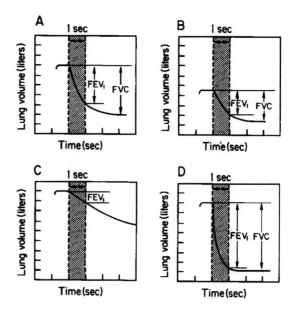

Figure 2–14

(A) Curve A

(B) Curve B

(C) Curve C

(D) Curve D

258. A patient asks you for advice about travel to the Himalayas. You recommend acetazolamide (a carbonic anhydrase inhibitor) for prevention of mountain sickness. Which of the following statements about the action of acetazolamide is correct? Acetazolamide

(A) causes metabolic alkalosis

(B) directly increases the respiratory drive

(C) directly suppresses the respiratory drive

(D) increases bicarbonate concentration in the urine

(E) increases hydrogen concentration in the urine

259. Figure 2–15 illustrates a plot of a blood protein electrophoresis from a 6-month-old boy with a suspected congenital immunodeficiency syndrome. Proteins in which of the electrophoretic fraction are responsible for humoral immunity?

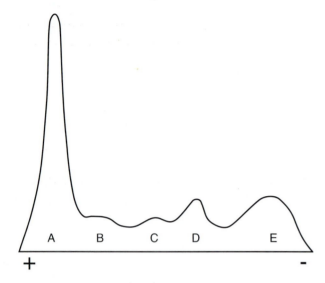

Figure 2–15

(A) Fraction A
(B) Fraction B
(C) Fraction C
(D) Fraction D
(E) Fraction E

260. In response to a small drop in blood pressure, homeostatic events are set in motion that restore and maintain both GFR and blood pressure. By what mechanism is GFR increased when the macula densa senses a decreased concentration of sodium in the renal tubular filtrate?

(A) Decreased hydrostatic pressure in the glomerular capillary
(B) Dilation of the afferent arteriole
(C) Increase in water channels to generate a concentrated urine
(D) Suppression of renin release from juxta-glomerular cells
(E) Upregulation of angiotensin II receptors

261. ADH secretion is most responsive to

(A) decreased plasma osmolarity
(B) decreased plasma volume
(C) hypothalamic-releasing factor
(D) increased plasma osmolarity
(E) increased plasma volume

262. One of your diabetic patients has a blood glucose level of 200 mg/dL. Surprisingly, a dipstick test is negative for urinary glucose. How could this finding be explained?

(A) Dipstick tests are more sensitive for reducing sugars other than glucose.
(B) The patient has defective tubular glucose transporters.
(C) The patient has diabetes insipidus.
(D) The patient has significantly reduced glomerular filtration rate.
(E) The patient is in a state of antidiuresis.

263. A 79-year-old patient with congestive heart failure and peripheral edema is given a diuretic. Which of the following diuretics promotes diuresis by opposing the action of aldosterone?

(A) Carbonic anhydrase inhibitor
(B) Loop diuretic
(C) Mannitol
(D) Potassium-sparing diuretic
(E) Thiazides

264. Liver glycogen content is affected by several hormones. Which of the following shows the correct effects of hormones on liver glycogen content?

	Catecholamines	Glucocorticoids	Glucagon
(A)	decreased	decreased	decreased
(B)	decreased	decreased	increased
(C)	decreased	increased	decreased
(D)	increased	decreased	increased
(E)	increased	increased	decreased

265. Endogenous opioid peptides are an important mechanism of relief from painful stimuli. However, when opiates are used as pharmacologic agents they may have a number of physiological side effects, including

   (A) difficulty sleeping
   (B) hypermotility of the GI tract
   (C) placebo effect
   (D) respiratory alkalosis
   (E) tolerance (need for higher dosage to achieve the same therapeutic effect)

266. Following an automobile accident a patient suffers a pelvic fracture and significant internal blood loss resulting in hemorrhagic shock. Which of the following organs has the largest specific blood flow (blood flow per gram of tissue) under resting conditions and is especially vulnerable during the shock phase?

   (A) Brain
   (B) Heart muscle
   (C) Kidneys
   (D) Skeletal muscle
   (E) Skin

267. A crucial dimension of the pathophysiology of liver disease is elevation of portal venous pressure. Normally blood percolates through the liver at low pressure in part due to specializations unique to liver vasculature, including

   (A) bulk phase endocytosis
   (B) fenestrations between hepatocytes and reticuloendothelial cells
   (C) lack of a typical basement membrane between endothelial cells and hepatocytes
   (D) the presence of asialoglycoprotein receptors
   (E) tight junctions between endothelial cells

268. Following an acute stroke, a patient denies the presence of paralysis of his left upper and lower extremities. The most likely cortical lesion in this patient is localized in the

   (A) posterior inferior gyrus of left frontal lobe

   (B) posterior superior gyrus of left temporal lobe
   (C) right postcentral gyrus
   (D) right posterior parietal cortex
   (E) right precentral gyrus

269. Which of the following is the primary site for salt and water reabsorption in the kidneys?

   (A) Collecting duct
   (B) Glomerulus
   (C) Juxtaglomerular apparatus
   (D) Proximal tubule
   (E) Thick ascending limb of Henle's loop

270. Which of the following renal sites is characterized by low water permeability under all circumstances?

   (A) Collecting duct
   (B) Glomerulus
   (C) Juxtaglomerular apparatus
   (D) Proximal tubule
   (E) Thick ascending limb of Henle's loop

Questions 271 and 272

271. A 58-year-old male visits your office and complains about impotence. Upon questioning you learn that he is capable of erections, but they do not last as long and are of lesser strength than previously. Which of the following neurotransmitters is primarily responsible for dilation of the penile artery during erections?

   (A) Acetylcholine
   (B) Epinephrine
   (C) GABA
   (D) Nitric oxide
   (E) Norepinephrine

272. Nitric oxide causes penile artery dilation by

   (A) decreasing cellular cAMP
   (B) decreasing cellular cGMP
   (C) increasing cellular cAMP
   (D) increasing cellular cGMP
   (E) increasing cellular inositol-trisphosphate (IP$_3$)

273. Creatinine clearance is used to estimate GFR in patients with chronic renal diseases. Which of the graphs in Figure 2–16 shows the correct relationships between renal rate of excretion and plasma concentration of creatinine?

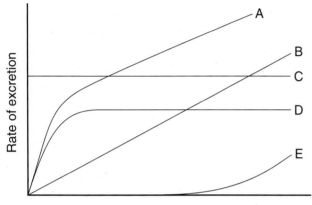

Figure 2–16

(A) Curve A

(B) Curve B

(C) Curve C

(D) Curve D

(E) Curve E

274. One of your obstetric patients is 5 months pregnant with her second child. Pregnancy and delivery of her first child were unremarkable. Which of the following combinations poses a significant risk of hemolytic anemia for her second child?

	Mother	First Child	Second Child
(A)	Rh negative	Rh negative	Rh positive
(B)	Rh negative	Rh positive	Rh positive
(C)	Rh positive	Rh positive	Rh negative
(D)	Rh positive	Rh negative	Rh positive
(E)	Rh positive	Rh positive	Rh positive

275. Which of the following statements about human chorionic gonadotropin (hCG) is correct?

(A) hCG can be detected in the urine prior to the first missed menstrual cycle.

(B) hCG directly suppresses fetal production of steroids.

(C) hCG is often negative in patients with ectopic pregnancy.

(D) hCG is usually negative in patients with choriocarcinoma.

(E) hCG levels are highest at the end of pregnancy.

276. You see a patient with damage to the left cervical sympathetic chain ganglia as a result of a neck tumor. Which of the following physical signs would be expected?

(A) Increased sweat secretion on the left side of the face

(B) Lateral deviation of the left eye

(C) Pale skin on the left side of the face

(D) Ptosis (hanging of the upper eye lid) on the left

(E) Pupil dilation of the left eye

277. Which of the following transmembrane proteins is mainly responsible for the resting membrane potential of vascular smooth muscle cells?

(A) Cl^- channels

(B) K^+ channels

(C) Na^+ channels

(D) Na^+/K^+ pump

(E) Nonselective cation channels

278. Functional zonation is the observation that the pattern of enzymatic activities displayed by hepatocytes varies depending on their location along the liver acinus from the portal vein to the central vein (Figure 2–17). Thus, zone 1 hepatocytes, closest to the portal vein, are particularly active in gluconeogenesis whereas zone 3 hepatocytes closest to the central vein are more active in glycolysis. What accounts for this difference?

(A) Hepatocytes of zone 1 are in association with reticuloendothelial cells.

(B) Hepatocytes of zone 1 are undergoing apoptosis.

(C) Hepatocytes of zone 3 are bathed in high concentrations of hormones in the portal vein.

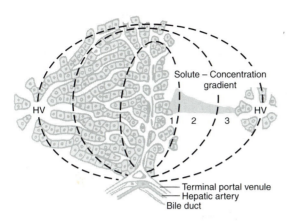

Figure 2–17. *(Reproduced with permission from Gumico, JJ: Hepatic transport. In: Textbook of Medicine. Kelley, WN. Lippincott, 1989.)*

(D) Hepatocytes of zone 3 are more active in urea synthesis.

(E) The gradient of oxygen from portal vein to central vein.

279. What are the insensible losses of water (e.g., via skin and lungs) over 24 hours in a typical adult at room temperature?

(A) 0 mL
(B) 100 to 250 mL
(C) 500 to 1000 mL
(D) 2500 to 3500 mL
(E) 5000 to 10,000 mL

Questions 280 to 282

A 79-year-old man with chronic renal failure and a GFR of 25 mL/min (normal 120 mL/min) is admitted to the hospital because of a spontaneous fracture of the left humerus. X-ray shows numerous subperiosteal erosions with low bone density.

280. The most likely cause of this patient's fracture is

(A) osteomalacia due to primary hyperparathyroidism
(B) osteomalacia due to secondary hyperparathyroidism
(C) osteoporosis due to lack of sex steroids
(D) osteoporosis due to old age
(E) rickets due to lack of dietary vitamin D

281. Which of the following statements about renal handling of phosphate is correct? In this patient

(A) increased urinary phosphate binds urinary calcium, resulting in a loss of both phosphate and calcium
(B) most of the filtered phosphate is excreted
(C) the filtration rate of phosphate is lower than normal, resulting in phosphate accumulation
(D) the tubular reabsorption rate is higher than normal, resulting in phosphate accumulation
(E) the tubular secretion rate is higher than normal, resulting in phosphate loss

282. Which of the following statements is correct? Phosphate reabsorption in the proximal tubule is

(A) due to active cotransport with calcium ions
(B) due to active cotransport with chloride ions
(C) due to passive diffusion down its electrochemical gradient
(D) inhibited by calcitonin
(E) inhibited by parathyroid hormone (PTH)

Answers and Explanations

156. (A) During pregnancy many physiologic changes take place in the mother's body. Maternal blood volume increases up to 40% due to elevated aldosterone and estrogen levels. GI tone and motility decrease because of the inhibitory effect of progesterone (choice B). Bone marrow production of erythrocytes also increases, but does not keep up with the plasma volume expansion, resulting in a decrease in hematocrit ("physiologic anemia of pregnancy") (choice C). Respiratory minute volume increases by about 50% because of the increased basal metabolic rate and oxygen consumption. This increase is largely due to an increase in tidal volume without increase in respiratory rate (choice E). Both residual volume and expiratory reserve volume decrease (choice D).

157. (C) The cerebellum is generally considered to play an important role in the coordination and smoothing out of voluntary movements. Intention tremor, which may be observed in cerebellar disease, is absent at rest (choice B) but appears at the onset of voluntary movements (choice A). This aspect of the tremor readily differentiates it from tremor observed with degeneration of the nigrostriatal dopaminergic tracts in Parkinson disease, which produces tremor that is present at rest. Frequency of tremor is a less reliable means to distinguish these types of tremor (choice E), and the amplitude of oscillations is not generally constant throughout a voluntary movement (choice D).

158. (B) The ADH system is utilized in two ways. On a minute-by-minute basis, it responds to extracellular fluid osmolality, as monitored at the hypothalamus. In sudden and severe volume depletion (e.g., in response to hemorrhage), the ADH system responds to volume. Thus, the amount of ADH secreted per unit rise in osmolarity is a function of volume status. In hypovolemia very small increases in osmolarity induce large amounts of ADH to be secreted. In hypervolemia, even very large increases in plasma osmolality induce only modest increases in ADH secretion.

159. (E) Urination occurs whenever bladder pressure exceeds sphincter tone. The external sphincter is a skeletal muscle innervated by motor neurons from the pudendal nerve, not by sympathetic fibers (choice D). Higher centers in the brainstem keep the micturition reflex inhibited except when micturition is desired (choice A). As the bladder fills, sensory signals from bladder stretch receptors elicit a micturition reflex via parasympathetic fibers originating in the sacral spinal cord. These transient contractions elicit an urge to urinate, but normally urination does not occur unless the external sphincter relaxes. If the lumbar spinal cord is damaged (choice B) while the sacral segments are intact, micturition reflexes occur, resulting in spontaneous and uncontrolled bladder emptying (automatic bladder). If the sacral spinal cord is damaged (choice C), micturition reflexes are lost and the bladder fills to capacity, resulting in overflow incontinence (atonic bladder).

160. (D) Figure 2–1 shows the endometrial changes expected during a textbook menstrual cycle of 28 days' length. Ovulation occurs on day 14, counting as day 1 the first day of the last menstrual period. Progesterone produced by the corpus luteum reaches its peak around day 21. In the absence of fertilization, the corpus luteum then degenerates and progesterone levels begin to drop.

161. **(C)** In contrast to progesterone, which is detectable in significant amounts only during the secretory phase, estrogen levels show a biphasic time course. Peak levels are secreted by the growing follicle about 36 hours prior to ovulation (which occurs on day 14), inducing the LH surge. A second but smaller increase of estrogen occurs during the luteal phase of the cycle.

162. **(E)** Pupil diameter is determined by the balance between sympathetic tone to the radial fibers of the iris and parasympathetic tone to the pupillary sphincter muscle. Phentolamine is a blocker of α-adrenergic receptors, which causes pupil constriction. Pupil dilation occurs during increased sympathetic activity (e.g., emotional excitement [choice C], decreased parasympathetic activity during darkness [choices B and D], or block of muscarinic receptors by atropine [choice A]).

163. **(A)** Water that is either higher or lower than body temperature when introduced into the external auditory meatus may set up convection currents within the endolymph of the inner ear. These currents may result in the stimulation of the semicircular canals by causing movements of the ampullar cristae. Conflicting information from the right and left sides may in turn result in vertigo and nausea. Decreased movement or immobilization of the otoliths (choice E) or the ampullar cristae (choice C) is not caused by such changes in temperature. Furthermore, changes in the discharge rate of vestibular afferents (choices B and D), which must occur with caloric stimulation, are most likely to be caused by the changes in the activity of the receptors, rather than being a direct response of the afferents to changes in temperature.

164. **(C)** The principle behind a radioimmunoassay involves using a purified sample of a hormone, and an antibody or other binding protein that recognizes that hormone, to generate a "standard curve" to which unknowns (e.g. blood samples whose level of hormone you wish to determine) can be compared. To generate a standard curve, a trace amount of the purified hormone is made radioactive, and the ability of a given amount of antibody to bind the radioactive hormone is compared in the presence of increasing amounts of purified nonradioactive hormone. When the unknown sample is substituted for non-radioactive hormone, the amount of radioactive hormone that binds to the antibody allows you to indirectly estimate how much hormone was likely present. This assay is reproducible (given the same antibody and purified hormone preparation), fast, and relatively inexpensive compared to bioassays (choices A and B). An antibody alone (choice D), without a sample of purified hormone, is insufficient to establish a radioimmunoassay. Column chromatography (choice E) to separate hormone isoforms might be a useful step in purification, and could be used to develop an alternate direct means of detection and measurement of the hormone, but does not, by itself, allow establishment of a radioimmunoassay.

165. **(D)** The primary change in the cochlea due to an increase in the frequency of a sound wave is a change in the position of maximal displacement of the basilar membrane. A low-pitched sound produces the greatest displacement toward the apex of the cochlea and produces the greatest activation of hair cells at that location. As pitch increases, the position of greatest displacement moves closer to the base of the cochlea. Increased amplitude of basilar membrane displacement (choice B) and increases in the number of hair cells that are activated (choice A) and in the frequency of discharge of units in the auditory nerve fibers (choice C), together with an increase in range of frequencies to which such units respond (choice E), are all more likely to be observed in response to increases

in the intensity of a sound stimulus rather than to increases in pitch. In the auditory cortex, sound frequencies are organized topographically so that a change in pitch may be represented by a change in the location of activated cortical units.

166. **(C)** Increased activity of phase I (e.g., due to enzyme induction in a patient drinking alcohol or taking phase I metabolized medications) combined with diminished activity of phase II (e.g., in nutritionally deficiency in cysteine, the rate limiting component in synthesis of glutathione, which is often used for drug conjugation), can result in accumulation of metabolites that are more toxic than the initial drug itself or the other options indicated (choices A, B, D, and E).

167. **(A)** The patient clearly has an increase in her state of insulin resistance. This could be due to increased obesity, less exercise, worsening of her diet, or more likely, given the magnitude of her increased insulin requirements, development of a high titer of anti-insulin antibodies that are preventing the injected insulin from lowering blood glucose effectively. An improved diet (choice B) and exercise program (choice C) or weight loss (choice E) each would have decreased her insulin requirements. Progression of macrovascular disease (choice D) is largely irrelevant to her insulin requirements, except to the extent that angina might decrease her ability to exercise.

168. **(E)** The stimulation of receptors in the Golgi tendon organs leads to the inverse stretch reflex. This reflex is responsible for the relaxation observed when a muscle is subjected to a strong stretch. Impulses from the organs travel in type Ib fibers to the spinal cord, where they activate inhibitory interneurons. These in turn suppress the activity of motoneurons and therefore lead to relaxation of the extrafusal muscle fibers (choice A) attached to the tendons. The state of contraction of intrafusal fibers (choice B), the gamma-efferent discharge rate (choice D), and the activity in group II afferent fibers (choice C) control the stretch reflex, which is

distinct from the inverse stretch reflex mediated by the Golgi tendon organs.

169. **(C)** Leukotrienes, like the prostaglandins and thromboxanes to which they are structurally related, are extracellular signaling molecules (and therefore can be considered hormones) derived from the lipid arachidonic acid. None of the other options are lipids. ACTH (choice A) is a 39-residue polypeptide. Catecholamines (choice B) are derived from modified amino acids. Nitric oxide (choice D) is released as a gas by metabolism of arginine. TRH (choice E) is a tripeptide.

170. **(C)** Fiber provides bulk, which promotes satiety through gastric distention and is not broken down by small intestinal digestive enzymes. It thus moves quickly through the GI tract, speeding the elimination of potentially carcinogenic substances. Some of the fiber is broken down by colonic microbes generating small-chain fatty acids that are an important source of nutrition for the healthy colonic epithelium and at the same time promote apoptosis (programmed cell death) of cells that have undergone malignant transformation. Fiber actually speeds GI transit time as opposed to slowing it (choice D). Fiber has no specific effects on GI blood flow (choice A), pancreatic bicarbonate secretion (choice B), or acid secretion (choice E).

171. **(A)** Significant aortic stenosis impairs flow out of the left ventricle, thus, should the patient have a repeat GI bleed, the ability to increase cardiac output would be impaired. Choices C and D are true of patients with severe aortic stenosis, but do not reflect protective mechanisms that would be called upon in the event of a repeat GI bleed. Choices B and E are not correct. Severe aortic stenosis is an indication for afterload reduction and surgical correction, but not anticoagulation, and has no direct effect on venous return.

172. **(A)** Two features that distinguish ventricular tachycardia from sinus tachycardia are that the QRS complex of the latter is normally nar-

row (a feature easily distinguished) and in fixed relationship to P waves (choice E), making them more difficult to see and measure, compared to the QRS complex in ventricular tachycardia. With bundle branch block, the conduction system defect makes the QRS complex as wide even though impulses originate from the sinus node. The other three options are not specifically relevant to distinguishing these two conditions. Heart rate > 100 (choice B) is necessary for the definition of sinus tachycardia. Inverted T waves (choice C) are seen in a number of conditions. Prolonged QT interval (choice D) is associated with increased risk of ventricular tachycardia, but is not a distinguishing feature between these conditions.

173. **(B)** Teleologically speaking, starvation is not a great time for the added burdens of raising young. Hence it is not surprising that the reproductive neuroendocrine axis is downregulated in response to stress in general and starvation in particular. All the other options (choices A, B, D, and E) are opposite of what is observed in starvation.

174. **(A)** The loss of insulin secretion that results in type 1 diabetes (insulin-dependent diabetes) leads to severely altered metabolism. Associated with loss of insulin is a concomitant elevation in glucagon secretion from the pancreas. One major effect of increased glucagon is an increased rate of fatty acid mobilization from adipose tissue. The fats are then taken up by other tissues, predominantly the liver, where they are oxidized to acetyl-CoA. The rate of fat oxidation exceeds the capacity of the liver to completely oxidize the acetyl-CoA to CO_2 and H_2O in the tricarboxylic acid cycle. The excess acetyl-CoA is converted into the ketones that are then delivered to the blood. Nonhepatic tissues cannot oxidize the excess ketones, which are highly acidic. Elevations in blood concentrations of these compounds result in the consumption of bicarbonate ion as well as other organic buffers. The net effect is a precipitous drop in blood pH. Glycogen synthesis (choice C), fatty acid synthesis (choice B), and pro-

tein synthesis (choice E) are processes that are typically suppressed in poorly controlled diabetes; they are metabolic responses to increased secretion of insulin. In addition to increased fatty acid oxidation, the lack of insulin secretion that is the cause of type 1 diabetes leads to pronounced increases in other catabolic reactions in the body (choice D). However, protein catabolism does not significantly contribute to the pool of excess acetyl-CoA that leads to ketoacidosis.

175. **(E)** The most rapid filling of the ventricles occurs in early diastole, immediately after opening of the atrioventricular valves. This happens after the repolarization phase (T wave) and resulting relaxation of the cardiac ventricular muscle. Excitation of the atria (choice A) also results in increased blood flow into the ventricles, occurring around choice B. However, the flow at that time is less than during early diastole. Ventricular contraction begins with the QRS complex (choice C) and lasts until the end of the T wave (choice D). During this time, the mitral and tricuspid valves are closed.

176. **(D)** Note that the end-diastolic volume of this patient is the same as that of a normal subject. Because the patient's stroke volume is larger than that of a normal subject, the force of contraction must also be larger. This could be due to increased sympathetic tone or to the fact that the patient took inotropic medications. The volume remaining after the ventricular contraction is correspondingly smaller compared to normal. Preload (choices B and E) equals end-diastolic volume and is the same in the patient and normal subjects. Afterload (choice A) is equal to arterial pressure. Both afterload and stroke volume (choice C) are larger in this patient compared to normal.

177. **(C)** Figure 2–18 shows the jugular vein pressure curve. Pressure in the jugular vein reflects atrial pressure and is highest during the atrial contraction (a wave). The v wave (choice A) represents the rise in atrial pressure before the tricuspid valve opens during

diastole. The y notch (choice B) is due to fall of atrial pressure during the ventricular filling phase. The c wave (choice D) is due to the rise in atrial pressure produced by the bulging of the mitral valve during isometric contraction of the left ventricle. The x notch (choice E) coincides with the ventricular ejection phase.

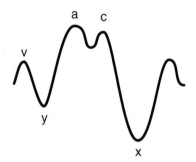

Figure 2–18

178. **(A)** Reticuloendothelial cells of the liver play a variety of important roles. A distinctive characteristic of quiescent, normal, Stellate cells is the presence of a droplet of vitamin A. Upon activation, this feature is lost, and is accompanied by a host of changes in gene expression, including overproduction of new forms of collagen, which contributes to hepatic fibrosis, the hallmark of cirrhosis. Whether loss of the vitamin A droplet reflects loss of function as a vitamin A storage cell or has other implications is unknown. Insulin receptors (choice D) and bile synthesis (choice C) are irrelevant. Stellate cells are not restricted to periportal location, either normally or in cirrhosis (choice E). Kupffer cells (choice B) are tissue macrophages of the liver and represent another member of the category of reticuloendothelial cells, but are not associated structurally or functionally with Stellate cells.

179. **(D)** Not only are there different prostaglandins, some of which are vasoconstrictive and some of which are vasodilatory, but different prostaglandins have different effects in one part of the kidney versus another. In the renal cortex, prostaglandins are local mediators that protect glomerular circulation under condi-

tions of volume depletion. The other options all decrease GFR, either locally (choices A, B, and C) or via the generation of angiotensin II (choice E).

180. **(C)** Erythropoietin serves to stimulate red blood cell production in the bone marrow. One of the consequences of chronic renal disease is loss of this hormone resulting in anemia that is responsive to erythropoietin injections. Aldosterone (choice A) is a steroid, secreted in part in response to angiotensin II, that acts on the kidney but is not synthesized by the kidney. Angiotensinogen (choice B) is a liver secretory protein that is the substrate for the kidney secreted hormone renin. Insulin (choice D) is cleared in part by the kidney, but is made by the β-cells of the endocrine pancreas. Parathyroid hormone (choice E) has effects on the kidney but is made in the parathyroid glands.

181. **(A)** Albumin, synthesized by the liver, is the major determinant of plasma oncotic pressure. Extravasation of fluid from the vasculature is determined by the balance between oncotic and hydrostatic pressures (choice B). Insufficient energy to maintain Na^+/K^+ ATPase (choice C) is incompatible with life. Certain parasitic infections (choice D) can cause portal hypertension and ascites (e.g., schistosomiasis), and malnutrition is a relatively immunosuppressed state, but neither is a necessary condition for ascites. In hepatic cirrhosis, hydrostatic pressure is elevated due to portal hypertension (choice E), but in protein–calorie malnutrition oncotic pressure is decreased due to insufficient albumin synthesis. The net effect in both cases is ascites formation.

182. **(D)** High-dose exogenous glucocorticoids suppress the adrenal neuroendocrine axis. Patients treated for longer than 2 weeks need to be tapered off glucocorticoids slowly to avoid adrenal insufficiency. In times of stress, they need to be treated with high dose glucocorticoids. Other complications of high-dose glucocorticoids include growth suppression in children (choice A) and volume overload (choice

E). Hyperkalemia (choice B) and hyponatremia (choice C) are observed in adrenal insufficiency due to loss of mineralocorticoid effects and are not relevant to glucocorticoid therapy, nor is acromegaly (choice A), a condition caused by excess of growth hormone in adults.

183. **(B)** Heart rate increases whenever sympathetic firing rate increases or parasympathetic firing rate decreases; the cardiac atria receive tonic input from both sympathetic and parasympathetic nerves. In humans, the ventricles are not innervated by parasympathetic nerves (choice D), and the strength of contraction increases with increasing preload (Frank-Starling mechanism), increasing sympathetic firing rate (choice E). With few exceptions, blood vessels are not innervated by parasympathetic nerves, and there is little effect of changes in parasympathetic tone on total peripheral resistance (choices A and C).

184. **(A)** Surfactant serves to lower surface tension allowing alveoli to remain open, thereby diminishing air trapping and decreasing the work of breathing. Neutrophil proteases (choice C) are released in the course of the inflammatory response. When these activities exceed protective mechanisms (e.g., antiproteases secreted from respiratory epithelia), lung injury can occur, leading ultimately to loss of elasticity and destruction of terminal airspaces. Smooth muscle relaxation (choice D) is an important parameter of ventilatory function and determinant of flow rates. Prostaglandins (choice E) are important mediators of airway smooth muscle tone. Antioxidants (choice B) can prevent tissue injury such as that caused by toxins in cigarette smoke. However, choices B, C, D, and E are not important determinants of atelectasis.

185. **(C)** About 40% of total plasma Ca^{2+} is bound to proteins and not filtered at the glomerular basement membrane. Therefore, the estimated daily filtered load is 1.5 mM/L · 160 L/day = 240 mM/day. The exact amount of free versus total Ca^{2+} depends on the blood pH: free Ca^{2+} increases during acidosis and decreases during alkalosis.

186. **(D).** Mucous gland hypertrophy and the resulting overproduction of mucus contribute to obstruction of airways that increases resistance to airflow. Other important contributors include smooth muscle constriction in medium-sized bronchioles, and collapse of airways (e.g., due to either a lack of surfactant or destruction of alveolar walls). Antioxidants (choice E) and smooth muscle relaxation (choice B) are protective against increased airway resistance to airflow. Diminished neutrophil infiltration (choice A) and increased pulmonary blood flow (choice C) are not relevant to the question.

187. **(D)** Normally, O_2 is transferred from air spaces to blood via a perfusion-limited process. Thus, O_2 moves across the alveolar–capillary membrane by a process of simple diffusion, and the amount of gas taken up depends entirely on the amount of blood flow. Processes that impair diffusion of O_2 transform the normal relationship to a diffusion-limited process. Thus, if O_2 must move a greater distance because of a thickened barrier, as would occur with increased extravascular lung water (pulmonary edema) or cell components (interstitial fibrosis or asbestosis), the diffusion process is limited. Breathing a hyperbaric gas mixture (choice A) would increase the driving force and may overcome diffusion limitation in patients with mild fibrosis or interstitial edema. Chronic obstructive lung diseases (choice B) have little effect on pulmonary diffusion capacity. Increasing the ventilatory rate (choice C) does not have this effect and only serves to maintain a high gradient of O_2 from air to blood. Strenuous, but not mild exercise (choice E), decreases passage time and may also favor diffusion limitation.

188. **(D)** Obesity is an insulin-resistant state for many reasons: The larger the mass of fat cells in the body, (1) the greater the baseline level of hormone sensitive lipase activity and hence of free fatty acids generated, which impairs insulin action; (2) the greater the amount of insulin needed to direct fat storage; and (3) the greater the level of cytokines

such as TNF-α produced by adipocytes, that counter insulin action. All the other options are opposite what is observed in most human obesity, which is typically a leptin resistant state (choice E) with elevated LDL (choice B), diminished HDL (choice C) and elevated blood estrogen (choice A). The latter is due in part to the increased aromatase activity that converts androgens to estrogens. Interestingly, not all fat is equal. A growing body of evidence suggests that visceral fat (deposited in the abdomen) is far worse in terms of insulin resistance and cardiovascular risk than peripheral fat.

189. **(A)** The action potentials illustrated must be those of cardiac nodal cells (SA node or AV node). The duration of these action potentials is too long for either motor axons (2 msec) (choice B) or skeletal muscle fibers (5 msec) (choice C). Also, the configuration is different. They cannot represent vascular smooth muscle cells (choice D), which have no appreciable action potential. They cannot be ventricular Purkinje action potentials (choice E) because these have a more negative diastolic component that does not gradually depolarize, a longer duration (200 msec), and a plateau region.

190. **(E)** Ventricular performance in normally enhanced (e.g. during exercise) by the effect of the sympathetic nervous system stimulating contractility via norepinephrine. The effect of the parasympathetic nervous system (choice D) is primarily to slow the heart rate. The number of myocardial cells induced to contract (choice A) is not a variable through which myocardial contractility is regulated, in contrast to skeletal muscle. Decreases in ATP levels (choice B) and systemic acidosis (choice C) diminish ventricular performance, the former by impeding myocardial relaxation and the latter by depressing left ventricular work at any given end diastolic volume.

191. **(E)** Depression of myocardial function can be due to pharmacologic depressants such as calcium antagonists, β-adrenergic blockers, or loss of myocytes. Myocyte loss can occur

through either necrosis (e.g., with myocardial infarction) or through cardiac remodeling through programmed cell death (apoptosis). Choices A, B, C, and D represent mechanisms that would improve ventricular contractility and performance at any given end diastolic volume.

192. **(B)** With arterial blood pH of 7.33, the patient clearly has an acidosis. The first question you should ask yourself is, "Is it respiratory or non-respiratory (metabolic)?" If it were respiratory (choices D and E), the Pa_{CO_2} would be above normal. Because it is lower than normal, this indicates the acidosis is metabolic with some respiratory compensation in response to the acidemia. Uncompensated metabolic acidosis (choice C) would show normal Pa_{CO_2}. It is unlikely that the metabolic acidosis is due to diabetic ketoacidosis (choice A); if this were the case, you would expect glucose to be present in the urine.

193. **(A)** In healthy subjects on a normal diet, about 70 mEq of hydrogen ion is produced each day (largely from oxidation of sulfur-containing amino acids). This produces a progressive metabolic acidosis if the H^+ is not excreted in the urine as NH_4^+ and $H_2PO_4^-$. Both are decreased in the later stages of renal failure (e.g., from chronic glomerulonephritis). Because NH_4^+ excretion plays the major role in disposing of daily H^+, a deficiency in ammonium excretion explains the metabolic acidosis (probably simply a reflection of the diminished number of functioning nephrons). Hyperventilation (choice D) or hypoventilation (choice E) are not the cause of this patient's acidosis. Excess β-hydroxybutyric and acetoacetic acids (i.e., ketoacidosis) (choice C) is unlikely in this patient. Decreased catabolism of methionine and cysteine (choice B) also could not account for the metabolic acidosis.

194. **(A)** Of the Starling forces determining fluid distribution across a membrane, the contributions of interstitial fluid hydrostatic and oncotic pressure are usually small. Hence edema

formation is largely determined by the difference between capillary hydrostatic and oncotic pressure. When this difference is sufficiently large to exceed the capacity of lymphatic drainage, edema develops. ADH (choice C) inserts water channels in the distal renal tubule, resulting in retention of free water that increases hydrostatic pressure. Elevated portal venous pressure (choice D) results in ascites, a form of edema fluid, but is not a necessary condition for edema formation. Like total body water overload, sodium depletion (choice E) with activation of ADH and resulting water retention can result in edema, but is not a necessary condition for its formation.

195. **(C)** Acidemia is the presence of excess H^+ ions in blood, which creates a driving force for their entry into cells. Because potassium is the major intracellular cation, electroneutrality is maintained in the face of entry of H^+ ions into cells by movement of K^+ out of cells and into blood. Choices A, B, D, and E are the opposite of what is observed in acidemia.

196. **(A)** This patient probably suffers from myopia (nearsightedness). Myopia is either due to eyeballs that are too long or a lens that is too strong. To focus a distant object onto the retina (far accommodation), the lens has to decrease its refractive power (i.e., increase its focal length). This is accomplished through relaxation of the ciliary muscles that oppose the pull of the sclera, resulting in a tightening of the zonula fibers and a flattening of the lens. Relaxation of the zonular fibers (choice E), rounding of the lens (choice C), and shortening of the focal length (choice B), all occur during near accommodation. The pupils also constrict during near accommodation (choice D), perhaps to increase depth of field.

197. **(D)** A fixed lesion of the renal artery results in impaired perfusion. When the kidney senses poor perfusion, it increases its secretion of renin in an effort to raise blood pressure and improve renal blood flow. Hence the appropriate treatment is surgical correction of the renal artery lesion. There is no clear relationship between adrenal insufficiency (choice A) or hyperparathyroidism (choice C) and hypertension. Estrogen deficiency (choice B) and volume depletion (choice E) are situations that tend to diminish blood pressure.

198. **(C)** Malignant hyperthermia is due to a genetic variation of the skeletal muscle ryanodine receptors (sarcoplasmic Ca^{2+} release channels). Halothane and several other drugs may trigger excessive Ca^{2+} release, leading to muscle contractures, increased muscle metabolism, and an enormous increase in heat production. This condition is fatal if not treated promptly with a ryanodine receptor antagonist such as dantrolene. Convectional heat loss (e.g., lack of appropriate clothing during winter) (choice A) would result in cooling of the body temperature. An increased hypothalamic temperature set point (choice D) occurs during febrile episodes of infectious diseases. Such change of set point is due to increased blood levels of interleukin-1 (choice B). Increased sweat production (choice E) is a consequence, but not the cause, of malignant hyperthermia.

199. **(D)** The A–a oxygen gradient is increased in either shunting or in ventilation-perfusion mismatch as occurs in airway, interstitial, alveolar or pulmonary vascular diseases. Hypoventilation caused by narcotic overdose (choice B) and neuromuscular disease (choice A) will lead to a high blood P_{CO_2}. Inspiration of low oxygen content air (choice C) will lead to a low blood P_{CO_2}. In all of these latter situations the difference between alveolar and arterial P_{O_2} is normal.

200. **(A)** Breathing is stimulated by a fall in Pa_{O_2}, a rise in Pa_{CO_2}, or a fall in arterial pH. Normally, the hydrogen ion concentration monitored by central chemoreceptors controls the drive to breathe, determined largely by Pa_{CO_2}. The carotid bodies at the bifurcation of the common carotid arteries are the peripheral chemoreceptors that sense arterial oxygenation. Their firing increases ventilation in response to hypoxia. Pulmonary stretch re-

ceptors are also located in the airway smooth muscle and monitor lung volumes. Increased lung volume decreases the rate of respiration by increasing the time of expiration. None of the other choices (B, C, D, and E) contribute to the control of breathing.

201. **(C)** Both Na^+ and K^+ excretion are tightly regulated. Thus, as GFR decreases in disease, the percentage of filtered Na^+ or K^+ excreted increases to maintain a normal amount of Na^+ or K^+ excretion (assuming Na^+ and K^+ intake remain the same). Substances like urea (choice A) (some reabsorption) and creatinine (choice D) (almost exclusively excreted by glomerular filtration) have no adaptive mechanisms to regulate plasma levels. Thus, a significant decrease in GFR results in significant increases in plasma creatinine and urea (assuming production of both substances remains constant). This is because the amount of substance x that is excreted ($U_x \cdot V$) equals the amount produced. Furthermore, $U_x \cdot V = $ GFR $\cdot P_x$. If GFR decreases, P_x increases. Because of the increase in percent filtered Na^+ and K^+ that is excreted, an increase in plasma Na^+ (choice B) or a decrease in plasma K^+ (choice E) would not be expected with a GFR that is 50% of normal. $U_x \div$ urine concentration of x; $P_x \div$ plasma concentration of x; $V \div$ urine volume.

202. **(C)** Normal sleep occurs in alternating cycles between slow-wave sleep (non-REM sleep) and rapid eye movement (REM) sleep, the latter characterized by high metabolic brain activity and desynchronization of the EEG. Enuresis (bedwetting) (choice A), night terrors (choice B) and somnambulism (sleep walking) (choice E) occur during slow-wave sleep or arousal from slow-wave sleep. During REM sleep there is hypotonia of all major muscle groups except the ocular muscles, due to a generalized spinal inhibition that prevents acting out of dreams. Dreams, nightmares, and penile erections in the male all occur during REM sleep. Sleep spindles (choice D) in the EEG are characteristic of the early sleep stages.

203. **(C)** The relationship between alveolar ventilation ($\dot{V}A$) and alveolar CO_2 pressure ($PACO_2$) is represented as

$$\dot{V}A = (\dot{V}CO_2/PACO_2) \cdot K$$

where K is a constant such that $PACO_2 = FACO_2 \cdot K$. ($FACO_2$ is the fraction of alveolar CO_2). Because $\dot{V}CO_2$ is constant if CO_2 production remains unchanged, $PACO_2$ will double if $\dot{V}A$ is halved. In normal persons, alveolar CO_2 pressure ($PACO_2$) is virtually identical to arterial CO_2 pressure ($PaCO_2$). Therefore, $PaCO_2$ will also double if $\dot{V}A$ is halved. On the other hand, alveolar CO_2 pressures ($PACO_2$) (choice A) would decrease if ventilation were increased. Unless inspired air is enriched with O_2, arterial O_2 pressure (PaO_2) (choices D and E) and alveolar O_2 pressure (PAO_2) (choice B) will decrease.

204. **(D)** The adrenogenital syndrome results from two consequences of this enzyme deficiency. First, failure to make cortisol results in an inability to provide negative feedback suppression of ACTH production. As a result, the adrenal glands are under constant stimulation to maximize steroidogenesis, including adrenal gland hypertrophy. Second, because the flow of substrates cannot reach cortisol due to the enzyme lack, the flow down other pathways, and by mass action, drives the massive overproduction of androgens that can also be peripherally aromatized to estrogens. No significant change in serum cholesterol is observed (choice E), probably because the cholesterol reservoir in the body is large compared even to the massive levels of steroids being synthesized in this syndrome. Cortical atrophy (choice A) and release of excess cortisol (choice C) are the opposite of what is observed. There is no mechanism to achieve selective hypertrophy of the adrenal medulla (choice B) because the action of ACTH to drive adrenal hypertrophy is limited to the cortex.

205. **(B)** Bed rest and immobilization cause stasis, which predisposes to formation of inappropriate clots. Anemia (choice A) is not a risk

factor for thrombosis. Heart failure due to low output states can result in back up of blood (and stasis) on the venous side. However this is not the case in *high*-output cardiac failure (choice C). Oral anticoagulant therapy (choice D) and strenuous activity (choice E) tend to *prevent* venous thrombosis by prevention of clot formation and prevention of stasis, respectively.

206. **(C)** Spermatogenesis requires extremely high concentrations of androgens. To achieve these high levels the seminiferous tubules contain an androgen binding protein (ABP). Under stimulation by gonadotropins, the testes produce androgens including testosterone. Initially, upon synthesis in the testes, these steroids are bound to ABP. Androgens spill over into the circulation only after the ABP "reservoir" in the testes has been saturated with androgen. At that point, androgen feedback inhibits GnRH and gonadotropins at the hypothalamus and pituitary gland. By injecting testosterone peripherally, the weightlifter bypassed his testicular ABP reservoir and shut off his hypothalamus and pituitary before adequate ABP saturation with androgens was achieved in the testes.

207. **(E)** Hyponatremia of this magnitude for any reason is likely to cause seizures and coma, especially if the deviation from normal occurred rapidly (e.g. over 1 or 2 days). Withdrawal from painful stimuli (choice A) is a normal reaction. If intact, it would have provided information on the intactness of sensation and motor reflexes on the tested side. However lack of withdrawal would be consistent with either a structural or a metabolic cause of coma, and therefore does not help. Blood in the cerebral spinal fluid (choice B) in a nontraumatic lumbar puncture suggests a structural rather than a metabolic cause of coma. Pupillary light responses (choice C) are typically preserved in metabolic encephalopathies. Posturing of limbs (choice D) is suggestive of a focal process involving the brainstem or midbrain rather than a metabolic encephalopathy.

208. **(A)** Insulin is normally secreted by the endocrine pancreas into the portal venous drainage; thus, under normal circumstances, it passes through the liver before being seen by the periphery. A certain fraction of insulin is extracted by the liver; thus, the concentration of insulin seen by the liver is normally higher than that seen by the periphery. However, with peripheral insulin injections exactly the opposite is true. Thus, undesired effects of insulin that may contribute to hypertension and cardiovascular disease in patients with diabetes and may be increased. Injected insulin is missing C peptide (choice D) and endogenous insulin is cosecreted with C peptide, whose physiologic functions, if any, remain unknown. Injected insulin is biologically active and not in the proinsulin form (choice E). Exogenous insulin generally used today in the United States is recombinant human insulin, not from animal sources (choice C). Anti-insulin antibodies that used to be a major problem with animal insulins is now rarer. Insulin resistance (choice B) is generally due to receptor downregulation or desensitization, or anti-insulin antibodies, and is generally equally true for both endogenous and exogenous insulin. However, the dose of the latter can be increased, although a patient with diminished β-cell reserve may not be able to increase endogenous insulin secretion sufficiently to overcome insulin resistance.

209. **(A)** Under normal circumstances, depolarization is initiated in the SA node and then propagates to the AV node. From there, action potentials are propagated through the bundle of His and through the Purkinje system to the ventricular muscle. Conduction in the AV node is slower than conduction from the SA node to the AV node (choice B), from the AV node to ventricular muscle (choices C and D), or conduction within the ventricular muscle (choice E). The AV nodal delay is typically on the order of 100 msec.

210. **(C)** Osteoporosis is one of the most feared complications of long-term high dose glucocorticoid therapy. This effect is compounded

by stimulation, not suppression, of osteoclast breakdown of bone (choice E); suppression, not activation, of osteoblast deposition of new bone (choice D); increased calcium loss, not readsorption (choice A), in the urine; and decreased, not increased (choice B), synthesis of bone matrix proteins.

211. **(C)** Increased pulmonary fibrosis is the hallmark of restrictive lung diseases. As a result of fibrosis, the diffusing capacity (choice B) is progressively reduced, total lung capacities (choice D) are decreased and the FEV_1/FVC ratio is increased (choice E), even as TLC, FEV1, and FVC are reduced in absolute terms. Bronchial wall thickening (choice A) due to mucous gland hypertrophy is a characteristic of chronic bronchitis and obstructive lung diseases, not of a pure restrictive disorder (Figure 2–19).

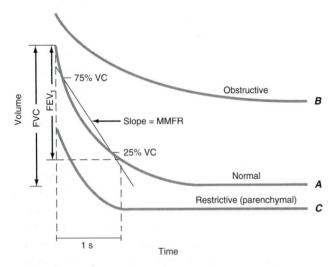

Figure 2–19. (*Reproduced with permission from Braunwald et al: Harrison's Principles of Internal Medicine, 15th ed., McGraw-Hill, 2001.*)

212. **(B)** Bile acid export occurs via transporters localized to the apical plasma membrane. Bile acid conjugation (choice A), like the related events of drug detoxification, takes place in the smooth endoplasmic reticulum. Bile acid synthesis (choice C) occurs in the cytoplasm. Protein synthesis (choice E) occurs throughout the hepatocyte and secretion of proteins into the bloodstream is largely across the basolateral plasma membrane that is contiguous with the hepatic sinusoids. The enzymes that carry out carbohydrate metabo-

lism (choice D) are also distributed throughout the hepatocyte cytosol (Figure 2–20).

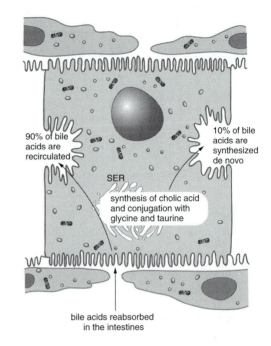

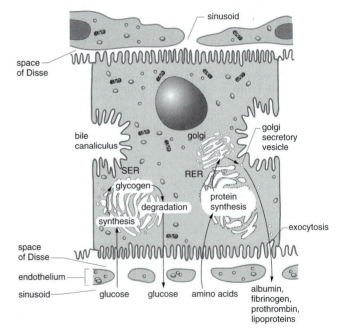

Figure 2–20. (*Modified with permission from Junquiera, LC et al.: Basic Histology, 9/e. McGraw-Hill, 1998.*)

213. **(C)** Chocolate, along with ethanol and fat, are common foods that diminish LES tone and thereby predispose to "heartburn" and its progression, due in part to acid-mediated injury and scarring, to a chronically incompetent LES and reflux esophagitis. All the other

agents and processes indicated (choices B, C, D, and E) have the opposite effect of *increasing* LES tone.

214. **(D)** Angiotensin II is the direct active product of the renin–angiotensin system and is produced under conditions of intravascular volume depletion and hypotension. Angiotensin II secretion leads to antidiuretic hormone (ADH) secretion and increased thirst to increase water absorption and intake, respectively. Production of angiotensin II is stimulated by rennin, angiotensin II does not enhance renin secretion (choice B). In addition to being a direct vasoconstrictor, angiotensin II acts to stimulate, not inhibit, aldosterone secretion (choice C) for sodium conservation.

215. **(C)** The primary control over prolactin secretion is inhibition by hypothalamic dopamine; all other anterior pituitary hormones are primarily controlled by hypothalamic hormone stimulation. Hence, with stalk transection, loss of connection of the hypothalamus to the pituitary is associated with decreased secretion of all pituitary hormones except prolactin, whose secretion increases in the absence of dopamine. Thus, secretion of GH (choice B), POMC (choice D) and TSH (choice E) all decrease. GnRH (choice A) is a hypothalamic hormone, and is not made in the pituitary gland.

216. **(B)** Thyroid hormone is crucial for proper adjustment of metabolic rate, with slowing of various functions including GI tract motility. In hypothyroidism patients typically manifest cold intolerance, weight gain, constipation, bradycardia. Heart palpitations (choice C), heat intolerance (choice D), and weight loss (choice E) are typical for hyperthyroidism. Some findings, such as menstrual irregularity, altered mental status, and weakness can be observed with *either* hypo- or hyperthyroidism. Abdominal pain (choice A) is a classical finding of adrenal insufficiency, not thyroid disease.

217. **(D)** Leptin is a hormone secreted by adipocytes that signals satiety at the hypothalamus. The Ob-Ob mouse that allowed leptin to be discovered is obese due to *lack* of leptin. Thus, its fat cells never signal the hypothalamus to *stop* eating. However, most obese humans have high rather than low leptin levels, reflecting leptin resistance. That is, the fat cells are trying to tell the hypothalamus to stop, but no one is listening. This illustrates the more general point that a clinical phenotype can result from many different molecular mechanisms of physiologic dysfunction. Cushing syndrome (choice A) is due to glucocorticoid excess secondary to ACTH excess, not resistance. These patients do have insulin resistance, primarily because glucocorticoids oppose insulin action. Addison disease (choice B) is due to a lack of glucocorticoids, not glucocorticoid resistance. Hypoparathyroidism (choice C) occurs when excessive parathyroid tissue is removed during surgery for a parathyroid adenoma. Graves disease (choice E) is hyperthyroidism due to the presence of an auto-antibody that mimics thyroid stimulating hormone (TSH) resulting in overproduction of thyroid hormone. None of the incorrect conditions are themselves due to hormone-resistant states.

218. **(C)** Because the liver is supplied by umbilical venous blood from the placenta, and the heart and head receive blood before it has mixed with significant amounts of desaturated blood, these important organs receive blood that is relatively high in saturated oxyhemoglobin. The high rate of blood flow at the placenta and the significant resistance of the placenta to diffusion of O_2 result in blood in the umbilical vein that has a lower P_{O_2} (30 mm Hg) than maternal mixed venous blood (choice A). However, the left shift in fetal oxyhemoglobin concentration (choice E) and the Bohr effect both act to increase the transport of O_2 to fetal tissues. A number of significant differences in circulating patterns are present in the fetus. The foramen ovale (choice B) remains open until after birth and a significant portion of inferior vena cava flow is shunted through it to the left. The major portion of right ventricular output is shunted through the ductus arteriosus to the aorta, not the lungs (choice D). The net effect of these shunts

in the presence of high fetal pulmonary vascular resistance is very low fetal pulmonary blood flow. At birth, these patterns normally are quickly changed to ex utero patterns with high pulmonary perfusion.

219. **(E)** The brain autoregulates, and consequently an increase in blood pressure is offset by an increase in local vascular resistance to maintain constant cerebral blood flow. Cerebral blood flow will increase when Pao_2 is decreased to < 50 mm Hg or when $Paco_2$ increases above normal. A decrease in arterial oxygen (choice D) or an increase in arterial CO_2 (choice A) would therefore cause vasodilation and decreased resistance to cerebral blood flow. A decrease in viscosity (choice C) would also increase blood flow. Cerebral blood flow is closely linked to brain parenchymal metabolism, and intense activity during a seizure (choice B) results in large, widespread increases in blood flow.

220. **(D)** P_{alv} is ambient atmospheric pressure, or zero reference pressure, and P_{pl} is a negative intrapleural pressure that becomes even more negative during inspiration. The lungs expand to a higher volume during inhalation as a result of an increase in the transpulmonary or distending pressure $(P_{alv} - P_{pl})$. Static compliance is measured under conditions of no airflow (stepwise changes in volume with no airflow during measurement of distending pressure). With each increase in distending pressure there is a corresponding increase in lung volume. Compliance is $\Delta V / \Delta P$. Distending pressure divided by change in lung volume (choice A) gives the lung elasticity. The lung volume divided by recoil pressure $(P_{alv} - P_{pl})$ (choice E) equals compliance only during the first linear part of the lung distention/pressure relationship. Generally speaking, V/P does not equal $\Delta V / \Delta P$. Change in elastic recoil pressure (choice C) is only part of the compliance calculation.

221. **(E)** Hyperthyroidism is associated with tremor, tachycardia, low serum cholesterol, and hyperreflexia. All of the other options are classical findings in hypothyroidism. Thick, rough skin (choice D) reflects glycosaminoglycan deposition; delayed reflexes (choice B) are due to impaired nerve conduction; and high serum cholesterol (choice C) is due to impaired lipid metabolism.

222. **(A)** Long-term stimulation of most endocrine gland target tissues results in hypertrophy and hyperplasia (Figure 2–21). ACTH stimulation of the adrenal cortex increases, not decreases, blood flow (choice B); increases, not decreases, conversion of cholesterol to pregnenolone (choice C); and increases, not decreases, glucocorticoid production (choice D). Glucocorticoids are counter-regulatory hormones to insulin. Thus the increased glucocortocoid secretion, in response to ACTH, increases insulin resistance rather than insulin sensitivity (choice E).

223. **(C)** Breathing a low-oxygen gas mixture is similar to being at high altitude, but if this is done for only a few minutes, there will be no time for renal compensation. The hypoxia stimulates hyperventilation, which lowers the Pco_2. The slightly lowered bicarbonate is due to buffering by nonbicarbonate buffers. Decreased Pco_2 results in decreased H_2CO_3. Decreased H_2CO_3 results in the following reaction being pulled to the right:

$$HCO_3^- + H^+ \rightarrow H_2CO_3 \rightarrow H_2O + CO_2$$

thus lowering the plasma bicarbonate HCO_3^- to slightly below normal. Had there been time for renal compensation, the bicarbonate would have been much lower. Severe chronic lung disease (choice A) or an overdose of heroin (choice E) would have caused respiratory acidosis due to abnormally high arterial Pco_2 (not low Pco_2, which this subject has). A lowlander at high altitude for 2 weeks (choice B) would have had both low Po_2 and low Pco_2 like this subject, but would have had an abnormally low plasma bicarbonate and a more nearly normal pH, due to renal compensation in the form of bicarbonate excretion. Acute aspirin overdose (choice D) in adults usually presents first with a respira-

A. Normal

B. After ACTH stimulation

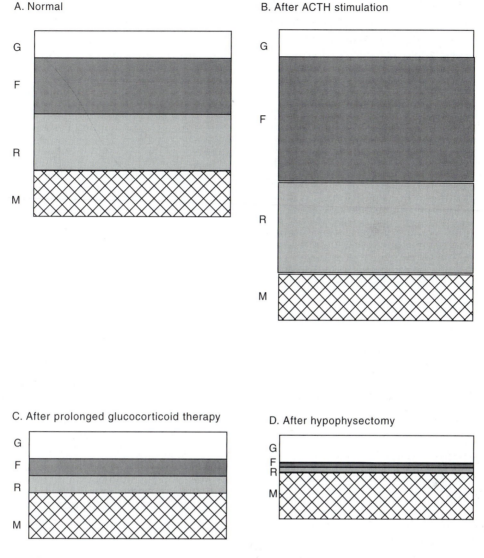

C. After prolonged glucocorticoid therapy

D. After hypophysectomy

Figure 2–21. (*Reproduced with permission from Lingappa and Farey:* Physiological Medicine, *McGraw-Hill, 2000.*)

tory alkalosis, which includes a low PCO$_2$, but not a low PO$_2$.

224. **(C)** Chlorpromazine is an antipsychotic drug and has significant anticholinergic action (i.e., it inhibits the effects of parasympathetic stimulation). Functions of the parasympathetic nervous system include increasing GI motility, decreasing GI sphincter tone, and emptying of the rectum and urinary bladder. Therefore, patients on chlorpromazine often complain about constipation and urinary retention. Parasympathetic fibers slow the heart rate and anticholinergic drugs cause tachycardia rather than bradycardia (choice

A). Increased motility (choice E), decreased sphincter tone (choice B), and bladder emptying (choice D) are not expected.

225. **(C)** Muscle tone is determined by the basal firing rate of the α-motor neurons and damage to these so-called lower motoneurons result in flaccid paralysis. In contrast, damage to the corticospinal tract (i.e., upper motoneuron lesions) (choice E) results in spastic paralysis because of hyperactive stretch reflexes. Activation of γ-efferent fibers (choice A) to muscle spindles also increases muscle tone due to reflex activation of the α-motor neurons (stretch reflex). Pathologically in-

creased γ-efferent discharge results in muscle clonus. Parkinson's disease (choice D) is characterized by muscle rigidity and tremors. Anxiety (choice B) is also associated with increased muscle tension.

226. **(D)** High dietary intake of calcium promotes calcium absorption, suppresses PTH release and bone dissolution, and is thus protective against osteoporosis. Choices A, B, C, and E are not risk factors for bone loss and in fact would protect bone from osteoporosis. Excessive alcohol intake, sedentary lifestyle, early menopause (due to decreased estrogen), and thin body habitus all promote bone loss.

227. **(D)** Shunted blood is blood that bypasses ventilated parts of the lung and directly enters the arterial circulation. In normal persons, this is largely due to mixing of arterial blood with bronchial venous and some myocardial venous blood, which drains into the left heart. Diffusion limitation (choice B), although finite, is usually immeasurably small, as is reaction velocity with hemoglobin (choice A). Unloading of CO_2 (choice C) may affect alveolar oxygen partial pressure, but would have no effect on the difference between alveolar and arterial P_{O_2}. A large ventricular septal defect (choice E) would result in a significantly lower arterial O_2 compared to alveolar O_2.

228. **(C)** The gene that is abnormal in cystic fibrosis encodes a cAMP-regulated Cl^- channel (CFTR). Because Cl^- flux via this channel plays different roles in different epithelia, it is not surprising that the symptoms of cystic fibrosis are quite diverse. The volume-absorbing airway epithelium in CF patients shows increased Na^+ reabsorption, probably because lack of CFTR increases the transepithelial potential difference. This results in a thick, dehydrated mucus and creates ionic conditions that inactivate antibacterial peptides of host innate immunity, thereby predisposing to airway infections. This is in contrast to sweat glands, where CF patients secrete nearly normal volumes of sweat into the acinus, but are unable to absorb NaCl from sweat as it moves through the sweat duct. Therefore, the Na^+ and Cl^- content of sweat are both elevated in CF patients (choice E). Lack of Cl^- and water secretion in GI epithelia can lead to severe constipation and small and large bowel obstruction. Impairment of the Cl^-/HCO_3^- exchange in pancreatic ductal epithelium results in water and enzyme retention, and may eventually destroy the pancreas. CF is more common in Caucasians than in African-Americans (choice B), and is one of the most common genetic disorders, occurring in 1 of 2000 Caucasian births. The abnormal gene is not located on the X chromosome (choice D), but on chromosome 7 (autosomal recessive). Sodium channels (choice A) are not defective in CF.

229. **(D)** With few exceptions, blood vessels are not innervated by parasympathetic nerves (choice E), and there is little effect of parasympathetic tone on total peripheral resistance. In contrast, sympathetic nerve activity contributes to the basal vascular smooth muscle tone, and cutting these nerve fibers results in immediate vasodilation of the affected extremity. Although hypersensitivity to circulating catecholamines (choice C) develops over time, this does not contribute to the vasodilation. Epinephrine and norepinephrine release from the adrenal medulla (choices A and B) is regulated by its direct sympathetic innervation (preganglionic cholinergic fibers from the splanchnic nerve), and not affected by sympathetic fibers to the extremities or circulating catecholamines.

230. **(C)** The initial segment of this EEG recording shows normal alpha brain wave activity. Alpha waves are indicative of a relaxed state, with eyes closed and the mind wandering freely. At the point marked by the arrow, the EEG becomes desynchronized (beta brain waves). Beta waves are seen when the patient performs specific mental tasks such as calculations or when he or she observes objects after opening the eyes. Closing one's eyes (choice A) would show the opposite pattern (EEG becomes synchronized). The EEG cannot discriminate thought content such as the

mind "wandering off" (choice D). Falling asleep (choice B) is associated with sleep spindles and increased synchronization of brain waves. Petit mal (absence seizures) (choice E) is characterized by a unique 3-per-second "spike and dome" pattern.

231. **(B)** Local inflammatory processes are often painful. This is due to sensitization of nociceptive nerve endings by PGE_2. Non-steroidal anti-inflammatory drugs (NSAIDs) inhibit prostaglandin synthesis and help to alleviate the pain. Thromboxane A_2 (choice E) and prostacyclin (PGI_2) are both derived from PGH_2, but have opposite effects on platelets and blood vessels. Thromboxane A_2, released from platelets, promotes vasoconstriction and platelet aggregation, and PGI_2, released from endothelial cells, is a potent vasodilator and inhibits platelet aggregation. Most prostaglandins have a large range of actions, and they may contract or relax smooth muscle cells depending on tissue source and species. In humans, $PGF_{2\alpha}$ (choice D) constricts bronchial smooth muscle and PGE_2 (choice A) relaxes it. An increase in prostaglandin production by fetal membranes is believed to be a major factor for onset of uterine contractions and labor in humans (choice C).

232. **(D)** In atrial fibrillation, the coordinated contraction of the atria to augment ventricular filling at the end of diastole is lost. Under normal conditions at rest, this accounts for a small fraction of cardiac output and is therefore not clinically significant. However, in a patient with a poor cardiac ejection fraction (e.g., due to disorders such as ischemic cardiomyopathy), loss of the "atrial kick" can substantially diminish cardiac output and be clinically significant (i.e., result in hypotension with dizziness or prerenal azotemia). Hyperthyroidism (choice A) is a common cause of atrial fibrillation as a result of increased sensitivity to catecholamines, but does not bear on the question asked. Hypotension (choice B) is the consequence of the loss of atrial contraction in some cases, not its cause. Left atrial clot formation (choice C) is a potentially devastating complication of atrial

fibrillation, and is why these patients are typically anticoagulated to prevent an embolic stroke. Patients with atrial fibrillation and a rapid heart rate are often treated with drugs to slow conduction through the AV node (e.g., digoxin) to improve ventricular filling, the opposite of the implication of the statement in choice E.

233. **(A)** Curve a shows the pattern expected for obstructive lung diseases such as asthma, chronic bronchitis or emphysema. Note the common physiologic findings of increased total lung capacity and greatly increased residual volume (due to air trapping). Curve c (choice C) shows the pattern expected for parenchymal restrictive lung disease (e.g., pulmonary fibrosis). Note the decreased total lung volume, decreased residual volume, and relatively preserved forced expiratory flow rates. Curve b (choice B) shows the pattern expected for extraparenchymal causes of restrictive lung disease such as obesity and neuromuscular disease whose hallmark is impaired inspiration with or without impaired expiration. The normal flow-volume curve is as indicated.

234. **(A)** Alert wakefulness and REM sleep are both characterized by beta waves, which indicate a high degree of brain activity. In the first stage of slow-wave sleep, which is associated with very light sleep (choice C), the EEG pattern shows very-low-voltage waves punctuated by occasional bursts of alpha activity, called sleep spindles. As sleep progresses, frequency of the EEG waveform decreases until it is approximately 2 to 3 cycles per second. This pattern, called delta waves, is characteristic of the deep sleep (choice B) of slow-wave stage 4. Quiet wakefulness is associated with alpha waves. If the patient woke up (choice D), her EEG would also show beta waves, but it is unlikely that she would still appear to be asleep. Central sleep apnea (choice E) is characterized by a sudden cessation of respiratory activity and drop in arterial oxygen saturation.

235. **(B)** Plasmin lyses fibrin and fibrinogen and is the active component of the fibrinolytic system. Plasminogen is a protein made in the liver. Cleavage of a single arginine–valine bond converts plasminogen to active plasmin. Streptokinase (choice C) has no direct effect on fibrin. Its action is due to formation of plasmin from its inactive precursor plasminogen. Neither plasmin (choice D) nor streptokinase (choice E) inhibit fibrinolysis. ε-Aminocaproic acid inhibits fibrinolysis by inhibiting the conversion of plasminogen to plasmin. Streptokinase does not act on tissue plasminogen activator TPA (choice A). Streptokinase, urokinase, and recombinant human TPA all activate plasminogen and are used clinically in early treatment of myocardial infarction.

236. **(C)** Compliance (stretchability) of the lung is the change in lung volume divided by the change in airway pressure ($\Delta V/\Delta P$) and is usually measured at the steepest portion of the pressure–volume curve. This patient's lungs have a compliance of 5 L/5 cm H_2O = 1 L/cm H_2O (Figure 2–22). Lung elasticity (choice B) equals 1 divided by compliance, and this patient's lungs have an elasticity of 1 cm H_2O/L.

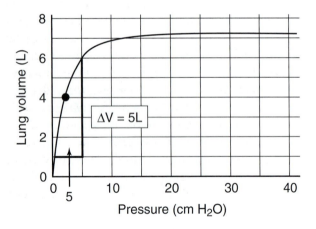

Figure 2–22

237. **(B)** Normal lung compliance is about 0.2 L/cm H_2O and this patient's lung compliance is significantly higher than normal. This occurs in emphysema resulting from chronic obstructive lung diseases or α_1-antitrypsin deficiency. Sarcoidosis (choice D) and tuberculosis (choice E) are chronic granulomatous lung diseases that have little effect on overall lung stretchability. Asbestosis (choice C) is a restrictive lung disease and would have a compliance less than normal (< 0.2 L/cm H_2O). Acute obstruction of the glottis (choice A) does not affect lung compliance, but would make this measurement difficult or impossible.

238. **(A)** Gout crystals directly activate complement and the kinin system, contrary to their suppression (choice D) and (choice E), respectively. Synovial macrophages phagocytose the crystals which triggers them to secrete pro-inflammatory products including cytokines IL-1, TNF, IL-8 and prostaglandin PGE_2 (contrary to choice C). These in turn trigger both endothelial activation, neutrophil chemoattraction and activation of neutrophil effector functions (Figure 2–23).

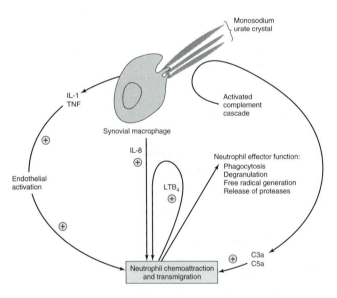

Figure 2–23. (*Reproduced with permission from McPhee et al: Pathophysiology of Disease: An Introduction to Clinical Medicine, McGraw-Hill, 2001.*)

239. **(E)** Although the early maturation of an ovarian follicle depends on the presence of FSH, ovulation is induced by a surge of LH. Although estrogens (choices A and B) usually have a negative feedback effect on LH and FSH secretion, the LH surge seems to be a response to elevated estrogen levels. In concert with FSH, LH induces rapid follicular swelling. LH also acts directly on the granulosa cells, causing them to decrease estrogen production, as well as initiating production of small amounts of progesterone. These changes lead to ovulation. FSH (choice C) causes follicle maturation, and is also required for Sertoli cells to mediate the development of spermatids into mature sperm cells. Inhibin (choice D) is a polypeptide secreted by the testes and ovaries that inhibits FSH secretion.

240.   **(C)** The brain depends on continuous blood flow and consciousness is lost after as little as 8 to 10 seconds of flow interruption. Dilation of cerebral blood vessels occurs during hypoxia, acidosis, and hypercapnia. Of these, hypercapnia (increased CO_2) is the main effector. Regional blood flow can increase by as much as 50% in response to the metabolic demands of cortical neurons and may be visualized by PET scan. However, these local increases in flow have little effect on overall cerebral blood flow (choice E). Barbiturates reduce neuronal oxygen demand (choice A). Blood flow through the brain is largely autoregulated, and increased systemic blood pressure has little effect on cerebral blood flow (choice D). Decreased arterial oxygen content also dilates cerebral vessels and increases cerebral flow; however, a decrease in arterial O_2 to 75 mm Hg (choice B) is less effective than an increase in arterial CO_2 to 45 mm Hg.

241.   **(B)** During strenuous physical exercise lactate is produced from anaerobic metabolism in skeletal muscle cells. This results in acidification of the blood (lactate acidosis). A right shift in oxygen binding occurs during acidosis, increased P_{CO_2}, increased 2,3-bisphosphoglycerate (2,3-BPG) concentration inside erythrocytes, and increased temperature. A right shift in oxygen binding also enhances release of oxygen from hemoglobin in peripheral tissues. A left shift in oxygen binding (choice A) occurs during alkalosis, decreased P_{CO_2}, decreased 2,3-BPG concentration inside erythrocytes, and decreased temperature. The oxygen-carrying capacity of the blood depends on hematocrit and erythrocyte hemoglobin concentration; however, oxygen saturation (choices C and D) ex-

pressed in percent is not affected by changes in oxygen-carrying capacity.

242.   **(D)** Intrinsic factor is a protein made in parietal cells of the stomach and secreted into the GI tract lumen. It binds vitamin B_{12} and is taken up via specific receptors in the terminal ilium. Gastrin (choice A) is a polypeptide secreted by endocrine cells in the stomach, but into the *bloodstream,* not the GI tract lumen. Histamine (choice B) is a paracrine product of amino acid metabolism released by enterocromaffin-like (ECL) cells into interstitial spaces of the GI tract. Hydrogen ions (choice C), in addition to the protein intrinsic factor, are also released into the GI tract lumen by parietal cells. Although intrinsic factor as a protein is released via the secretory pathway, hydrogen ions are pumped against a huge concentration gradient by H^+/K^+ ATPase, a transporter localized to the apical plasma membrane of the parietal cell. Transferrin (choice E) is secreted by the liver into the bloodstream for the purpose of iron uptake from the bloodstream into cells.

243.   **(A)** The renal tubular acidosis (RTA) refers to related conditions that are disorders of urine acidification even though other renal functions are not impaired. In type IV RTA, distal nephron dysfunction is due to either inadequate aldosterone production or aldosterone resistance resulting from intrinsic renal disease. Thus, patients develop hyperchloremic acidosis with hyperkalemia, due to impaired distal tubular secretion of both potassium and hydrogen ions. Treatment of patients is directed at controlling serum potassium. Choices B, C, D, and E are inconsistent with the known actions of aldosterone.

244.   **(A)** Acute dehydration results in decreased plasma volume and increased plasma osmolarity (choice B), because more water than salt is lost in sweat. The decrease in plasma volume leads to an inhibition of the baroreceptors and a lower firing rate. The increase in plasma osmolarity leads to increased ADH secretion (choice D) and high plasma ADH

levels, which increases water permeability of collecting duct cells (choice E). Therefore, more water is reabsorbed by the kidneys and renal water excretion is low (choice C).

245. **(A)** The hallmark of poorly controlled diabetes mellitus is elevated blood glucose. When glucose is chronically elevated, nonenzymatic glycosylation of various proteins occurs. Of these, modification of hemoglobin A to form hemoglobin A_{1c} is most commonly measured. Such so-called Amadori reaction products go on to form complex crosslinks called advanced glycosylation end products, the accumulation of which may be a cause of some of the devastating chronic complications of diabetes mellitus. Albumin (choice C) is the most abundant plasma protein, but is not significantly affected by glycosylation. Sorbitol (choice E) is another sugar derivative, unrelated to hemoglobin A_{1c} that is believed important in causing other diabetic complications such as cataracts and peripheral neuropathy. Myoinositol (choice D) is a signaling molecule whose decrease in response to elevated sorbitol has been suggested as a complication of diabetes. Lipoprotein (a) (choice B) is a lipoprotein particle implicated in atherosclerosis and thrombosis.

246. **(B)** Respiratory alkalosis is due to hyperventilation, which lowers CO_2. Decreasing tidal volume will reduce alveolar ventilation and correct the respiratory alkalosis. Assuming a dead space of 150 mL, alveolar ventilation in this patient is 450 mL · 12/min = 5400 mL/min. If the tidal volume were decreased from 600 to 300 mL and the frequency increased from 12 to 24 per minute, then the alveolar ventilation would decrease to 150 · 12/min = 1800 mL/min even though the minute ventilation (12 · 600 mL/min = 24 · 300 mL/min) remains unchanged. The fraction of O_2 (choice D) in the respiratory air does not affect respiratory volumes or frequencies in a mechanically ventilated patient. Increasing minute ventilation (choice C) or decreasing dead space (choice A) would increase alveolar ventilation and worsen respiratory alkalosis. PEEP (choice E) is positive pressure applied during the expira-

tory phase to prevent the collapse of alveoli and to increase functional residual capacity of the lungs. It is used primarily to improve arterial oxygenation in severely hypoxic patients.

247. **(E)** This patient has increased extra- and intracellular volumes and a decreased osmolarity. SIADH results in inappropriately low water permeability of the renal collecting duct tubular cells and inappropriate water retention. As a result, patients with SIADH often present with hypotonic overhydration. Adrenal insufficiency (lack of aldosterone) (choice A) and chronic vomiting (choice B) lead to dehydration. Fluid overload with isotonic NaCl (choice C) results in volume expansion without change in osmolarity. Fluid overload with hypertonic solution (choice D) results in volume expansion with increased osmolarity.

248. **(A)** Myoglobins and hemoglobins are oxygen-carrying proteins that differ in their O_2 affinity. These differences reflect their functional adaptation. HbA, which accounts for 95% of normal adult hemoglobin, consists of two alpha chains and two beta chains, each carrying one molecule of heme. Initial binding of oxygen to hemoglobin facilitates further binding of additional oxygen, resulting in a characteristic sigmoidal binding curve (curve C). Fetal hemoglobin HbF consists of two alpha chains and two gamma chains and differs from HbA in two important respects: (1) it does not bind organic phosphates including 2,3-bisphosphoglycerate (2,3-BPG) as effectively as HbA, and (2) its oxygen-binding curve is shifted to the left (curve B). Therefore, the oxygen content of umbilical vein blood is higher than that of placental vein blood, even though the Po_2 of umbilical blood is slightly lower than that of the placental veins. Myoglobin resembles hemoglobins but binds only one molecule of O_2 rather than four molecules. Its oxygen-binding curve therefore is not sigmoidal but has a higher affinity compared to hemoglobins, resulting in a transfer of oxygen from arterial blood to skeletal muscle fibers. Percent saturation should always top at 100% because it is a normalized measure and not at 50%

(curve D). Physically dissolved O_2 in plasma shows a linear relationship (curve E).

249. **(C)** The photoreceptor cell membrane is relatively depolarized in darkness due to Na^+ entry through nonselective cation channels. Openings of these channels are maintained by the high intracellular cGMP levels in photoreceptors during darkness, and the Na^+ inward current through these channels is usually called "dark current." Illumination causes a conformational change in the photosensitive pigment rhodopsin, which is linked via a G protein to a cGMP specific phosphodiesterase. Activation of phosphodiesterase lowers cGMP levels and, because cGMP is required to maintain openings of the nonselective cation channels, results in membrane hyperpolarization with light exposure. Chloride channels (choice A) or nonselective anion channels (choice B) do not contribute to the dark current of photoreceptors. Ryanodine receptors (choice E) are located on the sarcoplasmic reticulum (SR) and when opened release stored Ca^{2+} from the SR. These channels are locked into the open state by the plant alkaloid ryanodine (hence the name). Like in most other cells, the Na^+/K^+ pump (choice D) is responsible for the high intracellular K^+ concentration in photoreceptor cells.

250. **(C)** Creatinine clearance is independent of plasma creatinine concentration; otherwise, creatinine would not be a useful measure of glomerular filtration rate. Clearance is defined as the amount of plasma that delivered the excreted substance, and for a substance that is neither actively secreted nor reabsorbed by the kidneys, its clearance equals the amount of plasma filtered through the glomerular membrane. All creatinine contained in that amount of plasma is excreted by the kidney, no matter what the concentration of creatinine in that plasma volume was. Because in the normal person a small amount of creatinine is secreted by the tubuli, clearance at low plasma concentrations is slightly higher than at elevated plasma concentration (slight initial upward bend of curve). Curve A describes the relationship between creatinine plasma concentration and renal excretion of creatinine. Note that excretion and clearance are not synonymous (also compare with question 273). Curves B and D describe the clearance of a substance that is secreted and filtered, or secreted and reabsorbed, respectively. At large plasma concentration the active transporters become saturated and the clearance of these substances approaches the creatinine clearance. Curve E depicts an improbable event with relatively increased clearance at both low and high concentrations of a substance, although there is an independent linear clearance at intermediate substance concentrations.

251. **(C)** Despite tremendous progress in understanding the role of cytokines in normal and pathologic processes, the therapeutic and research potential of these substances has just begun to be explored. Interferons, by definition, elicit a nonspecific antiviral activity by inducing specific RNA synthesis and protein expression in neighboring cells. Common interferon inducers are viruses, double-stranded RNA, and microorganisms. INF-γ (choice C) is produced mainly by CD4- and CD8-positive T cells, and to a lesser extent by B cells and natural killer cells. INF-γ has antiviral and antiparasitic activity and is synergistic with INF-α and INF-β, but its main biological activity appears to be immunomodulatory. Among its many functions are activation of macrophages and enhanced expression of MHC-II proteins (DP, DQ, and DR) on macrophages. The other two common human interferons are INF-α (choice A) and INF-β (choice B), derived from leukocytes and fibroblasts, respectively. INF-α is currently in clinical use against hairy cell leukemia, Kaposi's sarcoma, and venereal warts (condyloma acuminata). In addition to the common inducers, INF-β production by fibroblasts is also elicited by TNF and IL-1. In contrast to INF-α, INF-β is strictly species specific. INF-β appears to be useful for treatment of squamous sarcomas, viral encephalitis, and possibly multiple sclerosis. Macrophages produce IL-1 (choice D) and TNF (choice E). The effects of IL-1 and TNF are widespread and include activation of T cells, B cells, fever induction, and many others.

252. **(B)** Trained athletes have a larger heart volume (muscular hypertrophy) compared to untrained persons. This results in a significantly higher stroke volume at rest and an increased cardiac reserve (maximal cardiac output during exercise). Under resting conditions, however, the cardiac output of trained and untrained persons is nearly the same (choice A), and this is due to a correspondingly lower resting heart frequency (choice C). It is not uncommon to find resting heart frequencies of 40 to 50 beats/min in trained athletes. Oxygen consumption (choice D) and respiratory frequency (choice E) at rest are little affected by athletic training.

253. **(B)** This patient suffers from an acute glaucoma attack. The aqueous humor leaves the eye in the anterior chamber, passes through a meshwork of trabeculae, and enters the canal of Schlemm which empties into extraocular veins. Pupil dilation tends to open the canal of Schlemm and to enhance outflow because of the proximity of the pupillary dilator muscle insertion at the sclera to the canal and trabeculae. Normal ocular pressure is around 15 mm Hg, and remains constant in a normal eye throughout the day, usually within about ± 2 mm Hg (choice E). The production rate of aqueous humor is approximately 2 to 3 μL/min, and intraocular pressure is mainly determined by the balance of rate of production and outflow (choice D). Closure of the ocular angle (canal of Schlemm) leads to an acute glaucoma attack. Because of the high risk of permanent damage to the retina and optic nerve, this medical emergency should be treated with drugs that dilate the pupils. Drugs of choice are antimuscarinics (pilocarpine) or β-blockers (timolol). In addition, carbonic anhydrase inhibitors reduce the rate of production of aqueous humor during acute attacks, but are not useful for long-term treatment. Corticosteroids (choice A) play no role in the emergency management of acute glaucoma. Glaucoma is not a rare cause of blindness in the United States (choice C), but rather one of the most common causes of acquired blindness.

254. **(A)** CCK is produced by the duodenum and reaches the pancreas via the bloodstream. It causes secretion of large quantities of digestive enzymes by the pancreatic acinar cells.

GIP (choice B) is produced in the duodenum in response to sugars and fat. This peptide inhibits gastric secretion and motility, but its main effect appears to be stimulation of insulin production in pancreatic beta cells. Gastrin (choice C) is produced by G cells in the stomach antrum following vasovagal reflexes, stomach distention, or chemical stimuli, in particular amino acid and protein-rich food. Together with histamine and acetylcholine, gastrin stimulates acid secretion from parietal cells. Secretin (choice D) is produced by duodenal mucosa glands when highly acidic food enters the small intestine. This hormone stimulates secretion of a bicarbonate-rich solution from pancreatic ductal epithelium, but does not stimulate pancreatic enzyme secretion. VIP (choice E) stimulates water and electrolyte secretion by intestinal mucosa.

255. **(B)** Parietal cells secrete an essentially isotonic solution of pure HCl containing 150 mM Cl^- and 150 mM H^+ (pH < 1). Intracellular $[H^+]$ of parietal cells is 10^{-4} mM/L (pH ≈ 7.0) and active transport is necessary to transport H^+ against this gradient. This is achieved by a H^+/K^+-ATPase in the apical membrane that exchanges H^+ for K^+. Chloride ion (choice A) is extruded passively down its electrical gradient through Cl^- selective ion channels rather than transported actively. Na^+/K^+-ATPase (choice D) constitutes the major active transport process at the basolateral, but not the apical, membrane of parietal cells. The Cl^-/HCO_3^- exchange (choice C) also takes place at the basolateral membrane of the parietal cell. HCO_3^- comes from H_2CO_3 (the product of carbonic anhydrase enzyme), and is extruded from the cell in exchange for Cl^- to maintain electroneutrality. Passive diffusion (choice E) occurs always down an electrochemical gradient, never against a gradient.

256. **(B)** Most patients with primary aldosteronism (Conn syndrome) have an adrenal adenoma. The increased plasma aldosterone concentration leads to increased renal Na^+ reabsorption, which results in plasma volume expansion. The increase in plasma volume suppresses renin release from the juxtaglomerular apparatus and these patients usually have low plasma renin levels. Salt restriction (choice D) and upright posture (choice E) decrease renal perfusion pressure and therefore increase renin release from the juxtaglomerular apparatus. Secondary aldosteronism is due to elevated renin levels and may be caused by heart failure (choice A) or renal artery stenosis (choice C).

257. **(C)** What is recorded in all of the examples is the forced expiratory volume in 1 second (FEV_1). The patient is connected to a spirometer, and after taking in as much air as possible (maximal inhalation), is asked to expire as forcefully as he or she can to exhale as much air as possible as rapidly as possible. The volume exhaled in the first second (shaded area of examples) is the FEV_1. The difference between the beginning total lung capacity (TLC) and the residual volume (RV) is the vital capacity. The forced vital capacity (FVC), shown in all but example C, is not always the same as in a less forced measurement. Curve C represents a patient with an obstructive disease that makes it difficult to force large volumes of air out at a high rate of flow. Thus, the slope is less steep than normal, and it takes a long time to reach the residual volume (it may take 20 or 30 seconds; this is why example C does not include FVC). Asthma, emphysema, and chronic bronchitis are common obstructive diseases. Both the TLC and the RV are higher than normal in such patients. At the bedside the same kind of information can be obtained by asking the patient to blow out a lighted match. Patients with obstructive disease have difficulty doing so. Curve A represents a normal, healthy adult. The flow rate is high at first (steep downward slope) near the beginning of TLC, but then becomes less and less steep as the lung volume decreases, until it plateaus (becomes flat) at residual volume and zero flow. Curve B represents the FEV_1 of a patient with restrictive lung disease (lungs are restricted in volume). Pulmonary fibrosis is a chronic condition that can follow pulmonary inflammation (pneumonitis) brought about by a number of conditions. Other examples of restrictive disease include problems with chest wall movement (Pickwickian syndrome, scoliosis, myasthenia

gravis) and loss of lung compliance (e.g., lack of surfactant, pulmonary edema, fibrosis). Although flow rates are quite good at any given volume (comparable to that of a normal subject at that same lung volume), the TLC, VC, and RV are all below normal. Curve D (increased flow rates with normal or larger than normal lung volumes) is not realistic.

258. **(D)** Acetazolamide is an inhibitor of carbonic anhydrase, an enzyme found in large quantities in the brush border of the proximal tubule. This enzyme has two important functions: In the tubular lumen it promotes the dissociation of H_2CO_3 into H_2O and CO_2 and thereby helps to recover filtered bicarbonate. Inside the epithelial cells it promotes the formation of H_2CO_3. Inhibition of this enzyme therefore increases bicarbonate concentration in the urine, and results in a mild metabolic acidosis that counteracts the effect of respiratory alkalosis caused by hyperventilation in an oxygen-poor environment. Metabolic alkalosis (choice A) would worsen the symptoms of mountain sickness. Acetazolamide has no direct effect on respiratory drive (choices B and C). Hydrogen concentration in the urine (choice E) plays only a minor role in acid–base regulation by the kidneys. Most of the excess hydrogen is excreted in the form of nontitratable acid (NH_4^+)

259. **(E)** Plasma proteins consist of albumin, globulins, and fibrinogen. These can be separated by their rate of migration in an electrical field (electrophoresis). The fractions shown in Figure 2–15 are (fraction A) albumin, (fraction B) α_1-globulins, (fraction C) α_2-globulins, (fraction D) β-globulins, and (fraction E) γ-globulins. The smallest of these proteins (albumins) are also the most numerous and are responsible for much of the oncotic pressure of plasma (about 25 mm Hg). Iron bound to transferrin and β-lipoproteins are transported in the β-globulin fraction, whereas bilirubin, fatty acids, and many drugs are transported adsorbed to albumin. Antibodies (immunoglobulins) constitute the bulk of γ-globulins.

260. **(B)** Dilation of the afferent arteriole results in decreased resistance to blood flow, increased

glomerular capillary hydrostatic pressure, increased filtration fraction, and therefore increased GFR. The other effect of the macula densa sensing decreased distal tubular sodium is increased renin secretion, which will result in increased generation of angiotensin II, which will raise blood pressure. Choices A, C, D, and E are incorrect.

261. **(D)** Increased plasma osmolarity is the most potent stimulus for ADH release. An increase in plasma osmolarity of only 1% is sufficient to increase ADH levels. Decreased plasma volume (choice B) also stimulates ADH release but is a less potent stimulus. Plasma ADH levels are not affected until blood volume is reduced by about 10%. Nevertheless the decreased blood volume and arterial pressure in patients with severe hemorrhage results in ADH secretion, causing increased water reabsorption by the kidneys that helps to restore blood pressure and volume. Hypothalamic releasing factors (choice C) control release of anterior pituitary hormones TSH, ACTH, FSH, LH, GH, and prolactin, but not the release of posterior pituitary hormones ADH and oxytocin.

262. **(D)** Glucose excretion by the kidneys depends on the glomerular filtration and tubular reabsorption rates. Glucose first appears in the urine when the capacity of the glucose transporters in the proximal tubuli cells is exceeded. This usually occurs at plasma glucose levels higher than 180 mg/dL. Patients with long-standing diabetes mellitus often have decreased renal function and reduced GFR. Under these circumstances the threshold (i.e., plasma level) for excretion of glucose is higher than in a healthy person. Urine dipsticks nowadays are both sensitive and specific for glucose, detecting as little as 100 mg/dL (choice A). Earlier dipstick tests were sensitive but not specific (they detected other reducing sugars in addition to glucose). A defect in glucose transporters (choice B) results in glucosuria even at normal plasma glucose concentration. Patients with diabetes insipidus (choice C) have a large urine output due to absence of ADH or defective renal ADH receptors, but should not have a plasma glucose

level of 200 mg/dL. Antidiuresis (choice E) increases the concentration of solutes in the urine and increases the sensitivity to detect urine glucose. Reabsorption of filtered glucose occurs in the proximal tubule by active transport.

263. **(D)** Potassium-sparing diuretics act by either antagonizing the action of aldosterone (spironolactone) or by inhibiting Na^+ reabsorption in the distal tubules (amiloride). Mannitol (choice C) is freely filtered at the glomerulus, but in contrast to glucose is not reabsorbed and produces an osmotic diuresis. Clinically it is used to treat cerebral edema, and in prerenal azotemia to convert oliguric acute renal failure. Thiazides (choice E) inhibit Na^+ and K^+ reabsorption in the distal tubule, and loop diuretics (choice B) (e.g., furosemide, ethacrynic acid) inhibit the Na^+/K^+/$2Cl^-$ cotransporter in the thick ascending loop of Henle. Carbonic anhydrase inhibitors (choice A) reduce H^+ secretion and HCO_3^- reabsorption in the proximal tubules. Because these are coupled with Na^+ reabsorption through the Na^+/H^+ countertransport in the luminal membrane, a decrease in HCO_3^- reabsorption also reduces Na^+ reabsorption, causing these ions to remain in the tubular fluid and act as an osmotic diuretic.

264. **(C)** Glycogen synthesis and breakdown depend on the balance of glycogen synthase activity (glycogen synthesis) and glycogen phosphorylase activity (glycogen breakdown). These enzymes are under the control of cAMP-dependent protein kinases. Phosphorylation of glycogen phosphorylase activates this enzyme and promotes glycogen degradation. This phosphorylation is carried out by an enzyme called glycogen synthase/phosphorylase kinase, which itself is activated by a cAMP-dependent protein kinase. Therefore, hormones that increase liver cell cAMP promote glycogen breakdown, and hormones that decrease liver cell cAMP promote glycogen synthesis. Epinephrine and glucagon stimulate the mobilization of glycogen by triggering the cAMP cascade. Cortisol, the main glucocorticoid, regulates the metabolism of proteins, fats, and carbo-

hydrates. On most organs cortisol acts catabolic, however on the liver it has anabolic effects, increasing glycogen synthesis and accumulation in the liver.

265. **(E)** Tolerance is commonly observed with many pharmacologic agents, including opioids. Difficulty sleeping (choice A), hypermotility of the GI tract (choice B), and respiratory alkalosis (choice D) are opposite to the expected effect of opiates. The placebo effect (choice C) is, at least in part, likely due to the release of endogenous opioid peptides in anticipation of pain relief, and is not a complication of therapy.

266. **(C)** During resting conditions, approximately 15% of the cardiac output goes to the brain, 15% to the muscles, 30% to the GI tract, and 20% to the kidneys. However, when normalized by organ weight, the kidneys receive the largest specific blood flow (400 mL/min · 100 g) at rest and are particularly vulnerable during hemorrhagic shock. The brain (choice A) also receives relatively high specific blood flow (50 mL/min · 100 g). Heart muscle (choice B) not surprisingly also has a relatively high resting specific blood flow (60 mL/min · 100 g), which may increase fivefold during exercise. Skeletal muscles (choice D) have low specific blood flow (2 to 3 mL/min · 100 g) at rest, which may increase up to 20-fold during strenuous exercise. Blood flow through the skin (choice E) varies between 1 and 100 ml/min · 100 g and serves temperature regulation.

267. **(C)** Lack of a typical basement membrane is key to the ability of blood to percolate through the liver at low pressure. Bulk phase endocytosis (choice A) is a general mechanism of transport of solute across endothelial cells and is not specific to the liver, or relevant to maintenance of the low pressure circuit. Fenestrations (choice B) are an important specialization that allow direct contact between plasma and hepatocytes, but they are between the endothelial cells that make up the sinusoid, and are not between reticuloendothelial cells and hepatocytes. Asialoglycoprotein receptors (choice D) are impor-

tant for the liver's clearance function, but have nothing to do with maintenance of low portal pressure. Tight junctions (choice E) represent exactly the opposite extreme from that of the fenestrated hepatic endothelium. In the presence of tight junctions, access of plasma to tissues is restricted

268. **(D)** Large injury to the nondominant parietal cortex may cause the patient to ignore the serious nature of his illness, and to neglect or even deny the presence of the paralysis affecting the side of the body opposite to the lesion. Occasionally this neglect may involve not only the patient's body but also the perception of the external world. Injury to the dominant hemisphere involving the posterior inferior gyrus of the frontal lobe (choice A) (Broca's area) produces an expressive or motor aphasia in which the patient's comprehension of language is preserved, but his ability to form words is impaired. Injury to the dominant hemisphere involving the posterior superior gyrus of the temporal lobe (choice B) (Wernicke's area) produces a sensory aphasia in which words are spoken fluently but without meaning. The patient does not understand his own word salad, either. Smaller injuries to the nondominant parietal cortex involving the precentral gyrus (primary motor cortex) (choice E) or postcentral gyrus (primary sensory cortex) (choice C) result in contralateral spastic paralysis or contralateral loss of tactile sensation, respectively.

269. **(D)** The proximal tubule reabsorbs the majority (about two-thirds) of filtered salt and water. This is done in an essentially iso-osmotic manner. Both the luminal salt concentration and the luminal osmolality remain constant (and equal to plasma values) along the entire length of the proximal tubule. Water and salt are reabsorbed proportionally because the water is dependent on and coupled with the active reabsorption of Na^+. The water permeability of the proximal tubule is high, and therefore a significant transepithelial osmotic gradient is not possible (a minute gradient of as little as 1 mosm/L may exist). Sodium is actively transported, mainly by basolateral sodium pumps,

into the lateral intercellular spaces; water follows. The collecting duct (choice A) reabsorbs only a small fraction of filtered Na^+. The glomerulus (choice B) is where solutes are filtered from the plasma. The juxtaglomerular apparatus (choice C) produces renin. The thick ascending limb of Henle's loop (choice E) actively transports Na^+ and Cl^- from lumen to the peritubular space using a $Na^+/K^+/Cl^-$ co-transporter. About 30% to 35% of filtered salt is reabsorbed here.

270. **(E)** Both the thin and the thick ascending limbs of Henle's loop have very low permeability to water. Because there are no regulatory mechanisms to alter its permeability, it remains poorly permeable to water under all circumstances. Sodium and chloride are transported out of the luminal fluid into the surrounding interstitial spaces where they are reabsorbed. Because water must remain behind (it is not reabsorbed), the solute concentration becomes less and less (the luminal fluid becomes more dilute). This is one of the principal mechanisms (along with diminution of ADH secretion) for the production of a dilute, hypo-osmotic urine (water diuresis). Water permeability of the collecting duct (choice A) is under control of ADH, allowing adjustment of the renal function according to the body's state of hydration. The glomerulus (choice B) is completely permeable to water, acting as a filter. The juxtaglomerular apparatus (choice C) produces renin. The proximal tubule (choice D) is characterized by high water permeability, preventing the establishment of an osmotic gradient across the proximal tubular epithelium, and reabsorption of any solute here is accompanied by reabsorption of water.

271. **(D)** Nitric oxide has recently been discovered to have important neurotransmitter-like functions. Its short half-life due to spontaneous decay limits its range and action. Nitric oxide acts on smooth muscle cells in a generally inhibitory manner; it relaxes the GI muscles and sphincters and dilates blood vessels. In blood vessels, nitric oxide is derived from endothelial cells and has been identified as the long-hypothesized endothelium-derived relaxing factor (EDRF). Acetylcholine (choice A) is the classic neurotransmitter of the parasympathetic nervous system. Although activation of the pelvic parasympathetic nerves leads to erection, it is nitric oxide and not acetylcholine that relaxes penile artery smooth muscle cells. GABA (choice C) is an inhibitory neurotransmitter found in the central nervous system. Epinephrine (choice B) and norepinephrine (choice E) play a role during the ejaculation phase of the male sexual act, but do not contribute to penile artery dilation during the erectile phase.

272. **(D)** Nitric oxide relaxes vascular smooth muscle by activating guanylate cyclase and increasing production of cGMP, which activates protein kinase G and possibly also protein kinase A. Sildenafil (Viagra) inhibits type V guanylate phosphodiesterase, increases cGMP levels and thereby supports the vasodilatory effect of nitric oxide. Increased cAMP levels (choice C) also relax vascular smooth muscle. Epinephrine binds to vascular β-receptors, which stimulate adenylate cyclase via a G protein, increasing cellular cAMP. A decrease in cAMP (choice A) or cGMP (choice B) promotes contraction of vascular smooth muscle, rather than dilation. Inositol-trisphosphate (IP_3) (choice E) is another important second messenger contributing to vascular smooth muscle contraction. For example, angiotensin II is a potent vasoconstrictor, whose action is mediated by AT_{1A} receptors coupled to phospholipase, leading to hydrolysis of PIP_2 to IP_3 and diacylglycerol (DAG).

273. **(B)** Measurement of GFR is a sensitive index of renal function. Clearance is defined as the amount of plasma that delivered the substance excreted. In the case of a substance like inulin or creatinine, which is filtered through the glomerular basement membrane, but neither reabsorbed nor secreted by renal tubular epithelial cells, this equals the amount of plasma filtered. Therefore the rate of excretion is a linear function of the substance's plasma concentration. Any deviation from linearity in the excretion versus plasma

concentration relation indicates active transport processes. Because creatinine is also slightly secreted by the tubular cells, the actual line should be slightly above line B. Substances like PAH and penicillins that are both filtered and actively secreted show a steep excretion rate at low plasma concentrations (choice A). When the active transporters are saturated, this relationship becomes parallel to the curve for inulin. Line C is impossible, simply because renal excretion has to be 0 at a plasma concentration of 0. Substances that are actively secreted by tubular cells, but are too big to be filtered through the glomerular basement membrane, show initially steep excretion rates (choice D). When the transporters become saturated no further increase in excretion rate is possible. Glucose is readily filtered through the glomerular basement membrane, but almost completely reabsorbed by tubular cells (choice E). Renal excretion of glucose typically occurs at venous plasma concentrations above 180 mg/dL.

274.   **(B)** The main difference between the ABO system of blood groups and the Rh system is the following: ABO antibodies are naturally occurring; a person missing an Rh antigen will not have antibodies against Rh in serum unless sensitized. Sensitization of Rh-negative persons can occur through massive blood transfusions or through a prior pregnancy with an Rh-positive child. Having a first Rh-negative child does not pose a risk of sensitization for the mother (choice A). However, the second Rh-positive child may still be at risk if the mother was sensitized by other means; for example, by previous transfusion with Rh-positive blood. Rh-positive mothers (choices C, D, and E) do not develop Rh antibodies and there is no risk of hemolytic transfusion reactions due to Rh incompatibility.

275.   **(A)** New generation pregnancy tests using an immunoconcentration method (ICON) can detect urine hCG as early as 4 to 5 days before the first missed period. hCG is a glycoprotein produced by the syncytiotrophoblast. It is composed of an α and a β subunit, and the α subunit is identical to the α subunits of

LH, FSH, and TSH. The role of hCG is to maintain the corpus luteum in the ovary and it has no direct effect on fetal production of steroids (choice B). hCG is usually positive in patients with ectopic pregnancy (choice C) or a choriocarcinoma (choice D). hCG has its highest levels at the end of the first trimester, not the end of pregnancy (choice E). Levels of estradiol, estriol, and progesterone, however, continue to rise until term.

276.   **(D)** The patient in question has Horner syndrome. Unilateral loss of sympathetic innervation of the face results in ptosis and pupil constriction, not dilation (choice E). Vasodilation of the skin vessels and loss of sweating results in dry, red skin, and not pale (choice C) or sweaty skin (choice A). Lateral deviation of the eye (choice B) suggests damage to cranial nerve III.

277.   **(B)** The resting membrane potential of excitable cells is largely due to the selective permeability of the cell membrane to potassium ions. The Na^+/K^+ pump (choice D) generates the ion gradient across the cell membrane (i.e., high intracellular K^+, high extracellular Na^+), but it is the back diffusion of K^+ ions through K^+ channels that are open at rest that charges the cell membrane. If the cell membrane were a perfect K^+ electrode, the membrane potential would equal the equilibrium potential for K^+ as predicted by the Nernst equation. In reality, the resting membrane potential is more positive because of small contributions by Na^+ channels (choice C), Cl^- channels (choice A), and nonselective cation channels (choice E).

278.   **(E)** Oxygen concentration in the portal vein is already diminished compared to that in freshly oxygenated arterial blood, hence the further diminution in oxygen concentration as blood flows from the portal vein to the central vein is significant and affects gene expression making hepatocytes in the two zones biochemically and physiologically "different." There is no difference in association to reticuloendothelial cells in different zones (choice A). Zone 1, not zone 3 (choice D), is more ac-

tive in urea synthesis because its hepatocytes see the highest concentration of ammonia, a substance that enters hepatocytes by diffusion. All hepatocytes see essentially the same concentration of hormones in the portal vein (choice C). There is no selective phenomenon of apoptosis (choice B) involving one zone over another.

279. **(C)** Normally, fluid balance is maintained by water intake that is equal to losses in urine, stool, sweat and insensible losses (through skin and lungs). The magnitude of insensible losses is often not realized and is a major contributor to dehydration in patients who are vomiting or simply too nauseated to maintain fluid intake.

280. **(B)** Osteomalacia in chronic renal failure is caused by decreased production of vitamin D and phosphate retention by the kidneys. The rise in serum phosphate causes increased binding of calcium, resulting in a decrease in ionized calcium concentration, which stimulates PTH secretion by the parathyroid glands (secondary hyperparathyroidism). PTH stimulates release of calcium from the bones, leading to demineralization. Osteoporosis (choice D) is a reduction in bone mass, particularly a decrease in cortical thickness. In contrast to osteomalacia, the ratio of mineral to organic phase is normal in osteoporosis. Bone loss occurs with age in both men and women at a rate of about 0.5% per year. Osteoporosis predominantly involves the spine, hip, and distal radius. In postmenopausal women, an accelerated loss of bone mass is superimposed on the age-related loss due to declining estrogen levels. In men, bone modeling is less dependent on sex steroids (choice C). Osteomalacia occurs with both primary (choice A) and secondary hyperparathyroidism. In patients with chronic renal failure, hyperparathyroidism is secondary to reduced ionized calcium concentration in the serum. Lack of active vitamin D also contributes to osteomalacia in this patient. In chronic renal failure the conversion of 25-hydroxycholecalciferol to the active 1,25-dihydroxycholecalciferol by the kidneys

is impaired. Lack of dietary vitamin D (choice E) is less likely in this patient.

281. **(C)** In the normal adult about 90% of the filtered phosphate is reabsorbed in the proximal tubule, and about 10% of filtered phosphate is excreted by the kidneys. Patients with chronic renal failure accumulate phosphate because of the low GFR. Binding of phosphate with calcium in the urine (choice A) does not result in increased serum phosphate. Depending on the activity of PTH, between 5% and 40% of filtered phosphate is excreted (choice B). Phosphate is not secreted by renal tubular epithelium cells (choice E), but is actively reabsorbed. Because the phosphate load to the proximal tubule is low in patients with a reduced GFR, the rate of reabsorption (in percent of filtered phosphate) is indeed higher than normal (choice D), but this is not the cause for the phosphate accumulation. It is the decreased GFR, and not the increased reabsorption rate, that is primarily responsible for phosphate accumulation in patients with chronic renal disease. Increased serum phosphate binds ionized calcium in the serum, leading to low serum calcium levels.

282. **(E)** Regulation of phosphate excretion is accomplished primarily by PTH, which inhibits phosphate reabsorption in the proximal tubule. At high PTH concentration, as much as 40% of filtered phosphate may be excreted. Reabsorption of phosphate by renal tubular cells occurs via a carrier cotransport of phosphate and sodium. This mechanism is similar to the reabsorption of glucose and amino acids and is driven by the Na^+ gradient built by the Na^+/K^+-ATPase at the basolateral membrane of the tubular epithelium. Cotransport with calcium (choice A) or chloride (choice B) does not occur. Reabsorption of phosphate occurs against its electrochemical gradient (choice C) and therefore cannot be passive. Calcitonin (choice D) has only minor effects on renal calcium and phosphate handling. It lowers serum calcium by suppressing bone osteoclasts, thus shifting the balance in favor of calcium deposition in the bone.

REFERENCES

Braunwald E, Fauci AS, Kasper DL, et al. *Harrison's Principles of Internal Medicine,* 15th ed. New York: McGraw-Hill; 2001.

Gerhart J, Kirschner M. *Cells, Embryos, and Evolution.* Malden, MA: Blackwell Science; 1997.

Guyton AC, Hall JE. *Textbook of Medical Physiology,* 10th ed. Philadelphia: Saunders; 2000.

Kandel ER, Schwartz JH, Jessel TM. *Principles of Neural Science,* 5th ed. Stamford, CT: Appleton & Lange; 2000.

Lingappa VR, Farey KF. *Physiological Medicine.* New York: McGraw-Hill; 2000.

McPhee SJ, Lingappa VR, Ganong WF, Lange JD, et al. *Pathophysiology of Disease: An Introduction to Clinical Medicine,* 4th ed. New York: McGraw-Hill; 2002.

Rose DB. *Clinical Physiology of Acid-Base and Electrolyte Disorders,* 6th ed. New York: McGraw-Hill; 2001.

Stites DP, Terr AI, Parslow TG, et al. *Medical Immunology,* 9th ed. Stamford, CT: Appleton & Lange; 1997.

Subspecialty List: Physiology

Question Number and Subspecialty

156. Pregnancy
157. Nervous system
158. Circulation
159. Urogenital system
160. Female reproductive physiology
161. Female reproductive physiology
162. Nervous system
163. Sensory system
164. Endocrinology
165. Sensory system
166. Liver physiology
167. Endocrine pancreas
168. Muscle
169. Endocrinology
170. Gastrointestinal
171. Cardiac
172. Cardiac
173. Metabolism
174. Metabolism
175. Cardiac
176. Cardiac
177. Cardiac
178. Liver physiology
179. Renal physiology
180. Endocrinology
181. Endocrinology
182. Endocrinology
183. Circulation
184. Respiratory physiology
185. Renal physiology
186. Respiratory
187. Respiratory
188. Metabolism
189. Cardiac
190. Cardiac
191. Cardiac
192. Acid/Base
193. Acid/Base
194. Fluid and electrolyte physiology
195. Fluid and electrolyte physiology
196. Sensory system
197. Cardiac
198. Thermoregulation
199. Respiratory
200. Respiratory
201. Renal
202. Sleep physiology
203. Respiratory
204. Adrenal physiology
205. Circulation
206. Male reproductive physiology
207. Nervous system
208. Endocrine pancreas
209. Cardiac
210. Endocrinology
211. Respiratory
212. Liver physiology
213. Gastrointestinal physiology
214. Endocrinology
215. Endocrinology
216. Thyroid physiology
217. Endocrinology
218. Circulation
219. Circulation
220. Respiratory
221. Thyroid physiology
222. Adrenal physiology
223. Respiratory
224. Nervous system
225. Muscle
226. Bone and mineral metabolism
227. Respiratory
228. Cell physiology
229. Circulation

230. Nervous system
231. Inflammation
232. Cardiac
233. Respiratory
234. Sleep physiology
235. Blood
236. Respiratory
237. Respiratory
238. Immunology
239. Endocrinology
240. Circulation
241. Exercise physiology
242. Endocrinology
243. Renal physiology
244. Circulation
245. Endocrine pancreas
246. Respiratory
247. Circulation
248. Cell physiology
249. Sensory system
250. Renal
251. Immunology
252. Exercise physiology
253. Sensory system
254. Gastrointestinal
255. Gastrointestinal

256. Renal
257. Respiratory
258. Acid/Base
259. Immunology
260. Renal physiology
261. Endocrinology
262. Renal
263. Renal
264. Gastrointestinal
265. Endocrinology
266. Circulation
267. Liver physiology
268. Nervous system
269. Renal physiology
270. Renal physiology
271. Cellular physiology
272. Cellular physiology
273. Renal
274. Blood
275. Endocrinology
276. Endocrine pancreas
277. Muscle
278. Liver physiology
279. Fluid and electrolyte physiology
280. Bone and mineral metabolism
281. Renal physiology
282. Renal physiology

CHAPTER 3

Biochemistry
Questions

Michael W. King, PhD

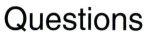
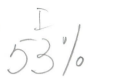

DIRECTIONS: (Questions 283 through 409): Each of the numbered items or incomplete statements in this section is followed by answers or by completions of the statement. Select the ONE lettered answer or completion that is BEST in each case.

283. A 22-year-old black man was given the anti-malaria drug primaquine to take while on an expedition to the Amazon River. After taking the drug, he developed an acute anemia. The anemia was secondary to an intravascular hemolytic crisis. This crisis was reversed when he discontinued taking the primaquine. This drug-induced hemolytic anemia arises in persons who have a deficiency in which of the following enzymes?

    (A) Glucose-6-phosphate dehydrogenase
    (B) Glyceraldehyde-3-phosphate dehydrogenase
    (C) Glycerol-3-phosphate dehydrogenase
    (D) Pyruvate dehydrogenase
    (E) Succinate dehydrogenase

284. There is but a single enzyme catalyzed reaction in the human body known to generate carbon monoxide (CO) as one of its products. The enzyme that catalyzes this CO producing reaction is

    (A) biliverdin reductase
    (B) coproporphyrinogen oxidase
    (C) heme oxygenase
    (D) protoporphyrinogen oxidase
    (E) uroporphyrinogen decarboxylase

285. The activity of the urea cycle enzyme, carbamoyl phosphate synthetase I (CPS-I), is absolutely dependent on which of the following allosteric effectors?

    (A) Argininosuccinate
    (B) Bicarbonate ion
    (C) Fumarate
    (D) N-acetylcysteine
    (E) N-acetylglutamate

286. A percentage of the population manifests the ABO blood group antigens in saliva and other mucous secretions and are thus referred to as "secretors," whereas those that do not are termed "nonsecretors." The difference between these two populations results from

    (A) ABO antigens on circulating lipids
    (B) ABO antigens present on circulating proteins
    (C) inappropriate activation of the ABO-specific glycosyltransferases in mucus-secreting tissues
    (D) mild hemolysis that releases cellular ABO antigens
    (E) the presence of a mutant glycosyl hydrolase that releases the ABO antigens from cell surfaces

287. The statin class of drugs that are currently used to control hypercholesterolemia function to lower circulating levels of cholesterol by

   (A) decreasing the absorption of dietary cholesterol from the intestines
   (B) increasing the elimination of bile acids leading to increased diversion of cholesterol into bile acid production
   (C) increasing the synthesis of apo-B100 resulting in increased elimination of cholesterol through the action of LDL uptake by the liver
   (D) inhibiting the interaction of LDLs with the hepatic LDL receptor
   (E) inhibiting the rate-limiting step in cholesterol biosynthesis

288. Which of the following represents the enzyme deficiency that leads to "essential fructosuria?"

   (A) Fructokinase
   (B) Fructose-1-phosphate aldolase (aldolase B)
   (C) Fructose-6-phosphate aldolase (aldolase A)
   (D) Hexokinase
   (E) Phosphofructokinase-1

289. There are many cancer chemotherapeutics, such as methotrexate, that target the synthesis of the pyrimidine nucleotide, thymidine monophosphate (dTMP). These drugs interfere with dTMP synthesis by

   (A) blocking the conversion of TMP to dTMP at the level of ribonucleotide reductase
   (B) blocking the conversion of thymidine to dTMP at the level of thymidine kinase
   (C) inhibiting the action of PRPP synthetase, the initial step in nucleotide synthesis
   (D) blocking the conversion of dUMP to dTMP at the level of dihydrofolate reductase
   (E) inhibiting the action of thymine phosphoribosyltransferase, which adds ribose-5-phosphate to thymine

290. There are numerous disorders that result from defects in hemoglobin. The class of hemoglobin disorders known as the thalassemias are caused by

   (A) a reduction in the level of synthesis of one or more of the globin proteins
   (B) increased synthesis of adult globin genes during fetal development
   (C) mutations in the globin genes resulting in structural variants of these proteins
   (D) synthesis of abnormal fetal globin genes during embryonic development
   (E) the presence of an abnormal fetal hemoglobin in the adult

291. The anticoagulant effect of aspirin (acetylsalicylate) occurs through its ability to inhibit which of the following activities?

   (A) Cyclooxygenase
   (B) Fibrin cross-linking by factor XIIIa
   (C) Phospholipase A_2
   (D) Thrombin binding to activated platelets
   (E) von Willebrand factor

292. An adult man suffered from stable angina pectoris for 15 years, during which time there was progressive heart failure and repeated pulmonary thromboembolism. Upon his death at age 63, autopsy disclosed enormous cardiomyopathy (1100 g), cardiac storage of globotriaosylceramide (11 mg lipid/g wet weight), and restricted cardiocytes. The lipid storage disease indicated by these results would most likely be

   (A) Fabry disease
   (B) Gaucher disease
   (C) Krabbe disease
   (D) Niemann–Pick disease
   (E) Tay–Sachs disease

293. The rate-limiting step in glycolysis occurs at the step catalyzed by

   (A) glyceraldehyde 3-phosphate dehydrogenase
   (B) phosphofructokinase-1 (PFK-1)
   (C) phosphofructokinase-2 (PFK-2)

(D) phosphoglycerate kinase

(E) pyruvate kinase

294. The primary positive control of gluconeogenesis is exerted by

(A) high acetyl-CoA levels

(B) high ATP levels

(C) high citrate levels

(D) low ATP levels

(E) low citrate levels

Questions 295 and 296

A 6-month-old who is failing to thrive is brought to your office. Tests reveal hepatosplenomegaly, muscle weakness and atrophy, hypotonia, and decreased deep tendon reflexes. Blood tests reveal that the infant has normal glucose levels. Biopsy of the liver reveals initial stages of cirrhosis due to the accumulation of an abnormal glycogen with few branch points whose structure resembles amylopectin.

295. The clinical and laboratory results presented are indicative of which glycogen storage disease?

(A) Andersen disease (type IV glycogen storage disease)

(B) Cori or Forbes disease (type III glycogen storage disease)

(C) McArdle disease (type V glycogen storage disease)

(D) Tarui disease (type VII glycogen storage disease)

(E) von Gierke disease (type I glycogen storage disease)

296. A deficiency in which of the following enzymes leads to this disorder?

(A) Amylo-1,6-glucosidase (glycogen debranching enzyme)

(B) Glucose-6-phosphatase

(C) Glycogen branching enzyme

(D) Liver phosphorylase

(E) Muscle phosphorylase (myophosphorylase)

Questions 297 and 298

A 9-month-old child is presented to the emergency room by his parents who report that he has been vomiting and has severe diarrhea. The episodes of vomiting began when the parents starting feeding their child cow's milk. The infant exhibits signs of failure to thrive. Laboratory tests show elevated blood galactose, hypergalactosuria, metabolic acidosis, albuminuria, and hyperaminoaciduria.

297. These clinical and laboratory findings are most consistent with

(A) alkaptonuria

(B) essential fructosuria

(C) hereditary galactosemia

(D) Menke disease

(E) von Gierke disease

298. The clinical symptoms result from a defect in which of the following enzymes?

(A) Galactose 1-phosphate uridyltransferase

(B) Ferrochelatase

(C) Fructokinase

(D) Glycogen phosphorylase

(E) Homogentisic acid oxidase

299. Under conditions of anaerobic glycolysis, the NAD^+ required by glyceraldehyde 3-phosphate dehydrogenase is supplied by a reaction catalyzed by

(A) glycerol-3-phosphate dehydrogenase

(B) α-ketoglutarate dehydrogenase

(C) lactate dehydrogenase

(D) malate dehydrogenase

(E) pyruvate dehydrogenase

300. Pyruvate dehydrogenase activity is regulated by its state of phosphorylation. The activity of the kinase which catalyzes the phosphorylation of pyruvate dehydrogenase is increased by

(A) acetyl-CoA

(B) AMP

(C) cAMP

(D) coenzyme A

(E) NAD^+

301. The eukaryotic translation initiation factor (designated Factor ? in Figure 3–1) required as a component of the eIF-2 cycle is

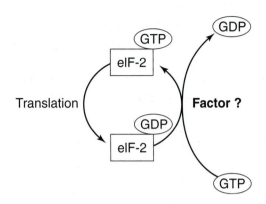

Figure 3–1

(A) eIF-1

(B) eIF-2B

(C) eIF-3

(D) eIF-4A

(E) eIF-4F

302. Attenuation is one mechanism by which the expression of genes is regulated in prokaryotic organisms. Attenuation is not possible in eukaryotes because

(A) eukaryotic mRNAs are not polycistronic as they are in prokaryotes

(B) eukaryotic mRNAs must be modified at the 5'-end by the cap structure prior to translation initiation

(C) introns, present in most eukaryotic genes, interfere with the process of attenuation

(D) there is always and excess of amino acid charged tRNAs in eukaryotes and thus is not limiting

(E) translation of eukaryotic mRNAs takes place in the cytosol, whereas transcription takes place in the nucleus

303. Excretion of the heme degradation product bilirubin into the bile depends on its conjugation to

(A) albumin

(B) cholesterol

(C) glucuronic acid

(D) glycine

(E) taurine

Questions 304 and 305

A 25-year-old man has experienced chronic blistering and scarring of his skin when exposed to sun light. This man is a smoker and drinks heavily, both of which exacerbate his responses to sun light. Analysis of his urine and plasma indicates a high accumulation of complex porphyrins, predominantly uroporphyrin.

304. The symptoms and clinical signs displayed by this patient indicate he is suffering from

(A) acute intermittent porphyria (AIP)

(B) hereditary coproporphyria (HCP)

(C) porphyria cutanea tarda (PCT)

(D) variegate porphyria (VP)

(E) X-linked sideroblastic anemia

305. This disorder results from a defect in which of the following enzymes?

(A) δ-Aminolevulinic acid dehydratase (ALAD)

(B) Coproporphyrinogen oxidase (CPO)

(C) Ferrochelatase

(D) Porphobilinogen deaminase (PBGD)

(E) Uroporphyrinogen decarboxylase (UROD)

306. Synthesis of glycogen is inhibited in hepatocytes in response to glucagon stimulation primarily as a result of a (an)

(A) decrease in the level of phosphoprotein phosphatase

(B) decrease in the level of phosphorylated phosphorylase kinase

(C) decrease in the levels of phosphorylated phosphoprotein phosphatase inhibitor-1

(D) increase in the level of the dephosphorylated form of glycogen synthase

(E) increase in the level of the phosphorylated form of glycogen synthase

307. Which of the following occurs in the lipidosis known as Tay–Sachs disease?

    (A) Ganglioside GM$_2$ is not catabolized by lysosomal enzymes.
    (B) Phosphoglycerides accumulate in the brain.
    (C) Synthesis of a specific ganglioside is decreased.
    (D) Synthesis of a specific ganglioside is excessive.
    (E) Xanthomas, due to cholesterol deposition, are observed.

308. In diabetes, the increased production of ketone bodies is primarily a result of

    (A) a substantially increased rate of fatty acid oxidation by hepatocytes
    (B) an increase in the rate of the citric acid cycle
    (C) decreased cyclic AMP levels in adipocytes
    (D) elevated acetyl-CoA levels in skeletal muscle
    (E) increased gluconeogenesis

309. Fragile X syndrome is characterized by

    (A) accumulation of copper leading to formation of Kayser–Fleischer rings in the eyes
    (B) hypoketotic hypoglycemia and metabolic acidosis
    (C) isovaleric acidemia, severe metabolic acidosis, and neonatal fatality
    (D) mental retardation of severity linked to the level of trinucleotide repeat expansion
    (E) very-long-chain fatty acid accumulation and myelin defects

310. A 4-year-old patient is presented in the pediatric clinic with microcytic anemia. An analysis of his blood by nondenaturing electrophoresis reveals the following composition of hemoglobin isoforms: HbF = 75%, HbA = 23%, HbA$_2$ = 2%, and HbS = 0%. Utilizing this data, it is possible to determine that the infant is most likely homozygous for a

    (A) complete deletion of the α-globin locus
    (B) complete deletion of the β-globin locus
    (C) mutation in the promoter of the β-globin genes
    (D) nonsense mutation in the α-globin genes
    (E) nonsense mutation in the β-globin genes

311. Hepatocytes deliver ketone bodies to the circulation primarily because they lack

    (A) β-hydroxybutyrate dehydrogenase
    (B) hydroxymethylglutaryl-CoA-lyase
    (C) hydroxymethylglutaryl-CoA-synthetase
    (D) succinyl-CoA-acetoacetate-CoA-transferase
    (E) the form of the β-ketothiolase necessary to hydrolyze acetoacetyl-CoA

Questions 312 and 313

A seemingly normal full-term infant exhibits increased lethargy and hypothermia, and begins vomiting during the evening of his second day in the hospital. The astute attending physician in the nursery suspects the infant may be suffering from hyperammonemia and orders tests to assay plasma ammonia. Indeed, the results confirm the physicians initial diagnosis. Additional blood and urine tests are ordered. The results indicate that the infant has no acidosis or ketosis and his citrulline levels are barely detectable. In contrast, urine orotic acid levels are greatly elevated.

312. These clinical findings indicate the infant is suffering from

    (A) carbamoyl phosphate synthetase I (CPS I) deficiency
    (B) methylmalonic acidemia
    (C) ornithine transcarbamoylase deficiency
    (D) propionic acidemia
    (E) Reye syndrome

313. The most effective treatment course for this infant involves administration of sodium phenylbutyrate in the diet. The biochemical reason for this treatment course is that the compound

    (A) induces intestinal bacteria to generate acidic byproducts that in turn promote ammonia excretion in the feces
    (B) interacts with glutamine diverting nitrogen to the product, phenylacetylglutamine
    (C) interacts with glycine diverting nitrogen to the excreted product, hippurate
    (D) is taken up by and kills intestinal ammonia-producing bacteria

314. One mechanism by which RNA tumor viruses can cause cancer is

    (A) by carrying into infected cells a protein that turns off the expression of tumor suppressor genes
    (B) by restricting the function of cellular DNA polymerase
    (C) that the action of reverse transcriptase induces overexpression of growth-promoting genes
    (D) to alter plasma membrane architecture upon infection
    (E) to integrate near a growth control gene and alter its expression

315. Patients who exhibit a prolonged mucocutaneous bleeding time with normal coagulation times, clot retraction, and platelet counts, but with reduced levels of plasma factor VIII, should be suspected to have a deficiency in

    (A) factor IX
    (B) fibrinogen (factor I)
    (C) prothrombin (factor II)
    (D) tissue factor (factor III)
    (E) von Willebrand factor

316. Figure 3–2 represents the electron-transport chain of oxidative phosphorylation. Which component of the chain is the site for the inhibitory action of cyanide?

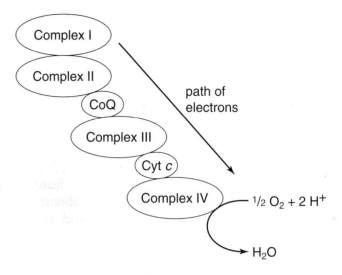

Figure 3–2

    (A) Coenzyme Q
    (B) Complex I
    (C) Complex II
    (D) Complex III
    (E) Complex IV

317. Which of the following is quantitatively the major contributor to routine clinical measurements of circulating plasma cholesterol concentrations?

    (A) Chylomicrons
    (B) High-density lipoproteins (HDLs)
    (C) Intermediate-density lipoproteins (IDLs)
    (D) Low-density lipoproteins (LDLs)
    (E) Very-low-density lipoproteins (VLDLs)

318. The activity of the urea cycle enzyme, carbamoylphosphate synthetase I depends on the allosteric activator N-acetylglutamate. N-acetylglutamate is synthesized through the action of N-acetylglutamate synthase, which is itself allosterically regulated by

    (A) arginine
    (B) carbamoyl phosphate
    (C) citrulline
    (D) fumarate
    (E) ornithine

319. Which of the following compounds serves as a source of waste nitrogen?

    (A) Arginine
    (B) Argininosuccinate
    (C) Asparate
    (D) Fumarate
    (E) Ornithine

320. An infant is characterized with the following clinical symptoms: course facial features, psychomotor retardation, skeletal abnormalities, impaired joint movement, and significantly elevated levels of lysosomal enzymes in the blood and other fluids. These symptoms result from impaired lysosomal targeting of lysosomal enzymes, which requires

    (A) attachment of mannose 6-phosphate to the enzymes
    (B) γ-carboxylation of glutamate residues in the enzymes
    (C) O-linkage of carbohydrate to the enzymes
    (D) prenylation of the enzymes
    (E) proteolytic activation following transport to the lysosome

321. Which of the following statements best characterizes ATP synthase?

    (A) It couples ATP export from the mitochondrial matrix to ATP synthesis.
    (B) It is a soluble protein found inside the mitochondrial matrix.
    (C) Its catalytic function is to synthesize ATP in a reaction driven by a chemiosmotic potential.
    (D) Oligomycin binds to ATP synthase, directly preventing ATP export.
    (E) The low H^+ ion concentration outside the inner mitochondria membrane establishes an electrochemical gradient that drives ATP synthesis.

322. Neonatal hyperammonemia associated with trace levels of plasma citrulline and trace levels of urinary orotic acid is the consequence of

    (A) arginase deficiency
    (B) argininosuccinate lyase deficiency
    (C) argininosuccinate synthetase deficiency

    (D) carbamoylphosphate synthetase I deficiency
    (E) ornithine transcarbamoylase deficiency

Questions 323 and 324

A 4-month-old boy presents with painful progressive joint deformity (particularly of the ankles, knees, elbows, and wrists), hoarse crying, and granulomatous lesions of the epiglottis and larynx leading to feeding and breathing difficulty. Biopsy of the liver indicates an accumulation of ceramides.

323. The observed symptoms and the results of the liver biopsy are indicative of which disease?

    (A) Farber's lipogranulomatosis
    (B) Fucosidosis
    (C) Gaucher disease
    (D) Metachromic leukodystrophy
    (E) Sandhoff–Jatzkewitz disease

324. Specific diagnosis of this disease requires assay of skin fibroblasts for a deficiency in

    (A) acid ceramidase
    (B) arylsulfatase A
    (C) galactocerebrosidase
    (D) hexosaminidase A
    (E) sphingomyelinase

325. Placement of eukaryotic mRNAs on the small ribosomal subunit during initiation of a functioning ribosome

    (A) depends on the interaction of cap-binding factor, eIF-4F, with met-tRNA^{met} after it first recognizes the cap structure of the mRNA
    (B) is random because the initiator met-tRNA^{met} invariably aligns with the first AUG
    (C) requires the cap-binding factor, eIF-4F to allow for correct alignment of the initiator AUG with the initiator met-tRNA^{met}
    (D) requires the interaction of eIF-2 with the initiator met-tRNA^{met} and subsequent interaction of this complex with the small subunit prior to engagement of the mRNA
    (E) requires the presence of fmet-tRNA^{fmet}

326. Muscle membrane depolarizes in response to acetylcholine binding its receptors at the neuromuscular junction. Associated with this depolarization is the following change in enzyme activity:

    (A) decreased glycogen phosphorylase kinase activity due to an increase in calcium binding to its calmodulin subunit
    (B) decreased phosphorylation of, and inhibited activity of glycogen phosphorylase kinase
    (C) increased glycogen phosphorylase kinase activity due to an activation of phosphoprotein phosphatase
    (D) increased glycogen phosphorylase kinase activity due to an increase in calcium binding to its calmodulin subunit
    (E) increased phosphorylation and inhibited activity of glycogen phosphorylase kinase

327. A 42-year-old man presents with hepatomegaly, jaundice, refractory ascites, and renal insufficiency. Peripheral leukocytes exhibit only 20% of normal glucocerebrosidase activity. Which of the following would explain his symptoms?

    (A) Fabry disease
    (B) Gaucher disease
    (C) Krabbe disease
    (D) Niemann–Pick disease
    (E) Tay–Sachs disease

328. The increased intracellular concentrations of 5-phosphoribosyl-1-pyrophosphate (PRPP) and urate in the genetic hyperuricemia called the Lesch–Nyhan syndrome is most likely a consequence of

    (A) allopurinol inhibition of xanthine formation
    (B) deficiency of hypoxanthine–guanine phosphoribosyltransferase (HGPRT)
    (C) elevated PRPP synthetase activity
    (D) elevated synthesis of hypoxanthine
    (E) increased purine synthesis

329. The net conversion of carbons from fat into carbons of glucose cannot occur in humans because

    (A) fat oxidation occurs in the mitochondria and gluconeogenesis occurs in the cytosol
    (B) states of catabolism and anabolism are never concurrently active
    (C) storage of fats occurs in adipose tissue and gluconeogenesis occurs in liver and kidney
    (D) the carbons of acetyl CoA from fat oxidation are lost as CO_2 in the TCA cycle
    (E) the carbons of acetyl-CoA from fat oxidation inhibit conversion of pyruvate to oxaloacetate

330. Numerous related inherited disorders result from defects in the synthesis and/or processing of connective tissue proteins. Which of the following disorders results from a defect in the synthesis of fibrillin?

    (A) Cutis laxa
    (B) Ehlers–Danlos syndrome
    (C) Marfan syndrome
    (D) Occipital horn syndrome
    (E) Osteogenesis imperfecta (OI)

331. Which important metabolic pathway is depicted in Figure 3–3?

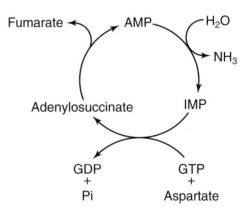

Figure 3–3

(A) Adenosine deaminase cycle

(B) Hypoxanthine–guanine phosphoribosyl-transferase cycle

(C) Nonoxidative cycle in pentose phosphate pathway

(D) Purine nucleotide cycle

(E) Urea cycle

332. Proofreading activity is necessary to maintain the fidelity of DNA synthesis and

(A) occurs after the synthesis has been completed

(B) occurs in prokaryotes but not eukaryotes

(C) is a function of the 3' to 5' exonuclease activity of DNA polymerases

(D) is independent of the polymerase activity in prokaryotes

(E) requires the presence of an enzyme separate from the DNA polymerase holoenzyme

333. Shown in Figure 3–4 is the nonstandard amino acid selenocysteine. This amino acid is incorporated into certain enzymes by a unique translational process. Selenocysteine is an important modified amino acid found in

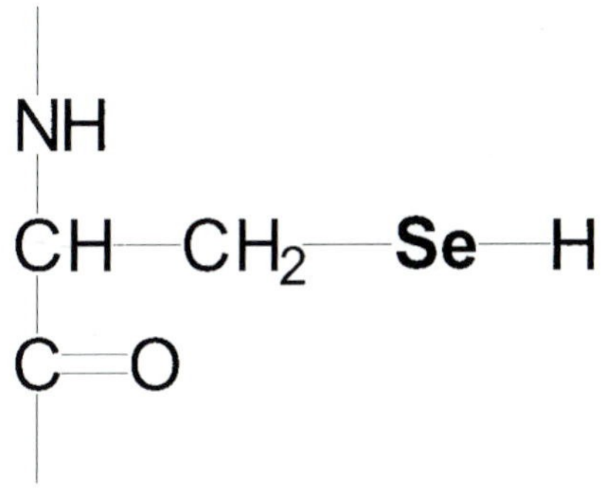

Figure 3–4

(A) alcohol dehydrogenase

(B) glutathione peroxidase

(C) heme oxygenase

(D) HMG-CoA reductase

(E) phosphoenolpyruvate carboxykinase

334. Patients with poorly controlled diabetes mellitus have elevated levels of blood glucose. This leads to an increase in the formation of glycosylated

(A) albumin

(B) cholesterol

(C) fatty acids

(D) hemoglobin

(E) transferrin

Questions 335 and 336

A child born and raised in Chicago planned to spend the summer on a relative's fruit farm and help with the harvest. The summer passed uneventfully, but several days after the harvest began the child became jaundiced and very sick. Upon admission to the hospital the following clinical findings were recorded: In addition to the expected hyperbilirubinemia, the patient was hypoglycemic, had a markedly elevated rise in blood fructose concentration, and was hyperlactic acidemic. Further history taking revealed that during the harvest it was customary for the family to indulge in fruit-filled meals and to snack freely on fruit while carrying out the harvest. The following conclusions were reached.

335. The elevated blood fructose was due to

(A) an allergic reaction to constituents in the fruit diet

(B) defective hepatic fructokinase

(C) defective hepatic fructose-1-phosphate aldolase (aldolase B)

(D) defective hepatic fructose-1,6-bisphosphate aldolase (aldolase A)

(E) defective hepatic glucokinase

336. The hyperlactic acidemia was attributed to

(A) a diet-induced insufficiency of niacin, leading to low cell levels of available NAD$^+$ and NADH

(B) an allergic reaction to a constituent in the fruit diet

(C) an inability to carry out liver oxidative phosphorylation and gluconeogenesis, secondary to a severe deficiency of available inorganic phosphate in hepatocytes

(D) an inability to metabolize pyruvate because of a dietary vitamin insufficiency, leading to inhibition of the pyruvate dehydrogenase complex

(E) excess production of pyruvate from dietary fructose sources

337. Stem cells

(A) are only found in the hematopoietic system in adults

(B) are only useful if derived from embryos

(C) can be stimulated to differentiate into multiple tissue types

(D) from adults can only differentiate into the tissue type from which they were derived

(E) have a very limited potential for self-renewal in culture

338. Which of the following symptoms can occur frequently in infants suffering from medium-chain acyl-CoA dehydrogenase (MCAD) deficiency if periods between meals are protracted?

(A) Bone and joint pain and thrombocytopenia

(B) Hyperammonemia with decreased ketones

(C) Hyperuricemia and darkening of the urine

(D) Hypoglycemia and metabolic acidosis with normal levels of ketones

(E) Metabolic alkalosis with decreased bicarbonate

339. A decrease in the level of heme leads to a reduction in globin synthesis in reticulocytes. Which of the following best explains this phenomenon?

(A) A heme-controlled phosphatase dephosphorylates cap-binding factor, which prevents recognition of globin mRNA by the ribosomes.

(B) A tRNA degrading enzyme is active in the absence of heme.

(C) Heme normally activates peptidyltransferase in reticulocytes.

(D) RNA polymerase activity is decreased in reticulocytes by low heme.

(E) The initiation factor eIF-2 becomes phosphorylated, reducing its level of activity.

340. Infants exhibiting profound metabolic ketoacidosis, muscular hypotonia, developmental retardation and who have very large accumulations of methylmalonic acid in their blood and urine suffer from a disorder known as methylmalonic acidemia. This disorder results from a defect in

(A) α-keto acid dehydrogenase

(B) homogentisic acid oxidase

(C) methylmalonyl-CoA mutase

(D) phenylalanine hydroxylase

(E) tyrosine aminotransferase

341. Following a minor respiratory illness, a seemingly healthy, developmentally normal 15-month-old boy exhibited repeated episodes of severe lethargy and vomiting following periods of fasting, such as during the middle of the night. The parents brought the infant to the ER following a seizure. The child was hypoglycemic and was administered 10% dextrose, but remained lethargic. Blood ammonia was high, liver function tests were slightly elevated, and his serum contained an accumulation of dicarboxylic acids. Only low levels of ketones were detectable in the urine. This infant suffers from

(A) glutaric acidemia type II

(B) Lesch–Nyhan syndrome

(C) medium-chain acyl-CoA dehydrogenase deficiency

(D) pyruvate dehydrogenase deficiency

(E) type III (Cori's) glycogen storage disease

342. A 28-year-old man has the following symptoms: diffuse grayish corneal opacities, anemia, proteinuria, and hyperlipidemia. Renal function is normal and serum albumin level is only slightly elevated. Plasma triglycerides and unesterified cholesterol levels are elevated, as are levels of phosphatidylcholine. These symptoms are indicative of which lipoprotein-associated disorder?

(A) Bassen–Kornzweig syndrome

(B) Familial hypercholesterolemia

(C) Familial hypertriacylglycerolemia

(D) Familial lecithin–cholesterol acyltransferase (LCAT) deficiency

(E) Wolman disease

343. Which of the following posttranslationally modified amino acids is found in several proteins of the blood clotting cascade?

(A) γ-Carboxyglutamate

(B) Hydroxylysine

(C) Hydroxyproline

(D) N-acetylmethionine

(E) Phosphoserine

344. I-cell disease (also identified as mucolipidosis type II) is characterized by the presence of inclusion bodies in fibroblasts (hence the derivation of the term I-cell), severe psychomotor retardation, corneal clouding, and dystosis multiplex. These symptoms arise from a defect in the targeting of lysosomal enzymes due to an inability to

(A) produce mannose-6-phosphate modifications in lysosomal enzymes

(B) recycle the lysosomal receptor for mannose-6-phosphate present on lysosomal enzymes

(C) remove mannose-6-phosphates from lysosomal enzymes prior to their transport to the lysosomes

(D) synthesize the mannose-6-phosphate receptor found in lysosomes

(E) transport mannose-6-phosphate receptors to lysosomes

345. A 30-month-old child presents with coarse facial features, corneal clouding, hepatosplenomegaly, and exhibiting disproportionate short-trunk dwarfism. Radiographic analysis indicates enlargement of the diaphyses of the long bones and irregular metaphyses, along with poorly developed epiphyseal centers. Other skeletal abnormalities typify the features comprising dystosis multiplex. The child's physical stature and the analysis of bone development indicate the child is suffering from

(A) Hunter syndrome

(B) Hurler syndrome

(C) Maroteaux–Lamy syndrome

(D) Morquio syndrome type B

(E) Sanfilippo disease type A

346. Which of the following is associated with type I diabetes?

(A) Decreased insulin receptor response to insulin binding

(B) Impaired glucagon-dependent inhibition of glycolysis leading to hyperglycemia

(C) Decreased glucagon secretion leading to hypolipidemia

(D) Elevated insulin secretion leading to severe hypoglycemia

(E) Elevated glucagon secretion leading to hyperlipidemia

347. Which of the following polypeptides is derived by posttranslational processing of the pro-opiomelanocortin (POMC) gene product?

(A) Atrial natriuretic factor

(B) Bradykinin

(C) Cholecystokinin

(D) β-Endorphin

(E) Oxytocin

348. A deficiency in the amino acid metabolizing enzyme α-keto acid dehydrogenase results in neonatal vomiting, lethargy, and poor suckling behavior. Progressive neurologic signs include decerebrate posturing. Which one of the following disorders corresponds to this defect?

(A) Alkaptonuria

(B) Homocystinuria

(C) Isovaleric acidemia

(D) Maple syrup urine disease

(E) Phenylketonuria

349. Which of the following glycosaminoglycans exhibits antithrombic activity when released into the circulation?

(A) Chondroitin sulfate

(B) Dermatan sulfate

(C) Heparin

(D) Hyaluronate

(E) Keratan sulfate

350. A 37-year-old man presents with tophaceous deposits within the articular cartilage, synovium, tendons, tendon sheaths, pinnae, and the soft tissue on the extensor surface of the forearms. These clinical observations suggest the patient is suffering from

(A) adenosine deaminase deficiency

(B) gout

(C) Lesch–Nyhan syndrome

(D) purine nucleotide phosphorylase deficiency

(E) von Gierke disease

351. Figure 3–5 represents the *de novo* pathway of pyrimidine biosynthesis. The enzyme represented as A in the figure is

(A) aspartate transcarbamoylase

(B) OMP decarboxylase

(C) phosphoribosylpyrophosphate (PRPP) amido transferase

(D) phosphoribosylpyrophosphate (PRPP) synthetase

(E) ribonucleotide reductase

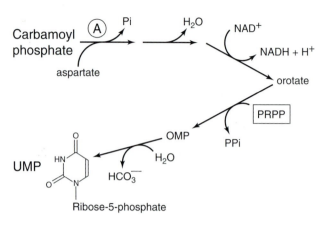

Figure 3–5

352. One important function of nitric oxide (NO) is the induction of vascular smooth muscle relaxation in response to acetylcholine. The production of NO requires which amino acid?

(A) Arginine

(B) Asparagine

(C) Cysteine

(D) Glutamine

(E) Lysine

353. In renal insufficiency, calcium absorption is reduced and leads to increased bone resorption, a condition referred to as renal osteodystrophy. Treatment with which of the following can ameliorate the symptoms of this condition?

(A) Antidiuretic hormone

(B) Calcitonin

(C) Calcitriol

(D) Growth hormone

(E) Parathyroid hormone (PTH)

354. A 32-year-old woman is diagnosed with hypertension, hypernatremia, hypokalemia, and alkalosis. Measurements of plasma glucocorticoid levels show them to be within the normal range; however, renin and angiotensin II levels are suppressed. Ultrasound indicates the possible existence of an adrenal cortical mass. These symptoms are likely due to excess production of

(A) aldosterone

(B) androstenedione

(C) dehydroepiandrosterone (DHEA)

(D) estradiol

(E) testosterone

355. The neurotransmitters epinephrine, norepinephrine, and dopamine are all derived from which amino acid?

(A) Arginine

(B) Asparagine

(C) Phenylalanine

(D) Tryptophan

(E) Tyrosine

356. A 17-year-old man who reports to his physician that he is incapable of obtaining an erection is also quite embarrassed by the apparent enlargement of his breasts (gynecomastia). These symptoms when present in males are associated with an excessive production of

(A) corticotropin-releasing hormone

(B) gonadotropin-releasing hormone

(C) growth hormone

(D) melanocyte-stimulating hormone

(E) prolactin

357. Numerous inherited disorders are the result of the expansion of trinucleotide (triplet) repeats either within the coding regions of genes or the untranslated regions of the resultant RNAs. Which of the following diseases has been shown to be caused by triplet expansion?

(A) Cystic fibrosis (CF)

(B) Duchenne muscular dystrophy (DMD)

(C) Familial hypercholesterolemia

(D) Huntington disease (HD)

(E) Menkes disease

358. Figure 3–6 represents a portion of the glycolytic pathway. Which lettered step in this pathway represents the rate-limiting reaction of glycolysis?

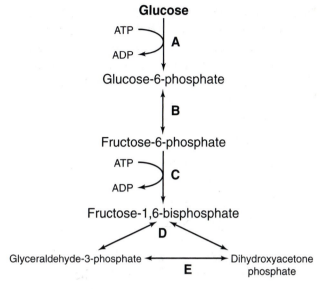

Figure 3–6

(A) A

(B) B

(C) C

(D) D

(E) E

359. Severe combined immunodeficiency disease (SCID) is characterized by a complete lack of cell-mediated and humoral immunity. This disorder results from a deficiency in

(A) adenosine deaminase (ADA)

(B) aspartate transcarbamoylase (ATC)

(C) hypoxanthine–guanine phosphoribosyl-transferase (HGPRT)

(D) orotic acid decarboxylase

(E) purine nucleoside phosphorylase (PNP)

360. The forensic analytical technique identified as DNA fingerprinting refers to

    (A) the establishment of a complete collection of cloned fragments of DNA
    (B) the identification of sequences of DNA to which specific proteins bind, thereby rendering them resistant to digestion by DNA degrading nucleases
    (C) the specific association of complimentary strands of DNA to one another
    (D) the synthetic oligonucleotide-directed enzymatic amplification of specific sequences of DNA
    (E) the use of repeat sequences to establish a unique pattern of fragments for any given individual

361. Glucagon binding to liver cells induces an increase in intracellular cAMP concentration. The rate-limiting step in cholesterol biosynthesis is regulated as a consequence of this glucagon-mediated rise in cAMP. The effect of increased cAMP on the rate of cholesterol biosynthesis occurs because

    (A) AMP-regulated kinase is activated and directly phosphorylates HMG-CoA reductase leading to an increase in the activity of the latter enzyme
    (B) cyclic AMP-dependent protein kinase (PKA) is activated and directly phosphorylates HMG-CoA reductase, reducing the activity of the latter enzyme
    (C) PKA is activated and phosphorylates AMP-regulated kinase, which then phosphorylates and activates HMG-CoA reductase
    (D) removal of phosphate from HMG-CoA reductase increases its activity; activated PKA results in a reduced level of phosphate removal from HMG-CoA reductase so that the latter enzyme is kept less active
    (E) the increased cAMP directly inhibits HMG-CoA reductase

362. The initial step toward the synthesis of triacylglycerols from free fatty acids and glycerol within hepatocytes requires which enzyme?

    (A) Glyceraldehyde 3-phosphate dehydrogenase
    (B) Glycerol 3-phosphate dehydrogenase
    (C) Glycerol kinase
    (D) Hormone-sensitive lipase
    (E) Lipoprotein lipase

363. A 3-month-old infant exhibits profound neurologic deficit in addition to being blind and deaf. Pathologic examination indicates renal cysts, hepatomegaly, and facial dysmorphism. Biochemical analysis reveals plasma accumulations of very-long-chain fatty acids, abnormal intermediates of bile acid synthesis, and a marked deficiency of plasmalogens. These physical and biochemical features are characteristic of

    (A) hyperpipecolic acidemia
    (B) infantile Refsum disease
    (C) neonatal adrenoleukodystrophy
    (D) rhizomelic chondrodysplasia punctata (RCDP)
    (E) Zellweger syndrome

364. Which of the following apoproteins is found exclusively associated with chylomicrons?

    (A) apo(a)
    (B) apo-B-48
    (C) apo-C-II
    (D) apo-D
    (E) apo-E

365. Which lettered reaction in Figure 3–7 (representing the nonoxidative portion of the pentose phosphate pathway) is catalyzed by transaldolase?

    (A) A
    (B) B
    (C) C
    (D) D
    (E) E

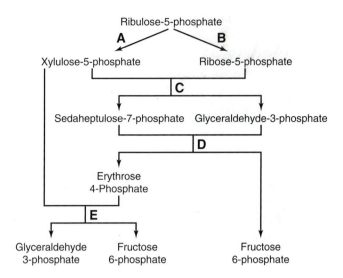

Figure 3–7

366. Acromegaly is characterized by protruding jaw, enlargement of the nose, hands, feet, and skull, and a thickening of the skin. This disorder is the result of excessive production of

(A) corticotropin-releasing hormone
(B) gonadotropin-releasing hormone
(C) growth hormone
(D) insulin-like growth factor II
(E) thyroid-stimulating hormone

367. The primary protein responsible for iron homeostasis is

(A) ceruloplasmin
(B) ferritin
(C) haptoglobin
(D) metallothionein
(E) transferrin

368. The signal transduction protein, ras, has been shown to play a role in the genesis of certain types of cancer. This effect is due to alterations in the sequence of this important regulatory protein. Ras belongs to the family of signal transduction molecules that are

(A) activated by GTPase activating proteins (GAPs)
(B) guanine nucleotide binding proteins, termed G-proteins

(C) nuclear transcription factors
(D) protein serine/threonine kinases
(E) receptor tyrosine kinases

369. A 3-month-old infant who otherwise appeared normal during the first 2 months of life except for a bout of hyperbilirubinemia is now clearly exhibiting developmental delay. In addition, the infant's hair has become grayish and dull and there is a stubble of broken hairs over the occiput and temporal regions. The facial appearance has also changed such that the infant has very pudgy cheeks, abnormal eyebrows, and sagging jowls. The occurrence of frequent convulsions was the stimulus for the parents to bring their child to the emergency room. These rapidly deteriorating symptoms are indicative of

(A) Crigler–Najjar syndrome type I
(B) Gilbert syndrome
(C) Hemochromatosis
(D) Menkes disease
(E) Refsum disease

370. Acute intermittent porphyria (AIP) is the major autosomal dominant acute hepatic porphyria. This disease is caused by a deficiency in porphobilinogen deaminase, an enzyme of heme biosynthesis. Patients afflicted with this disease would be expected to excrete excess amounts of

(A) δ-aminolevulinic acid (ALA)
(B) coproporphyrinogen III
(C) hydroxymethylbilane
(D) protoporphyrin IX
(E) uroporphyrinogen type III

371. The phosphorylase kinase-associated regulatory protein identified by the letter A in Figure 3–8 is a calcium-binding protein. This subunit of phosphorylase kinase is

(A) calmodulin
(B) fructose-2,6-bisphosphate
(C) glycogen synthase kinase-3
(D) phosphoprotein phosphatase
(E) phosphoprotein phosphatase inhibitor-1

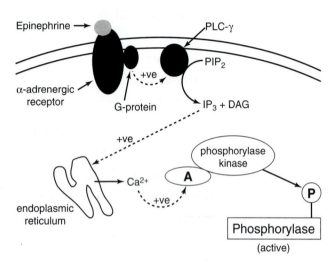

Figure 3–8

372. Mosaicism refers to a condition in which an individual has two or more genetically distinct cell types, derived from a single zygote, but that differ because of mutation or chromosomal aberration. Mosaicism occurs with a frequency of approximately 30% in females who are phenotypically normal but harbor gonadal dysgenesis, sexual immaturity, and infertility. These affected females also are short in stature, have webbing of the neck, and swelling of the hands and feet, as well as cardivascular and renal abnormalities. These symptoms are associated with

(A) achondroplasia
(B) Duchenne muscular dystrophy (DMD)
(C) fragile X syndrome
(D) Kleinfelter syndrome
(E) Turner syndrome

373. An 18-month-old boy is referred to the pediatrics clinic because of persistent anemia and associated failure to thrive. Laboratory analysis confirmed a microcytic anemia and revealed blood lead levels of 50 mg/dL (two times normal) and high levels of coproporphyrinogen III in the urine. The child was put on chelation therapy and recovered uneventfully. The cause of the child's difficulty was most likely due to the effects of lead inhibiting which of the following enzymes of heme biosynthesis?

(A) δ-Aminolevulinic acid (ALA) dehydratase
(B) Ferrochelatase
(C) Porphobilinogen (PBG) deaminase
(D) Uroporphyrinogen decarboxylase
(E) Uroporphyrinogen III cosynthase

374. Pyruvate dehydrogenase is a complex multisubunit enzyme. The activity of this complex is positively affected by

(A) acetyl-CoA
(B) ATP
(C) dephosphorylation
(D) NADH
(E) phosphorylation

375. Vitamin K is required for which of the following amino acid modifications?

(A) Aspartate to β-carboxyaspartate
(B) Glutamate to γ-carboxyglutamate
(C) Lysine to hydroxylysine
(D) Lysine to β-methyllysine
(E) Proline to hydroxyproline

376. Steroid hormones interact with specific receptors within target cells. The steroid–receptor complexes then regulate the rate of

(A) posttranscriptional processing of specific mRNAs
(B) posttranslational processing of specific proteins
(C) replication of DNA
(D) transcription of specific genes
(E) translation of specific mRNAs

Questions 377 and 378

A 5-month-old girl is presented to her pediatrician because her parents are frightened by the infants' hypersensitivity to auditory, visual, and tactile stimulation. They have noted a regression in her capacity for movement and she has repeated episodes of vomiting. While in the exam room, the child suffers a massive seizure that results in her death. Upon post mortem examination, it is noted that there is significant demyelination in the brain and presence of numerous multinucleated globoid cells of the macrophage lineage. Analysis of the content of these globoid cells finds the ratio of galactosylceramide to sulfatide to be abnormally high.

377. The physical and clinical symptoms exhibited by this infant are indicative of

   (A) Farber lipogranulomatosis
   (B) fucosidosis
   (C) Gaucher disease
   (D) Krabbe disease (globoid leukodystrophy)
   (E) metachromic leukodystrophy

378. The enzyme that is deficient in this disorder is

   (A) acid ceramidase
   (B) arylsulfatase A
   (C) α-L-fucosidase
   (D) galactocerebrosidase
   (E) glucocerebrosidase

Questions 379 and 380

A 12-year-old boy has suffered from chronic sinopulmonary disease including persistent infection of the airway with *Pseudomonas aeruginosa*. He has constant and chronic sputum production as a result of the airway infection. Additionally, he suffers from GI and nutritional abnormalities that include biliary cirrhosis, meconium ileus, and pancreatic insufficiency.

379. The described symptoms are classical for

   (A) congenital adrenal hyperplasia
   (B) cystic fibrosis
   (C) renal Fanconi syndrome
   (D) sickle cell anemia
   (E) Tay–Sachs disease

380. The described disease is genetically transmitted as a (an)

   (A) autosomal dominant disorder
   (B) autosomal recessive disorder
   (C) X-linked dominant disorder
   (D) X-linked recessive disorder
   (E) Y-linked disorder

381. Acetyl-CoA enhances the rate of gluconeogenesis by acting as an allosteric activator of

   (A) acetyl-CoA carboxylase
   (B) phosphoenolpyruvate carboxykinase
   (C) pyruvate carboxylase
   (D) pyruvate dehydrogenase
   (E) pyruvate kinase

382. A reaction important in oxygen transport is catalyzed by carbonic anhydrase. This reaction is

   (A) carbamoylation of hemoglobin
   (B) ionization of carbonic acid
   (C) production of CO_2 from carbonic acid
   (D) protonation of hemoglobin
   (E) transport of chloride ion in exchange bicarbonate ion

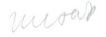

383. An observation that has been made over the past several decades is that certain dominantly inherited disorders exhibit earlier age of onset along with increasing severity in successive generations. This phenomenon is referred to as anticipation. A most striking example of this genetic trait is characterized by muscle wasting beginning with the face, neck, and hands gradually becoming generalized and by the inability of muscles to relax after contraction. These symptoms and the phenomenon of anticipation are associated with

(A) Becker muscular dystrophy (BMD)
(B) Duchenne muscular dystrophy (DMD)
(C) Marfan syndrome
(D) Myotonic dystrophy
(E) osteogenesis imperfecta

384. The accumulation of an oxygen debt during strenuous physical exercise may be accompanied by a (an)

(A) decrease in pyruvate in blood
(B) increase in ATP in muscle
(C) increase in citrate in muscle
(D) increase in lactate in blood
(E) increase in NAD$^+$ in muscle

385. Dietary triacylglycerols are transported in the plasma as

(A) albumin conjugates
(B) chylomicrons
(C) HDLs
(D) LDLs
(E) VLDLs

386. The analytical technique identified as DNA footprinting refers to the

(A) establishment of a complete collection of cloned fragments of DNA
(B) identification of sequences of DNA to which specific proteins bind, thereby rendering them resistant to digestion by DNA degrading nucleases
(C) specific association of complimentary strands of DNA to one another

(D) synthetic oligonucleotide-directed enzymatic amplification of specific sequences of DNA
(E) use of repeat sequences in genomic DNA to establish a unique pattern of fragments for any given individual

For questions 387 refer to Figure 3–9

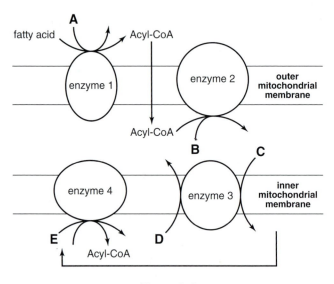

Figure 3–9

387. Carnitine, a zwitterionic compound derived from lysine, is involved in fatty acid metabolism and is required at which two points in the transport of fatty acids from the cytoplasm to the mitochondria?

(A) A and E
(B) A and C
(C) B and C
(D) B and D
(E) E and D

Questions 388 and 389

A male infant, delivered at 38 weeks' gestation, presents with severe bowing of long bones, blue sclera, and craniotabes at birth. Radiographs show severe generalized osteoporosis, broad and crumpled long bones, beading ribs, and poorly mineralized skull. Histologic examination of the long bones revealed the trabecula of the calcified cartilage with an abnormally thin layer of osteoid, and the bony trabeculae are thin and basophilic.

388. The symptoms observed in the infant are characteristic of which disease?

(A) Ehlers–Danlos syndrome
(B) Marfan syndrome
(C) Occipital horn syndrome
(D) Osteogenesis imperfecta
(E) Scurvy

389. The disease with the symptoms described results from the defective biosynthesis of

(A) α-collagen
(B) cytokeratin
(C) desmin
(D) fibrillin
(E) vimentin

390. A 2-month-old infant suffering from increased vomiting and diarrhea is seen in the hospital and observed to have significant abdominal distension due to hepatosplenomegaly. Unfortunately, the infant does not survive. Autopsy reveals calcification of the adrenals and massive accumulation of cholesteryl esters and triglycerides in most tissues. Analysis of enzyme activity in fibroblasts and lymphocytes demonstrates a significant acid lipase (cholesteryl ester hydrolase) deficiency. These clinical findings are indicative of

(A) hyperlipoproteinemia, type I (familial liproprotein lipase deficiency)
(B) I-cell disease (mucolipidosis type II)
(C) Maroteaux–Lamy syndrome
(D) Sanfillipo syndrome
(E) Wolman disease

391. Which of the following statements best describes the structure of a nucleosome?

(A) Each nucleosome encompasses around 50 to 100 base pairs of DNA.
(B) Histone H2A and H2B are disulfide bonded to histone H1 to stabilize the core.
(C) Histone H4 is also known as the linker histone.
(D) The core consists of an octamer of histones H2A, 2B, 3, and 4.
(E) The DNA of the core is encapsulated within the histone proteins.

392. Cockayne syndrome is a rare disorder that leads to sun sensitivity (without increased frequency of skin cancer), short stature, progressive neurologic degeneration, mental retardation, and progressive deafness. This disease is the result of a deficiency in which process?

(A) DNA repair
(B) DNA replication
(C) RNA processing
(D) Transcription
(E) Translation

393. In the presence of arsenate, which of the following may or may not occur during glycolysis?

(A) 1,3-Bisphosphoglycerate is formed.
(B) NADH is formed.
(C) P_i reacts with glyceraldehyde-3-phosphate.
(D) 3-Phosphoglycerate is not formed.
(E) Pyruvate is not formed.

394. In analyzing a sample of double-stranded DNA, it has been determined that the molar ratio of adenosine is 20%. Given this information, what is the content of cytidine?

(A) 10%
(B) 20%
(C) 30%
(D) 40%
(E) 60%

395. Measurement of the rate of creatinine clearance is used as a key determinant of renal function. In which of the following tissues is creatinine generated?

(A) Adipose
(B) Kidney
(C) Liver
(D) Lung
(E) Skeletal muscle

396. Numerous cancers are caused by a genetic phenomenon termed "loss of heterozygosity." This phenomenon led to the identification of genes termed tumor suppressors, because it is the loss of their function that leads to cancer. Which of the following has been shown to result from defects in a tumor suppressor gene?

(A) Creutzfeldt–Jakob disease (CJD)
(B) Crouzon syndrome
(C) Huntington disease (HD)
(D) Li–Fraumeni syndrome (LFS)
(E) Prader–Willi syndrome (PWS)

397. Following a relatively normal early developmental period, a 6-month-old boy becomes pale and lethargic and begins to show signs of deteriorating motor skill. The infant has severe megaloblastic anemia; however, serum measurements of iron, folate, and vitamins B_{12} and B_6 are within normal ranges. Urine samples were clear when fresh, but when left to stand for several hours showed an abundant white precipitate that was composed of fine, needle-shaped crystals. Analysis of the crystals identified them as orotic acid. Significant improvement is observed in the infant following oral administration of a nucleoside. Which of the following is most likely the nucleoside used?

(A) Adenosine
(B) Cytidine
(C) Guanosine
(D) Thymidine
(E) Uridine

398. Using the DNA shown as a template, what would be the sequence of the resultant mRNA following transcription?

5'-CATTCCATAGCATGT-3'

(A) 5'-ACAUGCUAUGGAAUG-3'
(B) 5'-CAUUCCAUAGCAUGU-3'
(C) 5'-GUAAGGUAUCGUACA-3'
(D) 5'-UGUACGAUACCUUAC-3'

Use the following codon table for Question 399

ACA	threonine	(T)	CAU	histidine	(H)
ACG	threonine	(T)	CUA	leucine	(L)
AUG	methionine	(M)	CGU	arginine	(R)
AAU	asparagine	(N)	CCU	proline	(P)
AGG	arginine	(R)	UGC	cysteine	(C)
AUA	isoleucine	(I)	UGU	cysteine	(C)
GGA	glycine	(G)	UAU	tyrosine	(Y)
GUA	valine	(V)	UAC	tyrosine	(Y)
GCA	alanine	(A)	UCC	serine	(S)
UGG	tryptophan	(W)			

399. If the RNA synthesized in Question 398 were translated in a eukaryotic *in vitro* translation system the composition of the resulting peptide would be

(A) C-T-I-P-Y
(B) H-S-I-A-C
(C) M-L-W-N
(D) T-C-Y-G-M
(E) V-R-Y-R-T

400. Which of the following statements most correctly reflects the effect of epinephrine stimulation of adipocytes?

(A) Enzyme-dependent addition of fatty acids to glycerol-3-phosphate
(B) Enzyme-dependent stepwise release of fatty acids from triglycerides
(C) Increases synthesis and activation of lipoprotein lipase
(D) Increases synthesis of HDL to transport fatty acids to peripheral tissues
(E) Release of glycerol-3-phosphate for gluconeogenesis in the liver

401. The "Bohr effect" is best described as the

(A) binding of O_2
(B) covalent attachment of CO_2 forming hemoglobin carbamate
(C) release of CO_2 from erythrocytes when they enter the high O_2 concentration of the alveoli
(D) release of O_2 from hemoglobin in response to the buffering of chloride ion by hemoglobin
(E) release of O_2 from hemoglobin in response to the buffering of H^+ by hemoglobin

402. Which of the following clotting factors forms an active complex with tissue factor (factor III) to initiate the extrinsic clotting cascade?

(A) Factor I (fibrinogen)
(B) Factor VII (proconvertin)
(C) Factor VIII
(D) Factor IX
(E) Protein S

403. The liver is the only body organ that is capable of

(A) ganglioside synthesis
(B) glycogen degradation
(C) medium-chain fatty acid catabolism
(D) nucleotide synthesis
(E) urea formation

404. When fatty acids with odd numbers of carbon atoms are oxidized in the β-oxidation pathway the final product is 1 mole of acetyl-CoA and 1 mole of the 3-carbon molecule, propionyl-CoA. To use the propionyl carbons, the molecule is carboxylated and converted ultimately to succinyl-CoA and fed into the TCA cycle. The vitamin cofactor required in one of the steps of this conversion is

(A) cobalamin (B_{12})
(B) pantothenic acid (B_5)
(C) pyridoxine (B_6)
(D) riboflavin (B_2)
(E) thiamine (B_1)

405. Mutant genes that affect several organ systems and bodily functions frequently show variable expressivity. A phenomenon referred to as phenotypic variation. The most striking example of phenotypic variability is manifest in an autosomal dominant condition characterized by the appearance of café-au-lait spots on the skin and cutaneous and subcutaneous neurofibromas. These symptoms are associated with

(A) familial adenomatous polyposis coli (FAP)
(B) familial hypercholesterolemia (FH)
(C) Li–Fraumeni syndrome
(D) von Hippel–Lindau (VHL) syndrome
(E) von Recklinghausen disease (type I neurofibromatosis)

406. Which of the following factors of blood coagulation is the major inhibitor of the extrinsic clotting cascade?

(A) Antithrombin III
(B) High-molecular-weight kininogen (HMWK)
(C) Lipoprotein-associated coagulation factor (LACI)
(D) α_2-Macroglobulin
(E) Protein C

407. Certain receptors function through the activation of phospholipase Cγ (PLCγ). Which of the following most accurately depicts the result of activated PLCγ?

(A) Activation of adenylate cyclase with increased production of cAMP
(B) Activation of phosphodiesterase, thereby decreasing the concentration of cAMP
(C) Decreased release of inositol phospholipids from the plasma membrane
(D) Increased cellular uptake of Ca^{2+} resulting in depolarization of the cell
(E) Increased release of diacylglycerol from plasma phospholipids

408. When adipose tissue is stimulated to release fatty acids to the circulation, these fatty acids are transported in the plasma associated with

(A) albumin
(B) chylomicrons
(C) α_2-macroglobulin
(D) β_2-microglobulin
(E) VLDLs

409. Protein synthesis requires each incoming amino acid be activated by attachment to a correct tRNA. During the formation of each aminoacyl tRNA

(A) a guanine nucleotide exchange factor is necessary to activate each tRNA by exchanging GTP for GDP

(B) a proofreading site on the aminoacyl tRNA synthetase selects the correct amino acid for attachment to the correct tRNA

(C) each amino acid residue is attached to a modified nucleotide at the 5'-end of the tRNA

(D) the amino acid is first activated through the formation of a high-energy covalent intermediate through interaction with ATP

(E) tRNAs that can bind to more than one codon may interact with multiple aminoacyl tRNA synthetases

Answers and Explanations

283. **(A)** Erythrocytes depend on the function of the pentose phosphate pathway to prevent permanent damage from the numerous reactive oxygen species that are present as a result of their role as oxygen transporters. The pentose phosphate pathway generates large quantities of NADPH through the actions of glucose-6-phosphate dehydrogenase and 6-phosphogluconate dehydrogenase. The need for NADPH stems from the fact that it is required for the action of glutathione reductase. Glutathione reductase converts oxidized glutathione (GSSG) to reduced glutathione (GSH). Red blood cells require GSH as a scavenger of reactive oxygen species to prevent oxidative damage. Deficiencies in glucose-6-phosphate dehydrogenase therefore lead to erythrocytes that are highly sensitive to oxidative damage with resultant hemolysis. The accelerated rate of hemolysis leads to anemia. Primaquine and related drugs are metabolized within erythrocytes to oxidative derivatives, which accelerate the rate of glutathione oxidation, as well as hydrogen transfer from NADPH and hemoglobin. Normally under these conditions, the rate of flux through the pentose phosphate pathway is greatly accelerated providing increased amounts of NADPH. In persons with glucose-6-phosphate dehydrogenase deficiencies this acceleration is not possible and oxidative stress leads to hemolysis. None of the other enzymes (choices B, C, D, or E) generates NADPH as a byproduct of their respective reactions and can therefore have no influence on erythrocyte oxidative management.

284. **(C)** Heme is oxidized, with the heme ring being opened by the endoplasmic reticulum en-zyme, heme oxygenase (see Figure 3–10). The oxidation step requires heme as a substrate, and any hemin (Fe^{3+}) is reduced to heme (Fe^{2+}) prior to oxidation by heme oxygenase. The oxidation occurs on a specific carbon producing the linear tetrapyrrole biliverdin, ferric iron (Fe^{3+}), and carbon monoxide (CO). This is the only reaction in the body that is known to produce CO. Most of the CO is excreted through the lungs, with the result that the CO content of expired air is a direct measure of the activity of heme oxidase in an individual. Biliverdin reductase (choice A) cat-

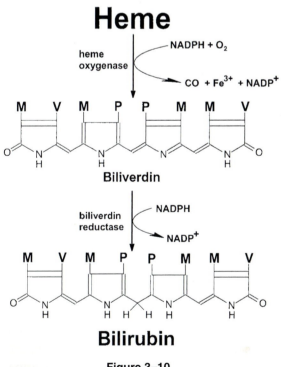

Figure 3–10

alyzes the conversion of biliverdin to bilirubin as shown in Figure 3–10. Coproporphyrinogen oxidase (choice B), protoporphyrinogen oxidase (choice D), and uroporphyrinogen decarboxylase (choice E) are all involved in the synthesis of heme and do not produce CO in the course of catalyzing their reactions.

285. **(E)** Carbamoylphosphate synthetase I (CPS-I) is absolutely dependent on the allosteric effector N-acetylglutamate for its activity. This allosteric effector is synthesized by the enzyme N-acetylglutamate synthetase, which is activated by the urea cycle amino acid arginine. None of the other compounds (choices A, B, C, and D) have any effect on CPS-I activity.

286. **(B)** The carbohydrates that constitute the ABO blood groups are covalently attached either to membrane sphingolipids or to circulating proteins. When present on the surface of cells, the ABO carbohydrates are linked to sphingolipid, and are therefore of the glycosphingolipid class (choice A). When the ABO carbohydrates are associated with protein in the form of glycoproteins, they are found in the serum and are referred to as the secreted forms. Some individuals produce the glycoprotein forms of the ABO antigens and others do not. This property distinguishes secretors from nonsecretors, a property that has forensic importance such as in cases of rape. Secretor/nonsecretor status is not due to any acute clinical situation (choice D) or to defects in any gene function (choices C and E).

287. **(E)** The statin class of cholesterol lowering drugs all exert their effects on the activity of HMG-CoA reductase. This enzyme carries out the rate-limiting step in cholesterol biosynthesis. The cholestyramine-based resins are used therapeutically to bind up intestinal bile salts which increases the excretion of bile (choice B). The net effect of increased bile excretion is increased diversion of cholesterol into bile acid synthesis, thereby lowering circulating cholesterol levels. No current therapy targets synthesis of apolipoprotein synthesis (choice C), decreasing intestinal absorption of cholesterol (choice A), or inhibition of LDL-receptor interactions (choice D).

288. **(A)** Essential fructosuria is an autosomal-recessive disorder manifesting benign asymptomology due to a lack of fructokinase. The principal clinical signs of essential fructosuria are hyperfructosemia and fructosuria. Deficiency in aldolase B (choice B) results in the clinically severe disorder, hereditary fructose intolerance. Symptoms include severe hypoglycemia and vomiting after ingestion of fructose. Prolonged fructose ingestion by infants with this disorder leads to poor feeding, hepatomegaly, vomiting, jaundice, and eventually hepatic failure and death. Aldolase A deficiency (choice C) is very rare, has only been observed associated with erythrocytes and fibroblasts, and leads to hemolytic anemia. Hexokinase deficiency (choice D) is also rare and associated with erythrocyte dysfunction leading to chronic hemolytic anemia. Deficiency in phosphofructokinase-1 (PFK-1) (choice E) results in the glycogen storage disease known as Tarui disease. Symptoms of PFK-1 deficiency include exercise induced cramping and pain, myoglobinuria, and hemolytic anemia.

289. **(D)** Methotrexate and related chemotherapeutics are structural analogs of folic acid and function by blocking the activity of dihydrofolate reductase (DHFR). DHFR is required during the synthesis of thymidine monophosphate (dTMP). Deoxyuridine monophosphate (dUMP) is converted to dTMP through the action of thymidylate synthase. The methyl group attached to dUMP during this reaction is derived from N^5-N^{10}-methylene-tetrahydrofolate. The byproducts of the thymidylate synthase reaction are dTMP and dihydrofolate. This is the only reaction in the body that utilizes a tetrahydrofolate compound and yields dihydrofolate. Regeneration of tetrahydrofolate is, therefore, necessary for the continued synthesis of dTMP, and subsequently DNA, and requires the action of DHFR. Thus, inhibition of DHFR blocks cell division by blocking the ability of cells to make DNA. None of the

other enzymatic processes of nucleotide synthesis (choices A, B, C, and E) are sites for chemotherapeutic drugs.

290. (A) The term *thalassemia* refers to a group of conditions in which the structures of the globin proteins (α and β) are normal but one or the other proteins are reduced in quantity through any of a number of mechanisms. This distinguishes these disorders from those hemoglobin disorders that are the result of structural defects in the globin proteins (choice C) (e.g., sickle cell anemia). The presence of an abnormal fetal globin protein in the adult (choice E) or the synthesis of abnormal fetal globin genes during embryonic development (choice D) would result in qualitative changes in the globin proteins and thus would not result in thalassemia. No disorder in globin production has been equated with adult globin gene expression during fetal development (choice B).

291. (A) The synthesis of the cyclic eicosanoids (the prostaglandins and the thromboxanes) begins with the cyclization of arachadonic acid. This reaction is carried out by the enzyme prostaglandin endoperoxide synthetase. This enzyme has two distinct activities, cyclooxygenase and a peroxidase. The activity of the cyclooxygenase domain is inhibited by a class of compounds referred to as nonsteroidal anti-inflammatory drugs (NSAIDs). Aspirin is of this class of drug and therefore inhibits the cyclooxygenase activity. The inhibition of prostaglandin synthesis has a negative effect on the process of coagulation through a reduction in the production of thromboxane A_2 (TXA_2), a potent activator of platelet function. Aspirin also reduces the production of prostacyclin (PGI_2) by endothelial cells. PGI_2 is a vasodilator and an inhibitor of platelet aggregation. Because endothelial cells regenerate active cyclooxygenase faster than platelets, the net effect of aspirin is more in favor of endothelial cell-mediated inhibition of the coagulation cascade. The action of the steroidal anti-inflammatory drugs occurs through the inhibition of phospholipase A_2 (choice C) and inhibition of this enzyme has

no direct effect on the coagulation process. The other choices (B, D, and E) are not targets for the action of aspirin.

292. (A) Fabry disease is an X-linked disorder that results from a deficiency in α-galactosidase A. This leads to the deposition of neutral glycosphingolipids with terminal α-galactosyl moieties in most tissues and fluids. Most affected tissues are heart, kidneys, and eyes. The predominant glycosphingolipid accumulated is globotriaosylceramide [galactosyl-(α1→4)-galactosyl-(β1→4)-glucosyl-(β1→1')-ceramide]. With advancing age, the major symptoms of the disease are due to increasing deposition of glycosphingolipid in the cardiovascular system. Indeed, cardiac disease occurs in most hemizygous males. Three types of Gaucher disease (choice B) have been characterized and are caused by defects in lysosomal acid β-glucosidase (glucocerebrosidase). Defects in this enzyme lead to the accumulation of glucosylceramides (glucocerebrosides), which leads primarily to central nervous system dysfunction and hepatosplenomegaly and skeletal lesions. Niemann–Pick disease (NPD) (choice D) comprises three types of lipid storage disorder, two of which (type A and B NPD) result from a defect in acid sphingomyelinase. Type A is a disorder that leads to infantile mortality. Type B is variable in phenotype and is diagnosed by the presence of hepatosplenomegaly in childhood and progressive pulmonary infiltration. Pathologic characteristics of Niemann–Pick are the accumulation of histiocytic cells that result from sphingomyelin deposition in cells of the monocyte–macrophage system. Tay–Sachs disease (choice E) results from a defect in hexosaminidase A leading to the accumulation of GM_2 gangliosides, particularly in neuronal cells. This defect leads to severe mental retardation, progressive weakness, and hypotonia, which prevents normal motor development. Progression of the disease is rapid and death occurs within the second year. Krabbe disease (choice C), also called globoid-cell leukodystrophy, results from a deficiency in galactosylceramidase (galactocerebroside β-galactosidase). This disease progresses rapidly and invariably leads to infantile mortality.

293. **(B)** There are three reactions of glycolysis that are thermodynamically irreversible. These are the hexokinase (glucokinase), phosphofructokinase-1 (PFK-1), and pyruvate kinase catalyzed reactions. Reactions that are essentially irreversible in most metabolic pathways are subject to complex regulatory controls and represent rate-limiting steps in the pathway. The primary site of regulation of glycolysis occurs at the level of the PFK-1 catalyzed step. Hence, this reaction is the rate-limiting step in glycolysis. PFK-1 is subject to allosteric control by numerous compounds. Citrate and ATP inhibit the activity of PFK-1, and AMP and fructose 2,6-bisphosphate (F2,6-BP) activate the enzyme. The principal control of PFK-1 activity is exerted by alterations in the level of F2,6-BP. This compound is synthesized from fructose 6-phosphate (F6-P) by the bifunctional enzyme, phosphofructokinase-2/fructose-2,6-bisphosphatase (PFK-2/F2,6-BPase). PFK-2 (choice C) contains two catalytic domains, one a kinase and the other a phosphatase, the activities of which are affected by the state of phosphorylation. The phosphatase domain is active when the enzyme is phosphorylated and converts F2,6-BP back to F6-P, thereby reducing the levels of this powerful activator of PFK-1. Thus, although the activity of PFK-2 determines the rate of activity of PFK-1, it is itself not the rate-limiting enzyme in glycolysis. Glyceraldehyde-3-phosphate dehydrogenase (choice A) and phosphoglycerate kinase (choice D) are not regulated enzymes of glycolysis. Pyruvate kinase (choice E) is regulated during glycolysis, but does not constitute a rate-limiting step.

294. **(A)** The first step in gluconeogenesis is the formation of oxaloacetate from pyruvate. The enzyme controlling this step is pyruvate carboxylase, an allosteric enzyme that does not function in the absence of its primary effector, acetyl-CoA, or closely related acyl-CoA. Thus, a high level of acetyl-CoA signals the need for more oxaloacetate. If there is a surplus of ATP, oxaloacetate is used for gluconeogenesis. Under conditions of low ATP, oxaloacetate is consumed in the citric acid cycle.

Citrate is the primary negative effector of glycolysis, and the primary positive effector of fatty acid synthesis. High levels of citrate (choice C), but not low levels (choice E), do positively affect the activity of fructose-1,6-bisphosphatase, one of the bypass enzymes of gluconeogenesis, but this is not the primary site of control; the carbon atoms must first go through the pyruvate carboxylase reaction. Low ATP levels (choice D) are reflected in an elevation in ADP levels, and ADP negatively affects the activity of pyruvate carboxylase. High ATP levels (choice B) are necessary for gluconeogenesis to proceed, and negatively affect glycolysis at the level of PFK-1, allowing for an increased net flow of carbon into glucose. However, increased levels of ATP do not directly regulate the enzymes of gluconeogenesis.

295. **(A)** Andersen disease (also referred to as type IV glycogen storage disease) manifests its symptoms as a result of the accumulation of glycogen with unbranched long outer chains in tissues. This structure of glycogen resembles that of plant amylopectin. Symptoms appear within the first year of life and lead to failure to thrive and pronounced hepatosplenomegaly. Hypoglycemia is rarely seen with this disorder. Cori disease (choice B) affects both liver and muscle with accumulations of glycogen that has short outer chains (resembles limit dextrin). Symptoms include hepatomegaly, hypoglycemia, hyperlipidemia, and retarded growth. McArdle disease (choice C) usually manifests in adulthood and characteristic symptoms include exercise intolerance, muscle cramping with exercise and myoglobinuria. The only affected tissue in this disease is skeletal muscle. Tarui disease (choice D) also affects skeletal muscle and as such manifests with clinical symptoms very similar to those of McArdle disease with the exceptions that Tarui patients also experience hemolytic anemia and myogenic hyperuricemia. Symptoms of von Gierke disease (choice E) result from the excessive accumulation of glycogen in liver, kidney, and intestinal mucosa. Symptoms include growth retardation, hypoglycemia, hepatomegaly, hyperlipidemia, lactic acidemia, and hyperuricemia.

296. **(C)** The long unbranched glycogen seen in Andersen disease is due to a defect in the glycogen branching enzyme. Defects in the glycogen debranching enzyme (choice A) result in Cori disease. Defects in glucose-6-phosphatase (choice B) result in von Gierke disease. Defects in liver phosphorylase (choice D) lead to Her disease (type VI glycogen storage disease). Defects in muscle phosphorylase (choice E) result in McArdle disease.

297. **(C)** Severe hereditary galactosemia presents in the first few months of life with symptoms that include poor feeding and associated weight loss, vomiting, diarrhea, lethargy, and hypotonia. Clinical findings include those presented in the case. The symptoms are aggravated by consumption of cow's milk and can be resolved provided proper diagnosis is made and treatment is started early. Alkaptonuria (choice A) results from the accumulation of homogentisic acid (a byproduct of tyrosine catabolism) in the urine and tissues. Oxidation of homogentisate in the urine causes it to turn dark and in the tissues results in ochronosis, which refers to the ochre color of the deposits in connective tissue, bones and other organs. Essential fructosuria (choice B) is a benign asymptomatic metabolic disorder manifesting with alimentary hyperfructosemia and fructosuria. Menke disease (choice D) results from a defect in intracellular copper transport and the symptoms of the disease are caused by loss of function of copper-dependent enzymes. Symptoms include abnormal (kinky) hair and pigmentation, cerebral degeneration, failure to thrive, and skin laxity. Symptoms of von Gierke disease (choice E) result from the excessive accumulation of glycogen in liver, kidney, and intestinal mucosa. Symptoms include growth retardation, hypoglycemia, hepatomegaly, hyperlipidemia, lactic acidemia, and hyperuricemia.

298. **(A)** Essential galactosemia results from a defect in the enzyme galactose 1-phosphate uridyltransferase. This enzyme is responsible for the interconversion of galactose-1-phosphate and UDP-glucose forming glucose-1-phosphate and UDP-galactose. This interconversion is required for humans to utilize galactose, consumed in the diet, as an energy source. Ferrochelatase (choice B) is responsible for inserting the iron atom into protoporphyrin IX yielding heme b. Fructokinase (choice C) catalyzes the phosphorylation of fructose so that it can be metabolized. Defects in fructokinase lead to essential fructosuria. Glycogen phosphorylase (choice D) is the enzyme responsible for the phosphorolytic removal of glucose units from glycogen. Homogentisic acid oxidase (choice E) is an enzyme involved in the pathway of tyrosine catabolism. A defect in this enzyme leads to the disorder known as alkaptonuria.

299. **(C)** When glycolysis (a cytoplasmic pathway) is proceeding under anaerobic conditions, the electrons transferred to NAD^+ (generating NADH) during the glyceraldehyde-3-phosphate dehydrogenase (G3PDH) catalyzed step cannot be transferred to mitochondrial NADH nor $FADH_2$, which would regenerate cytoplasmic NAD^+ levels. This would lead to a deficiency in the NAD^+ required by G3PDH and an eventual cessation of glycolysis. Therefore, under anaerobic conditions, tissues such as skeletal muscle reduce pyruvate (the end product of anaerobic glycolysis) to lactate catalyzed by lactate dehydrogenase (LDH). This reaction requires electrons to be donated from NADH and thereby regenerate NAD^+, which can be used by G3PDH. If pyruvate dehydrogenase (choice E) were to utilize any NAD in the oxidation of pyruvate to acetyl-CoA, there would be reduced levels available for G3PDH and glycolysis would cease, hence pyruvate is reduced by LDH. The citric acid cycle enzymes, α-ketoglutarate dehydrogenase (choice B) and malate dehydrogenase (choice D) require NAD^+, as well as being found in the mitochondria, and therefore would not be able to supply glycolysis with NAD^+. Although there is a cytoplasmic malate dehydrogenase and glycerol-3-phos-

phate dehydrogenase (choice A) is cytoplasmic, these enzymes are involved in the transfer of cytoplasmic electrons from NADH into the mitochondria, a process that is restricted by the lack of O_2 during anaerobic metabolism.

300. (A) Pyruvate dehydrogenase (PDH) activity is regulated both allosterically and by the state of phosphorylation. When phosphorylated the activity of PDH is reduced. The PDH kinase is associated with the PDH complex and is itself regulated by allosteric factors. High activity of PDH is observed under conditions of reduced energy charge to supply the TCA cycle with acetyl-CoA. As the level of ATP rises, the rate of flux through the TCA cycle begins to decline, leading to a buildup of acetyl-CoA. The increased acetyl-CoA in turn allosterically activates the PDH kinase, leading to an increased level of phosphorylation of PDH and a concomitant decline in its activity. Cyclic AMP (choice C) and AMP (choice B) have no effect on the activity of PDH kinase. Both NAD^+ (choice E) and coenzyme A (choice D) are negative regulators of the activity of PDH kinase.

301. (B) The eIF-2 cycle consists of the translation initiation factors, eIF-2A and eIF-2B (also called guanine nucleotide exchange factor, GEF). The cycle involves the binding of GTP by eIF-2A, forming a complex that then interacts with the initiator methionyl-tRNA. When the initiator methionyl-tRNA is placed into the correct position of the 40S ribosomal subunit, the GTP is hydrolyzed to provide the energy necessary to correctly position the incoming mRNA such that the initiator AUG codon and the initiator methionyl-tRNA anticodon are aligned. To regenerate an active eIF-2A for subsequent translation initiation events, the GDP must be exchanged for GTP. The exchange reaction is catalyzed by eIF-2B (GEF). The initiation factor, eIF-1 (choice A) facilitates the correct positioning of the initiator methionyl-tRNA and the mRNA. eIF-3 (choice C) binds to the 40S ribosomal subunit and acts as a ribosome anti-association factor. This interaction is necessary to induce disso-

ciation of the 40S and 60S subunits following completion of translation. Factor eIF-4A (choice D) binds to the mRNA and is required to "melt" any secondary structure that may exist at the 5'-end of the mRNA. Factor eIF-4F (choice E) binds to the cap structure that is added posttranscriptionally to all mRNAs.

302. (E) The process of attenuation in bacteria is a mechanism that controls the rate of transcription of specific RNAs through a coupled interaction between the processes of transcription and translation. A typical example is the regulation of the *trp* operon, the gene cluster responsible for tryptophan biosynthesis in *Escherichia coli*. The *trp* RNA contains an attenuator region, which is composed of sequences found within the transcribed RNA. The attenuator region of sequences of the RNA are found near the 5'-end of the RNA, termed the leader region of the RNA. The leader sequences are located prior to the start of the coding region for the first gene of the operon (the *trpE* gene). The attenuator region contains codons for a small leader polypeptide that contains tandem tryptophan codons. This region of the RNA is also capable of forming several different stable stem loop structures. Depending on the level of tryptophan in the cell, and hence the level of charged trp-tRNAs, the position of ribosomes on the leader polypeptide and the rate at which they are translating allows different stem loops to form. If tryptophan is abundant, the ribosome prevents a particular stem loop from forming and favors formation of another. The latter is found near a region rich in uracil and acts as the transcriptional terminator loop. Consequently, RNA polymerase is dislodged from the template. Because the process of attenuation couples transcription and translation it is not possible for eukaryotic cells to utilize this regulatory scheme; these two processes are separated by the nuclear membrane. Modification of the 5'-end of eukaryotic mRNAs (choice B), intron removal (choice C), and the monocistronic nature of eukaryotic mRNAs (choice A) would not have any impact on the ability of attenuation to occur in eukaryotes, nor would the level of charged tRNAs (choice D).

303. **(C)** Porphyrin (primarily from the iron-free protion of heme of red blood cells) is degraded and yields bilirubin (see Figure 3–10), a product that is nonpolar and therefore insoluble. Bilirubin, not generated in the liver, is transported to the liver in the plasma bound to albumin. In hepatocytes, bilirubin is solubilized by conjugation to glucuronate. The soluble conjugated bilirubin diglucuronide is then secreted into the bile. An inability to conjugate bilirubin, for instance in hepatic disease or when the level of bilirubin production exceeds the capacity of the liver, is a contributory cause of jaundice. Although bilirubin is transported in the plasma bound to albumin (choice A) it is not excreted this way. Bilirubin does not bind to any of the other molecules (choices B, D, and E).

304. **(C)** Porphyria cutanea tarda (PCT) is the most common porphyria. Symptoms of PCT include cutaneous involvement and liver abnormalities. Cutaneous features include chronic blistering lesions on sun-exposed skin. These lesions lead to skin thickening, scarring, and calcification. Symptoms usually develop in adults and are exacerbated by excess hepatic iron, alcohol consumption, and induction of cytochrome P_{450} enzymes as occurs in smokers. Symptoms of acute intermittent porphyria (AIP) (choice A) usually appear after puberty and are more common in women than in men. The majority of AIP carriers (> 80%) do not exhibit symptoms; those that do, manifest intermittent neurologic complications with no cutaneous photosensitivity. Hereditary coproporphyria (HCP) (choice B) has clinical features and precipitating factors that are essentially identical to those of AIP with the addition of occasional skin photosensitivity. Variegate porphyria (VP) (choice D) symptoms are also very similar to those of AIP and HCP, but photosensitivity is more common than in HCP. X-linked sideroblastic anemia (choice E) is due to a defect in erythoid-specific porphyrin synthesis. The reduction in heme synthesis in affected individuals leads to ineffective erythropoiesis. This results in nonferritin iron accumulation in the mitochondria of erythroblasts giving rise to the characteristic ring sideroblasts.

305. **(E)** PCT results from a decrease in the activity of uroporphyrinogen decarboxylase (UROD). Deficiencies in δ-aminolevulinic acid dehydratase (ALAD) (choice A) lead to δ-aminolevulinic acid dehydratase porphyria (ADP). Deficiencies in coproporphyrinogen oxidase (CPO) (choice B) lead to hereditary coproporphyria. Ferrochelatase (choice C) is the enzyme that inserts the iron atom into protoporphyrin IX generating heme b. Deficiencies in ferrochelatase are the cause of erythropoietic protoporphyria (EPP). Deficiencies in porphobilinogen deaminase (PBGD) (choice D) result in acute intermittent porphyria, the most common acute hepatic porphyria.

306. **(E)** Glucagon is released from the pancreas in response to low blood glucose and stimulates hepatocytes to synthesize glucose for delivery to the blood. Therefore, it would be counterproductive for hepatocytes to divert any of the gluconeogenically derived glucose into glycogen. This is accomplished by inhibition of glycogen synthase. Glucagon exerts its effects on the liver through the glucagon receptor. When glucagon binds, the receptor activates adenylate cyclase leading to increased production of cAMP. In turn, cAMP activates cAMP-dependent protein kinase (PKA), which then phosphorylates a number of substrates. Glucagon has no effect on the level of phosphoprotein phosphatase (choice A). One of the substrates of PKA is glycogen synthase/phosphorylase kinase. Therefore, there would not be a decrease in the level of phosphorylated phosphorylase kinase (choice B). In turn, synthase/phosphorylase kinase phosphorylates glycogen phosphorylase and glycogen synthase. Therefore, there is no increase in the level of dephosphorylated glycogen synthase (choice D). The effects of phosphorylation on glycogen synthase activity are inhibitory and on phosphorylase activating. In

addition PKA itself can phosphorylate glycogen synthase. The net effect is an increase in the rate of glucose phosphorolysis from glycogen and a reduced incorporation of glucose into glycogen. An additional PKA substrate is phosphoprotein phosphatase inhibitor-1, and therefore there would not be a decrease in the level of the phosphorylated form of this enzyme (choice C).

307. **(A)** In the genetic disorder known as Tay–Sachs disease, ganglioside GM_2 is not catabolized. As a consequence, the ganglioside concentration is elevated many times higher than normal. The functionally absent lysosomal enzyme is β-N-acetylhexosaminidase. The elevated GM_2 results in irreversible brain damage to infants, who usually die before the age of 3 years. Under normal conditions, this enzyme cleaves N-acetylgalactosamine from the oligosaccharide chain of this complex sphingolipid, allowing further catabolism to occur. The cause of most lipidoses (lipid storage diseases) is similar. That is, a defect in catabolism of gangliosides causes abnormal accumulation. None of the other choices (B, C, D, and E) result in glycosphingolipidoses such as is characteristic of Tay–Sachs disease.

308. **(A)** In fasting or diabetes, lipolysis predominates in adipocytes because of the inability of these cells to obtain glucose, which is normally used as a source of glycerol 3-phosphate. Glycerol 3-phosphate is necessary for the esterification of fatty acids into triacylglycerides. Circulating fatty acids become the predominant fuel source, and β-oxidation in the liver becomes substantially elevated. This leads to an increased production of acetyl-CoA. Although gluconeogenesis is increased (choice E) in the liver as a result of the persistent elevation of glucagon levels, this pathway does not supply acetyl-CoA for the production of ketone bodies. The increased gluconeogenesis predisposes oxaloacetate and reduces (not increases, choice B) the flow of acetyl-CoA through the citric acid cycle. As a consequence, acetyl-CoA is diverted to

the formation of ketone bodies. The persistently elevated levels of glucagon also increase the levels of cAMP in responsive tissues, such as adipocytes (choice C). This effect in adipocytes leads to persistently increased release of fatty acids to the circulation. Because skeletal muscle lacks receptors for glucagon, there is no diabetes-mediated increase in muscle metabolism, and thus no elevation in acetyl-CoA levels in skeletal muscle (choice D).

309. **(D)** Fragile X syndrome is the most common form of inherited mental retardation. The symptoms of this disorder are caused by a disruption in the FMR1 gene. The disruption occurs as a result of the expansion of a trinucleotide repeat sequence in the 5′ untranslated region of the FMR1 gene. The severity of mental retardation in fragile X syndrome is proportional to the level of expansion of the trinucleotide repeat. Copper accumulation leading to Kayser–Fleisher rings in the eyes (choice A) is indicative of Wilson disease which results from impaired biliary copper excretion. The symptoms of hypoketotic hypoglycemia and metabolic acidosis (choice B) are indicative of glutaric acidemia type II, which results from deficiencies in mitochondrial ubiquinone oxidoreductase. Isovaleric acidemia (choice C) is a severe neonatal disorder resulting from a deficiency in one of the enzymes of branched-chain amino acid metabolism, isovaleryl-CoA dehydrogenase. Accumulation of abnormally high levels of very long chain fatty acids and defects in myelin formation (choice E) are symptoms associated with X-linked adrenoleukodystrophy (X-ALD).

310. **(C)** An individual with a normal profile of hemoglobin would have the largest percentage in the form of HbA reflecting normal expression from the α- and β-globin genes. All individuals carry a small percentage (1% to 2%) of the fetal form, HbF, and the form that contains the δ-globin chains in place of the β-globin of HbA. This latter hemoglobin is termed HbA_2. The increase in the level of the

fetal hemoglobin in this patient, along with the presence of a reduced level of the adult form, indicates that there is a defect in the ability to express normal levels of the β-globin genes. This would be due to a promoter defect in the β-globin gene. A complete deletion of the α-globin locus (choice A) leads to the condition known as hydrops fetalis and is incompatible with life. Complete loss of the β-globin genes (choice B) results in the condition referred to as β⁰-thalassemia and there would be no HbA present in the blood. Nonsense mutations in the α-globin (choice D) or β-globin (choice E) genes would result in phenotypes similar to those of gene deletions at these loci.

311. **(D)** Ketogenesis occurs in the liver from acetyl-CoA during high rates of fatty acid oxidation and during early starvation. The principal ketone bodies are acetoacetate and β-hydroxybutyrate, which are reversibly synthesized in a reaction catalyzed by β-hydroxybutyrate dehydrogenase. The liver delivers β-hydroxybutyrate to the circulation where it is taken up by nonhepatic tissue for use as an oxidizable fuel. The brain derives much of its energy from ketone body oxidation during fasting and starvation. Within extrahepatic tissues, β-hydroxybutyrate is converted to acetoacetate by β-hydroxybutyrate dehydrogenase. Acetoacetate is reactivated to acetoacetyl-CoA in a reaction catalyzed by succinyl-CoA-acetoacetate-CoA-transferase (also called acetoacetate:succinyl-CoA CoA transferase), which uses succinyl-CoA as the source of CoA. This enzyme is not present in hepatocytes. The acetoacetyl-CoA is then converted to 2 moles of acetyl-CoA by the thiolase reaction of fatty acid oxidation. Each of the other enzyme choices (A, B, C, and E) are found within hepatocytes.

312. **(C)** There are three hallmark symptoms associated with disorders in enzymes of the urea cycle. These are hyperammonemia, encephalopathy, and respiratory alkalosis. Thus, elevated serum ammonia is not, in and of itself, indicative of a specific defect in the urea cy-

cle. An analysis of the levels of various amino and organic acids in the plasma and urine is the primary key to determining which defect led to the elevation in serum ammonia. Deficiency in ornithine transcarbamoylase (OTC) results in elevations in urine orotic acid in addition to serum ammonia. A distinction between deficiencies in urea cycle enzymes in the absence of knowledge of inheritance patterns (because OTC deficiency is the only X-linked urea cycle disorder) can be made by analysis of specific amino acid levels in the serum. Deficiency in arginase leads to elevated serum arginine as well as ammonia. In addition, arginine, lysine, and ornithine are elevated in the urine. Deficiency in argininosuccinate lyase is distinguishable by elevation in plasma argininosuccinate. Deficiency in argininosuccinate synthetase results in plasma and urine citrulline levels 100 to 500 times normal. This disorder is also called citrullinemia for obvious reasons. Because citrulline is a byproduct of the carbamoylphosphate synthetase I (CPS I) (choice A) and OTC, defects in either of these enzymes would lead to undetectable levels of citrulline. To distinguish defects in these two enzymes one needs to analyze the urine level of orotic acid. As indicated, a deficiency in OTC leads to elevations in urine orotate, whereas in CPS I deficiency, there is little urinary output of orotate. Methylmalonic acidemia (choice B) can result from deficiencies in several different enzymes associated with methylmalonyl-CoA metabolism, including methylmalonyl-CoA mutase and methylmalonyl- CoA racemase or defects in the synthesis of adenosylcobalamin. Affected individuals experience severe methylmalonic acidemia but not hyperammonemia. Propionic acidemia (choice D) is another disorder of organic acid metabolism and is due to deficiencies in propionyl-CoA carboxylase. Major symptoms include propionic acidemia and ketotic hyperglycemia but not hyperammonemia. Reye syndrome (choice E) is characterized by fatty liver, hyperammonemia, and hypoglycemia. The onset of this disorder has been associated with aspirin intake after a viral infection. Only choices A and C are disorders that appear severe in the first day after birth. Both are associated with severe hyperammonemia, but can be distinguished by plasma organic acid analysis as indicated.

313. **(B)** In the treatment of urea cycle defects, in particular deficiency in OTC, it is most important to reduce the level of ammonia. This can be accomplished by reducing protein in the diet, administration of compounds to reduce the level of ammonia, and administration of urea cycle intermediates that are missing due to enzyme defects. Phenylbutyrate reduces ammonia levels by interaction with glutamine forming phenylacetylglutamine. This prevents the release of ammonia from glutamine. Administration of levulose reduces ammonia through its action of acidifying the colon. Bacteria metabolize levulose to acidic byproducts, which then promote excretion of ammonia in the feces as ammonium ions (NH_4^+) (choice A). Administration of sodium benzoate reduces ammonia by complexing with glycine (choice C). Antibiotics can be administered to kill intestinal ammonia-producing bacteria (choice D).

314. **(E)** RNA tumor viruses have been shown to induce cancer in cells by several mechanisms. One mechanism is related to the insertion of the viral genome into the host genome during the life cycle of the virus. The viral sequences contain strong transcriptional promoter elements that, if inserted near a growth-control gene, can lead to enhanced, or unregulated, expression of the gene, which can lead to the transformed phenotype. None of the other choices (A, B, C, and D) represent viable mechanisms for virus-mediated cellular transformation.

315. **(E)** Any patient who exhibits mucocutaneous bleeding but possessing a normal platelet count should be suspected of having von Willebrand disease (vWD). Because factor VIII binds to von Willebrand factor (vWF) and is thus stabilized by this interaction, loss or reduction in vWF will lead to reduction in the circulating levels of factor VIII. Factor IX

deficiency (choice A) is the cause of hemophilia B, which is characterized by prolonged coagulation times. Disorders in fibrinogen (choice B) include afibrinogenemia (a complete lack of fibrinogen), hypofibrinogenemia (reduced levels of fibrinogen), and dysfibrinogenemia (presence of dysfunctional fibrinogen). Afibrinogenemia is characterized by neonatal umbilical cord hemorrhage, ecchymoses, mucosal hemorrhage, internal hemorrhage, and recurrent abortion. Hypofibrinogenemia is characterized by fibrinogen levels ≤ 100 mg/dL (normal, 250 to 350 mg/dL). Symptoms of hypofibrinogememia are similar to, but less severe than, afibrinogenemia. Dysfibrinogenemias are extremely heterogeneous, affecting any of the functional properties of fibrinogen. Clinical consequences of dysfibrinogenemias include hemorrhage, spontaneous abortion, and thromboembolism. Deficiencies in thrombin (choice C) are extremely rare and bleeding complications include gingival hemorrhage, menorrhagia, and postoperative hemorrhage. Tissue factor (choice E) is the only coagulation factor for which a congenital defect has not been identified.

316. **(E)** Cyanide causes a rapid inhibition of the mitochondrial electron transport chain at the cytochrome oxidase step, which constitutes complex IV of this process. Complex IV is composed of three atoms of copper and the hemes of cytochromes a and a_3. Cyanide binds to the Fe^3 in the heme of the cytochromes preventing oxygen from reacting with them. None of the other complexes or coenzymes (choices A, B, C, and D) are sites for cyanide interaction.

317. **(D)** LDLs are the primary carriers of blood cholesterol. Routine plasma lipid measurements are carried out after a 12-hr fast. In this way, the major endogenous plasma lipoproteins, VLDLs (choice E), and the major exogenous plasma lipoproteins (chylomicrons, choice A) have been cleared from the blood of normal individuals. LDLs, which are the end products of VLDL delipidation, and HDLs (choice B), which are protein rich, are the only lipoproteins circulating after a 12-hr

fast. LDLs are rich in cholesterol, being composed of about 45% cholesterol or cholesterol esters. In both dietary and familial hypercholesterolemia, circulating LDL levels are increased. IDLs (choice C) represent an intermediate in the pathway of delipidation of VLDLs, and their concentration would be minimal following a 12-hr fast.

318. **(A)** The urea cycle associated enzyme, N-acetylglutamate synthase, is allosterically regulated by the urea cycle intermediate arginine. None of the other urea cycle intermediates (choice B, C, D, and E) have any effect on N-acetylglutamate activity.

319. **(C)** Urea is the molecule humans use to excrete ammonia as a waste product of metabolism. Urea contains 2 moles of nitrogen and is synthesized in the urea cycle (see Figure 3–11). One mole of nitrogen is incorporated from free ammonia, the other is contributed from aspartate and is incorporated into citrulline to form argininosuccinate. Each of the other choices (A, B, D, and E) represent compounds that are intermediates in the urea cycle but that do not contribute nitrogen into urea and, therefore, do not serve as sources of waste nitrogen.

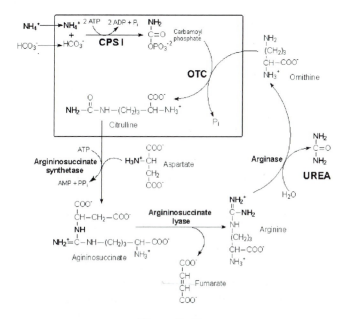

Figure 3–11

320. **(A)** Enzymes that are targeted to the lysosomes undergo a specific two-step modification in the Golgi complex. The first step in the modification involves the attachment of an α-N-acetylglucosamine 1-phosphate residue to the six position of a mannose residue on the high mannose carbohydrate portion of lysosomal enzymes. The second step involves removal of the N-acetylglucosamine residue exposing the mannose 6-phosphate marker. The presence of mannose 6-phosphate is necessary for targeting lysosomal enzyme to the lysosomes and deficiencies in the enzyme responsible for the first reaction in the modification lead to severe developmental abnormalities. Carboxylation of glutamate residues (choice B) is necessary to the function of several enzymes of the coagulation cascades. Lysosomal enzymes are not modified by attachment of carbohydrate though O-linkage (choice C). Many membrane-anchored proteins undergo lipid modification by prenylation (choice D) such as the protein product of the proto-oncogene *Ras*. Although many enzymes are activated by proteolytic processing (choice E), this is not required for targeting lysosomal enzymes to the lysosome.

321. **(C)** As electrons flow through the various carrier proteins of the oxidative-phosphorylation chain, protons are pumped out of the inner mitochondrial space into the outer mitochondrial space (between the inner and outer mitochondrial membranes). This leads to a chemiosmotic (electrochemical) potential difference across the inner mitochondrial membrane. This electrochemical potential difference is what drives the activity of the membrane-associated ATP synthase to phosphorylate ADP yielding ATP. ATP export (choice A) from the mitochondria is not coupled to ATP synthesis and is the function of ATP/ADP translocate (also called adenine nucleotide transporter). ATP synthase is a complex of proteins embedded in the inner mitochondrial membrane, not as a soluble complex inside the matrix (choice B). Oligomycin (choice D) binds to ATP synthase and inhibits the passage of protons through

ATP synthase, not the export of ATP. Transport of electrons through the complexes of oxidative-phosphorylation is coupled to the generation of a high concentration of H^+ outside the inner mitochondrial membrane, not a low concentration (choice E).

322. **(D)** Deficiency in carbamoylphosphate synthetase I (CPS I) results in severe hyperammonemia in the neonate. In this disorder there is no to trace level of citrulline in the plasma and extremely low levels of orotic acid in the urine. A distinction between deficiencies in urea cycle enzymes in infants with hyperammonemia can be made by analysis of specific amino and organic acid levels in the serum and urine. Deficiency in arginase (choice A) leads to elevated serum arginine as well as ammonia. In addition, arginine, lysine, and ornithine are elevated in the urine. Deficiency in argininosuccinate lyase (choice B) is distinguishable by elevation in plasma argininosuccinate. Deficiency in argininosuccinate synthetase (choice C) results in plasma and urine citulline levels 100 to 500 times normal. This disorder is also called citrullinemia for obvious reasons. Because citrulline is a byproduct of CPS I and ornithine transcarbamoylase, OTC (choice E) defects in either of these enzymes leads to undetectable levels of citrulline. To distinguish defects in these two enzymes, one needs to analyze the urine level of orotic acid. A deficiency in OTC leads to elevations in urine orotate, whereas in CPS I deficiency there is little urinary output of orotate.

323. **(A)** Farber's lipogranulomatosis is characterized by painful and progressively deformed joints and progressive hoarseness due to involvement of the larynx. Subcutaneous nodules form near the joints and over pressure points. Granulomatous lesions form in these tissues and there is an accumulation of lipid-laden macrophages. Significant accumulation of ceramide and gangliosides is observed, particularly in the liver. If these compounds accumulate in nervous tissue, there may be moderate nervous dysfunction. The illness often leads to death within the first few years of life, although milder forms of the disease have been identified. Fucosidosis (choice B) is characterized by the accumulation and excretion of glycoproteins, glycolipids, and oligosaccharides containing fucoside moieties. Symptoms of fucosidosis include psychomotor retardation, dystosis multiplex (a term referring to multiple skeletal abnormalities), growth retardation, and coarse facial features. Gaucher disease (choice C) is characterized by an accumulation of glucosylceramide (glucocerebroside). Several forms of the disease have been identified and vary in severity. Typical symptoms include hepatosplenomegaly, bone lesions, and central nervous system involvement. Occasionally the lungs and other organs may be involved. Metachromic leukodystrophy (choice D) is a disorder of myelin metabolism. It is characterized by the accumulation of galactosyl sulfatide (cerebroside sulfate). Symptoms may appear at any age and include mental regression, urinary incontinence, blindness, loss of speech, peripheral neuropathy, and seizures. Sandhoff–Jatzkewitz disease (choice E) is a disorder related to Tay–Sachs disease. It is characterized by a defect in the degradation of GM2 gangliosides with symptoms of severe mental retardation, blindness, and early mortality.

324. **(A)** Farber's lipogranulomatosis results from the defective function of acid ceramidase. Three biochemical pathways have been identified for the synthesis of ceramides: (1) a brain-specific ceramide synthetase; (2) microsomal synthesis from fatty acyl-CoA derivatives and sphingosine; and (3) the reversal of the reaction catalyzed by ceramidases (enzymes responsible for the degradation of ceramide). Acid ceramidase catalyzes the conversion of ceramides to sphingosine and a fatty acid. Arylsulfatase A deficiency leads to metachromic leukodystrophy (choice B). Deficiency in galactocerebrosidase (choice C) results in Krabbe disease (also termed globoid leukodystrophy). Tay–Sachs disease results from a deficiency in hexosaminidase A (choice D). Sphingomyelinase (choice E) deficiencies lead to Niemann–Pick disease.

325. **(D)** Translational initiation begins with the formation of the preinitiation complex. This complex is formed by interaction a binary complex of GTP and the initiation factor eIF-2 with the activated initiator tRNA, met-tRNA^met forming a ternary complex. The ternary complex then binds to the small ribosomal (40S) subunit forming the preinitiation complex. An incoming mRNA then associates with the preinitiation complex. The cap-binding factor eIF-4F (choice A) is necessary for mRNAs to be engaged by the preinitiation complex but does not facilitate recognition of the initiator AUG codon by met-tRNA^met. Alignment of the initiator met-tRNA^met over the initiator AUG codon does not occur randomly (choice B) but requires the interaction of the specific initiation factor eIF-1. Cap-binding factor eIF-4F (choice C) is necessary for interaction of mRNAs with the preinitiation complex but are not responsible for alignment of the initiator tRNA over the initiating AUG. The latter event requires initiation factor eIF-1 as indicated. Eukaryotic translation does not utilize a formylmethionine-tRNA (choice E) for initiation; this is a function of the prokaryotic translational machinery.

326. **(D)** The binding of acetylcholine to its receptor at the neuromuscular junction results in depolarization of the muscle membrane. This event triggers the release of calcium ions from the sarcoplasmic reticulum. The increase in intracellular calcium concentration leads to many changes in enzyme activity. One effect of calcium is that it is bound by various calcium-regulated binding proteins. One of the subunits of glycogen phosphorylase kinase is calmodulin, a calcium-binding protein. The interaction of calcium with calmodulin alters the conformation of calmodulin, which leads to an activation of glycogen phosphorylase kinase activity in the absence of phosphorylation. The activity of glycogen phosphorylase kinase is increased not decreased (choice A) by calcium interaction with calmodulin present in the enzyme complex. Increases in intracellular calcium (as in response to acetylcholine binding at the neuromuscular junction) do not affect the level of phosphorylation of glycogen phosphorylase kinase (choices B and E) nor does it affect the activity of phosphoprotein phosphatase (choice C).

327. **(B)** Numerous severe disorders are associated with the inability to properly degrade the complex carbohydrate moieties of glycosaminoglycans, proteoglycans, and glycoproteins. These disorders fall into a broad category of diseases termed the lysosomal storage diseases. Several of the lysosomal storage diseases result in hepatosplenomegaly, renal dysfunction, and skeletal defects, and therefore these symptoms are not diagnostic in themselves of a particular lysosomal storage disease, but only indicative of such disorders. However, disorders such as Niemann–Pick disease (choice D) and Tay–Sachs disease (choice E) are of such severity that early childhood mortality occurs and thus would not present in a 42-year-old patient. It is necessary to evaluate enzyme function in skin fibroblasts or white cells of the blood. Gaucher disease is caused by a defect in glucocerebrosidase activity and hence an assayable decrease in the activity of this enzyme would be diagnostic of this disease. Fabry disease (choice A) results from a defect in α-galactosidase A. Niemann–Pick disease (choice D) results from a defect in sphingomyelinase. Tay–Sachs disease (choice E) results from a defect in hexosaminidase A. Krabbe disease (choice C) results from a defect in galactocerebrosidase.

328. **(B)** The biochemical deficiency of the enzyme HGPRT results in mental retardation and compulsive self-destructive behavior seen in Lesch–Nyhan syndrome. This X-linked recessive disease also results in gout because of elevated levels of urate. However, unlike gout alone, allopurinol treatment of patients with Lesch–Nyhan syndrome does not increase the rate of synthesis of purines because it does not lower the level of PRPP. In genetically normal individuals, HGPRT allows the salvage synthesis of guanosine 5′-monophosphate (GMP) or inosine 5′-monophosphate (IMP) from guanine or hypoxanthine plus PRPP, thus there is less catabolism of these nucleotides to uric acid and gout symptoms do not occur. None of the other alterations in nucleotide metabolic pathways listed (choices C, D, and E) lead to disease states. Allopurinol (choice A) works principally to inhibit xanthine oxidase–mediated catabolism of xanthine to urate.

329. **(D)** When the carbons of fatty acids are oxidized for energy production, the byproduct of that process is the two-carbon compound, acetyl-CoA. Acetyl-CoA can then enter the TCA cycle for complete oxidation. Although several compounds of the TCA cycle can be directed into the gluconeogenic pathway of glucose synthesis the carbons of acetyl-CoA cannot provide a net source of carbon in that latter pathway. This is due to the fact that, following entry of the two carbons of acetyl-CoA into the TCA cycle, two carbons are lost as CO_2 during the subsequent reactions of the cycle. The subcellular compartmentalization of fat oxidation and gluconeogenesis (choice A) has no bearing on net carbon deposition into glucose. Anabolic and catabolic reactions (choice B) are always occurring concurrently in cells but at different rates dependent on cellular status. The site of fat storage (choice C) has no bearing on net incorporation of carbon into glucose. Acetyl-CoA does not inhibit conversion of pyruvate to oxaloacetate (choice E) but acts as an allosteric activator of pyruvate carboxylase, a gluconeogenic enzyme.

330. **(C)** Marfan syndrome results in cardiovascular, musculoskeletal, and ophthalmic abnormalities as a result of a defect in the fibrillin gene. Fibrillin is a structural protein of the 10-nm microfibrils of cells. This class of microfibrils is primarily associated with amorphous elastin and is thought to serve at least three functions: linking elastin to other matrix structures, serving as scaffolds for elastin deposition, and performing structural functions in tissues lacking elastin. Osteogenesis imperfects (OI) (choice E) consists of a group of at least four types (mild, extensive, severe, and variable). Symptoms of OI arise due to defects in two α-collagen genes, the COL1A1 and COL1A2 genes. There have been over

100 mutations identified in these two genes. The mutations lead to decreased expression of collagen or abnormal proα1 proteins. The abnormal proteins associate with normal collagen subunits, which prevents the triple helical structure of normal collagen from forming. The result is degradation of all the collagen proteins both normal and abnormal. Cutis laxa (choice A) is a disorder affecting connective tissue either through defective elastin metabolism or collagen metabolism. The latter mechanism is due to poor copper distribution as in occipital horn syndrome. However, cutis laxa is not X-linked as is occipital horn syndrome. Occipital horn syndrome (choice D), a disorder that manifests with symptoms similar to cutis laxa, results from defects in copper metabolism. The molecular basis for Ehlers–Danlos syndrome (choice B), which comprises at least 10 defined types of related symptoms, is heterogeneous. These related disorders are due to either defects in type III collagen metabolism, lysyl hydroxylation, or N-terminal procollagen protease.

331. **(D)** The synthesis of AMP from IMP and the salvage of IMP via AMP catabolism have the net effect of deaminating aspartate to fumarate. This process has been termed the purine nucleotide cycle and is very important in muscle cells. Increases in muscle activity create a demand for an increase in the TCA cycle, to generate more NADH for the production of ATP. However, muscle lacks most of the enzymes of the major anapleurotic reactions. Muscle replenishes TCA cycle intermediates in the form of fumarate generated by the purine nucleotide cycle. There is no HGPRT or ADA cycle; thus, choices A and B do not represent valid options. Choices C and E constitute pathways that do not involve nucleotides.

332. **(C)** The process of proofreading during DNA replication serves to ensure that the incorporation of mismatched nucleotides is corrected before the polymerase holoenzyme complex continues to move along the template strand. Proofreading involves a 3′ to 5′

exonuclease activity of the polymerase holoenzyme. This activity serves to remove a newly incorporated nucleotide that does not form a normal Watson-Crick base pair with the template strand of DNA. The ability to proofread cannot take place after DNA synthesis is complete (choice A), does occur in both prokaryotes and eukaryotes (choice B), is dependent on polymerase activity (choice D), and does not require an enzyme activity separate from the holoenzyme (choice E).

333. **(B)** Glutathione peroxidase is an enzyme involved in the protection of cells, particularly erythrocytes, from damaging peroxides. The enzyme utilizes 2 moles of glutathione (GSH) in a reaction that reduces hydrogen peroxide (H_2O_2) to 2 moles of H_2O and generates oxidized glutathione (GSSG). Subsequently, glutathione reductase reduces GSSG to 2 moles of GSH, utilizing NADPH as the electron donor. Alcohol dehydrogenase (choice A) catalyzes the reduction of ethanol to acetaldehyde. Heme oxygenase (choice C) is required in the metabolism of heme to bilirubin (Figure 3–10). HMG-CoA reductase (choice D) is the rate-limiting enzyme of cholesterol biosynthesis. Phosphoenolpyruvate carboxykinase (choice E) is a gluconeogenic enzyme involved in the GTP-dependent decarboxylation of oxaloacetate to phosphoenolpyruvate.

334. **(D)** The formation of glycosylated hemoglobin occurs spontaneously (i.e., nonenzymatically through a reaction known as the Amadori rearrangement) in red blood cells. The amino terminal groups of the β-chains of hemoglobin complex with the aldehyde groups of glucose to form an amino ketone linkage. This form of hemoglobin is known as HbA_{1c}. Measurement of the circulating level of glycosylated hemoglobin is a diagnostic tool used to determine the relative length of hyperglycemia and can be used as a measure of treatment effectiveness. Glucose does not form covalent bonds with any of the other choices (A, B, C, and E).

335. **(C)** Patients with hereditary fructose intolerance have defective function in hepatic fruc-

tose-1-phosphate aldolase (also called aldolase B). This enzyme hydrolyzes fructose-1-phosphate to glyceraldehyde and dihydroxyacetone phosphate. The reaction is the second in the hepatic pathway of fructose metabolism, the initial one being the phosphorylation of fructose at the 1 position by fructokinase (choice B). When fructose is high in the diet (as in the consumption of large quantities of fruit), the capability of diverting the fructose into the glycolytic pathway is severely impaired. Fructose becomes trapped in the liver as fructose-1-phosphate. Due to the lack of aldolase B, the capacity to phosphorylate fructose becomes limiting due to feedback inhibition of fructokinase, resulting in an elevation in serum fructose levels. Hepatic glucokinase (choice E) and aldolase A (choice D) are not involved in the metabolism of fructose. An allergic reaction (choice A) would not manifest with elevated serum fructose, hyperbilirubinemia, or hyperlacticacidemia.

336. **(C)** Fructose enters the liver and is phosphorylated to fructose-1-phosphate by fructokinase. This reaction requires ATP. The inability to further metabolize fructose in patients lacking aldolase B essentially traps hepatic energy in the form of fructose-1-phosphate. Gluconeogenesis requires a large input of energy and is severely impaired by the trapping of phosphate energy in fructose. Because lactate is a major gluconeogenic substrate, the impaired ability to carry out gluconeogenesis leads to hyperlacticacidemia. In the absence of aldolase B, fructose is not metabolized by pyruvate; therefore, one would not have elevated levels of pyruvate (choice E). A vitamin insufficiency capable of leading to an inhibition of pyruvate dehydrogenase (choice D) requires a longer period of development than that seen in the patient. Additionally, symptoms would be more characteristic of beriberi, reflecting a niacin deficiency (choice A), than those of hyperbilirubinemia and hyperlacticacidemia. As indicated in the answer to Question 335, an allergic reaction (choice A) would not lead to the symptoms observed.

337. (C) Stem cells are defined as cells that have the capacity for self-renewal and multilineage differentiation. This means that when stem cells divide, the progeny that result are composed of two distinct populations instead of two identical daughter cells. The consequence of stem cell division is a multipotent progenitor and another self-renewable stem cell. Stem cells have been isolated from numerous locations including the early embryo (embryonic stem cells), from umbilical vein, and from adult tissues. Stem cells from adults have been isolated from several tissues, not only from the hematopoietic system (choice A). Stem cells derived from adult tissues have a somewhat limited yet wide utility (choice B) for differentiation into numerous cell types and are not restricted to the lineage of the tissue from which they were isolated (choice D). Stem cells have near unlimited potential for self-renewal in culture (choice E).

338. (D) In infants, the supply of glycogen lasts less than 6 hours and gluconeogenesis is not sufficient to maintain adequate blood glucose levels. Normally, during periods of fasting (in particular during the night) the oxidation of fatty acids provides the necessary ATP to fuel hepatic gluconeogenesis as well as ketone bodies for nonhepatic tissue energy production. In patients with MCAD deficiency there is a drastically reduced capacity to oxidize fatty acids. This leads to an increase in glucose utilization with concomitant hypoglycemia. The deficit in the energy production from fatty acid oxidation, necessary for the liver to use other carbon sources, such as glycerol and amino acids, for gluconeogenesis further exacerbates the hypoglycemia. Normally, hypoglycemia is accompanied by an increase in ketone formation from the increased oxidation of fatty acids. In MCAD deficiency there is a reduced level of fatty acid oxidation and thus near-normal levels of ketones are detected in the serum. None of the other choices (A, B, C, and E) reflect symptoms related in any way to MCAD deficiency and are not in themselves indicative of any specific disorder per se.

339. (E) One mechanism by which initiation of translation in eukaryotes is effected is by phosphorylation of a ser(S) residue in the α subunit of eIF-2. The factor eIF-2 requires activation by interaction with GTP. The energy of GTP hydrolysis is used during translational initiation, thereby allowing eIF-2 to have GDP bound instead of GTP. To reactivate eIF-2, the GDP must be exchanged for GTP. This requires an additional protein of the guanine-nucleotide exchange factor (GEF) family known as eIF-2B. The phosphorylated form of eIF-2, in the absence of the eIF-2B, is just as active an initiator of translation as the nonphosphorylated form. However, when eIF-2 is phosphorylated, the GDP-bound complex is stabilized and exchange for GTP is inhibited. When eIF-2 is phosphorylated it binds eIF-2B more tightly thus slowing the rate of exchange. It is this inhibited exchange that affects the rate of initiation. Within reticulocytes the phosphorylation of eIF-2 is the result of an activity called heme-controlled inhibitor (HCI) (Figure 3–12). The presence of HCI was first seen in an *in vitro* translation system derived from lysates of reticulocytes. When heme is limiting, it is a waste of energy for reticulocytes to make globin protein because active hemoglobin cannot be generated. Therefore, when the level of heme falls, HCI becomes activated, leading to the phosphorylation of eIF-2 and reduced globin synthesis. Removal of phosphate is catalyzed by

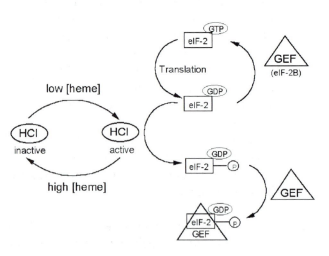

Figure 3–12

a specific eIF-2 phosphatase, which is unaffected by heme. There is no heme-controlled phosphatase activity (choice A) in any cell. No tRNA-specific degrading enzymes (choice B) are present in cells. There is no effect of heme levels on peptidyltransferase activity (choice C) or RNA polymerase activity (choice D).

340. **(C)** Defects in methylmalonyl-CoA mutase activity comprise four distinct genotypes whose clinical symptoms are remarkably similar. Characteristic findings in methylmalonyl-CoA mutase deficiency include failure to thrive leading to developmental abnormalities, recurrent vomiting, respiratory distress, hepatomegaly and muscular hypotonia. In addition, patients have severely elevated levels of methylmalonic acid in the blood and urine. Unaffected individuals have nearly undetectable levels of methylmalonate in their plasma, whereas, affected individuals have been found to have levels ranging from 3 to 40 mg/dL in their blood. Deficiency in α-ketoacid dehydrogenase (choice A) results in maple syrup urine disease, so named because of the characteristic odor of the urine in afflicted individuals. Mental retardation in maple syrup urine disease is extensive. Deficiency in homogentisic acid oxidase (choice B) results in alkaptonuria. Alkaptonuria results from the accumulation of homogentisic acid, a byproduct of tyrosine catabolism, in the urine and tissues. Oxidation of homogentisate in the urine causes it to turn dark and in the tissues results in ochronosis, which refers to the ochre color of the deposits in connective tissue, bones, and other organs. Deficiency in phenylalanine hydroxylase (choice D) results in phenylketonuria (PKU), which results in severe mental retardation if not detected and treated properly. Deficiency in tyrosine aminotransferase (choice E) results in eye, skin, and neurologic symptomology. The neurologic symptoms are similar to those seen in PKU.

341. **(C)** Deficiency in medium-chain acyl-CoA dehydrogenase (MCAD) is the most common inherited defect in the pathways of mitochondrial fatty acid oxidation. The most common presentation of infants with this disorder is episodic hypoketotic hypoglycemia following periods of fasting. Although the first episode may be fatal, and incorrectly ascribed to sudden infant death syndrome, patients with MCAD deficiency are normal between episodes and are treated by avoidance of fasting and treatment of acute episodes with intravenous glucose. Accumulation of acylcarnitines (dicarboxylic acids) is diagnostic, in particular octanoylcarnitine. Glutaric acidemia type II (choice A) results from a defect in electron transfer of flavoprotein-ubiquinone oxidoreductase and presents with symptoms of hypoketotic hypoglycemia as in the case of MCAD deficiency. However, this disorder manifests within the first 24 to 48 hours after birth and is frequently associated with congenital anomalies. Lesch–Nyhan syndrome (choice B) results from a defect in hypoxanthine-guanine phosphoribosyltransferase (HGPRT), an enzyme involved in nucleotide metabolism. Symptoms of Lesch–Nyhan syndrome include hyperuricemia, bizarre neurobehavioral manifestations, growth retardation, and anemia. Deficiency in pyruvate dehydrogenase (choice D) results in lactic acidemia, which can be quite severe at birth leading to neonatal fatality. Milder deficiency results in lactic acidemia associated with profound psychomotor retardation. Cori disease (choice E) results from a defect in the glycogen debranching enzymes. Clinical features include hepatomegaly, hypoglycemia, skeletal myopathy, short stature, and cardiomyopathy.

342. **(D)** Two familial syndromes directly involve defects in LCAT. Familial LCAT deficiency is characterized by near complete absence of the enzyme activity from the plasma. Fish eye disease is characterized by an absence of LCAT activity toward high-density lipoproteins (HDLs), but presence of activity toward low-density lipoproteins (LDLs). Clinical features of familial LCAT deficiency include corneal opacities, anemia, and proteinuria. Due to the lack of LCAT activity, the plasma level of esterified cholesterol is lower than

normal and phosphatidylcholine (the principal source of fatty acid for esterification to cholesterol) levels are higher than normal. The profile of all classes of plasma lipoproteins in patients with familial LCAT deficiency is abnormal. Bassen–Kornzweig syndrome (choice A), also identified as abetalipoproteinemia, is due to a defect in apo-B expression. Clinical symptoms include retinitis pigmentosa, ataxic neuropathy, and thorn-appearing erythrocytes (acanthocytosis). Familial hypercholesterolemia (choice B) is characterized by reduced LDL clearance, which leads to severe hypercholesterolemia. Major clinical symptoms are arterial deposition of LDL cholesterol which leads to atherosclerosis and coronary artery disease. Deposition of LDL cholesterol is also seen in tendons and skin resulting in xanthomas. Familial hypertriacylglycerolemia (choice C), also identified as hyperlipoproteinemia type IV, is a form of lipoprotein lipase deficiency. The defect leads to increased levels of circulating VLDLs and is associated with glucose intolerance and hyperinsulinemia. This disorder is frequently associated with type II diabetes. Wolman disease (choice E) is cholesterol ester storage disease that leads to massive accumulation of cholesteryl esters and triglycerides in most tissues. This disease is almost always fatal within the first year of life and thus would not be present in a 28-year-old patient.

343. **(A)** Several proteins of the clotting cascade are posttranslationally modified by a vitamin K–dependent reaction that incorporates carboxy groups onto the R-groups of intrachain glutamates generating γ-carboxyglutamate residues (gla residues). Proteins of the cascade so modified include prothrombin, factors VII, IX, and X, as well as protein S. The incorporation of gla residues is absolutely required for biological activity of these factors. The gla residues allow the clotting factors to chelate calcium ions. Because the carboxylation reaction requires vitamin K, agents that competitively block vitamin K action, such as warfarin and dicumarol, act as anticoagulants. Hydroxyproline (choice C) and hydroxy-

lysine (choice B) are found in the collagens. Many proteins are phosphorylated and this occurs primarily at serine residues (choice E). Acetylation of N-terminal residues of proteins is a common posttranslational modification, and if this occurred when methionine remained as the N-terminal amino acid, N-acetylmethionine would be seen (choice D).

344. **(A)** Enzymes that are destined for the lysosomes (lysosomal enzymes) are directed there by a specific carbohydrate modification. During transit through the Golgi apparatus a residue of N-acetylglucosamine-1-phosphate is added to carbon 6 of one or more specific mannose residues that have been incorporated into these enzymes. The N-acetylglucosamine is activated by coupling to UDP, and is transferred by an N-acetylglucosamine phosphotransferase, yielding N-acetylglucosamine-1-phosphate-6-mannose-protein. A second reaction removes the N-acetylglucosamine, leaving mannose residues phosphorylated in the 6 position. A specific mannose-6-phosphate receptor is present in the membranes of the Golgi apparatus. Binding of mannose-6-phosphate to this receptor targets proteins to the lysosomes. Defects in the proper targeting of glycoproteins to the lysosomes can also lead to clinical complications. Deficiencies in N-acetylglucosamine phosphotransferase lead to the formation of dense inclusion bodies in fibroblasts. Two disorders related to deficiencies in the targeting of lysosomal enzymes are termed I-cell disease (mucolipidosis II) and pseudo-Hurler polydystrophy (mucolipidosis III). I-cell disease is characterized by severe psychomotor retardation, skeletal abnormalities, coarse facial features, painful restricted joint movement, and early mortality. Pseudo-Hurler polydystrophy is less severe; it progresses more slowly, and afflicted individuals live to adulthood. Each of the other choices (B, C, D, and E) represent other potential pathways that are not affected in the processing, delivery, or presentation of lysosomal enzymes or the receptors that recognize the properly processed enzymes.

345. **(B)** Although multiorgan involvement, liver and spleen enlargement, and skeletal abnormalities are common to all the mucopolysaccharidotic (MPS) diseases, each encompasses features that allow for specific diagnosis. Hurler syndrome is characterized by progressive multiorgan failure and premature death. Hallmark features include enlargement of the spleen and liver, severe skeletal deformity, and coarse facial features (which are associated with the constellation of defects referred to as dystosis multiplex). The disease results from a defect in α-L-iduronidase activity, which leads to intracellular accumulations of heparan sulfates and dermatan sulfates. The accumulation of these GAGs in patients with Hurler syndrome severely affects development of the skeletal system leading, primarily, to defective long bone growth plate disruption. Hunter syndrome (choice A) has features similar to those of Hurler with a lack of corneal clouding. Additionally, symptoms progress more slowly, with onset of symptoms occurring between 2 and 4 years of age. Maroteaux–Lamy syndrome (choice C) encompasses symptoms similar to Hurler syndrome but with normal mental development. Morquio syndrome (choice D) comprises two related disorders, both of which are characterized by short-trunk dwarfism, fine corneal deposits, and a skeletal dysplasia (spondyloepiphyseal) distinct from other MPS. Sanfilippo syndrome (choice E) comprises four recognized types characterized by severe central nervous system degeneration with only mild involvement of other organ systems. Symptoms do not appear until 2 to 6 years of age.

346. **(E)** Type I diabetes results from the autoimmune destruction of the β-cells of the pancreas. The result is that patients can no longer produce and secrete insulin; thus, the disease is also referred to as insulin-dependent diabetes mellitus (IDDM). Patients with IDDM can be treated with injections of insulin indicating that receptor-mediated responses are normal and not due to decreased binding of insulin by the insulin receptor (choice A). The responses of the body to glucagon in a person

with IDDM are unaffected by loss of insulin production (choice B). Secretion of glucagon is actually increased, not decreased (choice C) in IDDM patients. Because IDDM is caused by a loss of insulin production, there could be no increased secretion (choice D).

347. **(D)** β-Endorphin is the only protein derived from the POMC gene. The POMC gene encodes an mRNA that can be processed to yield at least eight separate proteins with distinct activities. Several act as hormones (adrenocorticotropic hormone [ACTH], β- and γ-lipotropins, α- and β-melanocyte-stimulating hormones [MSH], and corticotropin-like intermediary peptide [CLIP]); others serve as neurotransmitters or neuromodulators (β-endorphin and met-enkephalin). The location of expression of the POMC gene dictates which of the biologically active proteins are made. Atrial natriuretic factor (choice A) is produced in the atria of the heart. Bradykinin (choice B) is derived from a plasma glycoprotein identified as high molecular weight (HMW) kininogen through the action of active plasma kallikrein. Cholecystokinin (choice C) is an intestinal peptide hormone. Oxytocin (choice E) is derived from prepro-oxytocin, a protein that is processed into oxytocin and neurophysin I.

348. **(D)** Deficiency in α-keto acid dehydrogenase leads to maple syrup urine disease, named because the odor of urine from patients resembles that of maple syrup or burnt sugar. Plasma levels of leucine, isoleucine, valine, and their α-keto acids are elevated. The defect is evident within the first week following birth. Diagnosis prior to this time is only possible by enzymatic analysis. Extensive brain damage results and infants die within the first year. Alkaptonuria (choice A) is characterized by the darkening, upon exposure to air, of urine from afflicted individuals. Homocystinurias (choice B) are defects in methionine catabolism, evidenced by elevated levels of homocysteine in the urine. Clinical symptoms include thromboses, osteoporosis, and frequently mental retardation. As the name implies, isovaleric acidemia (choice C) is elevated serum levels of isovaleric acid, a byproduct of leucine catabolism. Symptoms are evident following ingestion of protein-rich foods. Phenylketonuria (PKU) (choice E) is characterized by excess production of alternative catabolites of phenylalanine (phenylpyruvate), phenylacetate, and phenyllactate. This disorder leads to mental retardation if left untreated. Routine neonatal screening for PKU is now compulsory.

349. **(C)** Heparin is a naturally occurring sulfated glycosaminoglycan (GAG) that plays an important role in the regulation of blood coagulation. It is found primarily in granules of mast cells and released when these cells are stimulated. Heparan sulfates present on the surfaces of vascular endothelial cells also have limited antithrombic activity. Heparin binds to the major thrombin inhibitor, antithrombin III, resulting in an altered conformation of antithrombin III. The altered conformation has a higher affinity for thrombin (as well as for the activated forms of factors IX, X, XI, and XII) resulting in a reduced capacity of thrombin to convert fibrinogen to fibrin. In addition to cartilage, chondroitin sulfates (choice A) are found in bone and heart valves. Dermatan sulfates (choice B) are found in skin, heart valves, and vessels. Hyaluronate (choice D) predominates in synovial fluid and vitreous humor. Keratan sulfate (choice E) is found in cornea and bone and in aggregates with chondroitin sulfates in cartilage. None of these GAGs exhibit antithrombic activity.

350. **(B)** Gout is characterized by elevated levels of uric acid in the blood and urine. Uric acid is the end product of purine catabolism and excess production results from a variety of metabolic abnormalities that lead to overproduction of purines via the de novo pathway. Uric acid is very insoluble and when generated in large amounts precipitates as uric acid crystals in the joints of the extremities and in renal interstitial tissue. These deposits are gritty or sandy in nature and thus are termed tophaceous deposits. Adenosine deaminase (choice A) and purine nucleotide phosphorylase (choice D) deficiencies result

in various degrees of immune dysfunction and are not associated with gouty episodes. Lesch–Nyhan disease (choice C) is due to loss of hypoxanthine–guanine phosphoribosyltransferase activity. Characteristic symptoms include severe mental retardation and self-mutilation. A much less severe symptom associated with Lesch–Nyhan disease is hyperuricemia, which leads to gouty episodes. However, other symptoms are of such severity that patients die very early in life. Deficiency in glucose-6-phosphatase results in von Gierke disease (choice E). Clinical symptoms include fasting hypoglycemia, lactic acidemia, and mild gouty episodes. The hyperuricemia of von Gierke disease is seldom severe enough to lead to the level of gouty deposits observed in this patient.

351. **(A)** The first reaction of *de novo* pyrimidine biosynthesis is catalyzed by aspartate transcarbamoylase. This reaction is also the rate-limiting step in this pathway. OMP decarboxylase (choice B) catalyzes the decarboxylation of OMP, yielding UMP. PRPP amido transferase (choice C) is an enzyme of the *de novo* purine biosynthesis pathway. PRPP synthetase (choice D) catalyzes the production of PRPP (used in the synthesis of purines and pyrimidines) from ribose-5-phosphate and ATP. Ribonucleotide reductase (choice E) is required for the reduction of ribonucleotides to deoxyribonucleotides.

352. **(A)** Nitric oxide (NO) is generated from arginine in a reaction catalyzed by NO synthase (NOS). The other product of the reaction is citrulline. None of the other amino acids (choices B, C, D and E) are substrates for NOS.

353. **(C)** Calcitriol [1,25-$(OH)_2$-D] is the hormonally active form of vitamin D and functions in concert with parathyroid hormone (PTH) and calcitonin to regulate serum calcium and phosphorous levels. The major function of calcitriol is the induction of synthesis of an intestinal calcium-binding protein, calbinden, which facilitates intestinal absorption of calcium. Oral administration of calcitriol increases intestinal calcium uptake, but the hor-

mone does not enter the peripheral circulation in significant amounts. Therefore, patients with renal osteodystrophy may need intravenous administration of calcitriol. Antidiuretic hormone (choice A) is responsible for renal water readsorption in response to increased extracellular Na^+ concentrations which lead to increased plasma osmolarity. Calcitonin (choice B) acts to block bone resorption when there are sufficient levels of calcium in the serum. Growth hormone (choice D) does not influence calcium homeostasis and is therefore not useful in the treatment of renal osteodystrophy. PTH (choice E) acts to increase bone resorption, in concert with calcitriol, when serum calcium levels fall.

354. **(A)** Primary aldosteronism (Conn syndrome) leads to elevated production of aldosterone and the symptoms presented by the patient. This disorder is due to small adenomas of the glomerulosa cells of the kidney. The associated hyperkalemia, hypertension, and hypernatremia lead to a reduction in renin release from the juxtaglomerulosa cells. Renin is required for the conversion of angiotensinogen (released from the liver) to angiotensin I (which is in turn converted to angiotensin II by converting enzyme), and so reduced levels of renin lead to reduced levels of angiotensin II. Androstenedione (choice B) is produced from pregnenolone via the 17α-hydroxylase pathway of androgen synthesis in the adrenal cortex or of estrogen synthesis in the ovary. Androstenedione is derived from DHEA (choice C) and is converted to estradiol (choice D) in the ovary or to testosterone (choice E) in the testis. Estrogens are responsible for maturation of the ovaries and testosterone for maturation of sperm. None of these steroids regulate sodium or potassium and therefore do not lead to the symptoms presented if elevated or reduced.

355. **(E)** Tyrosine is the precursor for each of these neurotransmitters. Tyrosine hydroxylase converts tyrosine to dopa, which is in turn converted to dopamine, then to norepinephrine, and finally epinephrine. None of the other amino acids (choices A, B, C, and

D) can serve as precursors for these neurotransmitters.

356. **(E)** Prolactin is necessary for initiation and maintenance of lactation. Physiologic levels act only on breast tissue primed by female sex hormones. Endocrine dysfunction leading to excessive prolactin production is associated with breast enlargement and impotence in males. Excessive production of corticotropin-releasing hormone (choice A) results in an increase in ACTH production, which leads to enhanced glucocorticoid and mineralocorticoid production. Excessive production of gonadotropin-releasing hormone (choice B) leads to increased production of luteinizing hormone (LH), follicle-stimulating hormone (FSH), and chorionic gonadotropin (hCG), with consequent effects on the female reproductive system. Excessive production of growth hormone (choice C) leads to gigantism if it occurs prior to epiphyseal plate closure. If excessive release occurs following epiphyseal plate closure acromegaly results, with characteristic facial changes (protruding jaw, enlarged nose) and enlarged feet, hands, and skull. Excessive production of melanocyte-stimulating hormone (choice D) would lead to hyperpigmentation of the skin.

357. **(D)** Huntington disease (HD) is an autosomal dominant disorder leading to progressive memory loss, personality changes, and peculiar motor problems such as involuntary movements of the arms and legs. The disease results from the expansion of a CAG triplet in the amino terminus of the HD protein, referred to as huntingtin. The repeats number from 10 to 30 in normal chromosomes and from 36 to 121 on the HD chromosomes. There is a general correlation between the length of the repeat and the age of onset of symptoms. Cystic fibrosis (CF) (choice A) is due primarily to a common mutation (in 70% of cases) that deletes three nucleotides in exon 10 of the CF gene, which codes for the CF transmembrane conductance receptor (CFTR). Over 600 other mutations have been identified in the CF gene. Duchenne muscular dystrophy (DMD) (choice B) results from

deletions in one or more of the exons of the DMD gene that encodes the protein referred to as dystrophin. Familial hypercholesterolemia (choice C) results from defects in the gene encoding the LDL receptor. These defects encompass insertions and deletions that can be found throughout the length of the LDL receptor gene. Menkes disease (choice E) is due to defects in copper absorption leading to defective function of numerous enzymes that need copper as a cofactor.

358. **(C)** The rate-limiting step in glycolysis occurs at the reaction catalyzed by phosphofructokinase-1 (PFK-1). This enzyme catalyzes the phosphorylation of fructose 6-phosphate to fructose 1,6-bisphosphate. PFK-1 is controlled by numerous allosteric effectors that act in either a positive or negative manner. The reaction depicted by choice A is catalyzed by glucokinase/hexokinase. This reaction is regulated by product inhibition, but does not constitute a rate-limiting step in glycolysis. The reactions catalyzed by phosphoglucose isomerase (choice B), fructose-1,6-bisphosphate aldolase or aldolase A (choice D), and triose phosphate isomerase (choice E) are freely reversible and are therefore not regulated reactions of glycolysis.

359. **(A)** Adenosine deaminase (ADA) catalyzes the deamination of adenosine to inosine during the catabolism of purines. Loss of ADA leads to significantly elevated levels of phosphorylated deoxyadenosine (in particular deoxyadenosine triphosphate [dATP]). Levels of dATP in ADA deficiency can reach 50 times normal. High concentrations of dATP inhibit ribonucleotide reductase, which is required for the generation of deoxynucleotides from ribonucleotides. The inhibition of ribonucleotide reductase leads to severely impaired cellular DNA synthesis. Because lymphocytes must be able to proliferate dramatically in response to antigenic challenge, the loss of ADA activity results in a near complete lack of immune function. Aspartate transcarbamoylase (ATC) (choice B) is a component of a multifunctional enzyme that catalyzes the rate-limiting reaction of pyrimidine biosyn-

thesis. No known deficiencies in this enzyme have been identified, likely due to the embryonic lethality predicted if the enzyme were defective. Hypoxanthine–guanine phosphoribosyl transferase (HGPRT) (choice C) catalyzes the salvage of hypoxanthine to IMP and guanine to GMP. Deficiency in HGPRT results in Lesch–Nyhan syndrome. Orotic acid decarboxylase (choice D) catalyzes the decarboxylation of OMP to UMP. Deficiency in this enzyme results in type II orotic aciduria. Purine nucleoside phosphorylase (PNP) (choice E) is also a purine catabolic enzyme that converts inosine to hypoxanthine and guanosine to guanine. Deficiency in PNP leads to a mild immunodeficiency.

360. **(E)** DNA fingerprinting refers to the process of using polymorphic repeat sequences to establish a unique pattern of DNA fragments for any given individual. The polymorphic repeats that are identifiable by the fingerprinting technique are hypervariable repeats such as variable number tandem repeats (VNTRs). The bands are detected by Southern blotting enzyme-digested chromosomal DNA and probing the blot with various different VNTR probes. The generation of a DNA library (choice A) refers to the establishment of a complete collection of cloned fragments of DNA, either from genomic sources or cDNA. DNA footprinting (choice B) refers to the identification of sequences of DNA to which specific proteins bind, thereby rendering the DNA at that site resistant to digestion by DNA-degrading nucleases. Hybridization (choice C) refers to the specific association of complimentary strands of DNA to one another. The PCR technique (choice D) uses synthetic oligonucleotides to direct the enzymatic amplification of specific sequences of DNA.

361. **(D)** Regulation of HMG-CoA reductase (the rate-limiting enzyme of cholesterol biosynthesis) activity is complex and involves a number of distinct enzyme activities. Because cholesterol biosynthesis consumes large amounts of energy it needs to be regulated in response to energy demands, particularly in hepatocytes. The principal site for the action of the hypo-

glycemic response hormone, glucagon, is the liver. Glucagon binding to hepatocytes triggers the liver to stop catabolizing carbohydrate and to divert carbon atoms into the gluconeogenesis pathway. This change in hepatic metabolism, in response to glucagon, comes about through a change in the phosphorylation state of numerous enzymes. One of these enzymes is HMG-CoA reductase. HMG-CoA reductase is most active when in the nonphosphorylated state. The enzyme is phosphorylated and rendered less active through the action of AMP-regulated kinase. AMP levels rise as the energy charge in the cell declines and thus the cell is able to recognize this change, at the level of HMG-CoA reductase activity, by inducing its phosphorylation and inhibition. To reverse the effect of HMG-CoA phosphorylation the phosphates must be removed. This occurs through the action of HMG-CoA reductase phosphatase. HMG-CoA reductase phosphatase is regulated through the action of protein phosphatase inhibitor-1 (PPI-1). In turn the activity of PPI-1 is regulated by its state of phosphorylation; it is more active when phosphorylated. When glucagon binds to hepatocytes the result is a glucagon receptor-mediated activation of adenylate cyclase, which in turn produces cAMP from ATP. The effect of cAMP is to activate cAMP-dependent protein kinase (PKA), which then phosphorylates a number of substrates. With respect to glucagon-mediated regulation of cholesterol metabolism, PKA phosphorylates PPI-1. Phosphorylated PPI-1 is more active at inhibiting HMG-CoA reductase phosphatase so that the removal of phosphate from HMG-CoA reductase is inhibited. This keeps HMG-CoA reductase in the phosphorylated and less active state. AMP-regulated kinase is not affected by glucagon-mediated increases in the levels of cAMP (choice A). Although glucogon action leads to an increase in PKA activity, the latter enzyme does not itself phosphorylate HMG-CoA reductase (choice B). The activity of AMP-regulated kinase is affected by its level of phosphorylation but it is not phosphorylated by PKA (choice C). Cyclic AMP itself does not have a direct effect on HMG-CoA reductase (choice E).

362. **(C)** The *de novo* synthesis of triacylglycerols in adipocytes from free fatty acids and glycerol requires that glycerol first be phosphorylated to glycerol 3-phosphate through the action of glycerol kinase. Glyceraldehyde-3-phosphate dehydrogenase (choice A) is an enzyme of glycolysis/gluconeogenesis and does not participate in the initial step triacylglyceride synthesis. Glycerol-3-phosphate dehydrogenase (choice B) is responsible for the interconversion of glycerol 3-phosphate and dihydroxyacetone phosphate. Hormone-sensitive lipase (choice D) is the adipocyte enzyme responsible for the hydrolysis of stored triacylglycerols in response to hormone signals. Lipoprotein lipase (choice E) is the enzyme present on the surface of vessel endothelial cells necessary for the hydrolysis of fatty acids from triacylglycerols carried by lipoprotein particles.

363. **(E)** Zellweger syndrome is the most severe of a group of diseases that result from defective assembly of the peroxisomes, leading to the characteristic symptoms observed in the patient. This syndrome is apparent at birth and leads to death within the first year. The cause of Zellweger syndrome is a failure to import newly synthesized peroxisomal proteins into peroxisomes. Hyperpipecolic acidemia (choice A), infantile Refsum disease (choice B), and neonatal adrenoleukodystrophy (choice C) are all much less severe disorders of the group that result from peroxisome dysfunction. Affected individuals with these disorders can survive into the third or fourth decade, albeit with deficits in vision, hearing, and cognitive function. It is suspected that the reduced severity of these three disorders, relative to Zellweger, relates to retention of partial gene function as opposed to complete loss. RCDP (choice D) is related to peroxisomal dysfunction at the level of their distribution and structure. The phenotype of RCDP differs from that of Zellweger syndrome in that patients have striking shortening of the proximal limbs, coronal clefts of vertebral bodies, and severely abnormal endochondrial bone formation.

364. **(B)** Apoprotein B-48 is found exclusively associated with chylomicrons and no other

lipoprotein particle. apo-B-48 is synthesized from an mRNA that is transcribed from the apo-B-100 gene. Following transcription the mRNA is edited within the intestinal epithelium yielding the B-48 transcript. apo(a) (choice A) is an apoprotein found disulfide bonded to apo-B-100. This then forms a complex with LDL, generating a novel lipoprotein particle identified as lipoprotein (a), Lp (a). Lp(a) has a strong resemblance to plasminogen and its presence in the circulation is highly correlated with premature coronary artery disease. apo-C-II (choice C) is present in chylomicrons, VLDLs, LDLs, IDLs, and HDLs and is necessary for the activation of endothelial cell lipoprotein lipase. apo-D (choice D) is found exclusively with HDLs and is also associated with cholesterol ester transfer protein (CETP) activity. apo-E (choice E) is found in chylomicrons, VLDLs, LDLs, IDLs, and HDLs. It is necessary for interaction of lipoprotein with the LDL-receptor (which is also referred to as the apo-B-100/apo-E receptor).

365.   **(D)** The nonoxidative portion of the pentose phosphate pathway performs carbohydrate remodeling reaction, interconverting 3, 4, 5, 6, and 7 carbon sugars. Transaldolase catalyzes the interconversion of erythrose-4-phosphate and fructose-6-phosphate into glyceraldehyde-3-phosphate and sedoheptulose-7-phosphate. Ribulose-5-phosphate 3-epimerase (choice A) interconverts ribulose-5-phosphate and xylulose-5-phosphate. Ribose-5-phosphate ketoisomerase (choice B) catalyzes the interconversion of ribulose-5-phosphate and ribose-5-phosphate. Transketolase (choices C and E) catalyzes the interconversion of xylulose-5-phosphate and ribose-5-phosphate into sedoheptulose-7-phosphate and glyceraldehyde-3-phosphate, as well as the interconversion of xylulose-5-phosphate and erythrose-4-phosphate into glyceraldehyde-3-phosphate and fructose-6-phosphate.

366.   **(C)** Acromegaly results when there is an excess production of growth hormone after epiphyseal closure and cessation of long bone growth. Excessive production of cortico-

tropin-releasing hormone (choice A) would result in an increase in ACTH production, which leads to enhanced glucocorticoid and mineralocorticoid production. Excessive production of gonadotropin-releasing hormone (choice B) leads to increased production of luteinizing hormone (LH), follicle-stimulating hormone (FSH), and chorionic gonadotropin (hCG), with consequent effects on the female reproductive system. Excessive production of insulin-like growth factor II (choice D) could lead to abnormal neonatal development because it is expressed only during this period. Excessive production of thyroid-stimulating hormone (choice E) leads to increased release of the thyroid hormones, leading to multisystemic involvement such as rapid heart rate, nervousness, inability to sleep, weight loss, excessive sweating, and sensitivity to heat.

367.   **(E)** Transferrin is a glycoprotein synthesized in the liver having a central role in the body's metabolism of iron. Each mole of transferrin can transport 2 moles of Fe^{3+} in the circulation to sites where iron is required. Free iron is toxic, but when associated with transferrin this toxicity is greatly diminished. When bound to transferrin, iron can be directed to cells where it is needed. Many cells have transferrin receptors and upon binding, the transferrin–receptor complex is internalized. The acidic pH of the lysosome causes the iron to dissociate from transferrin. Iron-free transferrin is then recycled to the cell surface along with its receptor, where it then reenters the circulation. Ceruloplasmin (choice A) is the major copper carrier of the body and is also synthesized in the liver. Ferritin (choice B) is an intracellular iron-binding protein. It does not play a role in iron metabolism or transport, and its function is to prevent ionized iron (Fe^{2+}) from reaching toxic levels within cells. Haptoglobin (choice C) is a plasma glycoprotein that binds extracorpuscular (free) hemoglobin. This function of haptoglobin is to prevent free hemoglobin from being lost through the kidneys, because the haptoglobin-hemoglobin complex is too large to pass through the glomerulus. Metallothioneins (choice D) are found in many cells

and can bind copper, zinc, cadmium, and mercury.

368. **(B)** Signal transduction begins when a signal is received at the surface of cells. This signal is usually a protein that interacts with specific receptors in the plasma membrane. The signals are then transmitted through the receptor to numerous intracellular signaling proteins. One of the first classes of intracellular signaling proteins to be affected by activated receptors are proteins that bind and hydrolyze guanine nucleotides, specifically GTP. The ras protein is of this latter class; it binds GTP and in response to receptor activation, hydrolyzes the GTP to GDP and then transfers the activation signal to other proteins in the cascade. The ability of ras to hydrolyze GTP requires the activity of another protein class termed GTPase activating proteins (GAPs) (choice A). The steroid hormone receptor class of signaling molecules reside within the cytoplasm. Upon ligand binding these receptors enter the nucleus and bind to specific DNA sequence elements and effect changes in gene expression (choice C). Several classes signal transducing receptors have intrinsic enzymatic activity. These activities can be either serine/threonine kinase (choice D) or tyrosine kinases (choice E).

369. **(D)** Menkes disease is an X-linked recessive disorder that is manifest by a defect in copper absorption. This defect leads to dysfunction of numerous enzymes that need copper as a cofactor, leading to the typical symptoms observed in this patient. In fact, Menkes disease is also referred to as steely hair disease, because of the characteristic brittleness of the hair, which is easily broken. Crigler–Najjar syndrome type I (choice A) is also due to defective bilirubin metabolism as a result of a loss of UDP-glucuronosyltransferase (UGT) activity. UGT is required to transfer 2 moles of glucuronic acid to bilirubin, generating bilirubin–diglucuronide, which makes bilirubin much more water soluble and therefore facilitates its excretion. Crigler–Najjar syndrome results in nonhemolytic icterus (jaundice) within the first few days of life and is generally fatal during neonatal life due to severe kernicterus. Gilbert syndrome (choice B) results from a defect in bilirubin metabolism. It is typically diagnosed in young adults and is characterized by mild, chronic, and unconjugated hyperbilirubinemia without associated hemolysis. Hemochromatosis (choice C) is the term applied when organ structure and function are impaired by the presence of excess amounts of iron. The liver, heart, pancreas, skin, joints, and endocrine organs are the principal tissues affected by iron accumulation. Symptoms include cirrhosis, cardiomyopathy, arthritis, abnormal skin pigmentation, and hypogonadism, as well as diabetes mellitus. Refsum disease (choice E) results from a defect in the metabolism of phytanic acid, a plant lipid which must be oxidized by a separate pathway from that of animal fats. Cardinal symptoms include retinitis pigmentosa, peripheral neuropathy, and cerebellar ataxia.

370. **(A)** Porphobilinogen (PBG) deaminase (also referred to as uroporphyrinogen I synthase) catalyzes the conversion of four moles of porphobilinogen to hydroxymethylbilane. Porphobilinogen is the product of the δ-aminolevulinic acid (ALA) synthase. Therefore, a deficiency in PBG deaminase leads to an elevation in the excretion of ALA and PBG. All products of the heme biosynthesis pathway from porphobilinogen on are produced at extremely reduced levels due to a deficiency in PBG deaminase. These include a coproporphyrinogen III (choice B), which is produced from type III uroporphyrinogen, hydroxymethylbilane (choice C), and protoporphyrin IX (choice D), which is produced in several steps from coproporphyrinogen and type III uroporphyrinogen (choice E), which is produced from hydroxymethylbilane.

371. **(A)** Phosphorylase kinase (also referred to as phosphorylase/synthase kinase, because it can phosphorylate both glycogen phosphorylase and glycogen synthase) contains calmodulin as a subunit. The presence of calmodulin allows phosphorylase kinase to be activated in the absence of a cAMP-mediated phospho-

rylation cascade. This is important when muscle is stimulated by epinephrine binding to α-adrenergic receptors (this function is diagrammed in Figure 3–8) or by acetylcholine release at the neuromuscular junction. Each of these events leads to increases in intracellular Ca^2. Each of the other proteins (choices B, C, D, and E) are independent activities not associated with phosphorylase kinase.

372. **(E)** Turner syndrome is characterized by phenotypically normal females who are sexually immature and have gonadal dysgenesis and a host of somatic abnormalities. These symptoms arise due to chromosomal abnormalities in one of the X chromosomes as well as monosomy for the X chromosome. Only around 5% of monosomy X fetuses survive to birth. Some 15% of Turner syndrome females are mosaic for the karyotype 45,X:46,XX and another 15% are mosaic for a 45,X cell line plus a 46,X, abnormal X cell line or a 47,XXX cell line. Achondroplasia (choice A) is the single most common form of dwarfism and results from two specific defects in the gene encoding fibroblast growth factor receptor 3 (FGFR3). Symptoms of achondroplasia include rhizomelic short stature, midface hypoplasia, short ribs and trident hand. Duchenne muscular dystrophy (DMD) (choice B) is an X-linked condition whose symptoms occur in affected males in early childhood and only very rarely affects females. DMD is caused by defects in the dystrophin protein which is involved in the contractile apparatus of muscle cells. Fragile X syndrome (choice C) is the most common form of inherited mental retardation. The symptoms result from the loss of a portion of the X chromosome due to a site of fragility caused by the amplification of a trinucleotide repeat sequence in the FMR1 gene (*Fragile X Mental Retardation-1*). Symptoms of fragile X are most severe in males (affected females have much milder symptoms) and include severe mental retardation and facial abnormalities such as prominent jaw, forehead and ears. Kleinfelter syndrome (choice D) is associated with males harboring two or more X chromosomes (e.g. 47,XXY). Symptoms appear in puberty and affected individuals have a greater than expected frequency of social pathology. Although significant mental retardation is not associated with most Kleinfelter patients, the more X chromosomes and individual harbors the higher likelihood of mental retardation.

373. **(B)** The enzymes ferrochetalase and δ-aminolevulinic acid (ALA) synthetase are extremely sensitive to lead poisoning, which leads to severe anemia and excretion of high levels of coproporphyrinogen and ALA. None of the other enzymes (choices A, C, D, and E) of heme biosynthesis are affected by lead ingestion.

374. **(C)** Regulation of the pyruvate dehydrogenase (PDH) complex is effected by both allosteric means and by phosphorylation (Figure 3–13). Allosteric effectors of the enzyme complex are of both positive and negative type. The complex is phosphorylated by a specific kinase identified as PDH kinase and phosphate is removed by PDH phosphatase. When in the unphosphorylated state the complex is much more active; therefore, the activity of PDH phosphatase is important for maintaining the PDH complex in the active state. Acetyl-CoA (choice A) and NADH (choice D) are both allosteric inhibitors of the nonphosphorylated form of the PDH complex and also serve to activate PDH kinase leading to phosphorylated and inhibited PDH. Like acetyl-CoA and NADH, ATP

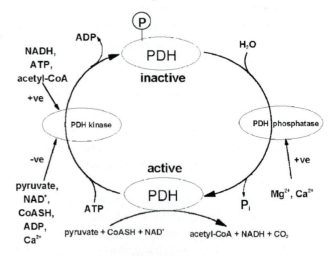

Figure 3–13

(choice B) allosterically activates the PDH kinase leading to phosphorylated and inhibited PDH. Phosphorylation (choice E) inhibits the activity of the PDH complex.

375. **(B)** Several enzymes of the blood clotting cascade (e.g., factors II, VII, IX, X, and protein C) bind calcium and are thus activated following cleavage of their zymogen forms. The ability of these proteins to bind calcium requires post-translationally modified glutamate residues. The modification is a γ-carboxylation yielding γ-carboxyglutamate (gla) residues. The carboxylation reaction has an absolute requirement for vitamin K as a cofactor. None of the other amino acid modifications (choices A, C, D, and E) requires vitamin K as a cofactor. Hydroxylation of proline (choice E) and lysine (choice C) is carried out by enzymes that require vitamin C as a cofactor.

376. **(D)** Steroid hormones are lipophilic and thus freely penetrate the plasma membrane of all cells. Within target cells, steroid hormones interact with specific receptors. These receptor proteins are composed of two domains; a hormone-binding domain and a DNA-binding domain. Following hormone–receptor interaction the complex is activated and enters the nucleus. The DNA-binding domain of the receptor interacts with specific nucleotide sequences termed hormone response elements (HREs). The binding of steroid–receptor complexes to HREs results in an altered rate of transcription of the associated gene(s). The effects of steroid–receptor complexes on specific target genes can be either stimulatory or inhibitory with respect to the rate of transcription. Complexes of steroid with receptor have no direct effect on posttranscriptional processing of RNA (choice A), posttranslational events (choice B), DNA replication (choice C), or translation (choice E).

377. **(D)** Krabbe disease is a rapidly progressing, invariably fatal disease of infancy whose symptoms begin around 3 months of age. The disease is also referred to as infantile globoid cell leukodystrophy. Earliest symptoms are neurologic in origin and progress to severe mental and motor deterioration; to decerebrate posturing, blindness, deafness; and ultimately death, often preceded by seizures. Farber lipogranulomatosis (choice A) is characterized by painful and progressively deformed joints and progressive hoarseness due to involvement of the larynx. Subcutaneous nodules form near the joints and over pressure points. Granulomatous lesions form in these tissues and there is an accumulation of lipid-laden macrophages. Significant accumulation of ceramide and gangliosides is observed, particularly in the liver. If these compounds accumulate in nervous tissue there may be moderate nervous dysfunction. The illness often leads to death within the first few years of life, although milder forms of the disease have been identified. Fucosidosis (choice B) is characterized by the accumulation and excretion of glycoproteins, glycolipids, and oligosaccharides containing fucoside moieties. Symptoms of fucosidosis include psychomotor retardation, dystosis multiplex (a term referring to multiple skeletal abnormalities), growth retardation, and coarse facial features. Three types of Gaucher disease (choice C) have been characterized and are caused by defects in lysosomal acid glucocerebrosidase. Defects in this enzyme lead to the accumulation of glucosylceramides (glucocerebrosides), which leads primarily to central nervous system dysfunction and also hepatosplenomegaly and skeletal lesions. Metachromic leukodystrophy (choice E) is a disorder of myelin metabolism. It is characterized by the accumulation of galactosyl sulfatide (cerebroside sulfate). Symptoms may appear at any age and include mental regression, urinary incontinence, blindness, loss of speech, peripheral neuropathy, and seizures.

378. **(D)** The enzyme deficiency in Krabbe disease is galactocerebrosidase. Deficiency in acid ceramidase (choice A) occurs in Farber lipogranulomatosis. Deficiency in arylsulfatase A (choice B) occurs in metachromic leukodystrophy. Deficiency in β-L-fucosidase (choice C) occurs in fucosidosis. Deficiency in gluco-

cerebrosidase (choice E) occurs in Gaucher disease.

379.   **(B)** Cystic fibrosis affects a number of organ systems including the lung and upper respiratory tract, liver, pancreas, and sweat glands. Classical symptoms of individuals with cystic fibrosis are chronic airway infection with *P. aeruginosa* and *Staphylococcus aureus*. Cystic fibrosis results from deficiencies in the gene encoding the cystic fibrosis transmembrane conductance regulator (CFTR). The protein encoded by this gene is a member of the ATP-binding cassette (ABC) transporter family of proteins. Although multiple organ systems are affected by defects in the CFTR gene, morbidity and mortality results primarily from impairment of the pulmonary defense system. Congenital adrenal hyperplasia (CAH) (choice A) is a group of diseases whose common features result from defects in the pathway leading to cortisol synthesis. The most frequent defects occur in the 21-hydroxylase gene (CYP21) that catalyzes the conversion of progesterone to 11-deoxycorticosterone and 17-hydroxyprogesterone to 11-deoxycortisol. Deficiency in CYP21 leads to loss of cortisol and aldosterone secretion and maximal secretion of the adrenal androgens. The effect on female development is masculinization of the external genitalia. Renal Fanconi syndrome (choice C) is acquired either through exposure to toxic agents or due to various inborn errors in metabolism that lead to generalized dysfunction of the proximal renal tubules. Affected individuals exhibit a characteristic vitamin D-deficient metabolic bone disease, polyuria, polydipsia, hypokalemia and acidosis. Sickle cell anemia (choice D) results from a mutation in the β-globin gene and is characterized by lifelong hemolytic anemia, an increased propensity to infection, and complications resulting from repeated vascular occlusions that result during cycling crises. Tay–Sachs disease (choice E) is a fatal disease of early childhood resulting from a deficiency in the hexosaminidase A enzyme. Hexosaminidase A is required for the catabolism of complex sphingolipids (G_{M2} ganglio-

sides) and defects in the enzyme lead to severe neurologic impairment.

380.   **(B)** Cystic fibrosis is one of the most common autosomal recessive disorders affecting white populations. The other choices (A, C, D, and E) are modes of inheritance not associated with cystic fibrosis.

381.   **(C)** The major substrates of gluconeogenesis are pyruvate and lactate. During gluconeogenesis lactate is oxidized to pyruvate. For pyruvate to be converted back to glucose, it must first be carboxylated to oxaloacetate; a reversal of the pyruvate kinase reaction of glycolysis cannot occur to convert the pyruvate to phosphoenolpyruvate. The carboxylation of pyruvate is catalyzed by the mitochondrial enzyme pyruvate carboxylase. The activity of pyruvate carboxylase absolutely depends on the presence of acetyl-CoA, which allosterically activates the enzyme. Of the enzymes listed, only pyruvate carboxylase and phosphoenolpyruvate carboxykinase (choice B) are involved in gluconeogenesis. Acetyl-CoA carboxylase (choice A) is involved in fatty acid synthesis and is not regulated by acetyl-CoA. Pyruvate dehydrogenase (choice D) is the entry point for pyruvate into the TCA cycle. It is also inhibited by acetyl-CoA via the acetyl-CoA–mediated activation of pyruvate dehydrogenase kinase, an enzyme that phosphorylates and inactivates pyruvate dehydrogenase. Pyruvate kinase (choice E) is a glycolytic enzyme and is inhibited by acetyl-CoA, not activated by it.

382.   **(C)** Carbonic anhydrase catalyzes the following reaction:

$$CO_2 + H_2O \leftrightarrow H_2CO_3$$

This reaction is freely reversible and proceeds in one direction or the other, depending on the relative partial pressures of CO_2 and O_2. In the lungs, where the partial pressure of O_2 is high, the O_2 leaves the alveoli and enters erythrocytes of the blood. There it is bound by hemoglobin for transport to the peripheral tissues. When O_2 is bound, hydrogen ions dissociate from hemoglobin and are titrated by bicarbonate ions to form carbonic acid (H_2CO_3). The increase in carbonic acid results in the carbonic anhydrase reaction proceeding to the right, relative to the equation above. The CO_2 thus formed flows out of the erythrocytes due to the relatively low partial pressure of CO_2 in the lungs. The CO_2 is then expelled from the lungs upon expiration. When erythrocytes enter the relatively high partial pressure of CO_2 in the tissues, the reverse process occurs, leading to release of the hemoglobin bound O_2. Carbamoylation of hemoglobin (choice A), ionization of carbonic acid (choice B), protonation of hemoglobin (choice D), and transport of chloride ion (choice E) all occur spontaneously, thus requiring no enzymes.

383. **(D)** Myotonic dystrophy is the most common muscular dystrophy affecting adults. Aside from the clinical manifestations of the disease described in the question, myotonic dystrophy affects cardiac and smooth muscle, and is associated with immune disorder, minor mental retardation, and cataracts. Myotonic dystrophy results from defects in the myotonin gene. These defects are associated with the expansion of a trinucleotide repeat sequence in the 3′-untranslated region of the gene. Becker muscular dystrophy (BMD) (choice A) and Duchenne muscular dystrophy (DMD) (choice B) both result from mutations in the DMD gene but the symptoms of BMD are milder than those of DMD. Transmission of these two diseases is X-linked. Marfan syndrome (choice C) and osteogenesis imperfecta (choice E) are disorders of connective tissue. Marfan syndrome results from defects in the fibrillin gene and osteogenesis imperfecta from defects in collagen. None of the other four diseases exhibits the inheritance phenomenon of anticipation.

384. **(D)** During strenuous physical exercise, the rate of production of pyruvate via glycolysis exceeds the capacity of the citric acid cycle to use it, and pyruvate accumulates. NADH also accumulates, and glycolysis cannot continue unless NAD^+ is regenerated. This is ac-

complished by the conversion of pyruvate to lactate by lactate dehydrogenase, which uses NADH as a cofactor and produces NAD^+. Pyruvate and lactate diffuse out of muscle into blood and are taken up by the liver, where lactate is converted to pyruvate, which is in turn converted to glucose. During strenuous (anaerobic) exercise), the NAD^+/NADH ratio is kept relatively constant through the linked activities of glyceraldehyde-3-phosphate dehydrogenase and lactate dehydrogenase, therefore NAD^+ (choice E) would not increase. As indicated, some pyruvate exits muscle cells and enters the blood, thus increasing (not decreasing) its relative concentration in that compartment (choice A). Anaerobic exercise inhibits the TCA cycle, so citrate would not accumulate (choice C). Exercise depletes the level of ATP, it does not increase it (choice B).

385. **(B)** Dietary triacylglycerols are hydrolyzed in the intestines by pancreatic lipase and pancreatic phospholipase A_2. The resultant free fatty acids and monoacylglycerols enter intestinal epithelial cells, where the triacylglycerols are reformed. These triacylglycerols are packaged into chylomicrons and delivered to the circulation via the lymphatic system. Chylomicrons are therefore the molecules produced by the body to deliver dietary triacylglycerols to the circulation. Albumin (choice A) does not transport triacylglycerols, but individual fatty acids. HDLs (choice C) are synthesized by the liver and intestine and are primarily involved in reverse cholesterol transport. LDLs (choice D) are by-products of intestinal VLDLs. VLDLs (choice E) are generated in the liver for transport of hepatic triacylglycerols to peripheral tissues.

386. **(B)** DNA footprinting is an analytical technique that takes advantage of the interaction of certain proteins with DNA. Many proteins interact with specific sequences of DNA (e.g., transcription factors) and these regions of protein-bound DNA are resistant to degradation by nucleases. The protected regions result in a "footprint" on the DNA when the radioactively labeled DNA is separately by

gel electrophoresis. The establishment of a complete collection of cloned DNA fragments (choice A) refers the technique of either cDNA or genomic DNA cloning. The association of complimentary strands of DNA with one another (choice C) is a process that is used for various nucleic acid hybridization assays. The polymerase chain reaction (choice D) uses oligonucleotide-directed enzymatic amplification of specific sequences of DNA. The human genome contains numerous types of repeated sequence elements (choice E) whose number varies from individual to individual. The phenomenon of variable numbers of tandem repeats (VNTRs) and an analysis of their numbers can be used in diagnosis.

387.   **(D)** Fatty acids are activated to the CoA derivatives at the outer mitochondrial membrane (catalyzed by enzyme 1 in Figure 3–9), but are oxidized inside the mitochondria. Long-chain fatty acyl-CoA molecules do not cross the mitochondrial membrane. A special transport system involving carnitine is used for movement of the activated fatty acids into the mitochondria. The fatty acyl moiety is transferred from the CoA to carnitine in a reaction catalyzed by carnitine acyltransferase I (enzyme 2 in Figure 3–9). Acyl carnitine thus formed is shuttled across the inner mitochondrial membrane (via enzyme 3 in Figure 3–9), where the fatty acyl group is transferred back to a CoA molecule within the mitochondrial matrix. The latter reaction is catalyzed by carnitine acyltransferase II (enzyme 4 in Figure 3–9). Medium-chain fatty acyl-CoAs can cross the mitochondrial membrane and do not require the carnitine transport system for entry into the mitochondria. The compound(s) at point A are ATP and CoA, point B is carnitine, point C is acylcarnitine, point D is carnitine, and E is acylcarnitine. Therefore, the requirements for carnitine occur on either side of the inner mitochondrial membrane at points B and D, which occur during the translocation process. All other combinations (choices A, B, C, and E) have a compound or compounds other than or in addition to carnitine.

388.   **(D)** Osteogenesis imperfecta consists of a group of at least four types (mild, extensive, severe, and variable). The disorder is characterized by brittle bones and abnormally thin sclerae, which appear blue owing to the lack of connective tissue. The symptoms arise due to defects in two α-collagen genes, the COL1A1 and COL1A2 genes. There have been over 100 mutations identified in these two genes. The mutations lead to decreased expression of collagen or abnormal proα1 proteins. The abnormal proteins associate with normal collagen subunits, which prevents the triple helical structure of normal collagen from forming. The result is degradation of all the collagen proteins, both normal and abnormal. Ehlers–Danlos syndrome (choice A) comprises at least 10 defined types of a related disorder. Characteristic clinical features are easy bruising, markedly soft hyperextensible skin, extreme joint hypermobility, and the formation of thin, atrophic, "cigarette-paper" scarring following injury. Marfan syndrome (choice B) results in cardiovascular, musculoskeletal, and ophthalmic abnormalities. Hallmark clinical manifestations are aortic dilation, mitral valve prolapse, dissecting aneurysms, arachnodactyly, and ectopia lentis. Occipital horn syndrome (choice C), a disorder that manifests with symptoms similar to other collagen metabolism disorders, results from defects in copper metabolism. Clinical features include loose skin and joints, hernias, and abnormally shaped bones. Scurvy (choice E), which is caused by a deficiency in vitamin C, is characterized by decreased wound healing and hemorrhaging, anemia, osteoporosis, soft swollen gums, and easily bruised skin.

389.   **(A)** Defective biosynthesis of α-collagen accounts for the clinical symptoms and signs observed with osteogenesis imperfecta. Marfan syndrome results from a defect in fibrillin (choice D) synthesis. Fibrillin is a component of the 10-nm microfibrils of the extracellular matrix. The biosynthesis of the intermediate filaments cytokeratin (choice B), vimentin (choice E), and desmin (choice C) are all unaffected in osteogenesis imperfecta.

390. **(E)** Wolman disease results from a deficiency in the lysosomal acid lipase enzyme (also called cholesteryl ester hydrolase) and is very nearly always a fatal disease of infancy. Symptoms of the disorder arise from massive accumulation of cholesteryl esters and triglycerides in most tissues. Clinical manifestations include hepatosplenomegaly leading to abdominal distension, GI abnormalities, steatorrhea and adrenal calcification. Type I hyperlipoproteinemia (choice A) results from a deficiency in lipoprotein lipase (LPL) activity. LPL is the enzyme found on the surface of vessel endothelial cells and is responsible for hydrolyzing fatty acids from the triglycerides found in circulating lipoprotein particles. This action allows cells to get fatty acids for energy production from lipoproteins in the plasma. This disorder leads to massive accumulation of chylomicrons and triglycerides in the plasma. Symptoms associated with type I hyperlipoproteinemia are usually detected in childhood and include eruptive cutaneous xanthomatosis, hepatosplenomegaly, and repeated episodes of abdominal pain. I-cell disease (choice B) results from a deficiency in the targeting of lysosomal enzymes to the lysosomes. Affected cells have dense inclusion bodies filled with storage material, hence the derivation of the disease name. There are elevated levels of lysosomal enzymes in the plasma and body fluids of I-cell patients. Symptoms include severe psychomotor retardation, coarse facial features and severe skeletal abnormalities. The rapidly progressing disease can lead to death between 5 and 8 years of age. Maroteaux–Lamy syndrome (choice C) results from a defect in the enzyme *N*-acetylgalactosamine-4-sulfatase (arylsulfatase B) responsible for the catabolism of complex glycosaminoglycans. There are three distinct forms of Maroteax–Lamy syndrome that range in severity. Symptoms include coarse facial features, skeletal abnormalities, corneal clouding, and aortic valve disruption. Sanfillipo syndrome (choice D) comprises at least four distinct genetic defects that result from deficiencies in enzymes required for the catabolism of complex glycosaminoglycans of the heparan sulfate class. In all cases the clinical symptoms are similar and include severe mental deterioration, hyperactivity, and disorders of the skin, lungs, heart, and skeletal muscle.

391. **(D)** The nucleosome is a structure formed by the interaction of histone proteins with chromosomal DNA. This structure comprises an octamer of histone proteins consisting of two copies each of histone H2A, H2B, H3, and H4. Wrapped around this core of histone proteins is stretch of roughly 140 to 150 base pairs of DNA. The histone H1 protein serves as a linking agent between two nucleosomes. None of the other choices (A, B, C, and E) constitutes an accurate description of the nucleosome.

392. **(A)** Cockayne syndrome results in patients harboring a defect in the ability to repair UV-damaged DNA. In particular, the defect is pronounced at the level of the repair of transcriptionally active genes, as opposed to overall excision repair in the total genomic DNA. Defects, if observed, in the other processes (choice B, C, D, and E) do not result in symptoms of Cockayne syndrome.

393. **(A)** Arsenate replaces the P_i that normally reacts with glyceraldehyde-3-phosphate (choice C) to form 1,3-bisphosphoglycerate. Instead, an unstable intermediate, 1-arseno-3-phosphoglycerate, is produced and immediately hydrolyzes to 3-phosphoglycerate (choice D). NADH is formed as usual (choice B). Thus glycolysis proceeds in the presence of arsenate, but the ATP usually produced in the conversion of 1,3-bisphosphoglycerate to 3-phosphoglycerate is lost. Because glycolysis proceeds, pyruvate is formed (choice E).

394. **(C)** The molar ratio of adenosine in any molecule of double-stranded DNA will be equivalent to that of thymidine, because these two nucleotides hydrogen bond to form base pairs. Therefore, the total amount of the DNA accounted for in A-T base pairs would be 40%. Because guanosine and cytidine hydrogen bond to form base pairs, they also contribute an equivalent molar ratio in double-stranded DNA. In double-stranded DNA with 40% A-T composition, the molar ratio of cytidine is half of the remaining 60% of the DNA, or 30%. No other molar ratio (choices A, B, D, and E) could account for the amount of cytidine in a double-stranded DNA with 20% adenosine.

395. **(E)** In cardiac and skeletal muscle, high-energy phosphate is stored through the transfer of a phosphate from ATP to creatine generating creatine phosphate. Creatinine is a nonenzymatic metabolite of creatine phosphate. When measured in the serum, levels of creatinine are remarkably constant from day to day and are proportional to muscle mass. In renal dysfunction, creatinine clearance is impaired and its levels therefore rise in the serum. Although creatine is synthesized in the liver (choice C) from guanidoacetate, which is produced in the kidneys (choice B), it is not used by these two tissues, or by the lung (choice D) or adipose tissue (choice A). Once synthesized, creatine is transported to cardiac and skeletal muscle where it is phosphorylated and stored for future energy needs.

396. **(D)** Li–Fraumeni syndrome (LFS) is a rare inherited form of cancer that involves breast and colon carcinomas, soft-tissue sarcomas, osteosarcomas, brain tumors, leukemia, and adrenocortical carcinomas. These tumors develop at an early age in LFS patients. The tumor suppressor gene found responsible for LFS is p53. Mutant forms of p53 are found in approximately 50% of all tumors. The normal p53 protein functions as a transcription factor that can induce either cell-cycle arrest or apoptosis (programmed cell death) in response to DNA damage. Creutzfeld–Jakob disease (CJD) (choice A) encompasses three forms—infectious, sporadic, and inherited—with the vast majority of cases being sporadic. Clinical abnormalities of CJD are confined to the central nervous system and result from a pathogenic protein identified as prion protein (PrP). Crouzon syndrome (choice B) is characterized by craniosynostosis (midface hypoplasia and ocular proptosis) and is the result of a mutation in one of the receptors for fibroblast growth factor (FGFR2). Huntington disease (HD) (choice C) is an autosomal dominant disorder resulting from expansion of the triplet CAG within the huntingtin gene. The exact function of the huntingtin protein is still unclear. Symptoms of HD include personality changes, memory loss, and involuntary leg and arm movements (chorea). The average age of onset is 37 years. Prader–Willi syndrome (PWS) (choice E) is a relatively common cause of genetic obesity and mental retardation. Symptoms of severe hypotonia and poor suckling are evident at birth. PWS is caused by a deletion of a portion of the long arm of chromosome 15 [del(15q11-q13)].

397. **(E)** Hereditary orotic aciduria results from a defect in the *de novo* synthesis of pyrimidines. The defect is in the bifunctional enzyme that catalyzes the last two steps in the de novo pathway, conversion of orotic acid to OMP and OMP to UMP. Administration of uridine allows afflicted individuals to produce sufficient levels of cytidine nucleotides via the salvage pathways. Treatment with uridine leads to a return of normal blood hemoglobin levels, and bone marrow will become normoblastic. Treatment with cytidine (choice B) has some limited ability to ameliorate symptoms of the disease, but not to the extent of uridine administration. None of the other nucleosides (choices A, C, and D) can be salvaged into cytidine or uridine nucleotides, and are therefore of no clinical value in the treatment of hereditary orotic aciduria.

398. **(A)** Transcription occurs in the 5' to 3' direction, and during this process RNA polymerase will move in the 3' to 5' direction relative to the template DNA strand. Therefore, the correct transcriptional product from the DNA template begins with its 5' ribonucleotide corresponding to the complementary deoxyribonucleotide of the 3' end of the template. None of the other RNA strands (choices B, C, D, and E) could be products generated from the template shown.

399. **(C)** Translation in a eukaryotic *in vitro* translation system would begin at an AUG codon residing near the 5'-end of the mRNA. Therefore, translation of the correct RNA product begins two nucleotides from the 5' end at the first AUG codon. This results in the translation of a protein of four amino acids. None of the other choices (A, B, D, and E) translate into a four-unit amino acid chain.

400. **(B)** When epinephrine stimulates adipocytes (by interaction with β-adrenergic receptors), the immediate response is the activation of adenylate cyclase, which in turn leads to an increase in cAMP. Increased levels of cAMP lead to activation of PKA, which in adipocytes phosphorylate and activate hormone-sensitive lipase. When hormone-sensitive lipase is active, it removes fatty acids in a step-wise manner from stored triacylglycerides. The released fatty acids then enter the blood and are bound by albumin for transport to peripheral tissues including the liver. Lipoprotein lipase (choice C) is present on the surfaces of vascular endothelial cells and is activated by apolipoprotein C-II present in VLDLs and chylomicrons. Epinephrine is a stimulus that leads to energy consumption and therefore does not lead to an increase in triacylglyceride synthesis (choice A). When triacylglyceride breakdown is activated in adipocytes, the glycerol backbone is released as free glycerol, not glycerol 3-phosphate (choice E) to the blood and delivered to the liver for gluconeogenesis. Fatty acids released from adipose tissue are transported in the blood bound to albumin, not within any lipoprotein particle (choice D).

401. **(E)** The pH of blood is maintained in a narrow range around 7.4. Even relatively small changes in this value of blood pH can lead to severe metabolic consequences. Therefore, blood buffering is extremely important in order to maintain homeostasis. Although the blood contains numerous cations and anions that can, as a whole, play a role in buffering, the primary buffers in blood are hemoglobin in erythrocytes and bicarbonate ion (HCO_3^-) in the plasma. Buffering by hemoglobin is accomplished by ionization of the imidazole ring of histidines in the protein. The formation of bicarbonate ion in blood from CO_2 and H_2O allows the transfer of relatively insoluble CO_2 from the tissues to the lungs, where it is expelled. The major source of CO_2 in the tissues comes from the oxidation of ingested carbon compounds. Carbonic acid (H_2CO_3) is formed from the reaction of dissolved CO_2 with H_2O, catalyzed by carbonic anhydrase. Formation of carbonic acid occurs predominately in the erythrocytes, since nearly all of the CO_2 leaving tissues via the capillary endothelium is taken up by these cells. Ionization of carbonic acid then occurs spontaneously yielding bicarbonate ion and a hydrogen ion (H^+). The resultant hydrogen ions are buffered by hemoglobin. Buffering of protons by hemoglobin results in a reduced affinity of hemoglobin for oxygen. This leads to a release of O_2 to the peripheral tissues. The phenomenon is termed the Bohr effect. Although the binding of O_2 (choice A) to hemoglobin in the lungs, CO_2 binding to form hemoglobin carbamate (choice B) in the periphery and release of CO_2 in the lungs (choice C) are events that can be affected by the ion concentration of the plasma and erythrocytes, these events do not comprise the Bohr effect. Hemoglobin does not buffer chloride ion (choice D). As CO_2 passes from the tissues to the plasma a minor amount of carbonic acid takes form and ionizes. The H^+ ions are then buffered predominantly by proteins and phosphate ions in the plasma. As the concentration of bicarbonate ions rises in erythrocytes, an osmotic imbalance occurs. The imbalance is relieved as bicarbonate ion leaves the erythrocytes in exchange for chloride ions from the plasma. This phenomenon is known as the chloride shift.

402. **(B)** The extrinsic pathway (see Figure 8–18) is initiated at the site of injury in response to the release of tissue factor (factor III). Tissue factor is a cofactor in the factor VIIa–catalyzed (lower case "a" refers to the active form of the coagulation factors) activation of factor X. The formation of a complex between factor VIIa and tissue factor is believed to be a principal step in the overall clotting cascade. Evidence for this stems from the fact that persons with hereditary deficiencies in the components of the contact phase of the intrinsic pathway do not exhibit clotting problems. Factor VIIa, a γ-glutamate (gla residue) containing serine protease, cleaves factor X to factor Xa in a manner identical to that of factor IXa of the intrinsic pathway. The activation of factor VII occurs through the action of thrombin or factor Xa. The ability of factor Xa to activate factor VII creates a link between the intrinsic and extrinsic pathways. An additional link between the two pathways exists through the ability of tissue factor and factor VIIa to activate factor IX. Fibrinogen (choice A) is cleaved by thrombin (factor IIa), yielding fibrin monomers that polymerize to form a fibrin clot. The activation of factor VIII (choice C) to factor VIIIa occurs in the presence of minute quantities of thrombin. Factor VIIIa is required for the activation of factor X, which represents the convergence of the intrinsic and extrinsic pathways. The activation of factor X to Xa requires assemblage of the tenase complex (Ca²⁺ and factors VIIIa, IXa, and X) on the surface of activated platelets. As the concentration of thrombin increases, factor VIIIa is ultimately cleaved by thrombin and inactivated. This dual action of thrombin upon factor VIII acts to limit the extent of tenase complex formation, and thus the extent of the coagulation cascade. Factor IX (choice D) functions only in the intrinsic cascade. When activated, factor IXa aids in the activation of factor X by functioning in the tenase complex as described above. Protein S (choice E) is a cofactor for protein C. Protein C is itself activated by thrombin and when active cleaves factors VIIIa and Va, thus limiting the extent of the coagulation cascade.

403. **(E)** The amino groups of amino acids are converted to urea for excretion via the urea cycle. The liver is the only organ capable of carrying this out. The human liver produces some 20 to 30 g of urea each day. Synthesis of gangliosides (choice A), which are components of all mammalian plasma membranes,

can be carried out in all cells. Glycogen can be degraded not only in the liver but also chiefly in muscle (choice B). Nucleotide biosynthesis (choice D) is also carried out by most cells, as is use of medium-chain fatty acids as an energy source (choice C).

404. **(A)** Propionyl-CoA is converted to succinyl-CoA in a series of reactions using three different enzymes. It is first carboxylated in an ATP-dependent reaction catalyzed by propionyl-CoA carboxylase, an enzyme the requires biotin as a cofactor. The product of the first reaction, D-methylmalonyl-CoA is then converted to L-methylmalonyl-CoA by methylmalonyl-CoA racemase. Finally, methylmalonyl-CoA is converted to succinyl-CoA by the cobalamin-requiring enzyme, methylmalonyl-CoA mutase. None of the other vitamins (choice B, C, D, and E) is required in this pathway.

405. **(E)** Von Recklinghausen disease (neurofibromatosis type I), an autosomal dominant disorder, is one of the most striking disorders that exhibits variable expressivity (phenotypic variation). Symptoms can range from the benign appearance of café-au-lait spots to severe disfiguring cutaneous neurofibromas, sarcomas, and gliomas. This disorder is caused by disruption in the neurofibromin gene whose protein product functions the catalysis of inactivation of the signaling protein ras. Familial adenomatous polyposis coli (FAP) (choice A) is a disorder that results the generation of numerous small polyps in the colon by the time an individual reaches age 20. Although the polyps are asymptomatic, they are a significant contributory factor to risk and likelihood of colon cancer. This disorder is caused by mutations in the adenomatous polyposis coli (APC) gene and is inherited in autosomal dominant fashion and whose penetrance is 100% in all afflicted individuals. Familial hypercholesterolemia (FH) (choice B) is caused by mutations in the gene for the LDL receptor. Inheritance is autosomal dominant with 100% penetrance. FH sufferers may be either heterozygous or homologous for a particular mutation in the receptor gene. Homozygotes

exhibit grossly elevated serum cholesterol (primarily in LDLs). The elevated levels of LDLs result in their phagocytosis by macrophages. These lipid-laden phagocytic cells tend to deposit within the skin and tendons, leading to xanthomas. A greater complication results from cholesterol deposition within the arteries, leading to atherosclerosis, the major contributing factor of nearly all cardiovascular diseases. Li–Fraumeni syndrome (choice C) is a rare form of autosomal dominant inherited cancer caused by mutations in the tumor suppressor gene, p53. The disruption in the function of p53 leads to aberrant cell cycle regulation and development of sarcomas, brain tumors, breast cancer, and leukemias. Cancer occurs in 50% of afflicted individuals by the time they are 30 years of age. von Hippel–Lindau (VHL) syndrome (choice D) is an inherited form of renal carcinoma that is caused by mutations in a tumor suppressor gene identified as the VHL gene.

406. **(C)** The major mechanism for the inhibition of the extrinsic pathway occurs at the tissue factor—factor VIIa—Ca^{2+}–Xa complex. The protein, lipoprotein-associated coagulation inhibitor (LACI, formerly named anticonvertin), specifically binds to this complex. LACI is composed of three tandem protease inhibitor domains. Domain 1 binds to factor Xa and domain 2 binds to factor VIIa only in the presence of factor Xa. Antithrombin III (choice A) is the most important of four thrombin regulatory proteins. This is because antithrombin III can also inhibit the activities of factors IXa, Xa, XIa, and XIIa. The activity of antithrombin III is potentiated in the presence of heparin. Heparin binds to a specific site on antithrombin III, producing an altered conformation of the protein, and the new conformation has a higher affinity for thrombin as well as its other substrates. This effect of heparin is the basis for its clinical use as an anticoagulant. The naturally occurring heparin activator of antithrombin III is present as heparan and heparan sulfate on the surface of vessel endothelial cells. It is this feature that controls the activation of the intrinsic coagulation cascade. High-molecular-weight kinino-

gen (HMWK) (choice B) is important for initiation of the intrinsic pathway. When prekallikrein, HMWK, factor XI, and factor XII are exposed to a negatively charged surface, they become active. This is termed the contact phase. Exposure of collagen to a vessel surface is the primary stimulus for the contact phase. In addition to antithrombin III, thrombin activity is also inhibited by α_2-macroglobulin (choice D). Protein C (choice E) is activated by thrombin when thrombin is bound to thrombomodulin. Active protein C functions with its cofactor, protein S, to degrade factors VIIIa and Xa.

407. **(E)** When receptor–ligand interaction stimulates the activity of PLCγ, an increase in membrane associated phospholipid degradation occurs (see Figure 3–8). The action of PLCγ is to hydrolyze polyphosphoinositides, in particular phosphatidylinositol-4,5-bisphosphate (PIP$_2$). The hydrolytic products of PLCγ action on PIP$_2$ is the release of inositol-1,4,5-trisphosphate (IP$_3$) and diacylglycerol (DAG). IP$_3$ interacts with intracellular membrane receptors resulting in the release of stored Ca^{2+}. DAG, in concert with Ca^{2+}, activates a specific kinase termed PKC (calcium, phospholipid-dependent kinase) that phosphorylates many substrates. As indicated, activation of PLCγ increases, not decreases (choice C), the release of membrane inositol lipids. PLCγ has no direct effect on the activity of adenylate cyclase (choice A) or on the activity of phosphodiesterase (choice B). The effect of PLCγ-mediated release of IP$_3$ is increased release of intracellular stores of calcium, not an increase in its uptake (choice D).

408. **(A)** When fatty acids are released from adipose tissue they are transported in the blood bound to albumin. Chylomicrons (choice B) are synthesized in the intestine as a means to deliver dietary lipid to the body. α_2-Macroglobulin (choice C) is an antiprotease that functions to regulate the activities of a number of proteinases, such as thrombin, of the coagulation cascade. β_2-Microglobulin (choice D) is involved in immune function. VLDLs (choice E) are synthesized by the liver as a means to trans-

port de novo synthesized fatty acids, in the form of triacylglycerides, to peripheral tissues.

409. (D) Activation of amino acids for protein synthesis is carried out by a two step process catalyzed by aminoacyl-tRNA synthetases. Each tRNA, and the amino acid it carries, is recognized by individual aminoacyl-tRNA synthetases. Activation of amino acids requires energy in the form of ATP and occurs in a two-step reaction catalyzed by the aminoacyl-tRNA synthetases. First the enzyme attaches the amino acid to the α-phosphate of ATP with the concomitant release of pyrophosphate. This is a high energy aminoacyl-adenylate intermediate. In the second step the enzyme catalyzes transfer of the amino acid to either the 2'- or 3'-hydroxyl of the ribose portion of the 3'-terminal adenosine residue of the tRNA generating the activated aminoacyl-tRNA. Although these reaction are freely reversible, the forward reaction is favored by the coupled hydrolysis of PP_i. None of the other choices (A, B, C and E) reflect the correct steps in amino acid activation.

REFERENCES

Baynes J, Dominiczak MH. *Medical Biochemistry.* New York: Mosby; 1999.

Devlin TM. *Textbook of Biochemistry: With Clinical Correlations,* 4th ed. New York: Wiley; 1997.

Murray RK, ed. *Harper's Biochemistry,* 25th ed. Stamford, CT: Appleton & Lange; 2000.

Voet D, Voet JG. *Biochemistry,* 2nd ed. New York: Wiley; 1995.

Subspecialty List: Biochemistry

Question Number and Subspecialty

283. Blood
284. Enzymes
285. Urea cycle
286. Blood
287. Cholesterol metabolism
288. Carbohydrate metabolism
289. Nucleotide metabolism
290. Hemoglobin
291. Coagulation
292. Errors in metabolism
293. Carbohydrate metabolism
294. Carbohydrate metabolism
295. Errors in metabolism
296. Errors in metabolism
297. Errors in metabolism
298. Errors in metabolism
299. Carbohydrate metabolism
300. Carbohydrate metabolism
301. Translation
302. Gene expression
303. Heme metabolism
304. Heme metabolism
305. Heme metabolism
306. Carbohydrate metabolism
307. Errors in metabolism
308. Diabetes
309. Congenital defects
310. Hemoglobin metabolism
311. Ketogenesis
312. Errors in metabolism
313. Errors in metabolism
314. Molecular biology
315. Coagulation
316. Oxidative phosphorylation
317. Lipoproteins
318. Urea cycle
319. Nitrogen metabolism
320. Post-translational modification
321. Oxidative phosphorylation
322. Urea cycle
323. Errors in metabolism
324. Errors in metabolism
325. Translation
326. Hormonal control of metabolism
327. Errors in metabolism
328. Nucleotide metabolism
329. Lipid metabolism
330. Proteins
331. Nitrogen metabolism
332. DNA synthesis
333. Translation
334. Diabetes
335. Carbohydrate metabolism
336. Carbohydrate metabolism
337. Cell biology
338. Fatty acid oxidation
339. Control of translation
340. Errors in metabolism
341. Errors in metabolism
342. Errors in metabolism
343. Coagulation
344. Errors in metabolism
345. Errors in metabolism
346. Diabetes
347. Hormones
348. Errors in metabolism
349. Coagulation
350. Errors in metabolism
351. Nucleotide metabolism
352. Amino acids
353. Hormones
354. Hormones
355. Hormones
356. Hormones

357. Inherited defects
358. Carbohydrate metabolism
359. Nucleotide metabolism
360. Molecular biology
361. Carbohydrate metabolism
362. Lipid metabolism
363. Errors in metabolism
364. Lipoproteins
365. Carbohydrate metabolism
366. Hormones
367. Iron metabolism
368. Signal transduction
369. Errors in metabolism
370. Errors in metabolism
371. Carbohydrate metabolism
372. Inherited defects
373. Heme metabolism
374. Carbohydrate metabolism
375. Vitamins
376. Hormones
377. Errors in metabolism
378. Errors in metabolism
379. Inherited defects
380. Inherited defects
381. Carbohydrate metabolism
382. Oxygen transport

383. Inherited defects
384. Carbohydrate metabolism
385. Lipoproteins
386. Molecular biology
387. Lipid metabolism
388. Errors in metabolism
389. Errors in metabolism
390. Errors in metabolism
391. Molecular biology
392. Inherited defects
393. Carbohydrate metabolism
394. Molecular biology
395. Muscle metabolism
396. Inherited defects
397. Nucleotide metabolism
398. Transcription
399. Translation
400. Lipid metabolism
401. Cancer biology
402. Coagulation
403. Hepatic metabolism
404. Fatty acid oxidation
405. Inherited defects
406. Coagulation
407. Signal transduction
408. Lipoproteins
409. Translation

CHAPTER 4

Microbiology
Questions

William W. Yotis, PhD and Nicholas J. Legakis, MD

137–101
100 — †

73%

DIRECTIONS (Questions 410 through 546): Each of the numbered items or incomplete statements in this section is followed by answers or by completions of the statement. Select the ONE lettered answer or completion that is BEST in each case.

410. A student has a genetic defect and cannot produce the J chain that is important in the structure of some immunoglobulin molecules. Most likely this student will have a (an)

    (A) decrease in mature B-cells
    (B) decrease in mature T lymphocytes
    (C) decrease in serum IgM
    (D) increase in IgA in the intestine
    (E) increase in serum IgM and decrease in IgE

411. A 37-year-old woman is suffering from acute diffuse otitis. The biochemical profile and blood counts were normal. The woman used to swim 4 times per week in the municipal swimming pool. Which one of the following microbes is most likely the causative agent of her otitis?

    (A) *Haemophilus ducreyi*
    (B) *Haemophilus influenzae*
    (C) *Pseudomonas aeruginosa*
    (D) *Staphylococcus aureus*
    (E) *Streptococcus pneumoniae*

412. Molecular amplification techniques like the polymerase chain reaction (PCR) can be used for the direct identification of *Mycobacterium tuberculosis* in clinical specimens because they

    (A) are always very sensitive and specific
    (B) are inexpensive

    (C) can be applied for nonrespiratory mycobacterial clinical specimens
    (D) can provide rapid results
    (E) have replaced the traditional culture techniques

413. To support the preliminary diagnosis of type I diabetes, an indirect immunofluorescent test has been suggested. A monolayer of pancreatic islet cells has been prepared, but you are not certain which reagent to add. On the advice of your supervisor you most likely will add

    (A) complement components C1qrs
    (B) fluorescein-labeled antibody specific for human Ig
    (C) fluorescein-labeled antibody specific for human Ig and the patient's serum
    (D) purified complement component C3
    (E) purified fluorescein dye

414. Treatment with certain antibiotics may stimulate the production of bacterial autolysins. Which one of the following antibiotics is most likely to stimulate autolysin production?

    (A) Aminoglycosides
    (B) Penicillins
    (C) Quinolones
    (D) Rifampins
    (E) Tetracyclines

415. Herpes simplex virus type I evades host immune responses most likely by using which one of the following mechanisms?

   (A) Antigenic drift
   (B) Antigenic masking
   (C) Antigenic shift
   (D) Antigenic variation
   (E) Latency

416. Major innate immune mechanisms that combat viral infections are the interferons that

   (A) are highly specific
   (B) are produced by most nucleated cells in the body
   (C) are strongly induced by bacterial proteins
   (D) exist in only two types, alpha and beta
   (E) inhibit viral growth by blocking the transcription of viral genes

417. A 25-year-old man with acquired immunodeficiency syndrome (AIDS) has malabsorption, chronic abdominal pain, low-grade fever, and nonbloody diarrhea. In fecal smears oocysts were detected. Which one of the following organisms is most likely the etiologic agent?

   (A) *Cryptosporidium parvum*
   (B) *Entamoeba histolytica*
   (C) *Giardia lamblia*
   (D) *Microsporidia*
   (E) *Taenia solium*

418. A 65-year-old woman, who had been healthy, develops abrupt fever. Empirical treatment with third-generation cephalosporins is ineffective. On examination, lobar pneumonia associated with pleurisy is diagnosed. The infection is treated successfully with penicillin. Which of the following microbes is most likely responsible for her illness?

   (A) *Chlamydia pneumoniae*
   (B) *Legionella pneumoniae*
   (C) *Mycoplasma pneunoniae*
   (D) *Pneumocystis carinii*
   (E) *Streptococcus pneumoniae*

419. Severe septic infections with encapsulated bacteria following splenectomy can occur because the spleen

   (A) inactivates rapidly many antimicrobial agents
   (B) is a source of IgM and IgG antibodies needed to opsonize encapsulated bacteria
   (C) is the main source of stem cells
   (D) is uniquely equipped to process capsular polysaccharides
   (E) readily metabolizes therapeutic doses of antibiotics

420. A 37-year-old man has back pain, fever, malaise, and lethargy. Following a series of tests, vertebral osteomyelitis is diagnosed. Physical examination reveals splenomegaly and hepatomegaly. The patient lives on a farm and was drinking unpasteurized goat milk. No immunosuppression is detected and the Mantoux skin test is negative. Which of the following microbes is the most likely etiologic agent?

   (A) *Actinomyces israelii*
   (B) *Aspergillus fumigatus*
   (C) *Brucella melitensis*
   (D) *Candida albicans*
   (E) *Mycobacterium tuberculosis*

421. A 72-year-old man has chest pain, difficulty breathing, and edema in the lower limbs. Upon examination, arrhythmias and cardiomegaly are found, and a diagnosis of viral myocarditis is made. Which of the following microorganisms is most likely responsible for this illness?

   (A) Adenovirus
   (B) Coronavirus
   (C) Coxsackie group B virus
   (D) Mumps virus
   (E) Rhinovirus

422. The main advantage of passive over active immunization is that passive immunization

(A) eliminates the risk of hypersensitivity reactions

(B) involves the injection of the specific antigen and antibody

(C) is very effective as a public health measure

(D) magnifies the specific immune response to the offending organism

(E) provides immediate protection

423. A 5-year-old child, known to suffer from sickle cell anemia, is presented to his pediatrician with fever, severe deep bone pain, and acute local bony tenderness. Following several laboratory tests, osteomyelitis of the right femur is diagnosed. Which of the following microbes is the most likely cause of this infection?

(A) *Bacteroides fragilis*

(B) *Haemophilus influenzae*

(C) *Pseudomonas aeruginosa*

(D) *Salmonella enteritidis*

(E) *Streptococcus pyogenes*

424. Which of the following statements concerning the application of acid-fast stains for the diagnosis of mycobacterioses is the most applicable?

(A) Acid-fast stains yield definitive results in less than 5 minutes.

(B) Cell wall proteins of mycobacteria are responsible for their acid-fast character.

(C) Discrimination between mycobacterial species is possible by these stains.

(D) These stains can be used to detect pathogenic mycobacteria.

(E) These stains replace the Gram stains because mycobacteria have large amounts of lipids in their cell walls.

425. A medical student has been immunized with hepatitis B virus (HBV) recombinant vaccine. The curve in Figure 4–1 represents the production of protective antibodies to the viral component present in the recombinant vaccine. This viral component most likely is

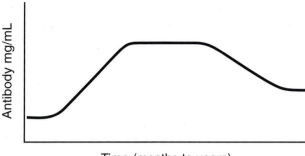

Figure 4–1

(A) nucleocapsid proteins of HBV

(B) RNA genome of HBV

(C) viral core antigen (HBcAg)

(D) viral e antigen (HBeAg)

(E) viral surface antigen (HBsAg)

426. A banker has been told by his physician that the rash on his arm is due to delayed-type hypersensitivity. If this is actually the case, which of the following statements is accurate?

(A) Delayed-type hypersensitivity can be transferred passively to volunteers by sensitized lymphocytes.

(B) Delayed-type hypersensitivity is suppressed by antihistaminic drugs.

(C) This allergy does not cause tissue damage.

(D) This allergy is due to IgE absorbed on mast cells.

(E) This type of allergy usually occurs after inhalation of grass pollens.

427. Ada had a catheter placed in her urethra. One week later she is experiencing suprapubic flank pain with urinary urgency and frequency. She also has chills and fever. After examining Ada and evaluating the sediment of her centrifuged urine, she is informed that she has acute ascending pyelonephritis. If the diagnosis is accurate and Ada's urine is cultured, what organism will most likely be isolated?

    (A) *Clostridium difficile*
    (B) *Escherichia coli* with pili
    (C) *Pseudomonas aeruginosa*
    (D) *Staphylococcus aureus*

428. Romeo, a 27-year-old electrician, has a sore throat with chills and fever. Within a week his throat has definitely improved, but he still has a fever and malaise. Suddenly he notices that his urine is gray-brown, and he visits his physician. If the doctor thinks that Romeo has acute glomerulonephritis, which one of the following tests is most likely to verify this diagnosis?

    (A) Evaluation of the number of T cells
    (B) Serum level of anti-DNA antibodies
    (C) Serum level of anti-H antibodies
    (D) Serum level of anti-streptolysin O antibodies
    (E) Serum level of IgE

429. A 22-year-old man complains to his family physician of fatigue, night sweats, and a dry unproductive cough. Until the past few months, he had apparently been in good health. A CBC and differential blood count reveal that he is lymphopenic. X-ray examination reveals interstitial pneumonia. Skin test reactions to a battery of materials are normal. The next step in evaluating this patient's illness should be

    (A) CH50 assay
    (B) chemotaxis assay
    (C) identification of the organism that is causing the pneumonia
    (D) intracellular killing assay
    (E) nitroblue tetrazolium reduction assay

430. A 2-year-old girl with recurrent pulmonary infections has been brought to the hospital with meningitis. Gram stain of the spinal fluid reveals numerous polymorphonuclear neutrophils and gram-positive cocci in grape-like clusters. The drug of choice to be employed until the antibiotic sensitivity report is received from the laboratory is

    (A) ampicillin
    (B) chloramphenicol
    (C) methicillin
    (D) penicillin
    (E) streptomycin

431. Which of the following statements concerning the Ouchterlony diagram in Figure 4–2 is true?

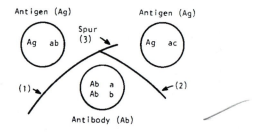

Figure 4–2

    (A) Line 1 will contain Ag ab and Ab b only.
    (B) Line 2 will contain Ag ac and Ab b.
    (C) The spur will contain Ab a and Ag ab.
    (D) The spur will contain Ag ab and Ab b.
    (E) The spur will contain Ag ac and Ab a.

432. Figure 4–3 depicts an electrophoretic pattern of serum proteins. This electrophoretic design is likely to be obtained from a 9-month-old infant with

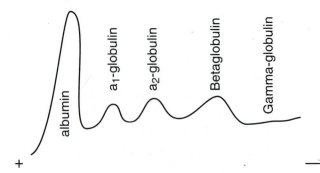

Figure 4–3

(A) Addison disease

(B) Bruton disease

(C) Goodpasture syndrome

(D) Grave disease

(E) myasthenia gravis

Questions 433 and 434

Mr. T., a 19-year-old college student, is experiencing intense burning during urination, and discharges a thick creamy urethral exudate. The exudate is composed of polymorphonuclear leukocytes with many intracellular, gram-negative, kidney-shaped diplococci. There are no lesions on the genital organ area.

433. The most likely presumptive diagnosis is

(A) chancroid

(B) gonorrhea

(C) lymphogranuloma venereum

(D) syphilis

(E) trichomoniasis

434. Which of the following approaches is likely to prevent future infection of Mr. T.?

(A) Frequent washing of the genital area

(B) Immunization with the appropriate toxoid

(C) Prophylactic use of 100 U oral penicillin

(D) Use of condoms

(E) Vaccination with heat-killed germs

435. A boy is attacked and bitten on the shoulder by a fox and suffers a slight wound. In addition to flushing the wound, cleaning it surgically, and giving anti-tetanus prophylaxis and antibiotics as indicated, the physician should immediately

(A) observe the boy very carefully

(B) order a search for the attacking fox for autopsy

(C) report the incident to the state epidemiologist

(D) start rabies vaccine

(E) start rabies vaccine and give anti-rabies serum

436. A laboratory worker is diagnosed with tuberculosis. He has been ill for 10 months with symptoms that include a productive cough, intermittent fever, night sweats, and a weight loss of 27.3 kg (60 lb). Numerous acid-fast bacilli are seen in a sputum examination, and more than 50 colonies of organisms grow out in culture. In a situation such as this, those contacts who have a positive skin test but no other signs of disease should

(A) be checked periodically by x-ray

(B) be immunized with bacillus–Calmette–Guerin (BCG) vaccine

(C) be vaccinated with purified protein derivative (PPD)

(D) receive a full course of isoniazid (INH) and ethambutol

(E) receive prophylactic isoniazid

437. A football player had gonococcal urethritis, and was treated with the appropriate doses of penicillin and probenecid. Three weeks later he had a relapse of gonococcal urethritis, and his physician administered another dose of penicillin. Within 2 minutes following the injection the football player experienced respiratory difficulties and collapsed. The most likely explanation for the difficulties in breathing and collapse is that

(A) he may have nongonococcal urethritis

(B) he might be reinfected

(C) the gonococcus that caused the initial infection became resistant to penicillin

(D) the patient developed a hypersensitivity to penicillin

(E) the patient developed gonococcal pneumonia

438. Ultraviolet light is used as an antimicrobial agent because it

(A) acts as an alkylating agent

(B) causes the formation of pyrimidine dimers

(C) disrupts the bacterial cell membrane

(D) is a common protein denaturant

(E) removes free sulfhydryl groups

439. A 5-year-old girl undergoing chemotherapy develops a disseminated varicella-zoster infection. The most likely reason for this viral infection is

(A) deficiency in the third component of complement

(B) hypogammaglobulinemia

(C) outgrowth of virus from varicella-zoster immunization

(D) synergism between varicella-zoster and chemotherapy

(E) T-cell deficiency

440. A zookeeper who had two seizures and is now semicomatose is brought to the hospital. His cerebrospinal fluid has normal glucose and protein levels, but 40 lymphocytes per cubic mm. A spherical, enveloped, double-stranded DNA virus has been isolated from clinical specimens and established as the etiologic agent of the viral infection. The most likely virus involved is

(A) echovirus

(B) herpesvirus

(C) poliovirus

(D) rabies virus

(E) St. Louis encephalitis

441. Which of the following statements concerning Figure 4–4 (showing the frequency of serologic reactivity after exposure to *Coccidioides immitis*) is true?

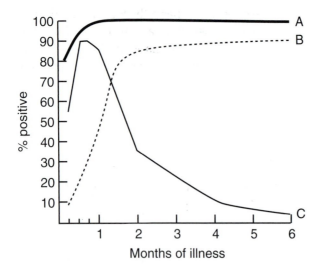

Figure 4–4

(A) Curve A represents the results of agglutination assays.

(B) Curve A represents the results of the precipitin assays.

(C) Curve B shows the results of the complement fixation assays.

(D) Curve C depicts the data of skin testing.

(E) Curve C shows the results of complement fixation assays.

442. Tetracycline antibiotics specifically inhibit protein synthesis in prokaryotes because they

(A) are transported by prokaryotes but not eukaryotes

(B) bind to prokaryotic and not eukaryotic DNA-directed RNA polymerase

(C) bind to prokaryotic but not eukaryotic membranes

(D) bind to prokaryotic but not eukaryotic ribosomes

(E) inhibit initiation of protein synthesis, which specifically requires formylmethionyl-tRNA

443. Figure 4–5 shows a quantitative precipitin curve of an antigen-antibody reaction. According to the figure, which of the following statements is correct?

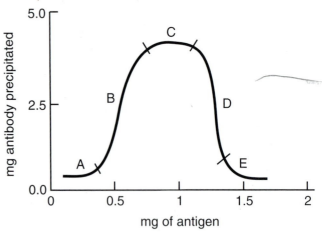

Figure 4–5

(A) Point A shows antigen excess.

(B) Point B shows that there is no antibody formation.

(C) Point C indicates that there is little, if any, free antigen and antibody in the reaction tube.

(D) Point D represents the area of antigen destruction.

(E) Point E indicates antibody excess.

444. A newborn boy appears to be lethargic and septic. A spinal tap is performed, and a Gram stain of the centrifuged spinal fluid revealed gram-positive bacilli resembling diphtheroids. Cultures of the spinal fluid on sheep blood agar plates, at a temperature of 22 to 25°C, yield gram-positive, catalase-positive, hemolytic rods that have a tumbling motion. Treatment with penicillin clears the infection. The most likely organism that caused this disease is

(A) *Bacillus cereus*

(B) *Bordetella pertussis*

(C) *Corynebacterium diphtheriae*

(D) *Listeria monocytogenes*

(E) *Neisseria meningitidis*

445. Secretory IgA consists of IgA dimer, secretory component (sc), plus

(A) e chain

(B) g chain

(C) J chain

(D) paraprotein

(E) sc epitope

446. Antigens can best be processed for presentation by

(A) B cells

(B) Kupffer cells

(C) macrophages

(D) suppressor T cells

(E) young erythrocytes

447. A medical student spending his summer in a dense forest as a tree cutter is bitten by infected ticks. In a week, he develops a high fever, headache, muscular aches, nausea, and splenomegaly. Five days later his symptoms subside. However, 1 week later all his previous symptoms return. Over the next 9 days, he goes through a recovery and another relapse, followed by a final recovery. The overall temperature curve of his illness is shown in Figure 4–6. The most likely etiologic agent is

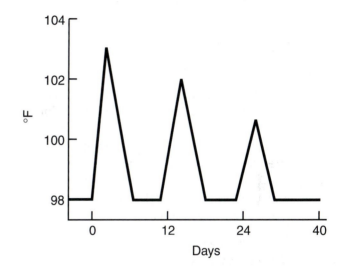

Figure 4–6

(A) *Borrelia burgdorferi*

(B) *Borrelia recurrentis*

(C) *Leptospira interrogans*

(D) *Treponema carateum*

(E) *Treponema pertenue*

448. A 7-year-old boy has a thick gray pseudomembrane over his tonsils and throat, and a clinical diagnosis of diphtheria is made. Which of the following is the most immediate course of action?

(A) Acid-fast stain of a throat specimen

(B) Culture of a throat specimen on blood agar

(C) Injection of diphtheria antitoxin

(D) Oral administration of sulfonamides

(E) Performance of a spinal tap

449. Patients with X-linked infantile agammaglobulinemia are known to

(A) be particularly susceptible to viral and fungal infections

(B) exhibit profound deficiencies of cell-mediated immunity

(C) have a depletion of lymphocytes in the paracortical areas of lymph nodes

(D) have normal numbers of B lymphocytes

(E) have very low quantities of immunoglobulin in their serum

450. During a routine pelvic examination, a woman is found to have vesicular lesions on the vagina. The patient states that she had similar lesions 12 months previously. The causative agent is most likely to be

(A) Coxsackie virus

(B) echovirus

(C) herpes simplex virus

(D) measles virus

(E) rubella virus

451. Antibodies against neural acetylcholine receptors are thought to be involved in the pathogenesis of

(A) acute idiopathic polyneuritis

(B) Guillain–Barré syndrome

(C) multiple sclerosis

(D) myasthenia gravis

(E) postpericardiotomy syndrome

452. A 7-month-old child is hospitalized for a yeast infection that does not respond to therapy. The patient has a history of acute pyogenic infections. Physical examination reveals that the spleen and lymph nodes are not palpable. A differential WBC count shows 95% neutrophils, 1% lymphocytes, and 4% monocytes. A bone marrow specimen contains no plasma cells or lymphocytes. X-ray reveals absence of a thymic shadow. Tonsils are absent. These findings are most compatible with

(A) chronic granulomatous disease

(B) multiple myeloma

(C) severe combined immunodeficiency disease

(D) Wiskott–Aldrich syndrome

(E) X-linked agammaglobulinemia

453. Figure 4–7 represents the

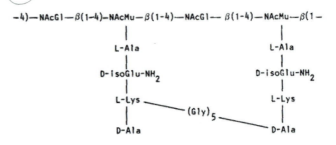

Figure 4–7

(A) C substance of *Streptococcus pneumoniae*

(B) H antigen of *Salmonella typhimurium*

(C) O antigen of *S. typhimurium*

(D) peptidoglycan of *Mycoplasma pneumoniae*

(E) peptidoglycan of *Staphylococcus aureus*

454. Immunity to whooping cough is

(A) acquired by active immunization

(B) conferred by antibody production to the Vi antigen of *Bordetella pertussis*

(C) of lifelong duration

(D) rarely acquired by natural infection with *B. pertussis*

(E) usually acquired during the third month of infancy

455. A mother is told that her 3-year-old child has an inherited deficiency in the inhibitor of the first component of complement. This deficiency is likely to lead to which one of the following conditions?

(A) Angioedema

(B) Bacteremia

(C) Decreased production of anaphylatoxins

(D) Enhancement of antibody production

(E) Increased susceptibility to pyogenic infections

456. A rabbit is repeatedly injected with a hapten. Two weeks later, its serum is subjected to a gel diffusion assay with the hapten and a carrier protein. It would be expected that

(A) a line of identity between serum and both the carrier and the hapten will be present

(B) a line of identity between the serum and carrier protein will be detected

(C) a line of nonidentity between serum, carrier, and hapten will be detected

(D) a line of partial identity between serum, carrier, and hapten will be detected

(E) no precipitin line will be present

457. A 19-year-old man who had not been vaccinated for any viral infection had fever and anorexia for 3 days. Then he developed a tender swelling of the parotid glands, which became very painful. The pain was exacerbated with fluid intake. Hemagglutination inhibition assays indicated a fourfold rise in antibody production against the etiologic agent. Which one of the following statements is correct about the etiologic agent?

(A) The genome of this virus is composed of DNA.

(B) The virus has been attenuated and used as a vaccine.

(C) This virus does not cause any complications.

(D) This virus is susceptible to antiviral therapy.

(E) This virus is transmitted to humans by insects.

458. A 6-year-old girl has been having recurrent pyogenic bacterial infections. The latest one has been caused by *Neisseria meningitidis*. The results of her diagnostic tests are as follows.

TEST	RESULT
White cell count	Normal
T-cell count	Normal
Production of IgM to polysaccharides	Normal
Production of anti-DNA antibodies	Not detected
Levels of complement components C3 and C5 to C8	Low
Levels of thyroid-stimulating hormone	Normal
Levels of immunoglobulins	Normal
Intracellular killing microbes by neutrophils	Normal

These results are consistent with a diagnosis of

(A) chronic granulomatous disease

(B) deficiency in the opsonization of microbes by phagocytes

(C) Grave disease

(D) systemic lupus erythematosus

(E) Wiskott–Aldrich syndrome

459. High-molecular-weight substances that possess both immunogenicity and specificity are termed

(A) adjuvants

(B) antigens

(C) complex haptens

(D) determinant groups

(E) simple haptens

460. A laboratory test used to identify *S. aureus* is based on the clotting of plasma. The microbial product that is responsible for this activity is

(A) coagulase

(B) coagulase reactive factor

(C) plasmin

(D) prothrombin

(E) thrombin

461. Which of the following is the best neutrophil and macrophage attractant?

(A) C5a

(B) HLA-A

(C) HLA-B

(D) J chain

(E) Variable region of the heavy chain of IgG

462. The most common medium used for the cultivation of fungi is

(A) Lowenstein–Jensen medium
(B) Sabouraud glucose agar
(C) selenite F medium
(D) SS agar
(E) tellurite medium

463. Congenital rubella syndrome is most prominent in an infant when a pregnant woman becomes infected

(A) during the first trimester of pregnancy
(B) during the third trimester of pregnancy
(C) hours before childbirth
(D) 1 month before a full-term delivery
(E) 1 week before a full-term delivery

464. The tolerance of facultative anaerobic bacteria to superoxide and hydrogen peroxide is due to the

(A) absence of catalase
(B) cytochrome oxidase
(C) inability to form oxygen
(D) presence of peroxidase
(E) presence of superoxide dismutase and catalase

465. A burn patient develops a wound infection, and a bacteriologic culture of the site indicates a gram-negative rod that is oxidase positive and produces a bluish-green pigment. The organism is relatively resistant to antibiotics, but susceptible to ticarcillin, gentamicin, and tobramycin. The organism is likely to be identified as

(A) Escherichia coli
(B) Klebsiella pneumoniae
(C) Proteus mirabilis
(D) Pseudomonas aeruginosa
(E) Serratia marcescens

466. Acute glomerulonephritis is a sequela of a previous infection by

(A) a few M types of group A streptococci
(B) all of the Lancefield groups of streptococci
(C) any M type of group A streptococci

(D) only encapsulated strains of Streptococcus pneumoniae
(E) only lysogenic group A streptococci

467. Cryptococcus neoformans differs from other pathogenic fungi in that it

(A) has a capsule
(B) has septate hyphae
(C) is an intracellular parasite
(D) is dematiaceous
(E) reproduces by binary fission

468. Diphyllobothrium latum causes anemia by

(A) competition with the host for vitamin B_{12}
(B) inhibition of the absorption of iron
(C) its blood-sucking activities
(D) occlusion of the common bile duct
(E) the production of a toxin that affects hematopoiesis

469. Which of the following zoonotic diseases is usually transmitted to humans by the bite of an arthropod vector?

(A) Anthrax
(B) Brucellosis
(C) Leptospirosis
(D) Plague
(E) Salmonellosis

Questions 470 and 471

Ms. Y. is sneezing and has a runny nose and watery eyes every summer. Her physician is convinced that Ms. Y. is suffering from an allergy and performs some skin tests. The results of these tests are shown below.

ALLERGEN USED FOR TESTING	RESPONSE TO ALLERGEN (WHEAL DIAMETER IN MM)
Cat dander	1
House dust	4
Kentucky blue grass	13
Pollen	7
Fungal spores	6
Solvent-only control	5

470. Which of the test allergens is most likely to be inducing the symptoms of Ms. Y.?

   (A) Cat dander

   (B) House dust

   (C) Kentucky blue grass

   (D) Mold

   (E) Pollen

471. Which of the following substances is most likely to prevent the attachment of the mold allergen to the sensitized mast cells of Ms. Y.?

   (A) Cromolyn sodium

   (B) Complement

   (C) Corticosteroids

   (D) Epinephrine

   (E) IgG anti-mold

472. A 64-year-old alcoholic man has fever, chills, cough, and pleuritic pain. His sputum is a dark brown color, and upon cultivation on blood agar, produces alpha hemolytic colonies. These colonies are composed of gram-positive, optochin-positive cocci. The microbes most likely are

   (A) *Enterococcus faecalis*

   (B) *Neisseria meningitidis*

   (C) *Staphylococcus aureus*

   (D) *Streptococcus pneumoniae*

   (E) *Streptococcus pyogenes*

473. According to Figure 4–8, the rate of growth of the bacterial culture for which it was ob-

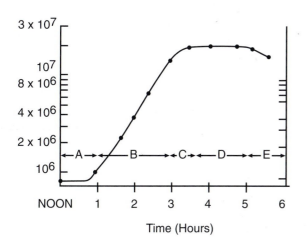

Figure 4–8

tained reaches its maximum rate of growth between

   (A) 12:00 PM and 1:00 PM

   (B) 1:00 PM and 3:00 PM

   (C) 3:00 PM and 3:30 PM

   (D) 3:30 PM and 5:00 PM

   (E) 5:00 PM and 6:00 PM

474. A 33-year-old woman may be suffering from a B-cell deficiency. What is the best method for assessing the total number of B lymphocytes of this patient?

   (A) E rosette assay

   (B) Fc receptor assay

   (C) Phytohemagglutinin A (PHA) mitogenicity

   (D) Quantitative immunoglobulin levels

   (E) Surface immunoglobulin (sIg) assay

475. A 21-year-old man has Lyme disease. Which of the following statements concerning Lyme disease is correct?

   (A) It does not respond to tetracycline treatment early in the acute illness.

   (B) It has not been associated with arthritis.

   (C) It is a disease in which the serum levels of IgM correlate with disease activity.

   (D) It is caused by *Leptospira interrogans*.

   (E) It is transmitted by mites.

476. A gram-negative bacterium is isolated from a patient's cerebrospinal fluid (CSF). It grows on enriched chocolate agar, but does not grow on blood agar, except adjacent to a streak of staphylococci. The organism most probably is

   (A) *Haemophilus influenzae*

   (B) *Listeria monocytogenes*

   (C) *Neisseria gonorrhoeae*

   (D) *Neisseria meningitidis*

   (E) *Streptococcus pneumoniae*

477. A laboratory worker died within a day following an accidental ingestion of a very small amount of a bacterial toxin. This toxin had the lowest 50% lethal dose (LD_{50}), and was most likely produced by

(A) *Clostridium botulinum*
(B) *Clostridium tetani*
(C) *Corynebacterium diphtheriae*
(D) *Salmonella typhi*
(E) *Yersinia pestis*

478. *Helicobacter pylori*

(A) appears to be important in the pathogenesis of peptic ulcer
(B) does not induce specific antibodies in gastritis patients
(C) is an obligate intracellular parasite
(D) is usually found in the oral cavity
(E) produces an abundant amount of coagulase

479. The immunoglobulin that passes the placental barrier in humans is

(A) IgA
(B) IgD
(C) IgE
(D) IgG
(E) IgM

480. A 27-year-old man is treated with penicillin for gonorrhea. Thirty-five days later he was reinfected with the same germ, and his physician administers an intramuscular dose of penicillin. Two minutes following the injection of penicillin the patient has respiratory difficulties and becomes unconscious. This reaction was most likely mediated by

(A) activation of the alternate complement pathway
(B) activation of the classical complement pathway
(C) IgD
(D) IgE
(E) IgG

481. A urine sample containing viable *E. coli* is inoculated into an appropriate medium to 500 cells per mL. Assuming the generation time of *E. coli* cells in this medium is 20 minutes, the number of viable cells per mL after 3 hours of incubation will be

(A) 8000
(B) 32,000
(C) 16,000
(D) 64,000
(E) 256,000

482. Viruses are attractive vectors for gene therapy because

(A) adenovirus vectors cannot be used to target gene transfer into cells of the respiratory tract
(B) retrovirus vectors can be produced in extremely small quantities from producer cell lines
(C) the genes inserted into viruses may be expressed in a regulated way
(D) they infect cells with much lower efficiency compared to chemical or physical means of gene transfer
(E) they work only in non-human diseases with multiple affected genes

483. An experiment is performed in which lawn bacteria is plated onto a nutrient plate and replica plated to four media, each containing an antibiotic. Results are shown in Figure 4–9. Which of the following statements is true concerning the interpretation of this experiment?

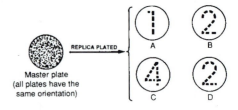

Figure 4–9

(A) Lamarckian theory is not supported.

(B) Mutation is not likely to occur in bacteria.

(C) Plates B and D likely contain the same antibiotics.

(D) Plates B, C, and D all contain different antibiotics.

(E) The replica plate technique is an inappropriate method to answer questions about spontaneous mutation.

484. Four hours after eating fried rice, a man develops diarrhea, vomiting, and nausea. Which of the following microorganisms is most likely involved?

(A) *Bacillus cereus*

(B) *Clostridium botulinum*

(C) *Clostridium tetani*

(D) *Proteus mirabilis*

(E) *Salmonella enteritidis*

485. X-linked agammaglobulinemic patients are most likely to present with repeated infections involving

(A) extracellular bacteria

(B) fungi

(C) intracellular bacteria

(D) *Pneumocystis carinii*

(E) viruses

486. Recent experiments in gene therapy have taken the approach of expressing tumor necrosis factor (TNF) in tumor-infiltrating lymphocytes (TIL). It is hoped that this approach will

(A) allow the TIL to return to the tumor and produce locally high levels of TNF

(B) generate high serum levels of endotoxin

(C) lyse tumor cells due to retrovirus infection

(D) stimulate natural killer (NK) cell activity

(E) stimulate T-cell proliferation

487. A 2-year-old boy who has not been vaccinated against any germ is experiencing se-

vere spasms in the muscles of the jaw and face. These spasms do not allow the child to open his mouth. Laboratory tests establish that a bacterial toxin is responsible for this boy's symptoms. The toxin involved was most likely produced by

(A) botulinum toxin

(B) cholera toxin

(C) clostridial alpha toxin

(D) diptherial toxin

(E) tetanus toxin

488. A college freshman has the typical symptoms of infectious mononucleosis. The most sensitive means of confirming this infection is

(A) antibody that reacts with Epstein–Barr virus–associated nuclear antigen

(B) antibody to hemagglutinin

(C) antibody to neuraminidase

(D) heterophile antibody that reacts with antigens on sheep erythrocytes

(E) nucleic acid hybridization assays for the presence of Epstein–Barr viral nucleic acid

489. A hemagglutination assay is performed with a sample of influenza virus. A fixed number of chicken red blood cells are mixed with increasing dilutions of the influenza virus. The results of the assay are shown in Figure 4–10. The hemagglutination titer of the virus is

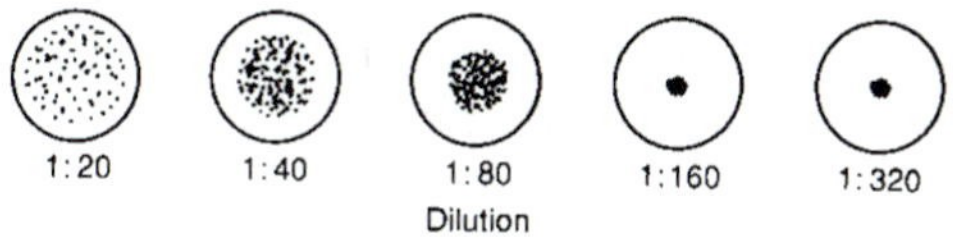

1:20   1:40   1:80   1:160   1:320
Dilution

Figure 4–10

(A) 20

(B) 40

(C) 80

(D) 160

(E) 320

490. The AIDS virus (HIV) differs from the RNA tumor viruses in that it

(A) contains the gag gene

(B) contains the pol gene

(C) contains two copies of single-stranded RNA in its virion

(D) does not require T4 receptor protein for adsorption to host cells

(E) lyses the host cells

491. A 24-year-old construction worker who had four injections of the DPT (diphtheria, pertussis, and tetanus) vaccine in his first year of life and boosters at ages 5 and 19 receives a deep laceration while excavating a building's foundation. The preferred treatment is

(A) equine tetanus immune globulin, because it will passively immunize him

(B) human tetanus immune globulin, because it will stimulate his anamnestic response

(C) penicillin

(D) streptomycin

(E) tetanus toxoid, because it will stimulate his anamnestic response

492. A 19-year-old student who spent a month removing bushes along the North Atlantic coast found a tick attached to his leg, and he crushed the tick with his fingers. A few days later he developed fever, chills, fatigue, and headache. In the area where he was bitten by the tick he noticed a spreading, circular rash with a clear center. The most likely diagnosis is

(A) epidemic typhus

(B) Lyme disease

(C) Q fever

(D) rickettsial pox

(E) trench fever

493. The structure in Figure 4–11 represents

(A) acyclovir, which inhibits the herpesvirus-encoded DNA polymerase

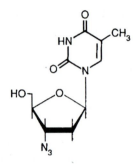

Figure 4–11

(B) azidothymidine (AZT), which inhibits the AIDS virus reverse transcriptase

(C) dideoxyinosine, which inhibits poliovirus replication

(D) enviroxine, which inhibits rhinoviruses

(E) idoxuridine, which inhibits herpesvirus thymidine kinase

494. A middle-aged nurse providing voluntary medical services in a very poor area is bitten by an infected arthropod vector and develops epidemic typhus. Which of the following vectors transmitted the disease?

(A) Flea

(B) Louse

(C) Mite

(D) Mosquito

(E) Tick

495. A young child develops staphylococcal scalded syndrome. Which of the following toxins is most likely responsible for this syndrome?

(A) Alpha toxin

(B) Erythrogenic toxin

(C) Exfoliatin

(D) Staphylococcal toxins A through D

(E) Toxic shock syndrome toxin

496. You are faced with the problem of controlling a virus infection in a community and are told that it has been determined it is a togavirus (arborvirus). You know then that your problem most likely is one of

(A) identifying and controlling an insect vector and identifying and controlling an animal reservoir

(B) improving the treatment of sewage

(C) preventing the use of arborvirus carriers as food handlers

(D) stopping spread by reducing the close contact of children in schools

(E) stopping the spread by respiratory droplets and dust of a virus that enters by the respiratory tract

497. Diagnosis of syphilis can be made using the treponemal and nontreponemal serologic tests. Which one of the following statements concerning the Venereal Diseases Regional Laboratory (VDRL) test is correct?

(A) It cannot be used to follow the efficiency of penicillin treatment.

(B) It does not require diphosphatidylglyc-erol (cardiolipin) as an antigen.

(C) It is a widely used nontreponemal test.

(D) It is basically a complement fixation test.

(E) It is not useful for screening large numbers of people for syphilis.

498. Jacklyn, a fashion model, had several teeth extracted because she had periodontal abscesses. Three months later, she develops a 40°C fever and lower abdominal pain. Anaerobic cultures of the biopsy material show small, spidery colonies in 2 to 3 days. The colonies contained gram-positive, non-acid-fast rods, and branching filaments. Pus from a liver abscess contains yellow granules. Administration of 6 million units of penicillin daily for 2 months brings complete remission of Jacklyn's illness. The most likely causative agent of her disease is

(A) *Actinomyces israelii*

(B) *Histoplasma capsulatum*

(C) *Mycobacterium kansasii*

(D) *Mycobacterium tuberculosis*

(E) *Nocardia asteroides*

499. A gardener pricks his toe while cutting rose bushes. Four days later, a pustule that changes to an ulcer develops on his toe. Then three nodules form along the local lymphatic drainage. The most likely agent is

(A) *Aspergillus fumigatus*

(B) *Candida albicans*

(C) *Cryptococcus neoformans*

(D) *Sporothrix schenckii*

(E) *Trichophyton rubrum*

500. The genome of which virus is a circular molecule of DNA having the structure diagrammed in Figure 4–12?

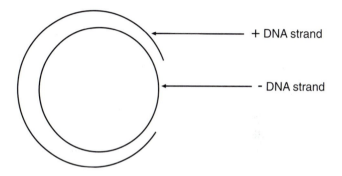

Figure 4–12

(A) Epstein-Barr virus

(B) Hepatitis A virus

(C) Hepatitis B virus

(D) J.C. virus

(E) Papillomavirus

501. A 19-year-old girl has smooth, annular, scaly, erythematous, vesicular lesions on her leg. Assuming that you suspect tinea corporis, what would be the most suitable laboratory diagnostic approach?

(A) Acid-fast staining on the vesicular fluid

(B) Culture of the vesicular fluid on agar

(C) Digestion of tissue biopsies with 10% to 25% KOH

(D) Serology for *Blastomyces dermatitidis*

(E) Silver staining of tissue scraping

502. A 46-year-old cattle rancher develops a low-grade fever 5 days after his 20th high school reunion, which included a rabbit hunt. Standard febrile agglutinin titrations reveal low levels of antibodies to the following organisms: *Francisella tularensis, Brucella suis, Brucella abortus, Salmonella typhi,* and *Proteus* OX-19. The differential diagnosis should include

    (A) brucellosis
    (B) Rocky Mountain spotted fever
    (C) tularemia
    (D) tularemia, brucellosis, typhoid fever, and Rocky Mountain spotted fever
    (E) typhoid fever

503. A child has fever, conjunctivitis, coryza, and sore throat. The clinical laboratory has isolated a nonenveloped, icosahedral DNA virus shown in Figure 4–13. This microorganism most likely is

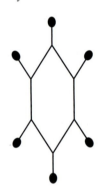

Figure 4–13

    (A) adenovirus
    (B) hepadnavirus
    (C) herpesvirus
    (D) parvovirus
    (E) poxvirus

504. An infant has congenital syphilis, which can best be detected by

    (A) dark-field examination
    (B) FTA-ABA IgM test
    (C) silver nitrate staining of spirochetes
    (D) use of Wassermann complement fixation test
    (E) x-rays

505. A 21-year-old man has been skin tested and had a positive test to purified protein derivative (PPD). This indicates that he has

    (A) active tuberculosis
    (B) been exposed to *Mycobacterium tuberculosis*
    (C) proper B-cell function
    (D) provided sound information on his health status
    (E) received BCG vaccine

506. Amantadine is used for the treatment of infections by

    (A) Epstein–Barr virus
    (B) herpes simplex virus
    (C) influenza virus
    (D) rabies virus
    (E) rhinovirus

507. Immunologic suppression for transplantation

    (A) cannot be achieved by cyclosporine administration
    (B) cannot occur by lymphoid irradiation
    (C) can occur by antilymphocyte globulin
    (D) is facilitated by gamma-interferon administration
    (E) is not likely to respond to steroid administration

508. A virus whose genome is a linear double-stranded DNA that contains a virus encoded protein covalently cross-linked to each 5'-end is

    (A) adenovirus
    (B) herpes simplex virus
    (C) SV40
    (D) vaccinia virus
    (E) varicella-zoster virus

509. Desirable properties of a vector plasmid for use in molecular cloning include

    (A) incorporation into host cell chromosome
    (B) low copy number
    (C) multiple sites for many restriction enzymes

(D) nonautonomous replication

(E) selectable phenotype

510. *Legionella pneumophila*

(A) cannot survive for months in tap water at 25°C

(B) has been found in air-conditioning systems

(C) is easily demonstrable in Gram stains of clinical specimens

(D) is not the major cause of legionellosis in humans

(E) is the cause of trench fever

511. A 19-year-old man has tuberculosis. Numerous acid-fast bacilli are seen in his sputum, and more than 70 colonies of *Mycobacterium tuberculosis* developed on the Lowenstein–Jensen medium. The individuals who have come into contact with this patient should

(A) be immunized by BCG vaccine

(B) not be checked periodically by sputum culture

(C) not be checked periodically by x-ray

(D) receive a full course of ethambutol and isoniazid (INH)

(E) receive prophylactic INH

512. Judging from the graph in Figure 4–14, which microorganism is likely to be the causative agent of food poisoning characterized by diarrhea, abdominal cramps, and severe vomiting?

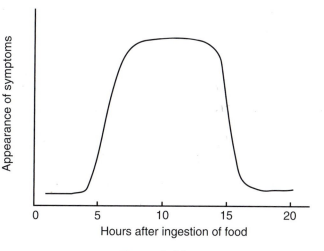

Figure 4–14

(A) *Campylobacter jejuni*

(B) *Salmonella typhimurium*

(C) *Staphylococcus aureus*

(D) *Vibrio parahaemolyticus*

(E) *Yersinia enterocolitica*

513. A boy with diphtheria, who has not been immunized against this disease, is given diphtheria antitoxin. Administration of the antitoxin may lead to

(A) development of serum sickness in 4 to 10 days

(B) elevation in the concentration of serum complement

(C) elimination of the need for immunization with the diphtheria toxoid

(D) lifelong immunity against diphtheria

(E) production of antibodies against diphtheria

514. Poliovirus type 2 is isolated from the stool of a 55-year-old patient who is clinically diagnosed as having poliomyelitis. There were no previous cases of polio reported. However, an infant grandchild was vaccinated about 3 weeks prior to onset of the disease. How can the laboratory determine whether the isolated virus is related to the vaccine strain or a wild-type virus?

(A) Determine the cytopathic effects of the virus.

(B) Inoculate the virus into mice to determine whether it kills them.

(C) Perform neutralization studies using the infant's serum.

(D) Perform oligonucleotide mapping of the unknown virus and compare with maps of wild-type and vaccine strains.

(E) Stain the virus with fluorescent antibody.

515. Two days following surgery to repair a defective valve, a patient develops an acute infection caused by a penicillin-resistant strain of *S. aureus*. Figure 4–15 shows the penicillin molecule. Select the most likely numbered site of penicillinase action.

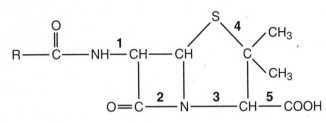

Figure 4–15

(A) 1
(B) 2
(C) 3
(D) 4
(E) 5

516. The laboratory diagnosis of tinea pedis (athlete's foot), caused by *Trichophyton rubrum*, may be made by finding characteristic conidia in cultures of skin scrapings. Which one of the drawings in Figure 4–16 shows the characteristic conidia of *T. rubrum*?

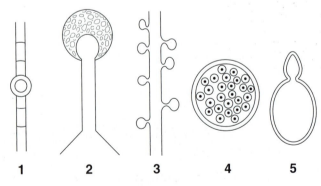

Figure 4–16

(A) 1
(B) 2
(C) 3
(D) 4
(E) 5

517. A 25-year-old man comes to your office experiencing inability to swallow and speech difficulty. The patient was in perfect health prior to the consumption of home-canned green beans. He also states that the can was swollen at the ends prior to its being opened. Which of the following is the most likely method of treatment?

(A) Administration of staphylococcal enterotoxin antiserum
(B) Administration of trivalent botulinum antitoxin
(C) Immunization with *Staphylococcus aureus* enterotoxin toxoid
(D) Penicillin administration
(E) Placement of the patient in a hyperbaric oxygen chamber

518. A patient is given an antifungal agent to inhibit the biosynthesis of fungal ergosterol. The agent most likely given is

(A) amphotericin B
(B) flucytosine
(C) griseofulvin
(D) ketoconazole
(E) nystatin

519. A 5-year-old child with a history of recurrent pulmonary infections is brought to the emergency room in respiratory distress. A Gram stain reveals numerous polymorphonuclear neutrophils and gram-positive cocci in grape-like clusters in his sputum. The antibiotic to be employed until antibiotic sensitivity tests are reported is

(A) ampicillin
(B) kanamycin
(C) methicillin
(D) penicillin
(E) streptomycin

Questions 520 through 522

Scott, a 10-year-old boy, was camping on the east coast during the summer when he was bitten by ticks. Seven days later he developed myalgia, a temperature of 102°C, macules, and petechiae. The rashes appeared first on his arms and legs, then spread over his body, and Scott became delirious.

520. Scott's pediatrician conducted the appropriate laboratory tests and became convinced that Scott had

  (A) epidemic typhus
  (B) Q fever
  (C) rickettsial pox
  (D) Rocky Mountain spotted fever
  (E) scrub typhus

521. Which of the following tests provided the most reliable information to establish the diagnosis of Scott's illness?

  (A) Complement fixation
  (B) Culture on blood agar
  (C) Culture on Saboraud agar
  (D) Gram stain
  (E) Weil–Felix reaction

522. It can be safely stated that the etiologic agent of Scott's disease

  (A) cannot be seen with a light microscope
  (B) has a cell wall resembling the cell wall of gram-negative bacteria
  (C) is resistant to tetracycline
  (D) lacks a cell wall
  (E) replicates with a distinct intracellular cycle

Questions 523 through 525

Miss T., upon her return from vacation in a tropical area with poor sanitary conditions, becomes ill. She experienced lower abdominal pain, colitis, tenesmus, flatulence, and bloody diarrhea caused by a protozoa.

523. The most likely diagnosis is

  (A) acute amoebic dysentery
  (B) malaria
  (C) toxoplasmosis

  (D) trichomoniasis
  (E) trypanosomiasis

524. The etiologic agent of Miss T.'s disease is usually transmitted by the ingestion of

  (A) cysts
  (B) gametocytes
  (C) larvae
  (D) ova
  (E) sporozoites

525. The drug(s) of choice for the treatment of Miss T.'s illness is(are)

  (A) chloroquine
  (B) metronidazole and iodoquinol
  (C) stibogluconate
  (D) sulfonamide and pyrimethamine
  (E) trimethoprim and sulfamethoxazole

Questions 526 through 528

Mr. X. has been feasting on raw oysters for the past 9 months. This 26-year-old man has been healthy all of his life. Suddenly, he develops fatigue, loss of appetite, nausea, vomiting, abdominal pain, and fever. Following a careful evaluation, his doctor informs him that he is suffering from a viral infection. This infection was caused by a small (20 to 30 nm), nonenveloped, single-stranded RNA virus.

526. This virus most likely is

  (A) adenovirus
  (B) hepatitis A virus
  (C) hepatitis B virus
  (D) rhinovirus
  (E) rotavirus

527. Diagnosis of the causative agent of Mr. X.'s illness can best be made by

  (A) a positive Tzanck smear
  (B) assays for specific viral cytopathic effects
  (C) detection of IgA antibodies against the specific virus
  (D) detection of IgM antibodies against the specific virus
  (E) detection of Negri bodies in Mr. X.'s tissues

528. Mr. X.'s viral infection can best be prevented by

(A) administration of human gamma globulin

(B) immunization with HBcAg

(C) immunization with the specific inactivated virus

(D) immunization with the specific subunit vaccine

(E) interferon

Questions 529 through 531

Neutrophils from a 3-year-old child who has been suffering from repeated staphylococcal infections show normal phagocytosis. However, intracellular killing of staphylococci by the neutrophils is severely impaired. Myeloperoxidase activity of neutrophils is normal. The child has no history of streptococcal infection.

529. The most likely disease affecting this patient is

(A) chronic granulomatous disease

(B) Graves disease

(C) rheumatoid arthritis

(D) severe combined immunodeficiency disease (SCID)

(E) systemic lupus erythematosus (SLE)

530. The reason the child has no history of streptococcal infection is that

(A) he has been administered antistreptolysin O

(B) he has been immunized with C-reactive protein (CRP)

(C) he has been injected with pooled human gamma globulin

(D) phagocytosis plays a minor role in the killing of streptococci

(E) streptococci are catalase negative

531. Diagnosis is made by the

(A) Coombs test

(B) India ink test

(C) methyl red test

(D) mixed lymphocyte reaction

(E) nitroblue tetrazolium test

532. The difficulty in the use of tumor necrosis factor-alpha (TNF-α) for cancer therapy is best described by which of the following statements?

(A) Cachexia is a complication.

(B) Suppression of cytotoxic T lymphocytes is a complication.

(C) TNF-α in low doses is an endogenous pyrogen.

(D) TNF-α is an anti-inflammatory agent.

(E) TNF-α suppresses production of interleukins 1 and 6.

533. A 39-year-old man with normal sexual behavior presents to his physician with mild fever (38.2°C). Upon physical examination, he is found to suffer from pharyngitis. This infection was not associated with tonsillitis, but conjunctivitis was also obvious. Which of the following microbes is the most likely cause of the infection?

(A) Adenovirus

(B) *Chlamydia pneumoniae*

(C) *Neisseria gonorrheae*

(D) *Streptococcus pyogenes*

(E) *Toxoplasma gondii*

534. 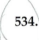 A 23-year-old student presents with intermittent fever, sweats, myaglias, and profound malaise for 15 days. Brucellosis is the most probable cause of this illness of unknown origin; he recently spent his vacation in Mexico where he consumed unpasteurized milk. Which of the following statements regarding this student's presumed brucellosis is most likely applicable?

(A) A routinely used skin test can rapidly confirm the diagnosis.

(B) After 5 to 7 days of aerobic incubation with 10% CO_2, blood cultures will grow small, gram-negative coccobacilli.

(C) If the patient were vaccinated, his disease would have been prevented.

(D) Only cultures can be used for the diagnosis of brucellosis because serology is not available.

(E) The patient will be treated with tetracycline for 5 days.

535. The most important initial clinical feature of systemic lupus erythematosus is the detection of

(A) a lesion known as erythema chronicum migrans

(B) a rash in a butterfly distribution on the face

(C) antibody to single-stranded RNA

(D) carditis

(E) pneumonitis

536. Patients tend to develop septicemia with hemorrhagic rash and shock more frequently with *Neisseria meningitidis* than with *Neisseria gonorrhoeae*. This is most likely due to

(A) absence of lipid A in the endotoxin of *N. gonorrhoeae*

(B) exotoxins produced by *N. meningitidis* but not by *N. gonorrhoeae*

(C) greater quantities of endotoxins released by *N. meningitidis*

(D) higher toxicity of endotoxins of *N. meningitidis*

(E) the larger capsule of *N. menigitidis* than that of *N. gonorrhoeae*

537. Bacterial resistance to rifampicin arises from mutations in

(A) dihydrofolate reductase

(B) DNA gyrase

(C) RNA polymerase

(D) rRNA methylase

(E) transpeptidase

538. Bronchial constriction and mucous formation contribute to the rapid, life-threatening symptoms of asthma. These physiologic changes are caused by mast cells, which release which one of the following substances?

(A) Eosinophil chemotactic factor of anaphylaxis

(B) Epinephrine

(C) Histamine

(D) Interleukin 1

(E) Interleukin 5

539. A 59-year-old immunocompromised man complains of headache, confusion, and neck stiffness. Computed tomography reveals multiple abscesses in the central nervous system. Which of the following microorganisms is the most likely etiologic agent?

(A) *Borrelia burgdorferi*

(B) *Cryptococcus neoformans*

(C) *Mycobacterium tuberculosis*

(D) *Treponema pallidum*

(E) *Treponema pertenue*

540. β-Lactam antibiotics are ineffective against *Mycoplasma pneumoniae* because this microorganism

(A) has a cell wall that is impermeable to these antibiotics

(B) has a membrane that contains large amounts of teichoic acids

(C) has a membrane that contains sterols

(D) lacks a rigid cell wall

(E) produces large amounts of β-lactamases

541. A pediatric immunologist informs you that your child has a severe deficiency in helper T-cell function. What is the most likely immunologic consequence?

(A) A deficiency in B-cell function

(B) A deficiency in serum complement

(C) Both a deficiency in B-cell and cytotoxic T-cell functions

(D) Only a deficiency in cytotoxic T-cell function

(E) Only a deficiency in T-helper cell function

542. A 45-year-old woman is seriously bitten by a dog. The wound is cleansed, and she was given tetanus toxoid as well as an injection of penicillin G. Several days later, the wound becomes infected and purulent. Cultures on blood agar yield gram-negative rods. The most likely organism isolated was

(A) *Clostridium botulinum*
(B) *Clostridium perfringens*
(C) *Clostridium tetani*
(D) *Pasteurella multicida*
(E) *Toxocara canis*

543. A housewife with a urinary tract infection caused by *Escherichia coli* was treated with sulfonamides. These antibiotics were administered because they are known to prevent synthesis of which one of the following bacterial constituents?

(A) Cytoplasmic membrane
(B) DNA
(C) Peptidoglycan
(D) RNA
(E) Tetrahydrofolic acid

544. A 25-year-old woman with non–X-linked agammaglobulinemia is 8 months pregnant. Her child most likely will be at risk for infection by which one of the following microorganisms?

(A) *Blastomyces dermatitidis*
(B) Encapsulated *Streptococcus pneumoniae*
(C) *Histoplasma capsulatum*
(D) *Leishmania donovani*
(E) *Mycobacterium tuberculosis*

545. An increase in the rates of ciprofloxacin resistance among enterobacteria most likely is due to

(A) an increase in the acquisition of an exogenous gene allowing efficient cell wall synthesis
(B) an increase in the number of strains with high rates of DNA polymerase synthesis
(C) an increase in the number of strains with high rates of protein synthesis
(D) an increase in the selection of strains mutated at genes encoding enzymes necessary for DNA replication
(E) the spread of a plasmid-carrying a ciproflaxacin-resistant gene

546. A 25-year-old man suddenly develops fever, rigors, lethargy, a stiff neck, difficulty breathing, tachycardia, and a petechial rash. Microscopic examination of the cerebral fluid shows a pyrogenic infection. Which of the following microbes is the most likely etiologic agent?

(A) *Borreria burgdorferi*
(B) *Neisseria meningitidis*
(C) *Staphylococccus aureus*
(D) *Streptococcus mitis*
(E) *Streptococcus mutans*

Answers and Explanations

410. (C) Deficiency in production of J chains for immunoglobulins could result in a decrease in serum IgA and IgM levels. These antibodies are dimers and pentamers of the basic immunoglobulin molecule, and require a J chain to join the immunoglobulin chains. There is no evidence to indicate that a deficiency in the production of J chains of IgA or IgM causes a decrease in mature B cells or T lymphocytes, an increase in serum IgM and decrease in IgE, or a decrease in IgA (choices A, B, D, and E).

411. (C) *Pseudomonas aeruginosa* is an oligotrophic bacterium which survives well in the water of the swimming pool. It also is not very susceptible to swimming pool disinfectants. Thus, it is a frequent cause of diffuse external otitis. *Haemophilus influenzae* (choice B), *Staphylococcus aureus* (choice D), and *Streptococcus pneumoniae* (choice E) are not as abundant as *P. aeruginosa* in swimming pools; they cannot grow in swimming pools because they require rich nutrients. Thus, although they can cause internal otitis their infective dose levels are well below those required for overinfections. *Haemophilus ducreyi* (choice A) is the causative agent of soft chancre transmitted venereally.

412. (D) Molecular amplification techniques provide fast diagnostic results when they are compared to traditional cultural procedures for *M. tuberculosis*, which has to be incubated for at least several weeks. They show an excellent specificity (more than 90%), but a low sensitivity (around 70%); therefore, they should not be applied to all specimens, only to specimens with a positive acid-fast stain

(choice A). Molecular amplification techniques can never replace mycobacterial cultures because the isolation of a mycobacterial strain is necessary for antibiotic sensitivity tests or additional verification (choice E). Molecular tests for the diagnosis of tuberculosis have been standardized only for respiratory tract mycobacterial specimens (choice C). Molecular amplification techniques like PCR are expensive (choice B).

413. (C) An indirect immunoassay, such as the immunofluorescent test, uses the patient's serum to detect antigen, and then an anti-human immunoglobulin, which is labeled to detect the binding of the patient's serum's antibody to the antigen. Fluorescein-labeled antibody is the final but not intermediate reagent (choice B). Similarly, fluorescein dye or complement components are not added as intermediate reagents (choices A, D, and E).

414. (B) β-Lactam–induced lysis of bacteria results from the inhibition of synthesis of cell walls and the hydrolysis of cells walls by cellular autolytic enzymes. Bacterial cells that lack or have suppressed autolysins are less susceptible to the bactericidal activity of β-lactams. Induction of autolysis occurs mostly from the increase in the amounts of cell wall metabolites. In that respect, only drugs directly involved in cell wall metabolism can exhibit this action. Quinolones (choice C) that inhibit DNA gyrase and the inhibitors of protein synthesis, such as aminoglycosides (choice A), and tetracyclines, or rifampins do not directly interfere with the synthesis of peptidoglycan (choices D and E).

415. **(E)** Induction of latent infection with herpes simplex virus type I is an effective mechanism of evading host defenses. Latency results in a drastic reduction of expression of all viral antigens, limiting the targets of the immune system. During latency, there are no cytopathic effects that would elicit an immune response. Antigenic variation is not encountered among herpes viruses (choice D). This mechanism is crucial for other viruses such as influenza, which also undergoes antigenic drifts and shifts (choices A and C). Antigenic masking (choice B) is actually the covering up of the viral antigens in a way so as to block access of antibodies, complement components, and cytotoxic cell. Masking is achieved by extensive glycosylation of the envelope proteins of viruses.

416. **(B)** Interferons are produced by most nucleated cells in the body, and inhibit the translation of viral proteins. There are three major types of interferons: α, β, and γ. These three types have many subtypes (choice D). Interferons are active against many viruses, and thus are not highly specific in their action (choice A). Interferons are strongly induced by viruses and double-stranded RNA, not microbial proteins (choice C). Interferons inhibit viral growth by blocking translation of viral proteins, not the transcription of viral genes (choice E).

417. **(A)** All five organisms are protozoa. There are two intestinal protozoa specifically associated with AIDS that can cause transient diarrhea in immunocompetent individuals, but can cause debilitating and potentially life-threatening, chronic diarrhea in AIDS patients. These organisms are *C. parvum* (choice A) (which has no effective drug therapy) and *Isospora belli* (which can be treated with folate antagonists, such as trimethoprim-sulfamethoxazole). *Entamoeba histolytica* (choice B) and *G. lamblia* (choice C) may cause diarrhea, but they are not closely associated with AIDS. *Microsporidia* (choice D) may cause severe, persistent, watery diarrhea in AIDS patients, but they produce spores rather than oocysts. *Taenia solium* (choice E) is the pork tapeworm that occasionally may cause diarrhea.

418. **(E)** *Streptococcus pneumoniae* is one of the principal germs associated with community-acquired pneumonia. This disease begins abruptly, it is usually lobar, and if it is not treated properly causes pleural effusion. *Streptococcus pneumoniae* is normally sensitive to penicillin, but refractory to third-generation cephalosporins. *Chlamydia pneumoniae* (choice A), *L. pneumophila* (choice B), and *M. pneumoniae* (choice C) produce atypical pneumonia; the disease begins gradually, often involves more than one segment, seldom produces pleurosy, and does not respond to penicillin. Therefore, atypical pneumonia is normally treated with macrolides. *Pneumocystis carinii* (choice E) is a significant cause of pneumonia in immunosuppressed individuals, such as AIDS patients.

419. **(B)** The spleen is important for the production of IgM and IgG antibodies needed to opsonize encapsulated bacteria. Involvement of the spleen in inactivation of antimicrobial agents (choice A), processing of capsular polysaccharides (choice D), or metabolism of microbial agents (choice E) is not considered important. The main source of stem cells is the bone marrow, not the spleen (choice C).

420. **(C)** *Brucella melitensis* is a gram-negative rod aerobic bacterium that grows well in the presence of 10% CO_2 as a coccobacillus. This microbe has a predilection for the cells of the reticuloendothelial system. This explains the frequent splenomegaly or hepatomegaly, which when present provide useful clues for the diagnosis of brucellosis. *Actinomyces israelii* (choice A) is a gram-positive branching rod bacterium that causes actinomycosis. *Aspergillus fumigatus* (choice B) is a branching, filamentous fungus that has been associated with invasive infections in immunocompromised hosts. *Candida albicans* (choice D) is a yeast that causes disseminated disease in immunosuppressed individuals. *Mycobacterium tuberculosis* (choice E) is a strictly aerobic acid-fast rod bacterium. It can cause tuberculosis and vertebral osteomyelitis. In these cases, and in the absence of immunosuppression, the Mantoux test is positive.

421. **(C)** Myocarditis is most commonly caused by Coxsackie group B viruses, and may be preceded by GI or respiratory symptoms. Adenovirus, coronavirus, mumps virus, and rhinovirus (choices A, B, D, and E) may be associated with influenza-like or GI symptoms, but they are not common causes of myocarditis.

422. **(E)** Passive immunization provides immediate protection against a microbe because the passively transferred serum contains preformed antibody from the donor. The transferred serum can induce a hypersensitivity reaction or allergic response to the foreign serum, but there is no evidence concerning magnification of the specific immune response to the microorganism by passively transferred antibodies, or that passive immunity with multiple injections are more expensive than direct vaccination (choices A, C, and D). Passive immunization involves only the injection of preformed, specific antibody (choice B).

423. **(D)** *Salmonella enteritidis* is a common cause of osteomyelitis in sickle cell anemia patients. *Streptococcus pyogenes* (choice E) and *H. influenzae* (choice B) may cause osteomyelitis in children, but the disease in this case is preceded by septicemia, very high fever, sweating, and rigors. Furthermore, these microbes are not the most common causes of osteomyelitis in sickle cell anemia patients. *Pseudomonas aeruginosa* (choice C) most frequently causes osteomyelitis in IV drug users, and *B. fragilis* (choice A) is a rare cause of osteomyelitis that is not associated with sickle cell anemia.

424. **(E)** The application of Gram stain to mycobacteria results either in the appearance of disfigured cells or the inability to stain the mycobacterial cells. The lipid-rich cell wall of mycobacteria is responsible for the acid-fast character of these bacteria (choice B). Acid-

fact stains cannot yield definitive results in less than 5 minutes, or be used to distinguish between pathogenic and nonpathogenic mycobacteria (choices A and D). Furthermore, acid-fast stains do not distinguish the various species of mycobacteria (choice C)

425. **(E)** The envelope of hepatitis B virus (HBV) contains an antigen known as hepatitis B surface antigen (HBsAg). This antigen is important because production of antibodies to HBsAg indicates immunity against hepatitis B virus, which resulted either from infection or vaccination with HBsAg. Treatment of HBV with a nonionic detergent removes the envelope and produces the viral core, which contains the hepatitis B core antigen (HBcAg). Antibodies to HBcAg are not protective (choice C). Treatment of the viral core with strong detergents results in the release of a soluble core antigen called hepatitis virus antigen e (HBeAg). Production of antibody to HBeAg signals active disease during which the patient is infectious (choice D). The DNA genome (choice B) and the nucleocapsid proteins of HBV (choice A) are not protective.

426. **(A)** Delayed-type hypersensitivity is mediated by helper CD4 lymphocytes, not antibody (choice D). Thus it can only be transferred by sensitized CD4 helper lymphocytes. Sensitization occurs via such substances as poison ivy, poison oak, some cosmetics, topically applied sulfonamides, or other drugs and simple chemicals, such as nickel and formaldehyde, but not inhalation of grass pollens (choice E). Part of the tissue destruction seen in tuberculosis is due to delayed-type hypersensitivity, so this type of hypersensitivity reaction may lead to tissue damage (choice C). Administration of antihistaminic drugs, epinephrine, or cromolyn sodium is used for the treatment of anaphylactic reactions resulting from type I hypersensitivity, but not delayed-type hypersensitivity (choice B).

427. **(B)** Piliated strains of *E. coli* move up the urethra to infect the bladder and kidney. Infections of the kidney cause pyelonephritis.

The vast majority of cases of bacterial pyelonephritis, cystitis, and other urinary tract infections are caused by *E. coli*. Introduction of catheters into the urethra has been associated with the occurrence of urinary tract infections. *Clostridium difficile* (choice A) is the cause of pseudomembranous colitis. *Pseudomonas aeruginosa* (choice C) is usually the cause of infections of skin and burns. It is also the major pathogen in cystic fibrosis, and can cause urinary infections, but not as commonly as *E. coli*. *Staphylococcus aureus* (choice D) is usually the cause of boils, skin sepsis, postoperative wound infections, scalded skin syndrome, food-borne infection, septicemia, endocarditis, toxic shock syndrome, osteomyelitis, and pneumonia.

428. **(D)** Acute glomerulonephritis appears as a complication only after pharyngeal infection with group A *Streptococcus pyogenes*. Patients with poststreptococcal acute glomerulonephritis develop high levels of antibodies against streptolysin O of *S. pyogenes*. Thus, the titer of antibodies to streptolysin O can be important in the diagnosis of poststreptococcal acute glomerulonephritis. Determination of serum levels of IgE (choice E) can be important in the diagnosis of immediate-type hypersensitivity, or in certain parasitic infections. Serum levels of antibodies against DNA (choice B) may be of value in the diagnosis of lupus erythematosus. Estimation of the number of T cells (choice A) is useful for the diagnosis of T-cell immunodeficiencies. *Streptococcus pyogenes* do not possess flagella, thus it lacks flagellar antigen H, which would be required for the production of anti-H antibodies (choice C).

429. **(C)** The patient described in the question probably has AIDS. Such individuals are lymphopenic and have greatly reduced immunity. AIDS victims commonly develop *P. carinii* pneumonia. The most important evaluative procedure is determining the cause of the pneumonia so the problem can be corrected. Identifying the infecting organism may assist in the overall diagnosis. Choices A, B, D, and E involve innate immunity, either complement activity or phagocytic cell functions, and would not be of much diagnostic assistance.

430. **(C)** The child appears to be suffering from meningitis due to *S. aureus*, which should always be assumed to be a β-lactamase–producing organism until the laboratory reports its antibiotic sensitivity. Methicillin is a β-lactamase–resistant penicillin that would be the drug of choice among those listed. It is also bactericidal and is not associated with toxicity, which is a feature of streptomycin (choice E) and chloramphenicol (choice B). Other antibiotics that might be used include the cephalosporins, gentamicin, or vancomycin, which may be injected intrathecally.

431. **(D)** In the Ouchterlony diagram, each antibody reacts with its homologous determinant group on the antigen molecule. Thus antibodies a and b will react with antigen ab, but only antibody a will react with antigen ac. Antibody b will diffuse through the line of precipitate formed by antibody a and antigen ac to bind to epitope band and precipitate with antigen ab, forming the spur at position 3. Line 1 will contain both antibodies. The spur (3) will contain antibody b, not antibody a. Line 2 will contain antigen ac and antibody a only.

432. **(B)** Bruton disease is an X-linked congenital agammaglobulinemia. Thus, electrophoresis of the serum of infants, after the passively transferred maternal antibodies have been eliminated, reveals the absence or very low levels of gamma globulin. In contrast to Bruton disease, all the other diseases listed reveal a gamma globulin peak. Addison disease (choice A) and Goodpasture syndrome (choice C) are caused by autoantibody production to basement membrane of kidney and adrenal cortex, respectively. Grave disease (choice D) is caused by autoantibody production to thyroid-stimulating hormone receptors. Myasthenia gravis (choice E) involves autoantibody production to acetylcholine receptor of the neuromuscular junctions.

433. (B) The most important presumptive diagnostic test for gonorrhea is the demonstration of gram-negative, kidney-shaped diplococci inside polymorphonuclear leukocytes obtained from a thick creamy urethral exudate. Chancroid (choice A), caused by *Haemophilus ducrei,* produces sharply circumscribed, non-indurated, painful ulcers. These ulcers are usually found in the genitalia and perianal regions. The ulcers have a soft base and thus are called soft chancres. Bacteria in chancres can be visualized by Gram stains, which reveal gram-negative rods. Lymphogranuloma venereum (choice C), caused by *Chlamydia trachomatis* immunotypes L1 to L3, produces abscesses in the lymph nodes. Diagnosis depends on the demonstration of cytoplasmic inclusions, which are visualized with Giemsa stain or immunofluorescence. Primary syphilis (choice D) produces painless ulcers on the genital organs, anal area, or mouth. These ulcers have well-defined, raised borders and a clean, hard base (hard chancre). The primary lesions usually contain spirochetes that cannot be demonstrated by conventional stains. However, the spirochetes can be visualized by silver stain with immunofluorescence, or with a dark-field microscope. Patients with gonorrhea experience an intense burning sensation during urination. Individuals with trichomoniasis (choice E) discharge a watery, foul-smelling urethral exudate, and staining of this discharge reveals pear-shaped trophozoites that have a jerky motion.

434. (D) Prevention of gonorrhea rests on the use of safe, properly worn condoms, and immediate treatment of symptomatic patients as well as their sexual partners. Ceftriaxone is the best treatment for uncomplicated cases of gonococcal infections. Frequent washing of the genital areas is not likely to prevent gonorrhea (choice A). Since 1976, penicillinase-producing strains of *Neisseria gonorrhoeae* have been isolated that show a high level of resistance to penicillin. Thus, use of 100 U penicillin will be of little if any value for the prevention of gonorrhea (choice C). There are no vaccines composed of either toxoids or killed germs available for the prevention of gonorrhea (choices B and E).

435. (E) If exposure to rabies virus appears definite, as in this case, treatment with human diploid cell live-derived vaccine and hyperimmune anti-rabies gamma globulin should be started immediately. Serum antibodies provide an immediate barrier to the growth of virus; meanwhile, antibodies are elicited by the vaccine. If the level of exposure is minimal (e.g., no skin puncture) and the animal probably is not rabid, vaccination is not recommended. Ordering a search for the attacking fox for autopsy (choice B) to determine if it has rabies is like searching for a needle in a haystack, and thus not the best approach to address a possible rabies infection, which requires immediate action. Initiation of rabies vaccine (choice D) will lead to production of antibodies against the rabies virus, but it will require approximately 2 weeks to develop protective antibodies. By that time, severe damage may have already occurred. Postexposure immunization and human rabies immunoglobulin is the best approach. Observation of the patient (choice A) or reporting of the incident to the state epidemiologist (choice C) do not address the real needs of an individual running the risk of rabies.

436. (E) Exposure to the TB bacillus does not assure disease, but a positive skin test makes the diagnosis more likely. Chemoprophylaxis with isoniazid (INH) is the treatment of choice for contacts of actively infected persons. Ethambutol is very effective against most mycobacteria, but is used in the therapy of TB, not in prophylaxis (choice D). The skin test is the most sensitive index of infection, and for individuals who have already shown a positive response, x-ray would not add much information. Sequential x-rays (choice A) months apart might indicate if the lesion were increasing in size, but that is certainly not a high priority procedure for the person described. Immunization with the live attenuated TB strain bacillus Calmette-Guerin (BCG) (choice B) is pointless because the contacts have already experienced an infection with *M. tuberculosis.* Immunization with purified protein derivative (choice C) does not induce protection against tuberculosis. It is used to determine exposure to *M. tuberculosis.*

437. **(D)** The most acute form of hypersensitivity is systemic anaphylaxis during which there is constriction of the bronchioles and hypotension. Anaphylaxis is mediated by such pharmacologically active substances as histamine, the slow-reacting substance eosinophil, chemotactic factor of anaphylaxis, serotonin, prostaglandins, and thromboxanes. Penicillin is known to be a sensitizing allergen. The patient was sensitized when he was given his first injection of penicillin to treat his urethritis. During the next 3 weeks, IgE formed and attached to receptors on the surface of mast cells. When the physician reinjected penicillin, it combined with the IgE and the mast cells released pharmacologically active substances, inducing constriction of bronchioles and collapse. Gonococcal pneumonia is an extremely rare infection caused by *N. gonorrhoeae* (choice E). Nongonococcal urethritis and reinfection of the urethra with penicillin-sensitive or -resistant strains of *N. gonorrheae* do not cause bronchoconstriction or collapse (choices A, B, and C).

438. **(B)** The mode of action of ultraviolet light on microorganisms is related to its absorption by the DNA. This absorption leads to the formation of covalent bonds between adjacent pyrimidine bases. These pyrimidine dimers alter the form of the DNA and thus interfere with normal base pairing during DNA synthesis. Disruption of the bacterial cell membrane (choice C), removal of free sulfhydryl groups (choice E), protein denaturation (choice D), and addition of alkyl groups to cellular components (choice A) are induced by detergents, heavy metals, heat or alcoholic compounds, and ethylene oxide or formaldehyde, respectively.

439. **(E)** An undesirable side effect of chemotherapy used to treat malignancies is the destruction of T cells, which play a key role in the development of immunity against viral infections. This is especially true for viral diseases in which the etiologic agent remains dormant in the body. Varicella-zoster is an excellent example of such a virus. Thus, flare ups of varicella-zoster infections are well-known occurrences in cancer patients who receive chemotherapy. The varicella-zoster virus is a single entity. It is a medium-sized (100 to 200 nm) double-stranded DNA virus of the herpesvirus group, with only one serologic type. Primary infection with the varicella-zoster virus causes chicken pox. Immunity develops, but the virus remains in the body. Deficiency in the third component of complement (choice A) is associated with enhanced susceptibility to pyogenic extracellular bacterial, but not viruses. Hypogammaglobulinemia has not been shown to cause disseminated varicella-zoster infection (choice B). Immunosuppression by chemotherapy reactivates the varicella-zoster virus and causes shingles (choices C and D).

440. **(B)** Herpes B virus is a spherical, enveloped, double-stranded DNA virus that causes a rare and often fatal encephalitis. Persons in close contact with monkeys (such as zookeepers) or tissue culture workers are at high risk for herpes B virus infection. St. Louis encephalitis virus (choice E) is a small (40-nm) spherical, enveloped, RNA flavivirus. Severe headache, vomiting, and nuchal rigidity are common symptoms, with tremors, convulsions, and coma developing in severe cases. The poliovirus (choice C) and the echovirus (choice A) are small (20 to 30 nm), nonenveloped, single-stranded viruses. Poliovirus causes flaccid paralysis, and echovirus usually induces a flu-like infection. Rabies virus (choice D) is a single-stranded RNA, bullet-shaped, enveloped virus. The pathognomonic symptoms of rabies are salivation, hydrophobia, and coma.

441. **(C)** Curve B depicts the frequency of serologic reactivity following exposure to *Coccidioides immitis* determined by the complement fixation test. Curve A shows the frequency in serologic reactivity following exposure to *C.*

immitis determined by the skin test. The skin test becomes positive approximately 2 weeks after the onset of coccidioidomycosis, precedes the appearance of precipitating complement-fixing antibodies, and tends to remain positive indefinitely (choices A and B). Curve C depicts the frequency of serologic reactivity following exposure to *C. immitis* determined by precipitin test. Precipitin antibodies can be detected in 90% of patients about 2 weeks after the appearance of the symptoms and disappear in approximately 4 to 5 months. Thus, a positive precipitin test suggests active primary or reactivated coccidioidomycosis (choices D and E).

442. **(A)** The specificity of the tetracycline antibiotics is attributable to an energy-dependent transport system present in prokaryotes, but not in eukaryotic cells. This transport system results in accumulation of the drug inside the bacterial cell, where it binds to the ribosome and interferes with binding of aminoacyl-tRNA to the acceptor site. Tetracyclines bind to the bacterial ribosome, but not to DNA-directed RNA polymerase (choice B), or prokaryotic membranes (choices C). Tetracyclines do not inhibit initiation of protein synthesis, which specifically requires formylmethionyl tRNA (choice E). Both prokaryotic and eukaryotic cells bind tetracyclines. However, the prokaryotic cells have much more effective tetracycline transport systems than eukaryotic cells. Thus, prokaryotic cells accumulate higher intracellular concentrations of tetracyclines than eukaryotic cells, which induces a significant inhibition of protein synthesis only in prokaryotic cells (choice D).

443. **(C)** Point C represents the zone of equivalence—that point of the antigen–antibody reaction when optimal concentrations of antigen and antibody combine. Thus, there is little, if any, free antigen and antibody, and as a consequence maximal amounts of antigen and antibody are found in the precipitate resulting from the antigen–antibody reaction. Points A and B represent areas in the antigen–antibody precipitin curve where there is an excess of antibody (choices A and B).

Points D and E show areas in the precipitin curve where there is an antigen excess in the antigen–antibody reaction mixture (choices D and E).

444. **(D)** *Listeria monocytogenes* causes meningitis and sepsis in newborns and patients whose immune systems have been compromised by irradiation or chemotherapy. When this microbe grows at a temperature of 22 to 25°C on blood agar it yields gram-positive rods, which move with a characteristic tumbling motion. A slight zone of hemolysis surrounds the colonies of *L. monocytogenes*. These characteristics are not applicable to *B. cereus* (choice A), *B. pertussis* (choice B), *C. diphtheriae* (choice C), or *N. meningitides* (choice E).

445. **(C)** Immunoglobulin A (IgA) is found in genital, intestinal, and respiratory secretions, and in saliva, tears, and colostrum. It inhibits contact of germs to mucous membranes. Secretory IgA consists of two heavy chains, two light chains, and a secretory component (sc) that allows IgA to pass to a mucosal surface and suppresses degradation of IgA in the intestinal tract. Secretory IgA also contains a J (joining) chain. IgA contains a secretory component but not an sc epitope (choice E). An epitope is defined as the antigenic determinant of a molecule. The heavy chains for IgG are designated g (choice B), for IgA are designated a, and for IgE are designated e (choice A). IgA does not contain paraprotein (choice D).

446. **(C)** There is evidence that antigens must be metabolically processed by macrophages before they can be recognized by the T-helper cells. For example, T-helper cells from F_1 hybrids between two inbred strains ($P_1 \times P_2$) that have been sensitized on antigen-pulsed macrophages from one parent (P_1) will proliferate in response to a second challenge of the antigen only if F_1 macrophages or macrophages from P_1 are present. B cells (choice A) may be involved in antigen processing, but are not the best antigen processors. Kupffer cells (choice B), young erythro-

cytes (choice E), or suppressor T cells (choice D) are not considered inducers of T-helper cell proliferation.

447. **(B)** The endemic form of relapsing fever is transmitted by ticks infected by *B. recurrentis.* Relapsing fever begins with headache, high fever, muscle aches, and splenomegaly. It has a unique fever curve owing to the emergence of various antigenic types of *B. recurrentis.* *Borrelia burgdorferi* (choice A) causes a distinct spreading circular rash with a clear center, called erythema chronicum migrans. *Leptospira interrogans* (choice C) is transmitted by rat urine and causes leptospirosis. This disease is associated with jaundice, uremia, and aseptic meningitis. *Treponema carateum* (choice D) is the cause of pinta, which is characterized by hyperpigmentation of the skin. *Treponema pertenue* (choice E) is transmitted by contact with infected persons and is characterized by the development of cauliflower-like skin lesions.

448. **(C)** A physician is justified in giving antitoxin on clinical evidence, or suspicion of diphtheria, without waiting for laboratory confirmation. The antitoxin dosage should be adjusted according to the weight of the patient and the severity of the infection. Antitoxin is given to neutralize free diphtheria exotoxin in the body fluids and timeliness is of extreme importance. Once the exotoxin is bound by the body cells and exerts its influence, diphtheria antitoxin is of little value. *Corynebacterium diphtheriae* localizes in the throat, and thus spinal taps (choice E) are useless. Tellurite agar, not blood agar, is used for the isolation of *C. diphtheriae* from throat swabs, because it is a selective medium for this germ, inhibiting the growth of other bacteria present in throat swabs (choice B). *Corynebacterium diphtheriae* is not an acid-fast microbe (choice A). Methylene blue is used to stain smears for the bacteriologic diagnosis of diphtheria. This initial treatment of choice for diphtheria is antitoxin. Treatment with penicillin G or erythromycin, but not sulfonamides (choice D), may be used. Penicillin G or erythromycin are not substitutes for diphtheria antitoxin.

449. **(E)** Bruton hypogammaglobulinemia is a B-cell immunodeficiency disorder. Affected patients are deficient in B cells in the peripheral blood and in B-dependent areas of lymph nodes and spleen. Most of the serum immunoglobulins are absent, and the IgG level is < 200 mg/L. Recurrent pyogenic infections usually begin to occur at 5 to 6 months of age, when maternal IgG has been depleted. Individuals with X-linked hypogammaglobulinemia have normally functioning T cells, and thus are not particularly susceptible to viral or fungal infections, which depend on proper T-cell–mediated immune responses (choice A). Individuals with Bruton syndrome have normal T-cell–mediated immune responses (choice B). Patients suffering from X-linked hypogammaglobulinemia do not have normal numbers of B lymphocytes, because the pre-B cells from which B cells are produced fail to differentiate into B cells. This is due to a gene mutation in pre-B cells, which does not allow pre-B cells to form tyrosine kinase (choice D). The number of lymphocytes in the paracortical areas of lymph nodes of patients with Bruton syndrome is normal (choice C).

450. **(C)** Recurrent vesiculating lesions in the genital region suggest human herpes virus type II, although type I is seen in some cases. Coxsackie virus (choice A) and echovirus (choice B) produce a wide variety of diseases, including meningitis, encephalitis, upper respiratory tract infections, and enteritis. A macular rash may accompany some of these conditions, but its presence has no particular diagnostic significance. Furthermore, they do not produce genital vesicular lesions. Rubella (choice E) and measles (choice D) are not closely associated with vesiculating genital lesions.

451. **(D)** Anti-acetylcholine receptor antibodies are found in more than 90% of myasthenia gravis patients. If the clinical symptoms are suggestive of myasthenia gravis, this finding alone is often considered diagnostic. Multiple sclerosis (choice C) patients tend to have high levels of measles virus antibodies in their spinal fluid.

However, the role of this agent in the disease is undetermined. Guillain–Barré syndrome (choice B), also called acute idiopathic polyneuritis (choice A), is a demyelinating disease of peripheral nerves. It commonly occurs after a viral infection or an injection, such as influenza immunization. The disease seems to be caused by a T-cell response to nervous tissue. Postpericardiotomy syndrome (choice E) is a term used to describe a disorder following surgery of the pericardium to remove cysts or tumors, or to correct a malformation.

452. **(C)** The patient described has a profound deficiency of both the B-cell and T-cell components of the immune response (i.e., severe combined immunodeficiency disease). The dramatic absence of lymphocytes and lymphoid tissue is not found in any of the other conditions listed. Chronic granulomatous disease (choice A) is the inability of the neutrophils to manifest intracellular microbicidal activity because they lack NADPH oxidase. Multiple myeloma (choice B) is a neoplasm of plasma cells characterized by excessive synthesis of myeloma proteins. Two-thirds of all myeloma proteins are IgG. Persons with Wiskott–Aldrich syndrome (choice D) are not able to synthesize IgM against bacterial capsular polysaccharides and thus suffer from recurrent pyogenic infections. The IgG and IgA levels are normal. However, the T-cell immune responses are variable. X-linked agammaglobulinemia (choice E) is a B-cell immunodeficiency disorder. Most serum immunoglobulins are absent, and the IgG level is < 200 mg/L. T cells are normal.

453. **(E)** Figure 4–7 represents the peptidoglycan of *S. aureus*. The C substance of *S. pneumoniae* (choice A) is part of the teichoic acid of *S. pneumoniae*. Pneumococci can be agglutinated with antisera against C substance, which is a polysaccharide. The H antigen of *S. typhimurium* is a flagellar protein, and not a part of the cell wall (choice B). The O antigen of *S. typhimurium* (choice C) is the outer moiety of the endotoxin (lipopolysaccharide) of *S. typhimurium*. It does not have the *N*-acetyl glucosamine-*N*-acetyl muramic acid units,

side peptides, or cross bridges of the bacterial peptidoglycan. *Mycoplasma pneumoniae* does not have a cell wall and is therefore devoid of peptidoglycan (choice D).

454. **(A)** Whooping cough can be prevented by vaccination with DPT (diphtheria, tetanus, pertussis) or DTaP (the acellular form of the pertussis vaccine). Immunization has drastically reduced the number of cases of whooping cough. The main immunogens used in the vaccines are either heat-killed cells (in DPT) or the toxoid of *B. pertussis* (in DTaP). Immunity is not acquired by the third month of infancy, but it can be induced by infection. Protection against whooping cough, whether achieved by infection or immunization, is not of lifelong duration, because infections have occurred in persons who either have been previously infected or vaccinated (choices C, D, and E). *Bordetella pertussis* does not possess Vi antigen; therefore, immunity to whooping cough cannot be conferred by antibody production to Vi antigen (choice B).

455. **(A)** Deficiency in the inhibitor of the first component of complement (C1) is associated with angioedema, because this condition leads to the production of anaphylatoxins C3a, C4a, and C5a. These anaphylatoxins act on mast cells, which release large amounts of histamine. Production of histamine increases capillary permeability, resulting in edema. Enhanced susceptibility to pyogenic infections has been attributed to C3 and C5 to C8 components of complement. Bacteremia (choice B) is a term used to indicate the presence of bacteria in the blood; it has nothing to do with C1. Inherited deficiencies of C3 and C5 to C8 have been associated with increased susceptibility to pyogenic infections, but not C1 complement (choice E). Complement can act synergistically with antibody to modify its action, but not its production (choice D). The conversions of the third (C3) and fifth (C5) components of complement by the C3 and C5 convertases to C3a and C5a anaphylatoxins lead to the increased production of anaphylatoxins (choice C) seen with C1 inhibitor deficiency.

456. (E) By definition a hapten is a substance of low molecular weight that by itself does not elicit the formation of antibodies. However, when attached to a carrier protein, antibody production becomes possible. The hapten-carrier approach has been employed to produce antibodies against penicillin, steroids, nucleotides, lipids, and even 2,4-dinitrophenol. Because the rabbit has been repeatedly injected with the hapten only, the serum cannot be expected to have antibodies against the hapten. It is clear that when the serum is subjected to a gel diffusion assay with the hapten and a carrier protein not used to complex the hapten during immunization, no antigen–antibody precipitin lines of either identity, partial identity, or nonidentity can be expected to form (choices A, B, C, and D).

457. (B) This patient has mumps, which can be prevented by immunization with a live attenuated vaccine. Immunization usually produces lifelong protection against mumps. The key diagnostic feature of mumps is tender swelling of the parotid glands, either bilaterally or unilaterally. Fever and anorexia usually precede the disease. Parotid gland swelling is accompanied by pain intensified by drinking citrus juices. There are no known antiviral agents to treat mumps (choice D). Two important complications of mumps are orchitis, which can lead to sterility, and meningitis (choice C). Mumps is an enveloped, nonsegmented, single-stranded RNA virus of negative polarity. The virus envelope has spikes that contain hemagglutinin and neuraminidase on each spike. The diagnosis of mumps is made clinically; however, confirmation rests on demonstration of a fourfold rise in antibody using hemagglutinin inhibition tests (choice A). The mumps virus is transmitted by respiratory droplets (choice E).

458. (B) The diagnostic tests ordered by the physician are consistent with a deficiency in the C3 and C5 to C8 components of complement. Individuals with these deficiencies have recurrent pyogenic infections, and show enhanced susceptibility to meningococcal in-fections. All other choices are inconsistent with the laboratory findings. Chronic granulomatous disease (choice A) entails a defect in the intracellular killing of microbes by neutrophils. Graves disease (choice C) involves autoantibody production to thyroid-stimulating hormone receptors. Lupus erythematosus (choice D) involves production of anti-nuclear antibodies. Wiskott–Aldrich syndrome (choice E) is associated with recurrent pyogenic infections, but is due to an inability of plasma cells to produce IgM against bacterial polysaccharides, and it occurs only in male infants.

459. (B) Antigens have the ability to induce an immune response (immunogenicity) and also react specifically with the products of that response, either humoral antibodies or specifically sensitized lymphocytes. Adjuvants (choice A) are substances that have the ability to enhance the immune response to antigens without necessarily being antigenic themselves. For example, *B. pertussis* causes the host to produce large amounts of IgE antibodies to antigens that normally do not induce the production of this antibody at all. Similarly, presence of mycobacterial cells in a vaccine encourage the development of cell-mediated immunity to other antigens in the vaccine. Haptens, whether simple or complex (choices C and E), are partial or incomplete antigens. They have specific reactivity, but are not immunogenic by themselves. Determinant groups (choice D) are the portions of the antigen molecule that determine its specificity.

460. (A) In a laboratory test used to identify *S. aureus*, coagulase reacts with a prothrombin-like compound in plasma to produce an active enzyme (a complex of thrombin and coagulase) that converts fibrinogen to fibrin. This activity of *S. aureus* has a very high correlation with the organism's virulence, although coagulase-negative organisms may cause less severe disease. Coagulase reactive factor (choice B) is a plasma protein with which coagulase reacts. This protein is presumably a modified derivative of prothrombin. Prothrombin (choice D) is the substrate from which coagulase splits a number of amino acids to convert it to thrombin. Thrombin (choice E) is the proteolytic enzyme that converts fibrinogen to fibrin, forming the plasma clot. Plasmin (choice C) is a plasma protein associated with the destruction of a plasma clot.

461. **(A)** C5a is a component of complement. Activation of complement by endotoxin, or antigen-antibody complexes produces C5a, which is a neutrophil and macrophage attractant. HLA-A and HLA-B are genes for the human leukocyte antigens (HLA), and they control the synthesis of class I antigens (choices B and C). The J moiety (choice D) of IgM and IgA does not possess chemotactic properties for neutrophils and macrophages. The variable region of the heavy chain of IgG (choice E) is not known as the best neutrophil or macrophage attractant.

462. **(B)** Cultivation of fungi requires a medium that is adjusted to the optimal pH of growth for fungi, a pH of 4.0 to 5.0. Such a medium is the one developed by Sabouraud. Lowenstein–Jensen medium (choice A) is used for the cultivation of *M. tuberculosis* and other mycobacteria. Selenite medium (choice C) is used to increase the number of *Salmonella* species that may be present in small numbers in fecal or other clinical specimens. The SS medium (choice D) is used to isolate bacterial species belonging to the genera *Salmonella* and *Shigella*. Tellurite medium (choice E) is used for the selective isolation of *Corynebacterium diphtheriae*, which is not as sensitive to the concentration of tellurite incorporated into the medium as other bacteria that may be encountered in specimens submitted for the microbiological diagnosis of diphtheria.

463. **(A)** The route of infection of rubella virus is the respiratory tract, with spread to lymphatic tissue and then to the blood (viremia). Maternal viremia is followed by infection of the placenta, which leads to congenital rubella. Many organs of the fetus support the multiplication of the virus, which does not seem to destroy the cells, but reduces the rate of growth of the infected cells. This leads to fewer than normal numbers of cells in the organs at birth. Therefore, the earlier in pregnancy infection occurs, the greater chance for the development of abnormalities in the infected fetus. Many maternal infections that occur during the first trimester of pregnancy result in such fetal defects as pulmonary stenosis, ventricular septal defect, cataracts, glaucoma, deafness, mental retardation, and other maladies.

464. **(E)** Superoxide, which is bactericidal, is generated during electron transport and in the autoxidation of hydroquinones, leukoflavins, ferredoxins, and flavoproteins. Superoxide dismutase, however, forms oxygen and hydrogen peroxide from superoxide radicals. When catalase is present, it destroys the bactericidal hydrogen peroxide, because catalase hydrolyzes hydrogen peroxide to water and oxygen. Thus, the presence of both enzymes allows aerobes, facultative anaerobes, and aerotolerant microbes to survive when they grow in the presence of oxygen. Obligate anaerobic bacteria generally lack superoxide dismutase, catalase, or both, and thus cannot grow in the presence of oxygen. Oxidase (choice B) is an enzyme that oxidizes a substrate by the addition of oxygen or the removal of hydrogen. It cannot oxidize the bactericidal radical superoxide. Catalase (choice A) is an enzyme that converts the bactericidal substance hydrogen peroxide to water and oxygen. It has no effect on the microbiocidal action of superoxide. Bacteria that lack catalase are likely to be suppressed by hydrogen peroxide. Peroxidase (choice D) is an enzyme that catalyzes the dehydrogenation of a substrate in the presence of hydrogen peroxide, which acts as hydrogen acceptor and becomes converted into two molecules of water. Thus, possession of peroxidase in a given microbe allows it to grow in the presence of hydrogen peroxide, but not in the presence of superoxide. There are no known pathogenic bacteria that form oxygen (choice C).

465. **(D)** *Pseudomonas aeruginosa* is a gram-negative, oxidase-positive, aerobic rod that produces a blue-green pigment called pyocyanin. This microorganism has been associated frequently with wound infections in burn patients, and it is the second leading cause of burn infections after *S. aureus*. *Pseudomonas aeruginosa* tends to develop resistance to various antibiotics. However, it may respond to ticarcillin, gentamycin, tobramycin, piperacillin, or azlocillin. *Escherichia coli* (choice A), *K. pneumoniae* (choice B), *P. mirabilis* (choice C), and *S. marcescens* (choice E) may cause urinary or pulmonary tract infections, but are not considered leading causes of burn infections. Furthermore, these bacteria are oxidase negative and do not produce blue-green pigments.

466. **(A)** There are two nonsuppurative sequelae of group A streptococcal disease: rheumatic fever and acute glomerulonephritis. Although rheumatic fever can follow pharyngeal infection with practically any group A streptococcal organism, the majority of nephritogenic strains belong to only six or seven M types. Types 1, 4, 12, 25, and 49 are the most commonly associated with acute glomerulonephritis. The preceding streptococcal infection need not be restricted to the upper respiratory tract to trigger this condition, and streptococcal erysipelas is a frequent cause.

467. **(A)** *Cryptococcus neoformans* is the only encapsulated yeast that is pathogenic for humans. Visualization of a capsule around yeast cells in an India ink preparation of spinal fluid is diagnostic for cryptococcal disease, although soluble capsular antigen could also be detected by countercurrent immunoelectrophoresis or latex agglutination. This organism is considered to be an opportunistic pathogen; more than 80% of the individuals who become clinically ill are immunosuppressed in some way or have compromised respiratory function. The organism is abundant in pigeon excreta-contaminated soil, which is most probably the source of human infections. *Histoplasma capsulatum* may occur as an oval budding yeast inside macrophages (choice C), and may exist in the soil as a mold that has septate hyphae (choice B). In general, fungi reproduce sexually by mating and forming sexual spores, or by forming asexual spores called conidia. The majority of medically important fungi reproduce by asexual spores (choice E). Fungi that contain brown-black pigments in their cell walls are called dematiaceous fungi. *Cryptococcus neoformans* does not possess these pigments (choice D).

468. **(A)** *Diphyllobothrium latum*, also known as the fish or broad tapeworm, is the biggest worm and can reach 10 m in size. Humans acquire the infection by eating raw fish containing the larvae of the tapeworm. The worm attaches to the small intestine and causes abdominal discomfort. Nausea, diarrhea, weight loss, and pernicious anemia can result. The anemia is induced by the tapeworm's tendency to compete with humans for vitamin B_{12}, which it easily accumulates from the intestinal contents. *Diphyllobothrium latum* does not possess blood-sucking organs (choice C). No one has demonstrated that *D. latum* toxin affects hematopoiesis (choice E) or the absorption of iron (choice B). *Schistosoma mansoni* tends to block the common bile duct (choice D).

469. **(D)** Plague, a zoonotic disease caused by the bacillus *Yersinia pestis*, is transmitted to humans from its animal reservoir (rats in urban plague, squirrels and other wild animals in sylvatic plague), by fleas (e.g., *Xenopsylla cheopis*, the rat flea). Anthrax (choice A) is an industrial disease, usually acquired by wool and leather workers. The spores contaminate the hides and raw wool and are inhaled by the workers during processing. Brucellosis (choice B) and salmonellosis (choice E) are acquired by ingestion of contaminated foods. Humans may develop leptospirosis (choice C) if they come in contact with groundwater that has been contaminated with urine from rodents who are harboring the agent in their normal flora, or through a subclinical infection. This disease occurs usually in campers and hunters. Veterinarians are particularly prone to developing zoonotic infections because of their constant contact with infected animals.

470. **(C)** Mrs. Y. is suffering from allergic rhinitis. The diagnosis of this allergy is made on the basis of clinical symptoms and the performance of a skin test, as well as a radioallergosorbent test (RAST). In a skin test, a battery of potential allergens are injected separately subcutaneously, and the area of the wheal and flare reaction is measured. The allergen inducing the greatest wheal and flare reaction when compared to solvent is usually the one causing the allergy. In this case, injection of Kentucky blue grass yielded the biggest wheal and flare reaction, and thus this is the allergen causing the Ms. Y's rhinitis. Allergens such as mold, cat dander, house dust, and pollen gave wheal and flare reactions that were either below or slightly above the skin test values of the allergen solvent. Therefore they are not likely to be causing allergy in Ms. Y. (choices A, B, D, and E).

471. **(E)** The IgG anti-mold-blocking antibody combines with the mold allergen and does not permit the mold allergen to reach the IgE anti-mold on the surface of the mast cells, thus inhibiting the allergic reaction. Cromolyn sodium (choice A) stabilizes the membrane of mast cells and thus prevents release of histamine from mast cells. Complement (choice B) is not fixed by IgE allergen complexes and plays no role in the attachment of mold allergen to sensitized mast cells. Corticosteroids (choice C) suppress inflammation, but do not prevent the attachment of the mold allergen to the sensitized mast cells. Epinephrine (choice D) reverses constriction of bronchioles and bronchi, and also has no effect on the attachment of mold allergen to sensitized mast cells.

472. **(D)** The main symptoms of pneumonia caused by *S. pneumoniae* are fever, chills, and cough that produces a dark brown sputum. Alcoholism predisposes an individual to pneumonia because it reduces phagocytic activity, and promotes aspiration of microbes.

In addition to *S. pneumoniae*, *S. pyogenes* (choice E), *S. aureus* (choice C), and *N. meningitidis* (choice B) can cause pneumonia. However, these other microbes do not produce alpha hemolysis and are not sensitive to optochin.

473. **(B)** By definition, the rate of growth of bacteria represents the change in the bacterial cell numbers over the change in time. From the choices given, the maximum rate of growth occurs between 2 PM and 3 PM, where, within 1 hour the number of bacteria increases approximately threefold. Between 12 PM and 1 PM (choice A) and from 3 PM to 6 PM (choices C, D, and E), there is no increase in the number of cells and the rate of growth is zero.

$$\frac{2 \times 10^7 - 2 \times 10^7}{5 - 4} = 0$$

474. **(E)** The best method for assessing the total number of B lymphocytes is performance of a surface immunoglobulin assay, because B lymphocytes have immunoglobulin on their surface. Quantitative immunoglobulin levels (choice D) reflect the secretory activity of B lymphocytes, and could be misleading as to the actual number of such cells; for example, in multiple myeloma or other B-cell malignancies, one would expect to find a marked hypergammaglobulinemia. B cells are not the only cells that have receptors for the Fc fragment of immunoglobulin. Phagocytic cells also have such receptors and thus could be included in an Fc receptor assay (choice B). E rosetting (choice A) is a property of T lymphocytes, as is PHA mitogenic response (choice C); neither of these assays would be appropriate for the enumeration of B lymphocytes.

475. **(C)** Lyme disease is a recently discovered illness caused by *B. burgdorferi*. The disease produces a unique annular skin lesion called erythema chronicum migrans (ECM). Diagnosis may be assisted by correlating the serum levels of IgM with Lyme disease activity, because patients develop IgM antibodies to *B. burgdorferi* 3 to 6 weeks after infection. Lyme disease

is transmitted by tick, not mite bites (choice E). Lyme disease is caused by *B. burgdorferi*, not *L. interrogans*, the organism that causes leptospirosis (choice D). Certain patients develop neurologic and cardiovascular symptoms and arthritis (choice B). Tetracyclines are the drugs of choice for the treatment of Lyme disease during its acute phase (choice A).

476. **(A)** The organisms of the genus *Haemophilus* are small, gram-negative, nonmotile, non-spore-forming bacilli with complex growth requirements. *Haemophilus influenzae* requires a heat-stable factor found in blood (X factor) that can be replaced by hematin, and nicotinamide adenine dinucleotide (V factor), which can be added to the medium as a supplement, or can be supplied by other microorganisms, such as staphylococci (satellite phenomenon). *Listeria monocytogenes* (choice B), *N. gonorrhoeae* (choice C), *N. meningitides* (choice D), and *S. pneumoniae* (choice E) are able to synthesize hematin and nicotinamide adenine dinucleotide; thus, they grow in culture media that do not contain these nutrients. They also do not rely on the production of hematin and nicotinamide adenine dinucleotide by *S. aureus* to grow. In contrast to *H. influenzae*, *S. pneumoniae* is a gram-positive, lancet-shaped diplococcus, not a gram-negative bacterium. *Listeria monocytogenes* is a gram-positive rod.

477. **(A)** By definition, LD_{50} is the dose of a microbe or its products that will kill 50% of the species into which it is injected. *Clostridium botulinum* produces one of the most powerful known bacterial toxins. It has been stated that the LD_{50} of *C. botulinum* exotoxin for humans is approximately 1 mg. *Clostridium tetani* (choice B) and *C. diphtheriae* (choice C) produce exotoxins that have an LD_{50} 6 to 10 times higher than *C. botulinum*. *Salmonella typhi* (choice D) and *Y. pestis* (choice E) are gram-negative bacteria, and as such produce endotoxins with a very high LD_{50}.

478. **(A)** Evidence now shows that *H. pylori* is associated with the pathogenesis of peptic ulcer. It is found in almost all patients with duodenal ulcers and more than 80% with stomach ulcers. *Helicobacter pylori* is a newly discovered curved and spiral-shaped gram-negative bacterium found in the human gastric mucosal layer, but not in the oral cavity (choice D). Patients infected with *H. pylori* develop IgM, IgG, and IgA, which can be used in its diagnosis (choice B). *Helicobacter pylori* produces an abundant amount of urease. It does not produce coagulase, which is elaborated by *S. aureus* (choice E). It is not an obligate intracellular parasite because it can be cultured on a number of artificial media in 2 to 7 days (choice C).

479. **(D)** There are five known classes of immunoglobulins: IgG, IgA, IgM, IgD, and IgE. IgG is the major immunoglobulin found in human serum and the only one that has been shown to pass the placental barrier in humans. IgA (choice A) is the major immunoglobulin of extracellular secretions. It has a molecular weight of 160,000 to 440,000, has modest agglutinating capacity, and its carbohydrate content is two to three times higher (7.5%) than that of IgG. IgD (choice B) constitutes a minor portion of serum immunoglobulins (1%). It contains higher amounts of carbohydrate (13%) than the other immunoglobulins, but it is an important B-cell receptor. No other biological functions have been described for IgD. IgE (choice C) is associated with anaphylactic hypersensitivity. It has a molecular weight of 190,000 to 200,000, contains 11% to 12% carbohydrate, and constitutes 0.002% of the total serum immunoglobulin. IgM (choice E) possesses higher agglutinating and complement-fixing capacity than IgG. IgM has a molecular weight of 900,000. Carbohydrates constitute 7% to 11% of its total weight.

480. **(D)** Anaphylaxis triggered by penicillin is an immediate hypersensitivity reaction, which is typically mediated by IgE antibodies. IgE antibodies bind to specific Fc receptors on the surface of mast cells and basophils. Upon cross-linking of the IgE antibodies with their specific antigen (penicillin in this case), mast cells and basophils release histamine within

minutes along with other pharmacologically active shock mediators that produce the characteristic symptoms of anaphylaxis. Activation of either the classical or the alternate complement pathway do not play any meaningful role in anaphylaxis (choices A and B). IgG and IgD are not involved in anaphylactic reactions (choices C and E).

481. **(E)** Bacteria divide by splitting into two equal parts (binary fission). The time required for bacteria to undergo binary fission is called the generation time. The given generation time of *E. coli* is 20 minutes. Thus, within three hours (180 minutes), *E. coli* will have undergone nine divisions. Therefore, the number of *E. coli* per mL if we start with 500 bacteria will be as follows: 1000 in 20 minutes, 2000 in 40 minutes, 4000 in 60 minutes, 8000 in 80 minutes, 16,000 in 100 minutes, 32,000 in 120 minutes, 64,000 in 140 minutes, 128,000 in 160 minutes, and 256,000 in 180 minutes.

482. **(C)** Gene therapy may be useful for acquired diseases such as cancer or infectious diseases. One of the problems encountered in gene therapy is the need of introducing the desired gene into the host cells. Viruses with weak pathogenic potential that are capable of entering host cells have been found to be useful gene carriers. One of the reasons viruses are attractive vectors in gene therapy is that the genes inserted into viruses can be expressed in a regulated way. Adenovirus vectors may be used to target gene transfer into cells of the respiratory tract (choice A). Retrovirus vectors can be produced in large quantities from producer cell lines (choice B). Viruses infect cells with a much higher efficiency compared to chemical or physical means of gene transfer (choice D). The concept of gene therapy is based on the assumption that definitive treatment for any genetic disease should be possible by directing treatment to the site of the defect itself, the mutant gene, and not to the secondary effects of that mutant gene. Because there are many hereditary diseases caused by defects in a single gene, there are many potential applications of this type of therapy to the treatment of human diseases (choice E).

483. **(C)** Mutation occurs in bacteria as in all other cells (choice B). After the initial observation that bacterial populations contain mutants (such as a mutant resistant to an antibiotic), the question is whether the mutation is directed (induced by the antibiotic) or random (spontaneous). This question is most easily answered by the use of the replica plate technique (choice E). A velveteen pad is used to press on the colonies of the master plate and then pressed to plates A, B, C, and D. When the bacteria are replica plated to plates A, B, C, and D, each containing a given antibiotic, the resistant colonies always appear in the same places. This is indeed the case in plates B and D, which contain the same antibiotic. This implies that resistant colonies existed before exposure to antibiotic. Hence, mutation is spontaneous. The Lamarckian theory states that acquired characteristics may be transmitted to descendants (choice A).

484. **(A)** The clinical features of food poisoning due to *B. cereus* include an incubation period of 2 to 8 hours during which nausea, vomiting, and diarrhea develop. Usually eating food containing preformed enterotoxin of *B. cereus* is the source of food poisoning. *Bacillus cereus* grows in the GI tract, leading to the production of enterotoxin that causes diarrhea and vomiting. Diplopia, dysphagia, dysphonia, and respiratory distress are the clinical features of food poisoning caused by *C. botulinum* (choice B). *Clostridium tetani* (choice C) infection is characterized by convulsive toxin contractions of voluntary muscles, leading to lockjaw, and opisthotonos (the spine and extremities are so bent that the body rests on the head and the heels). The incubation period of tetanus is 5 days to several weeks. *Proteus mirabilis* (choice D) is a normal inhabitant of the gut, and it may cause occasional urinary tract infections when the bacteria leave the intestinal tract. Diarrhea, vomiting, or nausea are not pathognomonic features of urinary tract infections. Gastroenteritis caused by *S. enteritidis* (choice E) has

an incubation period of 10 to 48 hours; vomiting is rare, but there is diarrhea and low-grade fever. The organisms grow in the gut, leading to superficial infection with little invasion and no enterotoxin production.

485. **(A)** Individuals who have been diagnosed as X-linked agammaglobulinemic lack B lymphocytes and are not able to produce immunoglobulins. The lack of immunoglobulins in X-linked agammaglobulinemia renders individuals susceptible to a succession of infectious diseases caused by extracellular bacteria. These infections may be partially controlled by the injection of specific gamma globulin as a supportive therapy. X-linked agammaglobulinemic patients have T cells that are the key players in cell-mediated immunity associated with graft rejection, intracellular parasites, viruses, and fungi. *Pneumocystis carinii* is now considered a fungus, causing infections in immunocompromised patients, such as those with AIDS (choices B, C, D, and E).

486. **(A)** Tumor necrosis factor (TNF) is cytotoxic to certain tumor cells. Recent experiments in gene therapy have taken the approach of expressing TNF in tumor-infiltrating lymphocytes (TIL), with the hope of allowing the TIL to return to the tumor and produce a high concentration of TNF and kill the tumor cells. Tumor necrosis factor is a mediator of endotoxin-induced shock and is involved in inflammation, but does not generate high levels of endotoxin (choice B). There is no evidence to support that TNF stimulates T-cell proliferation (choice E). TNF is cytotoxic to certain tumor cells, but it does not lyse tumor cells by retroviral participation (choice C). NK cells can destroy tumor cells; however, they cannot be stimulated by TNF (choice D).

487. **(E)** Tetanus toxin produced by *Clostridium tetani* is a protease that often first affects the masseter muscles. Patients so affected cannot open their mouths and have what is called trismus. Trismus provides an explanation for the term *lockjaw* used to describe tetanus. Botulinum toxin (choice A) cleaves the pro-

teins involved in the release of acetylcholine. This leads to paralysis of ocular, pharyngeal, and respiratory muscles. Cholera toxin causes fluid and electrolyte loss that leads to severe diarrhea (choice B). The clostridial alpha toxin (choice C) kills cells and produces necrosis. Diphtheria toxin (choice D) is an inhibitor of protein synthesis affecting heart, kidney, and other cells. Protein synthesis is inhibited because diphtheria exotoxin polyADP ribosylates elongation factor 2 (eEF-2).

488. **(E)** Infectious mononucleosis is caused by Epstein–Barr virus (EBV), which is a member of the herpesviruses. Nucleic acid hybridization assays for EBV DNA are the most sensitive means of diagnosing infectious mononucleosis. Important antigens that also may be used, but which are less sensitive for diagnostic purposes, include the viral capsid protein (VCA), the early proteins (EA), and the Epstein–Barr virus–associated nuclear antigen (EBNA). Infectious mononucleosis patients develop antibody titers exceeding 1:320 and 1:20 against VCA and EA, respectively, during the acute phase of infectious mononucleosis. Antibodies to EBNA develop 1 to 2 months after acute infection (choice A). Hemagglutinins (choice B) and neuraminidases (choice C) are associated with orthomyxoviruses and paramyxoviruses. The majority of patients with infectious mononucleosis develop what is known as heterophile antibody—antibodies that cross-react with unrelated antigens, such as those found on sheep and horse erythrocytes. The heterophile antibody test (choice D) is used for the diagnosis of infectious mononucleosis, but because it is not a very specific test, it is not as good as the nucleic acid hybridization assays for the presence of Epstein–Barr viral nucleic acid.

489. **(C)** The ability of certain viruses, such as influenza, mumps, and parainfluenza viruses, to agglutinate red blood cells is used to diagnose these viruses. In general, chicken or human type O red blood cells are used to identify influenza and other viruses. Red blood cells have receptors for the surface compo-

nent of the influenza virus called hemagglu-tinin, a glycoprotein. In a hemagglutination assay, a fixed number of red blood cells is mixed with increasing dilutions of the influenza virus. Following incubation at 4°C for 2 hours, the tubes containing the red blood cells and the virus are examined for hemagglutination. Cells agglutinated by the virus form a lattice that covers the entire bottom of the test tube (virus dilutions 1:20; 1:40; 1:80). The hemagglutination titer of the virus is the highest dilution of virus that forms a lattice. In this case, the hemagglutination titer is 1:80. Unagglutinated cells form a dark bottom (virus dilutions 1:160; 1:320) (choices D and E).

490. **(E)** An important difference between the AIDS (HIV) virus and the RNA tumor viruses is that HIV lyses the host cells; RNA tumor viruses transform the cells they invade, but they lack cytolytic activity. The HIV virus is a retrovirus. The genomic RNA molecule of HIV contains the gag, pol, and env genes. Thus, HIV does not differ from RNA tumor retroviruses (choices A and B). HIV contains one copy, not two, of single-stranded RNA in its virion (choice C). The tropism of the HIV virus for T4 lymphocytes depends on the presence of the T4 protein (choice D) on the surface of the lymphocytes. This protein serves as the receptor for the adsorption of HIV to T4 lymphocytes.

491. **(E)** Because there are memory lymphocytes primed by a previous tetanus toxoid injection, booster immunization with tetanus toxoid will lead to rapid production of adequate levels of protective antibody. This is the routine procedure followed by physicians for trauma patients who have been vaccinated against tetanus and received booster immunization within the last 5 to 7 years. The antibody titer to tetanus toxoid remains at protective levels for 5 to 10 years. Aminoglycosides such as penicillin (choice C) or streptomycin (choice D) are not effective against the spores or vegetative cells of *Clostridium tetani.* Human tetanus immune globulin (choice B) only provides antibodies

to tetanus exotoxin for a short time and cannot induce an anamnestic response because an injection of tetanus exotoxin or toxoid is required. Individuals who have been vaccinated against tetanus require injections of the tetanus toxoid to induce rapid production of adequate levels of protective antibody. Treatment with equine tetanus immunoglobulin (choice A), which will only provide antitetanus antibody for a short time, is not the preferred method of treatment for this patient.

492. **(B)** This patient's symptoms point to a diagnosis of Lyme disease, caused by *B. burgdorferi,* and transmitted to humans by ticks that harbor this organism. The initial symptoms of Lyme disease are fever, chills, fatigue, and headache, but the pathognomonic feature is a spreading, circular rash with a clear center. The rash begins 3 to 18 days after the tick bite and is called erythema chronicum migrans. Epidemic typhus (choice A), Q fever (choice C), rickettsial pox (choice D), and trench fever (choice E) do not produce erythema chronicum migrans.

493. **(B)** The antiviral drug currently used against the immunodeficiency virus is AZT, or 3-azido-3-deoxythymidine (azidothymidine). Its structure is shown in Figure 4–11. The structures of related compounds idoxuridine (choice E) and dideoxyinosine (choice C) are shown in Figure 4–17. Acyclovir (choice A) and enviroxine (choice D) differ chemically from the structure depicted in Figure 4–11.

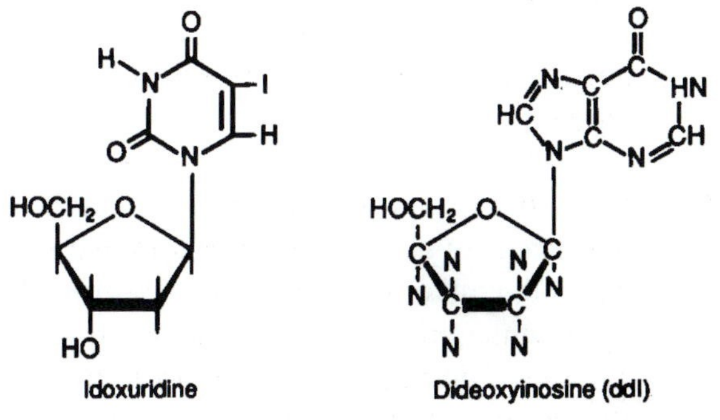

Figure 4–17

494. **(B)** Epidemic typhus is caused by *Rickettsia prowazeki*. It is transmitted from one individual to another by human body louse bites. The louse becomes infected when it takes a meal from an individual that harbors *R. prowazeki*. Fleas (choice A) transmit endemic typhus and plague. The mite (choice C) is the biological vector of rickettsial pox and another rickettsial disease called scrub typhus. Mosquitoes (choice D) transmit such diseases as malaria, yellow fever, St. Louis encephalitis, eastern equine encephalitis, western equine encephalitis, and California encephalitis. Ticks (choice E) are the biological vectors of many diseases, such as Lyme disease, Rocky Mountain spotted fever, and tularemia.

495. **(C)** Exfoliatin toxin is produced by certain strains of *S. aureus* belonging to phage group II. This exotoxin divides the epidermis between the stratum granulosum and the stratum spinosum. The end result of exfoliatin action is the exfoliation of the skin, known as the staphylococcal scalded skin syndrome. Alpha toxin (choice A) is produced by *S. aureus* and causes necrosis and hemolysis of blood cells. Erythrogenic toxin (choice B) is produced by *S. pyogenes* and is associated with scarlet fever. Staphylococcal enterotoxins A through F (choice D) are responsible for food poisoning. The toxic shock syndrome toxin (TSST) (choice E) causes multisystem involvement with shock that can be lethal. TSST is a super antigen that releases large concentrations of IL-1, IL-2, and tumor necrosis factor (TNF).

496. **(A)** Togaviruses contain viral species that cause encephalitis. They are transmitted via mosquito vectors with birds serving as reservoirs of infection. Western and eastern encephalitis viruses cause infections that have high mortality in children and aged individuals. These viruses enter the bloodstream from insect inoculation. The virus is removed by the reticuloendothelial cells and multiplies in the spleen and lymph nodes. From these tissues, a secondary viremia is established, spreading the virus to the central nervous system by passage through the blood–brain junction (virus grows through the vascular endothelium or in some way is passively transported across the blood–brain barrier). The brain and spinal cord become edematous and show vascular congestion and small hemorrhages. There are no human vaccines, and control is limited to controlling the insect vectors (choices B, C, D, and E).

497. **(C)** The most widely used nontreponemal test for syphilis is the glass slide flocculation Venereal Disease Research Laboratory (VDRL), or the card rapid plasma reagin (RPR) test. In the VDRL test, the antigen is an alcoholic extract of beef heart containing cardiolipin (diphosphatidyl glycerol), which also appears to be a component of the cytoplasmic membrane of *Treponema pallidum* that causes syphilis (choice B). The VDRL is a rapid serologic test that is very useful for screening large numbers of people for syphilis (choice E). The VDRL is a slide flocculation, and not a complement fixation test (choice D). The VDRL titer reflects the activity of the disease. Such titers reach a level of 1:32 or higher in secondary syphilis. A persistent fall in titer following penicillin or other antibiotic treatment indicates an adequate response to therapy (choice A).

498. **(A)** The detection of yellow sulfur granules in pus obtained from the liver abscess suggests hepatic actinomycosis, because the sulfur granules represent colonies of *A. israelii* or other oral *Actinomyces* species. The *Actinomyces* associated with hepatic actinomycosis, which may follow teeth extractions, especially in patients with paradental abscesses, are usually *A. israelii, A. bovis,* or *A. odontolyticus*. All these fail to grow aerobically, but can be cultured anaerobically on brain heart infusion agar where in 2 to 3 days at 37°C, *A. israelii* produces small, white, spidery colonies containing gram-positive rods and filaments. In pus, *A. israelii* is found as sulfur granules representing colonies of the microorganism. When the sulfur granules are washed, crushed between two glass slides, and gram stained, under the microscope they show a twisted aggregation of filaments which break up into bacilli, cocci, or small gram-positive, nonacid-fast filaments. *Mycobacterium tuberculosis* (choice D), *M. kansasii* (choice C), and *N. asteroides* (choice E) are aerobic, acid-fast microorganisms. *Actinomyces israelii* and *N. asteroides* are sensitive to penicillin, whereas *M. tuberculosis, M. kansasii*, and the fungus *H. capsulatum* (choice B) are resistant to it.

499. **(D)** *Sporothrix schenckii* is found on thorns, and it is introduced into the skin of extremities through trauma. A regional lesion begins as a pustule, abscess, or ulcer, and then nodules and abscesses are formed along the lymphatics. The history and the symptoms described in this patient are consonant with a diagnosis of sporotrichosis. *Aspergillus fumigatus* (choice A) and *C. albicans* (choice B) are associated with deep opportunistic infections in immunocompromised patients, such as those with AIDS. Aspergillosis is basically a pulmonary infection. Candidiasis can be associated with pathologic conditions of the mucous membranes of the respiratory, genital, and GI tract, where it is found as a normal inhabitant. *Cryptococcus neoformans* (choice C) causes meningitis. *Trichophyton rubrum* (choice E) causes dermatophytosis ringworm of skin, scalp, and especially nails. The nails thicken and are discolored.

500. **(C)** The genome of hepatitis B virus is composed of a circular, double-stranded DNA. It has a negative strand of 3200 nucleotides and another positive, incomplete strand of 1700 to 2600 nucleotides. Papilloma (choice E) and polyomaviruses belong to the family of *Papoviridae*, which lacks envelopes and have a double-stranded, circular DNA genome. Both strands are complete and thus differ from the genome of hepatitis B virus that has one incomplete positive strand. Hepatitis A virus (choice B), the cause of infectious hepatitis, has a linear, single-stranded RNA genome, and as such it is a member of the enteroviruses. Epstein–Barr virus, EBV (choice A) is a member of the herpesviruses and as such has a double-stranded, linear DNA genome. EBV has been associated with infectious mononucleosis, Burkitt lymphoma, and nasopharyngeal carcinoma (choice C). J.C. virus (choice D) is a member of the polyomaviruses.

501. **(C)** The most appropriate laboratory diagnostic procedure for cases of suspected tinea corporis is digestion of tissue biopsies with 10% to 20% KOH and a search for hyaline, branched septate hyphae on squamous epithelial cells. A 10% to 20% potassium hydroxide solution dissolves the tissue without destroying the fungal cytology, thus allowing easy visualization of the fungal cells. Acid-fast stain (choice A) is used to identify mycobacteria. Culture of the vesicular fluid (choice B) on nutrient agar does not permit growth of the fungal cells. Fungi are grown on Sabouraud nutrient agar, which contains peptones, carbohydrates, vitamins, minerals, and water; it has a pH of 5.3, which is optimal for fungal growth. Serology for *B. dermatitidis* (choice D) is inappropriate, because *T. rubrum* is the causative agent of tinea corporis. Furthermore, serology is of marginal value for the diagnosis of tinea corporis. Silver staining (choice E) is used for the detection of spirochetes.

502. **(D)** The history of the patient described in the question would require careful consideration of all of the diseases listed, and the serology would not serve to rule out any. In the acute phase of the illness, an elevation of antibodies specific for the causative agent might not occur. Usually the rise in antibody levels does not occur until the second or third week of the infection, thus the significance of paired (acute and convalescent) serum samples, which allow the observation of an increase in the antibody specific for the causative agent of the infection. Identifying the cause of most bacterial infections is ideally accomplished by culture of the organism. Serology is used to confirm these identifications and is also used when the agent is slow growing or very expensive to culture, or when the agent cannot be grown at all.

503. **(A)** Adenoviruses are the only ones that produce spikes extending from each one of the vertices of the capsid. These microbes are DNA, nonenveloped, icosahedral viruses. Adenoviruses cause upper respiratory infections associated with coryza, sore throat, fever, and conjunctivitis.

504. **(B)** The best way to detect congenital syphilis is by the use of fluorescent treponema antibody-absorption IgM (FTA-ABA-IgM). All newborn infants of mothers with reactive VDRL, or reactive FTA-ABA tests, will themselves have reactive tests, whether or not they have actually acquired syphilis, because of the passive placental transfer of maternal immunoglobulins. However, if IgM antisyphilitic antibody is present in the infant's serum, it reflects fetal antibody production in response to intrauterine infection (congenital syphilis) because maternal IgM antibody does not penetrate a healthy placenta. It is difficult to detect *T. pallidum* in infants by dark-field examinations (choice A) or by silver staining (choice C). Furthermore, sampling of an infant's blood or other body fluids entails risk for the infant. Use of the Wassermann complement fixation test (choice D) is not as specific as the FTA-ABA-IgM test for the detection of congenital syphilis. X-rays (choice E) do not reveal congenital syphilis in an infant.

505. **(B)** A positive PPD skin test indicates that the individual has experienced mycobacterial infection at some time. A positive PPD skin test is usually obtained in individuals who have been vaccinated with the attenuated strain of *Mycobacterium bovis* produced by Calmette–Guerin, who named the vaccine bacillus–Calmette–Guerin (BCG). However, as indicated, any individual who had contact with *M. tuberculosis* usually has a positive PPD test (choice E). The PPD skin test does not necessarily indicate current disease or give any information on the health status of the individual (choices A and D). The PPD skin test may be used to assess proper T-cell function, but not B-cell function (choice C).

506. **(C)** Amantadine (Symmetrel) inhibits an early event in the multiplication cycle of influenza virus, as well as arenaviruses. It blocks the uncoating process. Mutations in the M protein genes result in the development of drug-resistant mutants. The drug is not used extensively in the United States because it seems impractical to control this type of infectious disease that is not ordinarily fatal. To protect individuals at high risk and in those in whom the infection is potentially dangerous, the choice is between this drug and the influenza vaccine. In most cases, the vaccine is usually preferred. Acyclovir has slight antiviral action for Epstein–Barr virus (choice A). Acyclovir is used to shorten the duration of herpes simplex virus episodes and also to limit the duration of viral shedding (choice B). There are no antiviral drugs for rabies (choice D). There is no antiviral agent against rhinovirus (choice E).

507. **(C)** There are various ways by which immunologic suppression for transplanted tissue can occur. One of these ways is administration of antilymphocyte globulin. Other means include destruction of B and T lymphocytes by irradiation (choice B). Cyclosporin (choice A) is also used to achieve immunologic suppression for transplantation. It is thought to inhibit interleukin-2, which drives antigen-activated cells to proliferate. Steroid administration (choice E) is an effective means of suppressing the immune system. Suppression of transplanted tissue cannot be obtained by interferon administration, because interferon inhibits translation of viral mRNA (choice D).

508. **(A)** Adenoviruses do not have an envelope. Their linear, double-stranded DNA is enclosed within a capsid with icosahedral symmetry. Spikes project from each of the 12 vertices. The viral DNA contains a virus-encoded protein that is covalently cross-linked to each 5′-end of the linear adenovirus genome. Herpesviruses (choice B) and varicella-zoster virus (choice E) belong to the same family of herpes viridae and have a linear, double-stranded DNA genome, in which the complementary strands are not covalently cross-linked at the termini of the genome. SV40 virus (choice C) is a member of the polyoma group of viruses, and possesses a circular, double-stranded DNA genome. Finally, the genome of the vaccinia virus (choice D) has linear, double-stranded DNA with inverted terminal repeats.

509. **(E)** To be useful as a cloning vector, a plasmid should possess several properties. It should code for one or more selectable markers (such as antibiotic resistance) to allow identification of transformants and to allow maintenance of the plasmid in a bacterial population. Plasmids, by definition, are pieces of DNA that replicate autonomously in the host cell cytoplasm, without incorporation into host cell chromosome (choice A). A plasmid vector should have a high, not a low, copy number (choice B). With high copy numbers, large amounts of a specific segment of foreign DNA can be obtained readily in pure form. Plasmid vectors should contain single sites for restriction enzymes in regions of the plasmid that are not essential for replication. Single sites for restriction enzymes allow for insertion of foreign DNA molecules that have been cleaved with the restriction enzymes (choice C). A plasmid vector should have autonomous, not nonautonomous, replication (choice D). Autonomous replication is necessary and allows a high copy number of plasmids to be obtained.

510. **(B)** *Legionella pneumophila* is spread from water reservoirs, contaminated air-conditioning units, nebulizers filled with water, or evaporative condensers. The organism can survive for over a year in tap water at room temperature (25°C) (choice A). Legionellosis, or legionnaire's disease, was first detected in 1976 when an outbreak of deadly pneumonia occurred in over 200 persons attending an American Legion convention. Epidemiologic investigations showed that the disease was caused by a gram-negative rod that was named *L. pneumophila* (choice D). *Legionella pneumophila* is difficult to stain with Gram stain (choice C) or other common bacterial

stains. It will stain faintly gram-negative when safranin is left on for an extended period. The organism can be demonstrated by the direct fluorescent antibody procedure or by the silver impregnation method. The cause of trench fever (choice E) is *Bartonella quintana* (previously known as *Rochalimaea quintana*), not *L. pneumophila*.

511. **(E)** Exposure to *M. tuberculosis* does not ensure contraction. Thus, chemoprophylaxis with INH should be the treatment of choice for contacts of actively infected persons. Individuals receiving INH should be checked periodically by sputum cultures (choice B) and x-ray (choice C). Immunization with the live attenuated tuberculosis strain bacillus–Calmette–Guerin (BCG) is pointless because the contacts have already experienced infection with *M. tuberculosis* (choice A). Ethambutol is very effective against most mycobacteria, but it is used in the therapy of tuberculosis, not in prophylaxis (choice D).

512. **(C)** The short incubation of four hours indicates staphylococcal food poisoning. This is a situation arising from the ingestion of preformed staphylococcal enterotoxin, which induces symptoms within 1 to 6 hours following consumption of contaminated food, including diarrhea, abdominal cramps, and severe vomiting. These symptoms last for 6 to 12 hours, and complete recovery usually occurs in less than 1 day. The incubation periods for *S. typhimurium* (choice B), *V. parahaemolyticus* (choice D), *Y. enterocolitica* (choice E), and *C. jejuni* (choice A) are 8 to 12, 24 to 96, 24 to 48, and 72 to 168 hours, respectively. These longer incubation periods in comparison to the incubation period of staphylococcal food intoxication are due to the need for these bacteria to invade the human intestinal tract, and then multiply and form the toxins responsible for the infective form of food poisoning.

513. **(A)** Administration of diphtheria antitoxin quickly provides large amounts of preformed antibodies. These antibodies neutralize unbound diphtheria exotoxin in body fluids, and thus reduce tissue damage. Diphtheria antitoxin is produced in horses, sheep, or goats. Persons sensitive to horse, sheep, or goat proteins may develop type III hypersensitivity reactions, a good example of which is serum sickness. Administration of diphtheria antitoxin most likely combines with diphtheria exotoxin and complement, and thus decreases, not increases, the concentration of serum complement (choice B). Injection of diphtheria antitoxin can lead to production of antibody against serum proteins of the animal used to produce diphtheria antitoxin, but not antibodies against diphtheria (choice E). Administration of diphtheria antitoxin does not eliminate the need for immunization with diphtheria toxoid. Because the protection afforded by antitoxin is of short duration, and prolonged protection against diphtheria is achieved by vaccination with diphtheria toxoid, diphtheria antitoxin alone will not confer lifelong immunity (choices C and D).

514. **(D)** To determine whether the poliovirus is a wild-type virus or if it is related to that used for vaccination, it will be necessary to prepare oligonucleotide maps of the isolated virus and compare them to those of the wild-type and vaccine strains. Many viruses may kill mice; thus, one cannot determine whether poliovirus strains are related or unrelated by mouse lethality studies (choice B). Cytopathology cannot be used for definitive diagnosis of poliovirus strains or other types of viruses (choice A). Viral neutralization assays using the grandchild's serum will only indicate whether the grandchild has been exposed to and vaccinated for the polioviruses in question, but will not establish whether the poliovirus isolated from the grandfather's stool is related to the poliovirus used to vaccinate his grandchild (choice C). Staining the virus with fluorescent antibody may detect the presence of poliovirus, but will not establish whether the poliovirus is a wild-type virus or if it is related to that used for vaccination (choice E).

515. **(B)** An important part of the penicillin molecule is the β-lactam group. This group is com-

posed of two carbon and two hydrogen atoms at the top of the group. The bottom part of the group contains one carbon, which is linked to one nitrogen atom and one oxygen atom. Penicillinase breaks the bond between the bottom carbon and nitrogen atoms, and destroys the antibacterial activity of penicillin, along with that of cephalosporin, which also possesses a β-lactam group.

516. **(C)** The laboratory diagnosis of tinea pedis (athlete's foot) caused by *T. rubrum* depends on the demonstration of typical pear-shaped microconidia, which develop on white-red colonies of *T. rubrum*. Number 1 shows a chamydospore (choice A); number 2, a sporangiospore of *Rhizopus* (choice B); number 4, a spherule filled with endospores of *Coccidioides immitis* (choice D); and number 5, a budding yeast cell of *Blastomyces dermatiditis* (choice E).

517. **(B)** The patient is showing the typical symptoms of botulism, which is commonly caused by types A, B, or E *Clostridium botulinum* toxin. Therefore, early administration of potent botulinum antitoxin containing antibodies to toxins A, B, and E constitutes the most appropriate treatment. Administration of staphylococcal enterotoxin antiserum (choice A) could have been helpful if the patient were suffering from staphylococcal food poisoning, but he is not. Immunization with staphylococcal enterotoxin toxoid (choice C), administration of penicillin (choice D), or placing this patient in a hyperbaric chamber are all useless (choice E).

518. **(D)** Ketoconazole inhibits the biosynthesis of ergosterol by blocking demethylation at the C14 site of the ergosterol precursor, lanosterol. This results in the accumulation of lanosterol-like sterols in the cell, which alters the properties of the cell membrane and permits the leakage of potassium ions. Amphotericin B (choice A) and nystatin (choice E) impair the permeability of the cell membrane by directly complexing with the membrane sterol. The target of griseofulvin (choice C) is microtubules. Flucytosine (5-fluorocytosine)

(choice B) is incorporated into RNA after being deaminated and then phosphorylated. It also interferes with DNA synthesis because it is a noncompetitive inhibitor of thymidylate synthetase.

519. **(C)** The child described appears to be suffering from meningitis due to *Staphylococcus aureus,* which should always be considered a β-lactamase-producing germ until the laboratory reports its antibiotic sensitivity. Methicillin is a β-lactamase–resistant penicillin, and would be the antibiotic of choice among those listed. Other antibiotics that might be used are cephalosporins or vancomycin, but not ampicillin (choice A), kanamycin (choice B), penicillin (choice D), or streptomycin (choice E).

520. **(D)** The patient contracted Rocky Mountain spotted fever; it is transmitted by tick bites and characterized by high fever, myalgia, macules, and petechiae. The rash appears first on the arms and feet, and then spreads to the trunk. Epidemic typhus (choice A) is transmitted by lice, not ticks, and is characterized by a maculopapular rash that begins on the trunk, not the arms and legs. It is associated with severe meningoencephalitis and delirium. Q fever (choice B) is an influenza-like illness that progresses to a pneumonitis. It is not associated with rash, and it is transmitted by respiratory droplets, not arthropod vector bites. Rickettsial pox (choice C) is transmitted by mite bite, and is a mild illness characterized by moderate fever, headache, and a vesicular rash that forms an eschar. Scrub typhus (choice E) is also transmitted by mite bite, and is characterized by mild fever, a rash, which may have an eschar, and lymphadenopathy.

521. **(A)** The most reliable test for the diagnosis of Rocky Mountain spotted fever is the complement fixation test employing specific antigens of the etiological agent *Rickettsia rickettsii.* The etiologic agent *R. rickettsii* cannot be cultured on Sabouraud or blood agar plates (choices B and C). Gram staining (choice D) only reveals the presence of small gram-negative rods, and thus cannot be very useful for the diagnosis of Rocky Mountain spotted fever. The Weil–Felix reaction (choice E) employs *Proteus vulgaris,* OX-2, OX-19, and OX-K to test for antibody production to rickettsia. *Proteus vulgaris* can be used instead of rickettsia in the Weil–Felix agglutination reaction because rickettsia and *P. vulgaris* have common antigens. Because the cultivation and handling of rickettsia is difficult and dangerous, *P. vulgaris* provides convenient, safe antigens for the presumptive diagnosis of rickettsial diseases. However, patients infected with *P. vulgaris* also give positive results.

522. **(B)** Rickettsia are gram-negative short rods, and as such have a cell wall that resembles that of gram-negative bacteria. The cell size of rickettsia is 0.6 × 0.3 microns. The limit of resolution of the light microscope is 0.2 microns, thus rickettsia can be seen with a light microscope (choice A). Tetracyclines and chloramphenicol are the drugs of choice for the treatment of Rocky Mountain spotted fever (choice C). Rickettsia have cell walls that resemble the cell wall of gram-negative bacteria (choice D). Rickettsia replicate by binary fission. *Chlamydia* replicate with a distinct intracellular cycle (choice E).

523. **(A)** The most likely diagnosis is acute amoebic dysentery; the classical symptomatology of acute amoebic dysentery is lower abdominal pain, cramping, colitis, tenesmus, flatulence, and bloody diarrhea. Malaria (choice B) is characterized by periodic fever, fatal cerebral episodes, lysis of red blood cells, nephritis due to immune complex formation, and is transmitted by mosquito bites. Toxoplasmosis (choice C) is a mild influenza-like disease with possible lymph node enlargement, which may be severe in immunocompromised patients. Congenital infections can damage the eyes or brain and may be fatal. Trichomoniasis (choice D) is limited to the vagina and is associated with a watery, foul-smelling, abundant, greenish-gray discharge. Trypanosomiasis (choice E) is transmitted by bites of the tsetse fly and the trypanosomes initially cause chancres at the site of the bite.

Then the trypanosomes reach the central nervous system, and the patient has lassitude, develops sleeping episodes, and tissue wasting or even death can occur.

524. **(A)** Cysts are the infective form of *Entamoeba histolytica* and are transmitted by ingestion of infected food or drink. The gametocyte (choice B) is the infective stage of malaria parasites for mosquitoes. Larval penetration of the skin (choice C) is the mode of transmission for hookworms, *Strongyloides*, and *Schistosoma*. Ingestion of ova (choice D) is the mode of transmission of such organisms as *Enterobius vermicularis, Ascaris lumbricoides,* and *Trichuris trichiura,* but not *E. histolytica.* Sporozoites (choice E) are the infective stage of malaria parasites spread to humans by mosquito bites.

525. **(B)** The drugs of choice for acute amoebic dysentery are metronidazole and iodoquinol. Chloroquine (choice A) is normally used for the treatment of malaria. Stibogluconate (choice C) is recommended for the treatment of leishmaniasis. Sulfonamide and pyrimethamine (choice D) are used for the treatment of toxoplasmosis. Trimethoprim and sulfamethoxazole (choice E) are the drugs of choice for the treatment of *Pneumocystis carinii* pneumonia.

526. **(B)** Hepatitis virus A is a small (20 to 30 nm), nonenveloped, single-stranded RNA virus. The virus is transmitted via the fecal–oral route, usually by eating contaminated foods, such as oysters grown in polluted waters. The symptoms of hepatitis A infection include fatigue, loss of appetite, nausea, vomiting, abdominal pain, fever, and jaundice. The urine excreted from patients with jaundice may be dark and the feces pale. Adenovirus (choice A) is a nonenveloped, double-stranded, linear DNA virus. It is transmitted by respiratory secretions, and causes pharyngitis, conjunctivitis, keratoconjunctivitis, pneumonia, and gastroenteritis. Hepatitis B (choice C) is an enveloped, partially double-stranded DNA virus with a circular genome. It is transmitted by infected blood or blood products, sexually or congenitally. Rhi-

noviruses (choice D) are members of the picornaviruses. Rhinoviruses cause the common cold, and are isolated from people with mild upper respiratory tract infections. Rotavirus (choice E) is a member of the retroviruses. Its genome is quite unusual in that it is composed of double-stranded RNA consisting of 10 segments. Rotavirus causes diarrhea in children mostly under the age of six.

527. **(D)** Diagnosis of Mr. X.'s infectious hepatitis can best be made by the demonstration of a fourfold rise of IgM against hepatitis A virus. A positive Tzanck test (choice A) is useful for the diagnosis of herpes virus, not hepatitis virus A. Hepatitis virus does not induce any pathognomonic cytopathic effects (choice B). Patients with hepatitis virus A do not show any meaningful rise of IgA (choice C). The detection of Negri bodies (choice E) is useful in the diagnosis of rabies, not hepatitis virus A.

528. **(C)** Hepatitis virus A infection can best be prevented by immunization with the intact inactivated virus. Administration of human gamma globulin (choice A) may provide only passive immunity, which will be of short duration; thus, it is not the best way to prevent hepatitis A viral infection. Hepatitis B core antigen (HbcAg) (choice B) is not effective for vaccination, even against the hepatitis B virus from which it is derived. Immunization with a subunit vaccine (choice D) is used to prevent hepatitis virus B infection, not hepatitis virus A infection. Interferons (choice E) act only in the early phase of a viral infection limiting the spread of virus, and are not recommended for long-term protection against viral diseases.

529. **(A)** This patient has chronic granulomatous disease. Children with this disease suffer chronic suppurative infections caused most frequently by *S. aureus.* The cause of chronic granulomatous disease is a genetic defect in NADPH oxidase. Neutrophils contain myeloperoxidase, which utilizes hydrogen peroxide and halide ions to produce hypochlorite, which is highly microbiocidal. Because of the

defective NADPH oxidase, the patient's phagocytes cannot generate sufficient hydrogen peroxide; thus, the myeloperoxidase–hydrogen peroxide–halide system cannot function normally. Neutrophils from these patients can phagocytize bacteria and fungi normally, but they cannot kill them because of the defective myeloperoxidase–hydrogen peroxide–halide system. Patients with Graves disease (choice B) produce autoantibodies to thyroid-stimulating hormone receptors. Rheumatoid arthritis (choice C) is another autoimmune disease. Patients with this disease produce IgM autoantibodies to the Fc moiety of IgG. Severe combined immunodeficiency disease (SCID) (choice D) is characterized by the absence of T and B cells, absence of thymus, and lack of in vitro lymphocyte proliferative response to mitogens, antigens, and allogeneic cells. Systemic lupus erythematosus (choice E) is an autoimmune disease (type III hypersensitivity or immune complex disease). Patients with lupus erythematosus produce anti-nuclear antibodies.

530.   (E) Streptococcal infections in chronic granulomatous disease are rare, because the defective myeloperoxidase–hydrogen peroxide–halide system can use hydrogen peroxide accumulated by phagocytosed streptococci, which are catalase negative and cannot convert hydrogen peroxide to water and oxygen. Administration of pooled gamma globulin (choice C) or antistreptolysin (choice A) is likely to provide only brief, but not chronic, protection against streptococci. C-reactive protein (CRP) (choice B) is a beta serum globulin that reacts with the C carbohydrate of the cell wall of *Streptococcus pneumoniae*. It is not an antibody and thus does not provide even brief protection against streptococci. Phagocytosis (choice D) plays a major, not a minor, role in the killing of streptococci.

531.   (E) The diagnosis of chronic granulomatous disease is made by the inability of phagocytes to reduce the dye nitroblue tetrazolium (NBT). During phagocytosis in normal phagocytes, when reactive oxygen intermediates are produced, the yellow dye is converted to purple-blue formazan. In patients with chronic granulomatous disease during phagocytosis, reactive oxygen intermediates are not produced and NBT remains yellow. The Coombs test (choice A) is used to detect antibody on a patient's erythrocytes. If antibodies are attached, the erythrocytes are agglutinated by antihuman immunoglobulin. The India ink test (choice B) is used to demonstrate the capsule of *Cryptococcus neoformans*. The methyl red test (choice C) is designed to detect use of carbohydrate by bacteria. The mixed lymphocyte reaction (choice D) is used to test the responsiveness of recipient lymphocytes to antigens present on donor cells.

532.   (A) Tumor necrosis factor-alpha (TNF-α) has potent biological activity, and causes cachexia, which presents a difficulty in its use for cancer therapy. TNF-α in high, not in low, doses causes fever (choice C). TNF-α does not complicate the function of cytotoxic T lymphocytes (choice B); it enhances the production of interleukin 1 and 6 (choice E); it often leads to inflammation (choice D); and it is synthesized upon stimulation.

533.   (A) Adenoviruses are a frequent cause of infection characterized by a triad of symptoms, namely, pharyngitis, conjunctivitis and fever. *Chlamydia pneumoniae* (choice B) causes generally primary atypical pneumonia which is not usually associated with conjunctivitis. *Neisseria gonorrhoeae* (choice C) normally causes gonorrhea. *Streptococcus pyogenes* (choice D) causes 25% of cases of pharyngitis. However, the disease is often accompanied by tonsillitis. The infection is usually associated with a fever higher than 39°C. *Toxoplasma gondii* (choice E) in AIDS patients or other immunosuppressed individuals can cause disseminated disease and encephalitis.

534.   (B) Brucellae are small, gram-negative coccobacilli that require a prolonged period of cultivation. Skin tests for brucellosis are not reliable (choice A). Prevention of human brucellosis is accomplished through control of livestock by identification and elimination of

infected herds, and animal vaccination. A vaccine for humans against brucellosis is not available (choice C). Cultures represent the gold standard of diagnosis, but they are not always positive and thus standard tube agglutination tests supplement cultural assays (choice D). Treatment for 6 weeks with either tetracycline with an aminoglycoside, or tetracyclin with rifampin, is used against brucellosis (choice E). A titer of 1:160 or higher against *Brucella melitensis* in a convalescent serum from the 25-year-old student is of diagnostic value.

535. **(B)** Systemic lupus erythematosus (SLE) is an autoimmune disease initially recognized clinically by a rash on the face with a "wolf"-like shape (thus the name *lupus*). Such a butterfly rash is considered a distinctive manifestation of SLE. The development of erythema chronicum migrans is a pathognomonic feature of Lyme disease (choice A). Detection of antibodies to double-stranded DNA are pathognomonic for SLE (choice C). Arthritis, but not carditis (choice D) or pneumonitis (choice E), occurs frequently in patients with SLE.

536. **(C)** *Neisseria meningitidis* is a gram-negative coccus that continuously releases outer membrane fragments during infection. These fragments are endotoxins, which initiate the production of proinflammatory cytokines, which lead to disseminated intravascular coagulation, hypotension, hemorrhage, and finally shock. The endotoxins of *N. menigitidis* and *N. gonorrhoeae* both contain lipid A, which is the toxic moiety of endotoxin (choice A). Neither *N. meningitidis* nor *N. gonorrhoeae* produce exotoxins (choice B). It is not known if the endotoxins of *N. meningitidis* are more toxic than those produced by *N. gonorrhoeae* (choice D). The capsule of *N. meningitidis* is more pronounced than that of *N. gonorrhoeae*; however, there is no definitive evidence that this capsular difference alone explains why *N. menigitidis* cause hemorrhagic rash and shock more frequently than *N. gonorrhoeae* (choice E).

537. **(C)** Rifampin is a semisynthetic antibiotic active against a broad spectrum of bacteria including gram-positive, gram-negative, and mycobacteria. It inhibits the bacterial DNA-dependent RNA polymerase. Bacterial resistance to rifampin is most frequently due to point mutations, and to small insertions and deletions in the *rpoB* gene that encodes the beta subunit of RNA polymerase. The mutants exhibit reduced affinity for rifampin. Dihydrofolate reductase is the target of trimethoprim (choice A). DNA gyrase is the target of quinolones (choice B). rRNA methylase in not an antibiotic target, but an enzyme that mediates resistance to macrolides (choice D). Transpeptidases are involved in the synthesis of the bacterial cell wall and have not been associated with resistance to rifampin (choice E).

538. **(C)** During an asthma attack, mast cells release a number of physiologically active substances, such as histamine, leukotrienes, and other pharmacologically active molecules that cause life-threatening symptoms. Eosinophil chemotactic factor of anaphylaxis (choice A) attracts eosinophils, the role of which is not precisely known. Epinephrine (choice B) is useful in the treatment of anaphylactic shock, and suppresses bronchoconstriction, one of the major life-threatening symptoms of an asthma reaction. Interleukins 1 (choice D) and 5 (choice E) promote the growth and differentiation of B cells.

539. **(B)** *Cryptococcus neoformans* causes meningitis and multiple abscesses in the central nervous system. *Borrelia burgdorferi* (choice A) is the etiologic agent of Lyme disease. Fluctuating meningitis or meningoencephalitis may occur, often with cranial or peripheral nerve lesions. Myelitis, arthritis, and carditis may develop later on. However, multiple abscesses in the CNS do not develop. *Mycobacterium tuberculosis* (choice C) causes pulmonary tuberculosis with localized masses called tuberculomata, but it is not associated with multiple abscesses in the CNS. *Treponema pallidum* (choice D) causes syphilis. In whatever stage of the disease, primary, secondary, and tertiary meningitis may develop, but it is not associated with multiple abscesses in the CNS. *Treponema pertenue* (choice E) cause yaws, which is characterized by the formation of cauliflower-like lesions on the skin.

540. (D) *Mycoplasma pneumoniae* lacks a murein-containing cell wall, and thus resists the action of antibiotics that interfere with the synthesis of the bacterial cell wall. *Mycoplasma pneumoniae* is not impermeable to β-lactam antibiotics (choice A), does not contain large amounts of teichoic acids in its cytoplasmic membrane (choice B), and does not produce β-lactamases (choice E). *Mycoplasma pneumoniae* contains sterols in its cytoplasmic membrane, but this is irrelevant with regard to the activity of β-lactam antibiotics (choice C)

541. (A) A severe deficiency in helper T-cell functions leads to a deficiency in B-cell function, because B cells require assistance from helper T cells to function properly. Children with severe helper T-cell dysfunction usually do not show a deficiency in serum complement (choice B). Cytotoxic T cells do not require the help of helper T cells, and their function remains intact (choices C, D, and E).

542. (D) *Pasteurella multocida* is a gram-negative rod that is part of the oral flora of many animals, particularly dogs and cats. It is transmitted to humans by animal bites and causes wound infections. *Clostridium botulinum* (choice A), *C. perfringens* (choice B), and *C. tetani* (choice C) are gram-positive, spore-forming rods, and thus can be excluded as etiologic agents. *Toxocara canis* (choice E), a common intestinal parasite of dogs, is a metazoan that causes visceral larval migrans.

543. (E) Sulfonamides are bacteriostatic antibiotics that interfere with the biosynthesis of folic acid, which is essential for the formation of purines, pyrimidines, and amino acids. Within the folic acid metabolic pathway, dihydropteroate synthase catalyzes the synthesis of 7,8-dihydropteroate from para-animobenzoate and pterin pyrophosphate.

Sulfonamides compete with para-aminobenzoate for this enzyme, and inhibit its activity. Thus, synthesis of DNA and RNA may be affected. However, synthesis of DNA or RNA usually does not occur (choices B and D). Sulfonamides are not the most likely antibiotics used to inhibit the synthesis of the bacterial cytoplasmic membrane (choice A). Synthesis of peptidoglycan is inhibited by penicillins, not sulfonamides (choice C).

544. (B) *Streptococcus pneumoniae* is one of the microbes most frequently responsible for acute ear infection and meningitis in infants. The host defense against the encapsulated bacterium relies heavily on phagocytes that can engulf and destroy it only when *S. pneumoniae* is covered with opsonin. In a patient with agammaglobulinemia, this opsonization may not occur optimally. Consequently, encapsulated *S. pneumoniae* may not be killed, resulting in infection. The resistance to other microorganisms listed in the question depends predominantly on cell-mediated immunity, which is not affected in this patient (choices A, C, D, and E).

545. (D) Ciprofloxacin and other fluoroquinolones inhibit the enzymes DNA gyrase and topoisomerase IV, which are required for the replication of bacterial DNA. Fluoroquinolone resistance arises when a bacterium mutates in the fluoroquinolone binding sites of these two enzymes. Therefore, an increase in the rate of ciprofloxacin resistance among enterobacteria is not due to a spread of plasmids carrying fluoroquinolone resistance genes, to high rates of protein synthesis, to acquisition of an exogenous gene, or to high rates of synthesis of DNA polymerase (choices A, B, C, and E).

546. (B) *Neisseria meningitidis* causes the most severe form of meningitis characterized by sepsis, petechiae throughout the body, hypotension, dyspnea, disseminated intravascular coagulation, and shock, which can be fatal in a few hours. The other bacteria listed may cause meningitis, but the infection is not as abrupt and severe (choices A, C, D, and E).

REFERENCES

Brooks GF, Butel JS, Morse SA, et al. *Medical Micro-biology,* 21st ed. Stamford, CT: Appleton & Lange; 1998.

Joklik WK, Willett HP, Amos BD, et al. *Zinser Micro-biology,* 20th ed. Norwalk, CT: Appleton & Lange; 1992.

Levinson WE, Jawetz E. *Medical Microbiology & Immunology,* 6th ed. New York: Lange Medical Books/McGraw-Hill; 2000.

Murray PR, Rosenthal KS, Kobayashi GS, et al. *Medical Microbiology,* 3rd ed. St. Louis: Mosby-Year Book; 1998.

Roitt I, Brostoff J, Male D. *Immunology,* 5th ed. London: Mosby-Year Book; 1998.

Subspecialty List: Microbiology

Question Number and Subspecialty

410. Immunology
411. Bacteriology
412. Bacteriology
413. Immunology
414. Antibiotics
415. Virology
416. Immunology
417. Parasitology
418. Bacteriology
419. Immunology
420. Bacteriology
421. Virology
422. Immunology
423. Bacteriology
424. Bacteriology
425. Virology
426. Immunology
427. Bacteriology
428. Immunology
429. Immunology
430. Antibiotics
431. Immunology
432. Immunology
433. Bacteriology
434. Bacteriology
435. Virology
436. Bacteriology
437. Bacteriology
438. Antimicrobial agents
439. Virology
440. Virology
441. Mycology
442. Antibiotics
443. Immunology
444. Bacteriology
445. Immunology
446. Immunology
447. Bacteriology
448. Bacteriology
449. Immunology
450. Virology
451. Immunology
452. Immunology
453. Bacteriology
454. Bacteriology
455. Immunology
456. Immunology
457. Virology
458. Immunology
459. Immunology
460. Bacteriology
461. Immunology
462. Mycology
463. Virology
464. Antimicrobial agents
465. Bacteriology
466. Bacteriology
467. Mycology
468. Parasitology
469. Bacteriology
470. Immunology
471. Immunology
472. Bacteriology
473. Bacteriology
474. Immunology
475. Bacteriology
476. Bacteriology
477. Bacteriology
478. Bacteriology
479. Immunology
480. Immunology
481. Bacteriology
482. Microbial genetics
483. Microbial genetics

484. Bacteriology
485. Immunology
486. Immunology
487. Bacteriology
488. Virology
489. Virology
490. Virology
491. Bacteriology
492. Bacteriology
493. Antiviral agents
494. Bacteriology
495. Bacteriology
496. Virology
497. Bacteriology
498. Mycology
499. Mycology
500. Microbial genetics
501. Mycology
502. Bacteriology
503. Virology
504. Bacteriology
505. Bacteriology
506. Antiviral agents
507. Immunology
508. Virology
509. Microbial genetics
510. Bacteriology
511. Bacteriology
512. Bacteriology
513. Immunology
514. Virology
515. Antibiotics

516. Mycology
517. Bacteriology
518. Antifungal agents
519. Antibiotics
520. Bacteriology
521. Bacteriology
522. Bacteriology
523. Parasitology
524. Parasitology
525. Antiparasitic drugs
526. Virology
527. Virology
528. Virology
529. Immunology
530. Immunology
531. Immunology
532. Immunology
533. Bacteriology
534. Bacteriology
535. Immunology
536. Bacteriology
537. Antibiotics
538. Immunology
539. Mycology
540. Antibiotics
541. Immunology
542. Bacteriology
543. Bacteriology
544. Bacteriology
545. Antibiotics
546. Bacteriology

CHAPTER 5

Pathology
Questions

James F. P. Dixon, PhD, Clive R. Taylor, MD, DPhil,
and Karen D. Tsoulas, MD

DIRECTIONS: (Questions 547 through 673): Each of the numbered items or incomplete statements in this section is followed by answers or by completions of the statement. Select the ONE lettered answer or completion that is BEST in each case.

547. A 28-year-old, recently divorced man with no significant past medical history presents to the emergency room with progressive lower abdominal pain and cramping over the past 4 days, which are relieved by defecation. He has suffered from substantial bloody and mucoid diarrhea during this time. His temperature is 102.8°F. Laboratory studies reveal an elevated white blood cell count and a high erythrocyte sedimentation rate. Sigmoidoscopy reveals extensive rectal and sigmoid hyperemia and edema, numerous superficial ulcerations, and small focal mucosal hemorrhages, many of which have suppurative centers. Significant intestinal narrowing is seen in the distal transverse colon. These findings most likely suggest a diagnosis of

(A) amebic colitis
(B) collagenous colitis
(C) cytomegalovirus enterocolitis
(D) pseudomembranous colitis
(E) ulcerative colitis

548. A 33-year-old woman suffers from weakness of her ocular and facial muscles that worsens with repeated use. She has antibodies to acetylcholine receptors in her serum. The likely diagnosis is

(A) conjunctivitis
(B) myasthenia gravis

(C) orbital inflammatory pseudotumor
(D) Parkinson disease
(E) polymyositis

549. A 45-year-old woman who has had a chronic demyelinating neurologic disorder since she was 27, dies in an automobile accident. At autopsy a number of plaques are observed in the central nervous system and oligoclonal immunoglobulins are identified in the cerebrospinal fluid. She most likely suffered from

(A) amyotrophic lateral sclerosis
(B) Huntington disease
(C) multiple sclerosis
(D) pemphigus vulgaris
(E) spinocerebellar degeneration

550. A 39-year-old woman undergoes a total hysterectomy. A section of her left fallopian tube is shown in Figure 5–1. The most likely diagnosis is

(A) chronic salpingitis
(B) ectopic tubal pregnancy
(C) endometriosis
(D) endosalpingosis
(E) serous papillary carcinoma

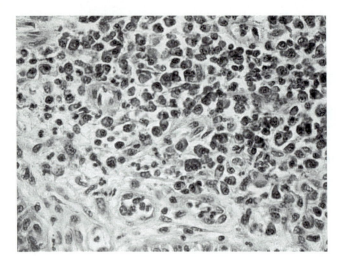

Figure 5–1. (See also Color Insert.) *(Courtesy of Dr. Parakrama Chandrasoma.)*

551. A 47-year-old gardener receives an insect sting while pruning some rose bushes. Within a few minutes the area around the sting is swollen and red. The swelling is mostly the result of

(A) decreased plasma oncotic pressure

(B) increased hydrostatic pressure

(C) increased vascular permeability

(D) lymphatic obstruction

(E) venous obstruction

552. A 24-year-old man complains of the gradual onset over the past year of dysphagia following the ingestion of either liquid or solid foods. He often has regurgitation after eating, particularly at night. Chest x-ray reveals an air–fluid level in an enlarged esophagus. The pathologic abnormality that is consistently present with this abnormality is

(A) decreased ganglion cells in the myenteric plexus

(B) fibrous stricture

(C) formation of one or more diverticulae

(D) *Helicobacter pylori* infection

(E) hiatal hernia

553. A 39-year-old man complains of the sudden onset of excruciating pain in the metatarsophalangeal joint in his right great toe. You find the joint to be extremely tender, hyperemic, and warm. Aspiration of synovial fluid from the joint reveals neutrophils containing

negatively birefringent crystals. The most likely diagnosis is

(A) acute bacterial pyarthrosis

(B) calcium pyrophosphate deposition disease

(C) ganglion cyst

(D) gout

(E) ochronosis

554. A 25-year-old woman complains that whenever she is in the sun for more than a few minutes she develops an erythematous rash on the sun-exposed skin by the next day. This is accompanied by joint pain and a feeling of fatigue. Laboratory tests reveal a Coombs-positive anemia and a urinary sediment containing red and white cells and some casts. To help you reach a diagnosis, you would next order a

(A) differential count on synovial fluid

(B) renal biopsy

(C) serum test for anti-nuclear antibodies

(D) skin biopsy

(E) urine test for porphyrins

555. A homeless, 43-year-old, chronic alcoholic develops pneumonia and is admitted to the County Hospital. Even though he has not been drinking during the past 24 hours, physical examination reveals difficulty walking without support, weakness of the ocular muscles, and global confusion. Based on these findings, you suspect that he suffers from a dietary deficiency of vitamin

(A) A

(B) B$_1$ (thiamine)

(C) B$_{12}$ (cyanocobalamin)

(D) C (ascorbate)

(E) D (calciferol)

(F) K

556. A 75-year-old chronically ill man with a long history of alcoholism suddenly develops dyspnea. A lung scan reveals a large segmental perfusion defect in the right lower lobe with normal ventilation. Of the following, what is the most likely factor that could have initi-

ated a sequence of events culminating in his dyspnea?

(A) Anemia due to chronic illness

(B) Cirrhosis of the liver due to alcoholism

(C) Pulmonary artery obstruction due to atherosclerosis

(D) Venous stasis due to inactivity

557. A 4-month-old baby boy who appeared normal at birth is now brought to you by the parents. They feel that he sleeps excessively, is relatively inactive, and rarely cries. Your examination reveals that he has abnormal deep tendon reflexes, hypothermia, jaundice, and muscular hypotonia. Of the following, the best therapy would be

(A) antibiotics

(B) growth hormone

(C) thiamine

(D) thyroxine

(E) vitamin D

558. A 41-year-old man with chronic hepatitis C viral infection has a chemistry profile performed. The serum analyte that is most likely to be decreased is

(A) alanine aminotransferase

(B) albumin

(C) aspartate aminotransferase

(D) gamma globulin

(E) lactate dehydrogenase

559. A 23-year-old man has been complaining of intermittent diarrhea, fever, and abdominal pain for several months. A radiograph of the small bowel reveals several separate areas of lumenal narrowing. A photomicrograph of this patient's ileal biopsy is displayed in Figure 5–2. The most likely diagnosis is

(A) abetalipoproteinemia

(B) adenocarcinoma

(C) carcinoid tumor

(D) Crohn disease

(E) ulcerative enterocolitis

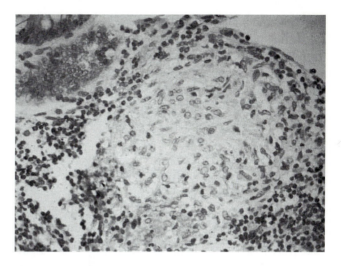

Figure 5–2. (See also Color Insert.) *(Courtesy of Dr. Parakrama Chandrasoma.)*

560. A 52-year-old woman has had rheumatoid arthritis for many years. She now comes to you complaining of the development in the past few months of redness, burning, and itching of her eyes and a dry mouth, making swallowing difficult. This newly developing condition gives the patient a greatly increased risk for

(A) esophageal carcinoma

(B) leukemia

(C) lymphoma

(D) melanoma

(E) pleomorphic adenoma

561. A laboratory test for a newly discovered infectious disease is found to have a sensitivity of 90% and a specificity of 90%. The disease has a prevalence of 1%. The test is run on one of your patients and yields a negative result. What is the probability (to the nearest whole number) of this result being a true negative rather than a false-negative result (what is the predictive value negative)?

(A) 1%

(B) 10%

(C) 50%

(D) 90%

(E) 100%

562. A 29-year-old woman presents with weakness, fatigue, easy bruising, and nosebleeds. Analysis of her blood reveals a reciprocal translocation between chromosomes 22 and 9, and low leukocyte alkaline phosphatase levels. These findings confirm a diagnosis of

(A) acute lymphoblastic leukemia
(B) Burkitt lymphoma
(C) chronic myelogenous leukemia
(D) follicular lymphoma
(E) Hodgkin lymphoma

563. A 35-year-old woman complains of stiffness of her hands and wrists in the morning which resolves during the day. Physical examination reveals slight swelling and tenderness of these joints. X-rays demonstrate only soft tissue swelling around the joints. Laboratory workup reveals the presence in the serum of an antibody to her own IgG. A biopsy of the synovium of the wrist would most characteristically show

(A) caseous necrosis
(B) fibrosis
(C) macrophages and multinucleated giant cells
(D) necrotizing vasculitis
(E) plasma cells and lymphocytes

564. About 6 months ago, a 59-year-old man developed a dull, continuous abdominal pain radiating to the right upper quadrant. He says the pain is relieved by bending forward. He has also had recurrent thrombophlebitis. He now develops jaundice. Of the following, the condition that would most likely explain all of these findings is

(A) alcoholic cirrhosis
(B) cholecystitis
(C) cholelithiasis
(D) pancreatic adenocarcinoma
(E) viral hepatitis

565. A 54-year-old man presents with a 3-month history of mild to moderate edema of the face and ankles. Past medical history is unremarkable except for an upper respiratory infection about a month ago, some mild osteoarthritis of both knees, and allergies to some grasses and pollens. He is not currently taking any medications. Blood pressure is 120/70 mm Hg. Serum creatinine is 1.1 mg/dL. The urine sediment contains some hyaline casts and oval fat bodies, and a 24-hour urine specimen contains 6.5 g protein. Based on this information, the most likely diagnosis is

(A) diabetic nephropathy
(B) Goodpasture syndrome
(C) membranous nephropathy
(D) minimal change disease
(E) postinfectious glomerulonephritis

566. While working in his garden, a 52-year-old man develops a severe substernal pain. This persists for the next 2 hours and radiates to his neck and jaw. Despite his protests, his wife calls 911 and he is transported to the emergency room 6 hours after the onset of his pain. Of the following laboratory tests run on his serum, the one that would be most likely to yield a useful result is

(A) bilirubin
(B) glucose
(C) lactate dehydrogenase
(D) lipase
(E) troponin I

567. A 67-year-old man is involved in a traffic accident and suffers a broken leg. An x-ray reveals a comminuted fracture of the right femur and a "railroad track" pattern of calcification of the femoral artery. This latter finding is best characterized as the result of

(A) dystrophic calcification
(B) metastatic calcification
(C) Mönckeberg sclerosis
(D) trauma from the accident

568. A 51-year-old man dies suddenly from a massive myocardial infarct. At autopsy, the lesion shown in Figure 5–3 is found in his stomach. This most likely represents

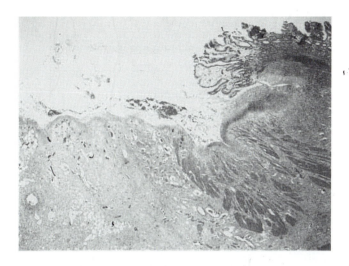

Figure 5–3. *(See also Color Insert.) (Courtesy of Dr. Parakrama Chandrasoma.)*

(A) adenocarcinoma
(B) adenomatous polyp
(C) Brunner gland adenoma
(D) leiomyoma
(E) peptic ulceration

569. A 67-year-old man complains of low back pain and generalized weakness, gradually worsening over the past 6 months. A physical examination reveals an individual in discomfort because of the back pain. Laboratory examination reveals an anemia with rouleaux formation of the erythrocytes on the peripheral smear. Urine shows proteinuria and hypercalciuria. X-rays reveal diffuse osteoporosis of the spine and small lytic lesions in the ribs. The diagnosis that most likely explains these findings is

(A) fibrous dysplasia
(B) iron-deficiency anemia
(C) metastatic prostatic carcinoma
(D) multiple myeloma
(E) osteosarcoma

570. A 49-year-old diabetic and arthritic man dies from severe congestive heart failure. An autopsy reveals that he has cardiomegaly, cirrhosis, and splenomegaly. Microscopic examination demonstrates a large amount of golden-brown granular pigment in most of his organs. The staining technique most useful in confirming the diagnosis is

(A) Congo red
(B) Gomori methenamine silver
(C) periodic acid-Schiff
(D) Prussian blue
(E) trichrome

571. A 24-year-old black woman notices a slowly growing firm nodule near the site of a recent ear piercing. Excision and microscopic examination of the nodule reveals it to be composed of densely collagenized fibrous tissue. The most probable diagnosis is

(A) Brenner tumor
(B) dermoid cyst
(C) hamartoma
(D) keloid
(E) teratoma

572. An 85-year-old man is hospitalized following a confirmed myocardial infarct. However, he develops intractable cardiogenic shock and dies on the third day. An autopsy is performed and a very hemorrhagic, wedge-shaped area is found in one of his organs. Microscopic examination shows this to be an area of coagulative necrosis. The lesion was most likely found in the

(A) brain due to a thromboembolus in the left cerebral artery
(B) heart due to a thrombus superimposed on coronary atherosclerosis
(C) kidney due to an embolized mural thrombosis
(D) liver due to cardiogenic shock
(E) lung due to an embolized deep vein thrombosis

573. An 8-year-old boy is diagnosed with glycogen storage disease. No one else in his family has the disease, but an investigation reveals that his 10-year-old brother and both parents are heterozygous for the defect but his 14-year-old sister is genotypically normal. The inheritance pattern is

(A) autosomal dominant
(B) autosomal recessive
(C) sex-linked dominant
(D) sex-linked recessive
(E) multifactorial

574. A 73-year-old man with congestive heart failure undergoes a thoracentesis, which yields about 200 mL of straw-colored watery fluid. A laboratory study of the fluid reveals:

Specific gravity	1.010
Total protein	0.4 g/dL
Cell count	very rare mesothelial cell present
Fat stain	negative

These pleural fluid findings are indicative of a(n)

(A) chylothorax
(B) empyema
(C) exudate
(D) hemothorax
(E) transudate

575. A 37-year-old man visiting a third world country drinks from a fecally contaminated source. During the next week he has gradually increasing fever, anorexia, myalgia, and headache. He subsequently develops a maculopapular rash on his abdomen and his fever increases to 104°F with abdominal pain and splenomegaly. During the third week, his condition rapidly deteriorates with intestinal bleeding, shock, and death. An autopsy reveals ulcerations overlying the Peyer patches of the small intestine, one of which is perforated. The most likely diagnosis is

(A) amebiasis
(B) cholera

(C) cryptosporidiosis
(D) giardiasis
(E) typhoid fever

576. During a routine pediatric visit, you discover a large abdominal mass in a 2-year-old boy. The mass is surgically removed and is illustrated in Figure 5–4. The most likely diagnosis is

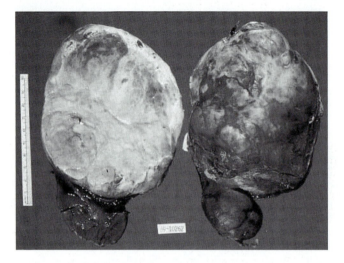

Figure 5–4. (See also Color Insert.) *(Courtesy of Dr. Nancy Warner.)*

(A) abscess
(B) neuroblastoma
(C) renal cell carcinoma
(D) tuberculosis
(E) Wilms tumor

577. A 76-year-old woman suffers a massive myocardial infarct and dies in cardiogenic shock 20 hours after its onset. Microscopic examination of her infarcted myocardium would be expected to demonstrate

(A) abundant neutrophils and monocytes
(B) coagulative necrosis without many neutrophils
(C) fibrosis and collagen deposition
(D) monocytes and neovascularization
(E) plasma cells and caseous necrosis

578. A 47-year-old man has had a cough that produces yellowish sputum for the past week.

He is found to have a total WBC count of 16,300/µL with a differential count of 75% segmented neutrophils, 11% band neutrophils, 9% lymphocytes, 4% monocytes, and 1% eosinophils. His temperature is 100°F and chest x-ray reveals a lesion in the right lower lobe that has a central cavity and an air-fluid level. The most likely diagnosis is

(A) bronchogenic carcinoma
(B) interstitial pneumonia
(C) lobar pneumonia
(D) pulmonary abscess
(E) pulmonary tuberculosis

579. A 2-day-old male infant has not passed any meconium and is now developing signs of obstruction. Of the following, you would most likely see

(A) absence of parasympathetic ganglion cells in the submucosal and myenteric plexus
(B) absence of the nerve fibers that innervate the wall
(C) atrophy of the mucosal lining of the wall
(D) hypertrophy of the muscle coat of the wall
(E) presence of multiple small polyps along the mucosal surface

580. Following a long and difficult labor, a 28-year-old woman gives birth to a healthy baby boy. Shortly thereafter, she develops severe dyspnea, cyanosis, and hypotensive shock. She becomes comatose and dies later that morning. These clinical manifestations are best explained by the development of

(A) bilateral adrenal necrosis
(B) disseminated intravascular coagulation
(C) preeclampsia
(D) pulmonary thromboembolism
(E) Sheehan syndrome

581. A 54-year-old construction worker collapses at his work site and is brought to the emergency room in a comatose state. His skin is dry and hot and his rectal temperature is 105°F. The most likely diagnosis is

(A) heat cramps
(B) heat exhaustion
(C) heat stroke
(D) malignant hyperthermia
(E) pyrexia

582. A 72-year-old alcoholic man is found dead at home during the winter. The medical examiner feels that the likely cause of death is lobar pneumonia. At autopsy this diagnosis is confirmed and is said to be at the "red hepatization" stage. What pathologic process within the lung is responsible for the gross abnormality termed "red hepatization?"

(A) Alcoholic toxic necrosis of the pulmonary tissue
(B) Desquamation of tracheal and bronchial epithelial cells
(C) Fibroblastic proliferation within the septal walls
(D) Leukocytes, erythrocytes, and fibrin filling the alveolar spaces
(E) Pleural deposits of fibrin and low-molecular-weight proteins

583. A 51-year-old alcoholic man comes to the emergency room complaining of severe midepigastric pain and persistent vomiting. An x-ray of the pancreas displays numerous, scattered, abnormal, small areas of calcification. The most likely histologic finding would be

(A) fat necrosis
(B) lipofuscin pigmentation
(C) liquefaction necrosis
(D) melanin pigmentation
(E) viral inclusion bodies

584. A 40-year-old black woman is admitted to County Hospital complaining of shortness of breath over the past 18 months, ankle edema for 9 months, ascites for 3 months, and a marked increase in these symptoms for the past 2 weeks. Chest x-ray shows nodular lesions through both lung fields associated with some pleural thickening. Her condition deteriorates, and she dies 2 days later. Autopsy reveals that her disease process also involved other organs, including heart, spleen, and liver. The photomicrograph in Figure 5–5 shows findings in the lungs that are similar to those of other organs. The most likely diagnosis is

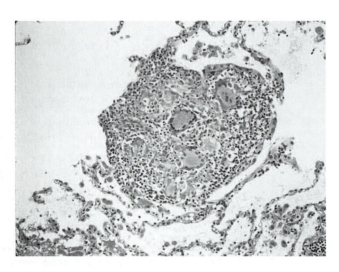

Figure 5–5. (See also Color Insert.) *(Courtesy of Dr. Nancy Warner.)*

(A) CREST syndrome
(B) metastatic lung carcinoma
(C) progressive systemic sclerosis
(D) sarcoidosis
(E) tuberculosis

585. A 61-year-old man has left atrial fibrillation that continues despite medical therapy. He has a massive stroke and dies the following day. Autopsy findings included left atrial hypertrophy with a large mural thrombus, and mitral stenosis. The history and autopsy findings are most compatible with a diagnosis of

(A) cardiac amyloidosis
(B) chronic interstitial lung disease

(C) dilated cardiomyopathy
(D) hypertrophic cardiomyopathy
(E) rheumatic heart disease

586. An autopsy heart specimen from a 58-year-old black man weighs 420 g. There are no anomalous connections between the ventricles or between the atria. The cardiac chambers are not dilated and all the valves appear unremarkable. The atrial walls and the right ventricle wall are of normal thickness. The left ventricle wall is hypertrophied to a thickness of 1.7 cm. The most likely cause of these cardiac findings is

(A) atrial septal defect
(B) Chagas disease
(C) chronic essential hypertension
(D) congestive heart failure
(E) tricuspid stenosis

587. A 36-year-old woman has a known history of alpha-1-antiprotease deficiency with a PiZZ genotype and micronodular cirrhosis. Her pulmonary reserve has been gradually decreasing over the past few years. The most likely pathologic process to be found on biopsy of her lung is

(A) alveolar proteinosis
(B) chronic viral pneumonia
(C) intralobar sequestration
(D) panacinar emphysema
(E) pulmonary hamartomas

588. Numerous previously healthy children in a day care center suddenly develop diarrhea. A culture of their stools is likely to grow which virus?

(A) Cytomegalovirus
(B) Herpes simplex virus
(C) Parvovirus B19
(D) Rotavirus
(E) Variola

589. A 5-week-old girl, who appeared to be healthy at birth, develops diarrhea and vomiting a few days after birth. Your current examination reveals that she has hepatomegaly, jaundice, and early cataract formation and is not meeting developmental milestones. You suspect that she has

(A) galactosemia
(B) Hurler syndrome
(C) pyloric stenosis
(D) Tay–Sachs disease
(E) type I glycogenosis

590. A 44-year-old alcoholic has a recent clinical history of prolonged vomiting and retching complicated by massive hematemesis. Endoscopy reveals a blood-coated mucosal tear of the gastric mucosa near the squamocolumnar junction. This syndrome is referred to as

(A) blind loop
(B) Conn
(C) Dubin–Johnson
(D) Letterer—Siwe
(E) Mallory–Weiss

591. An 81-year-old man who contracted syphilis while serving in World War II is now found to have a saccular aneurysm of the thoracic aorta. The pathogenesis of this is best explained as

(A) endarteritis obliterans of the vasa vasorum with subsequent mural ischemia
(B) hypersensitivity reaction with multinucleate giant cells and fibrinoid mural necrosis
(C) immune complex formation and complement activation
(D) intimal fibroplasia and lipid deposition
(E) medial cystic necrosis

592. The bone marrow biopsy depicted in Figure 5–6 was obtained from an infant with hepatosplenomegaly and mental retardation. The pathologic basis of this disorder is

(A) deficient cellular immunity that permits continued intracellular bacterial proliferation
(B) exposure to excessive radiation during embryogenesis

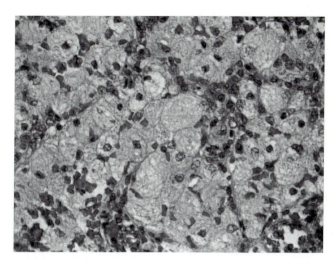

Figure 5–6. (See also Color Insert.)

(C) hereditary deficiency of catabolic enzyme that leads to abnormal intracellular accumulation of lipids
(D) oncogenic viral integration into host's DNA that initiates unregulated cellular proliferation
(E) traumatic injury during delivery

593. A 54-year-old male smoker notices a slowly enlarging mass over the past 2 years within his right parotid gland. At the time of surgical excision the mass measures 2.8 cm in diameter and was focally cystic. Microscopic examination reveals a tumor composed of benign papillary oncocytic epithelial fronds supported by benign lymphoid stroma. The most likely diagnosis is

(A) acute suppurative sialoadenitis
(B) adenoid cystic carcinoma
(C) mucoepidermoid carcinoma
(D) pleomorphic adenoma
(E) Warthin tumor (adenolymphoma)

594. A routine Pap smear on a 27-year-old woman is reported as low-grade squamous intraepithelial lesion with prominent koilocytosis. The most likely etiology for this finding is a

(A) hereditary disorder of squamous epithelium

(B) hormonal imbalance

(C) human papillomavirus

(D) normal intermenstrual reaction

(E) protozoan infection or infestation

595. A 13-year-old boy notices slowly progressive enlargement of his left breast. Surgical removal of the button-shaped subareolar mass confirms the clinical suspicion of gynecomastia. What is the usual pathogenesis of these changes?

(A) Clonal neoplastic proliferation

(B) Dietary deficiency

(C) Hyperestrinism

(D) Ionizing radiation

(E) Subacute inflammation

596. A 36-year-old man is now in his third year of steroid therapy since being diagnosed with a systemic vasculitis. Prior to initiating treatment in the acute phase of the disorder he underwent a biopsy of a medium-sized artery. This biopsy specimen displayed fibrinoid necrosis of the media accompanied by a transmural acute inflammatory infiltrate. Significant negative clinical findings included a normal aortic arch, absence of giant cells in the artery biopsy, normal upper airway examination, and no history of tobacco use. The disorder that best fits these findings is

(A) Kawasaki disease

(B) polyarteritis nodosa

(C) Takayasu disease

(D) temporal arteritis

(E) thromboangiitis obliterans

597. A 57-year-old woman is trapped in a burning house. When the firemen responding to the emergency eventually rescue her she is still alive but she dies on the way to the hospital. The most likely cause of her death is

(A) hypovolemia

(B) smoke inhalation

(C) stroke

(D) thermal burns

(E) vascular thrombosis

598. A 52-year-old man has a 6.4-cm tumor removed from the retroperitoneum. The frozen section report states that the tumor is malignant. Immunochemistry is positive for vimentin but not for keratin. Of the following, the most likely diagnosis is

(A) chondroma

(B) hemangioma

(C) hepatocellular carcinoma

(D) liposarcoma

(E) serous cystadenoma

599. A 24-year-old pregnant woman is diagnosed with Budd–Chiari syndrome. You explain to her that this is

(A) agenesis of a hepatic lobe

(B) a congenital inability to fully metabolize bilirubin

(C) a dietary deficiency of an essential nutrient

(D) a malignant transformation of the biliary epithelium

(E) an occlusion of the hepatic venous drainage

600. A 74-year-old man dies after a 4-day hospital course with a clinical diagnosis of adult respiratory distress syndrome. At autopsy a pathologic diagnosis of diffuse alveolar damage is rendered. The expected microscopic findings of the lung tissue at autopsy are

(A) alveolar hyaline membrane formation

(B) eosinophilic inflammatory infiltrates

(C) hemorrhagic infarction

(D) pleural effusion and fibrous pleuritis

(E) pulmonary vasculature occluded by microthrombi

601. A 28-year-old woman has an ultrasound examination during the second trimester of her

third pregnancy. She is found to have greatly decreased amniotic fluid but the fetus appears to be the appropriate size for the gestational age. Her two previous pregnancies produced normal term infants. The family history is otherwise unremarkable. Of the following, the condition that most likely explains these findings is

(A) bilateral cystic renal dysplasia
(B) bronchopulmonary dysplasia
(C) hypoplasia of the lungs
(D) Klinefelter syndrome
(E) placenta previa

602. A 46-year-old woman with a 30-year history of juvenile diabetes undergoes a left renal allograft for advanced diabetic nephropathy. The transplant is initially successful. However, 3 months later she develops an unproductive cough with associated arthralgia, malaise, diarrhea, and fever of 101.6°F. Upon hospital admission, she is found to be leukopenic. The patient continues to decompensate and dies 3 days following admission. A section of her right kidney taken at autopsy is shown in Figure 5–7. This indicates an infection with

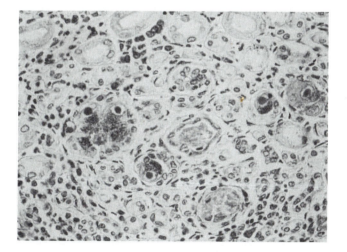

Figure 5–7. (See also Color Insert.) *(Courtesy of Dr. Parakrama Chandrasoma.)*

(A) cytomegalovirus
(B) Epstein–Barr virus
(C) human immunodeficiency virus

(D) *Pneumocystis carinii*
(E) *Staphylococcus epidermidis*
(F) *Streptococcus pyogenes*

603. A 63-year-old woman has a routine chest x-ray that reveals a suspicious subpleural lesion. The lesion is resected and sectioned, and reveals all (choices A through F) of the following microscopic findings. The one that would most strongly indicate to you that the lesion is a malignant neoplasm is

(A) hyperchromatism
(B) increased nuclear/cytoplasmic ratio
(C) invasion
(D) mitoses
(E) necrosis
(F) pleomorphism

604. A 68-year-old man with advanced atherosclerosis involving the circle of Willis suffers a thrombotic occlusion of the left cerebral artery resulting in an ischemic infarct. Microscopic examination of the affected area of the brain would show an area of necrosis that is

(A) caseous
(B) coagulative
(C) enzymatic
(D) fibrinoid
(E) liquefactive

605. A 57-year-old man seeks medical attention for the recent appearance of numerous, large, fluid-filled, cutaneous blisters. These involve the face, scalp, neck, and axillae. Manual pressure to the skin results in epidermal separation. These changes are most likely the result of

(A) autoimmune disorder
(B) bacterial infection
(C) dietary deficiency
(D) exposure to a chemical toxin
(E) local ischemia

606. A 5-year-old boy is diagnosed with an inherited disease. It is found that his 8-year-old brother and both parents are heterozygous for this disease. Of the following, the boy most probably has

(A) cystic fibrosis
(B) Duchenne muscular dystrophy
(C) galactosemia
(D) Klinefelter syndrome
(E) Tay–Sachs disease

607. A 56-year-old man is noted to have episodic hypertension, a mass in his adrenal gland, and elevated catecholamines. The most likely diagnosis is

(A) adrenal cortical carcinoma
(B) adrenal cortical hyperplasia
(C) ganglioneuroma
(D) neuroblastoma
(E) pheochromocytoma

608. A 67-year-old woman has lymphocytosis. The white blood count is elevated at 43,000/μL with 92% of the cells appearing as small, morphologically normal lymphocytes. Flow cytometry studies characterize almost all of the lymphocytes as CD5 positive, CD20 positive, κ light chain positive, and λ light chain negative. What is the most likely reason for her lymphocytosis?

(A) Adult T-cell leukemia
(B) Castleman disease
(C) Chronic lymphocytic leukemia
(D) Plasma cell leukemia
(E) Reactive lymphocytosis

609. A 15-month-old girl presents with a large abdominal mass, weight loss, and fever. At surgery, a large infiltrative tumor with areas of hemorrhage and necrosis is removed. A photomicrograph of a section from this tumor is shown in Figure 5–8. The most likely diagnosis is

(A) embryonal rhabdomyosarcoma
(B) malignant lymphoma
(C) neuroblastoma

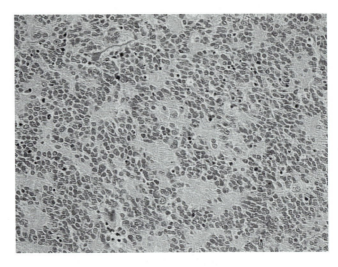

Figure 5–8. (See also Color Insert.)

(D) teratoma
(E) Wilms tumor

610. An autopsy heart from a 4-year-old boy with a premortem history of cyanotic congenital heart disease displays right ventricular hyperplasia, pulmonary stenosis, ventricular septal defect, and dextroposition of the aorta. What term best defines this disorder?

(A) Anomalous pulmonary venous drainage
(B) Dextrocardia
(C) Ebstein malformation
(D) Transposition of the great arteries
(E) Tetralogy of Fallot

611. A 5-year-old girl has had numerous childhood fractures. She is also found to have blue sclera, hearing abnormalities, and misshapen teeth. The cause of these findings is most likely

(A) abnormal intestinal receptors for calcium
(B) an inability to metabolize vitamin D
(C) inadequate mineralization of bone matrix
(D) renal inability to conserve phosphorous
(E) synthesis of abnormal type I collagen

612. A 21-year-old overweight woman suffers from amenorrhea and hirsutism. On laparoscopic biopsy her ovary is enlarged due to

the presence of a thickened cortex containing numerous benign small follicular cysts. These findings are compatible with a diagnosis of

(A) hereditary multiple endocrine neoplasia type 2A

(B) hereditary multiple endocrine neoplasia type 2B

(C) pseudomyxoma peritonei

(D) Stein–Leventhal syndrome

(E) true hermaphroditism

613. A 43-year-old woman has numerous bone marrow emboli within the pulmonary vasculature at autopsy. What is the likely premortem clinical history?

(A) Acute leukemia

(B) Anomalous venous drainage

(C) Idiopathic thrombocytopenia

(D) Pulmonary fibrosis

(E) Trauma

614. A 9-year-old girl living in rural South Carolina is noted by her physician to be anemic. An examination of her stool reveals hookworm eggs. She is infected with

(A) *Ascaris lumbricoides*

(B) *Dracunculis medinensis*

(C) *Entamoeba coli*

(D) *Enterobius vermicularis*

(E) *Necator americanus*

615. A 67-year-old woman notices a lump in her left supraclavicular area. It is excised and a section of it is shown in Figure 5–9. The microscopic appearance is most consistent with a diagnosis of

(A) adenocarcinoma

(B) carcinoid

(C) fibroadenoma

(D) fibrosarcoma

(E) malignant fibrous histiocytoma

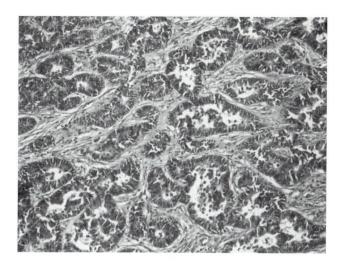

Figure 5–9. (See also Color Insert.) *(Courtesy of Dr. Nancy Warner.)*

616. A 61-year-old man develops fulminant diarrhea following extensive antibiotic therapy for osteomyelitis. Endoscopic biopsies of his large bowel demonstrates pseudomembranous colitis. The organism most likely to be isolated from his colon is

(A) *Clostridium difficile*

(B) *Helicobacter pylori*

(C) *Shigella* species

(D) *Salmonella* species

(E) *Yersinia* species

617. A 10-year-old girl develops sudden onset of hematuria and hypertension. She had a severe sore throat 2 weeks earlier, from which *Streptococcus pyogenes* was cultured. Her laboratory studies now demonstrate an elevated antistreptolysin, elevated antihyaluronidase, and elevated serum creatinine. The pathologic renal changes will be found at the

(A) afferent arteriole

(B) calyx

(C) distal convoluted tubule

(D) glomerulus

(E) proximal convoluted tubule

618. A 27-year-old hiker slips and falls down a steep rocky slope. When he is discovered several hours later and transported to the emergency room, he is found to be in hypotensive shock and to have a broken leg, multiple contusions and lacerations, and internal bleeding. The internal hemorrhage is very difficult to control; despite receiving several units of blood, it is another 6 hours before his blood pressure can be normalized. On the second day of hospitalization, he becomes oliguric, which can best be explained by the occurrence of

(A) acute tubular necrosis
(B) bone marrow embolization
(C) glomerulonephritis
(D) interstitial nephritis
(E) pyelonephritis

619. A 59-year-old woman dies following a 6-year history of a slowly progressive dementia marked by the early onset of behavioral changes with alterations in personality and language disturbances. Gross examination of her brain reveals severe atrophy of the frontal and temporal lobes. Microscopically, the affected lobes show a severe loss of neurons. Surviving neurons have a ballooned appearance and some contain cytoplasmic inclusions that are strongly positive with silver stains. The most likely cause of the dementia is

(A) Alzheimer disease
(B) Creutzfeldt–Jacob disease
(C) Huntington disease
(D) Krabbe disease
(E) Pick disease

620. A 33-year-old woman suffering from severe depression takes a fatal overdose of acetaminophen. The coroner's autopsy would be expected to find

(A) acute renal tubular necrosis
(B) hepatic necrosis
(C) infarction of the spleen
(D) meningeal inflammation
(E) pulmonary necrosis

621. A 3-day-old girl develops numerous skin lesions followed soon thereafter by severe encephalitis. Despite extensive treatment, she dies a few days later. An autopsy examination reveals that the infant has a systemic infection involving all major organs. The photomicrograph in Figure 5–10 is taken from a section of adrenal gland. The infectious agent is

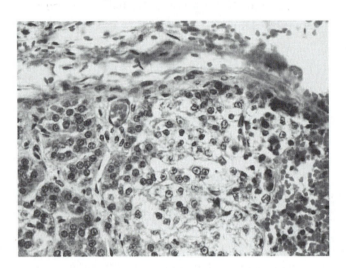

Figure 5–10. (See also Color Insert.) *(Courtesy of Dr. Nancy Warner.)*

(A) cytomegalovirus
(B) herpes
(C) rubella
(D) syphilis
(E) toxoplasma

622. A 58-year-old man has a 5-year history of progressively worsening heart failure. An autopsy limited to the heart reveals extensive replacement of the myocardium by an acellular eosinophilic material. This material is most likely to be

(A) amyloid
(B) calcium salt deposition
(C) cholesterol
(D) myocyte fibrinoid necrosis
(E) postinfarctive cicatrix

623. A 56-year-old man employed in a cotton mill has an asthma-like pulmonary disorder due to prolonged inhalation of dust at the mill. This condition is

(A) anthracosis
(B) berylliosis
(C) byssinosis
(D) silicosis
(E) stannosis

624. A 67-year-old retiree was employed for many years in the plastics industry where he was exposed to vinyl chloride. This industrial exposure has increased his likelihood of developing

(A) focal nodular hyperplasia
(B) hepatic adenoma
(C) hepatic angiosarcoma
(D) hepatic fibroma
(E) hepatocellular carcinoma

625. A 21-year-old woman presents with a 6-hour history of left-sided lower abdominal pain and is hypotensive. A hemorrhagic mass is discovered in her left fallopian tube during laparoscopy. The tube is surgically excised. A photomicrograph of the tubal contents is displayed in Figure 5–11. The most likely diagnosis is

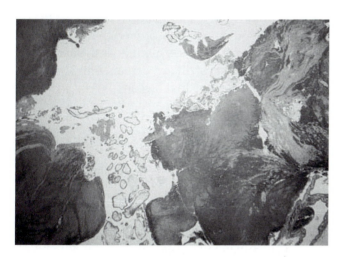

Figure 5–11. (See also Color Insert.) *(Courtesy of Dr. Juan Felix.)*

(A) chorioadenoma destruens
(B) choriocarcinoma
(C) ectopic tubal pregnancy
(D) granular cell tumor
(E) leiomyoma

626. A 1-year-old child has unilateral cryptorchidism. The pediatrician strongly recommends performing an orchiopexy. This procedure is recommended because cryptorchidism is associated with an increased risk of testicular

(A) feminization syndrome
(B) hemorrhage
(C) infarction
(D) infection
(E) neoplasia

627. A 35-year-old man with cirrhosis and a Parkinsonian tremor is found to have a reduced level of ceruloplasmin. You suspect that he has

(A) congenital hepatic fibrosis
(B) peliosis hepatis
(C) primary sclerosing cholangitis
(D) Reye syndrome
(E) Wilson disease

628. A 34-year-old woman who has been taking oral contraceptives for many years presents with acute abdominal pain and fullness. Paracentesis harvests 200 mL of bloody fluid. Imaging studies show a 6-cm mass in the liver that is subsequently resected. Histologic examination of this specimen would most likely reveal this to be a (an)

(A) angiosarcoma
(B) cholangiosarcoma
(C) focal nodular hyperplasia
(D) hepatocellular carcinoma
(E) liver cell adenoma

629. A 13-year-old girl presents with clinical symptoms suggestive of acute appendicitis. At surgery the appendix appears uninflamed and an alternative diagnosis of acute mesenteric adenitis with enterocolitis is made. The likely etiology of this entity is

(A) bacterial infection
(B) fungal infection
(C) local vascular compromise
(D) parasitic infection
(E) viral infection

630. A 34-year-old woman has a history of menorrhagia. Within the wall of her uterus are several solid whitish nodules. The histologic appearance of one of the nodules is depicted in Figure 5–12. These nodules represent

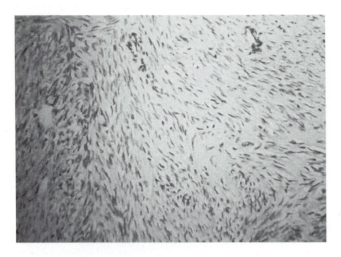

Figure 5–12. (See also Color Insert.) *(Courtesy of Dr. Juan Felix.)*

  (A) adenomyosis
  (B) Krukenberg tumors
  (C) leiomyomas
  (D) metastatic malignancy
  (E) ovarian ectopias

631. A 39-year-old man who has had ulcerative colitis for many years now presents with pruritis and jaundice. Laboratory tests reveal increased levels of total bilirubin and alkaline phosphatase. Endoscopic retrograde cholangiopancreatography (ERCP) shows a characteristic beading of the bile ducts. A liver biopsy shows a lymphocytic infiltrate, some bile duct proliferation with periductal fibrosis, and some destruction. The most likely diagnosis is

  (A) ascending cholangitis
  (B) choledochal cysts
  (C) polycystic liver disease
  (D) primary biliary cirrhosis
  (E) primary sclerosing cholangitis

632. A 55-year-old man has recently been discovered to be affected with Sézary syndrome. You would describe this as

  (A) adult T-cell leukemia due to infection with HTLV-1
  (B) gastric B-cell lymphoma
  (C) large B-cell lymphoma arising from chronic lymphocytic leukemia
  (D) leukemic variant of mycosis fungoides
  (E) lymphoma arising secondary to HIV-1 infection

633. A 69-year-old woman complains of a recent erosive eczematous change on her left nipple. A biopsy demonstrates intraepidermal adenocarcinoma. This histologic finding supports a diagnosis of

  (A) Bowen disease
  (B) dermatitis herpetiformis
  (C) desmoid tumor
  (D) epidermolysis bullosa
  (E) Paget disease of the nipple

634. A 33-year-old man is diagnosed with duodenal carcinoma. A large number of hamartomatous polyps are found throughout his GI tract and he is also observed to have pigmented macules on his lips and buccal mucosa. The most likely explanation for all of these findings is that he has

  (A) familial polyposis coli
  (B) Gardner syndrome
  (C) juvenile retention polyps
  (D) Peutz–Jeghers syndrome
  (E) Turcot syndrome

635. A 33-year-old man comes to you complaining of a slowly enlarging mass on the left side of his face at the angle of his jaw. You find that the mass is firm and movable but does not elicit any pain. The mass is surgically excised and found to arise in the left parotid gland. Microscopic examination reveals that it is composed of myoepithelial cells with ducts and acini intermixed with areas having a chondroid or myxoid appearance. Based upon these findings, your diagnosis is

(A) acinic cell carcinoma

(B) adenoid cystic carcinoma

(C) mucoepidermoid carcinoma

(D) pleomorphic adenoma

(E) Warthin tumor (adenolymphoma)

636. A 62-year-old woman has a history of repeated urinary tract infections. Her physician requests a cystoscopy, which reveals scattered soft yellow plaques in the bladder mucosa. Biopsy of a plaque contains a mixed chronic inflammatory infiltrate and numerous microcalcospherites. This disorder is

(A) chronic interstitial cystitis

(B) endometriosis

(C) exstrophy

(D) malakoplakia

(E) polypoid cystitis

637. A 31-year-old woman complains of an insidious onset of fatigue, sore tongue, and tingling and numbness of her extremities. When you examine her, you note that she is pale and has some scleral icterus. Laboratory analysis reveals anemia with a high MCV, leukopenia with hypersegmented neutrophils, and increased indirect bilirubin. Based on these findings, you suspect that she is suffering from a deficiency of

(A) folic acid

(B) iron

(C) vitamin B_1 (thiamine)

(D) vitamin B_{12} (cyanocobalamin)

(E) vitamin K

638. A 25-year-old woman complains of pelvic pain. Pelvic examination revealed a left cystic, mobile, adnexal mass measuring 7×7 cm. The mass is surgically removed and is found to be cystic and to contain hair. Microscopically, it is composed predominantly of dermal elements but also contains some squamous and glandular epithelium, muscle, and cartilage, all of which have normal morphology. This most likely represents

(A) choristoma

(B) hamartoma

(C) mixed tumor

(D) myxoma

(E) teratoma

639. A 54-year-old man presents with a productive cough and weight loss over the past 8 months. Chest x-ray reveals a large hilar mass, and sputum cytology shows round to oval cells with hyperchromatic nuclei, little cytoplasm, and inconspicuous nucleoli. These malignant cells most likely originated from a

(A) Clara cell

(B) metaplastic bronchial epithelial cell

(C) neuroendocrine cell

(D) type I alveolar pneumocyte

(E) type II alveolar pneumocyte

640. A 64-year-old man presents to his family physician with hematuria and flank pain. A radiology study identifies a renal mass. A photograph of this renal lesion's histology is displayed in Figure 5–13. The kidney mass is most likely a (an)

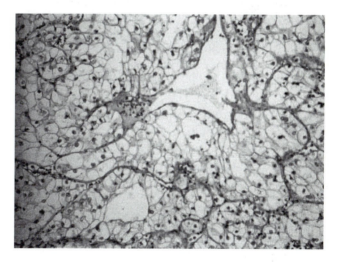

Figure 5–13. (See also Color Insert.) *(Courtesy of Dr. Nancy Warner.)*

(A) angiomyolipoma

(B) oncocytoma

(C) renal cell carcinoma

(D) transitional cell carcinoma

(E) xanthogranulomatous pyelonephritis

Questions 641 through 643

A baby boy is delivered without complications at 31 weeks gestational age. However, soon after birth, he develops progressive respiratory distress, hypoxemia, and cyanosis, and requires artificial ventilation and oxygen.

641. The prenatal laboratory test that could have predicted these developments is

(A) alpha-fetoprotein levels in the mother's blood

(B) chromosomal analysis of the fetal amniotic cells

(C) cytomegalovirus antibody levels in the mother's blood

(D) lecithin:sphingomyelin ratio in the amniotic fluid

(E) toxicology screen of the mother's urine

642. Histologic examination of the infant's lungs would reveal

(A) coagulated protein lining damaged alveoli and respiratory bronchioles

(B) foreign body granulomas and pulmonary interstitial fibrosis

(C) interstitial lymphocytes and plasma cells with early fibrosis

(D) intra-alveolar neutrophils and fibrin with hyperemia

(E) intranuclear and intracytoplasmic inclusions in type II pneumocytes

643. A potential complication of the use of oxygen in this infant is the development of

(A) asthma

(B) bronchopulmonary dysplasia

(C) cystic fibrosis

(D) panacinar emphysema

(E) sequestrated lung

Questions 644 and 645

A 27-year-old bank security guard is shot in the head during a robbery attempt. He survives in a comatose state for several days and then contracts bronchopneumonia from which he dies.

644. The manner of death in this case is

(A) accident

(B) gunshot wound to the head

(C) homicide

(D) natural

(E) pneumonia

645. The death certificate should list the underlying (proximate) cause of death as

(A) bronchopneumonia

(B) cardiopulmonary arrest

(C) cerebral edema with tonsillar herniation

(D) gunshot wound to the head

(E) intracerebral hemorrhage

Questions 646 through 648

A 26-year-old woman complains of the acute onset of anuria, purpura, and mental confusion. Her peripheral blood film displays marked thrombocytopenia and abundant schistocytes. Laboratory studies reveal elevations of bilirubin, creatinine, and lactose dehydrogenase. A skin biopsy shows numerous intravascular thrombi within the dermal microvasculature.

646. What is the likely diagnosis?

(A) Acute idiopathic thrombocytopenia purpura

(B) Bernard–Soulier syndrome

(C) Glanzmann thrombasthenia

(D) May–Hegglin anomaly

(E) Thrombotic thrombocytopenic purpura

647. The recommended treatment for this disorder is

(A) antibiotics

(B) antiviral therapy

(C) immunosuppressive agents

(D) plasmapheresis

(E) renal transplant

648. If appropriate and rapid treatment is instituted, the expected 1-year survival rate with this disorder is about

(A) 10%

(B) 25%

(C) 40%
(D) 60%
(E) 90%

Questions 649 and 650

A 14-year-old boy of normal stature and intelligence has recently been told that he has ichthyosis.

649. What histologic feature evident on a skin biopsy supports this diagnosis?

(A) Dermal fibrosis
(B) Hyperpigmentation of the epidermal basal layer
(C) Increased thickness of stratum corneum
(D) Perivascular chronic inflammation
(E) Subepidermal blister formation

650. This disorder is usually due to a

(A) bacterial infection
(B) hereditary condition
(C) hormonal imbalance
(D) type IV hypersensitivity
(E) viral infection

Questions 651 and 652

For the past 6 months, a 67-year-old white woman has been aware of a small, flesh-colored papule on her lower eyelid. More recently, it showed ulceration. A photograph of this papule's microscopic anatomy is shown in Figure 5–14.

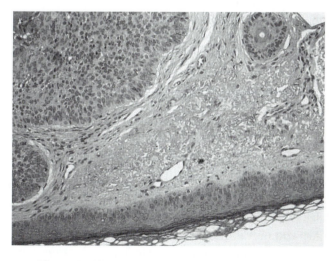

Figure 5–14. (See also Color Insert.) *(Courtesy of Dr. Parakrama Chandrasoma.)*

651. What is the appropriate diagnosis?

(A) Basal cell carcinoma
(B) Bowen disease
(C) Epidermal cyst
(D) Molluscum contagiosum
(E) Verruca vulgaris

652. What is the primary pathologic process that leads to the development of this lesion?

(A) Actinic damage
(B) Focal lumenal occlusion with subsequent cyst formation
(C) Fungal infection
(D) Papillomavirus infection
(E) Poxvirus infection

Questions 653 through 655

A 47-year-old woman has a 3-month history of fatigue and pruritus. A percutaneous liver biopsy reveals a nonsuppurative, granulomatous distention of medium-sized intrahepatic bile ducts.

653. The most likely diagnosis is

(A) alcoholic hepatitis
(B) hepatitis C
(C) primary biliary cirrhosis
(D) primary sclerosing cholangitis
(E) schistosomiasis

654. What is the most common etiology of this disorder?

(A) Acquired vascular abnormality
(B) Alcohol abuse
(C) Autoimmune disease
(D) Parasitic infection
(E) Viral infection

655. Which serum chemistry panel typifies the later stages of this disorder?

	ALKALINE PHOSPHATASE	BILIRUBIN	CHOLESTEROL
(A)	decreased	decreased	decreased
(B)	decreased	decreased	elevated
(C)	decreased	elevated	decreased
(D)	decreased	elevated	elevated
(E)	elevated	elevated	elevated

Questions 656 and 657

A 53-year-old woman recently noticed a firm, 2-cm nodule in her right breast during monthly self-examination. The histology of her breast biopsy tissue is displayed in Figure 5–15.

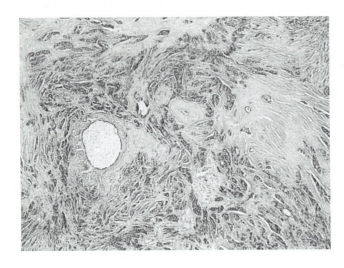

Figure 5–15. (See also Color Insert.) *(Courtesy of Dr. Nancy Warner.)*

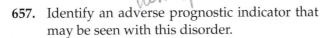

656. Identify a known risk factor that favors the development of this change.

(A) Asian ethnicity

(B) Early age of first pregnancy and multiparity

(C) Early menopause

(D) Family history of this disorder

(E) Late menarche

657. Identify an adverse prognostic indicator that may be seen with this disorder.

(A) Estrogen receptor positive

(B) Low S phase

(C) Overexpression of Her2/neu oncogene

(D) Progesterone receptor positive

(E) Well-differentiated histology, grade I of III

Questions 658 and 659

An overweight, 46-year-old man has complained of heartburn for the past 2 years. A biopsy of his lower esophagus is displayed in Figure 5–16.

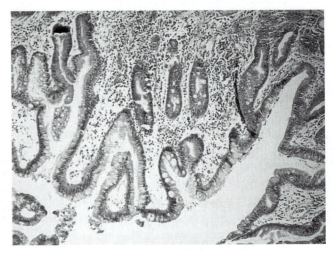

Figure 5–16. (See also Color Insert.) *(Courtesy of Dr. Parakrama Chandrasoma.)*

658. What is the diagnosis?

(A) Barrett esophagitis

(B) *Candida* esophagitis

(C) Granulomatous esophagitis

(D) Plummer–Vinson syndrome

(E) Viral esophagitis

659. If left untreated this lesion may predispose to the development of

(A) adenocarcinoma

(B) esophageal varices

(C) fungal septicemia

(D) squamous cell carcinoma

(E) viral encephalitis

Questions 660 through 662

An abdominal mass is discovered in a 2 year-old child during a routine physical examination. The pediatrician suspects that the mass is a Wilms tumor and refers the child to a regional medical center for further therapy.

660. During the course of this child's therapy the abdominal mass is excised and pathologic examination confirms the diagnosis of Wilms tumor. The expected microscopic morphology of this neoplasm is malignant

   (A) adrenal neural crest cells
   (B) endothelial cells forming abortive vascular structures
   (C) gland-forming epithelium with glycogen-containing clear cytoplasm and abundant vascularity
   (D) osteoid or cartilage
   (E) primitive renal tissue

661. If chromosomal analysis were performed on the surgical tissue the most likely abnormality would be

   (A) deletion
   (B) inversion
   (C) ring formation
   (D) translocation
   (E) trisomy

662. The 5-year survival rate of children with this tumor, if given appropriate combined surgical, radiation, and antineoplastic therapies, is about

   (A) 5%
   (B) 20%
   (C) 40%
   (D) 60%
   (E) 90%

Questions 663 and 664

A 6-year-old child has a long history of a hereditary bleeding disorder characterized by spontaneous nontraumatic hemorrhages into joint spaces, skeletal muscle, and mucous membranes. Laboratory studies reveal a normal prothrombin time, elevated partial thromboplastin time, very low factor VIII, normal factor X, normal factor XI, and normal platelet aggregation studies with ristocetin.

663. The likely diagnosis is

   (A) Christmas disease
   (B) hemophilia A
   (C) hemophilia B
   (D) Rosenthal syndrome
   (E) von Willebrand disease

664. The usual mode of inheritance of this disorder is

   (A) autosomal codominant
   (B) autosomal dominant
   (C) autosomal recessive
   (D) X-linked dominant
   (E) X-linked recessive

Questions 665 and 666

A 72-year-old man has radiographic evidence of multiple bony lytic areas. A fine-needle aspiration of one of these areas demonstrates clumps of atypical plasma cells. His lymph nodes are not enlarged. His total protein is elevated to 10.6 g/dL and his serum albumin is low.

665. The most likely disease is

   (A) malignant lymphoma
   (B) metastatic adenocarcinoma
   (C) metastatic melanoma
   (D) mononucleosis
   (E) multiple myeloma

666. A serum or urine electrophoresis will probably demonstrate

   (A) bisalbuminemia
   (B) hypogammaglobulinemia
   (C) monoclonal paraprotein
   (D) polyclonal hypergammaglobulinemia
   (E) reduced alpha fractions

Questions 667 and 668

A 49-year-old woman had a total hysterectomy 5 years ago for uterine prolapse. Her current vaginal Pap smear demonstrates clusters of benign glandular cells suggestive of vaginal adenosis.

667. Researching this patient's past history would likely reveal an in utero exposure to

   (A) aspirin

   (B) diethylstilbestrol

   (C) methotrexate

   (D) radiation

   (E) rubella virus

668. The most serious long-term complication of vaginal adenosis is the potential to develop

   (A) clear cell adenocarcinoma

   (B) endometrial adenocarcinoma

   (C) serous papillary carcinoma

   (D) uterine leiomyomas

   (E) vaginal sarcomas

Questions 669 through 671

A 14-year-old, severely physically disabled individual is now on a respirator. His first 4 years of life were medically uneventful. Over the last 10 years, he has suffered from increasing symmetric muscle weakness that first affected the pelvic girdle and now involves almost all muscle groups. Several years ago, the calf portion of his legs appeared enlarged and on biopsy demonstrated fatty pseudohypertrophy with random alternating muscle fiber atrophy and hypertrophy.

669. The most likely diagnosis is

   (A) cerebral palsy

   (B) muscular dystrophy

   (C) myositis ossificans

   (D) poliomyelitis

   (E) trichinosis

670. The disorder is

   (A) due to *Trichinella spiralis* infestation

   (B) hereditary

   (C) neoplastic

   (D) secondary to neonatal trauma

   (E) virus induced

671. Which serum chemistry panel typifies this disorder?

	CREATINE KINASE	ALDOLASE	LACTATE DEHYDROGENASE
(A)	decreased	decreased	decreased
(B)	elevated	elevated	elevated
(C)	elevated	normal	low
(D)	low	normal	elevated
(E)	normal	normal	normal

Questions 672 and 673

A 66-year-old man undergoes an elective right colectomy for stage III adenocarcinoma of the cecum.

672. What is the most likely set of preoperative laboratory findings?

	SERUM CEA	STOOL OCCULT BLOOD	HEMO-GLOBIN
(A)	elevated	negative for blood	normal
(B)	elevated	positive for blood	low
(C)	normal	negative for blood	elevated
(D)	normal	negative for blood	normal
(E)	normal	positive for blood	normal

673. Several months postoperatively, if distant non-nodal metastases are discovered, which organ is likely to first be affected?

   (A) Adrenal

   (B) Appendix

   (C) Brain

   (D) Liver

   (E) Lung

Answers and Explanations

547. **(E)** Ulcerative colitis (UC) is a recurrent acute and chronic inflammatory bowel disease of unknown etiology, although immunologic hypersensitivity is suspected and psychological stress is frequently recognized as a precipitating factor of attacks (this patient's recent divorce). Onset of disease peaks between 20 and 30 years of age and the incidence is slightly higher in women. Ulcerative colitis involves the rectum in virtually all cases; disease extends proximally in a continuous manner without skip lesions to include variable lengths of the colon. The region and continuity of the lesions in UC grossly differentiate it from Crohn disease, which typically involves the small and large intestines in a segmental manner with intervening "skip" areas (the rectum is uninvolved in greater than 50% of cases). The sigmoidoscopy findings, including the suppurative mucosal hemorrhages, are typical of the acute phase of UC. (Findings in the chronic phase include flat areas of atrophic mucosa due to reepithelialization of the ulcers, whereas the presence of inflammatory pseudopolyps indicates regenerated or nonulcerated mucosa). The clinical and laboratory features are indicative of severe acute disease with substantial volume and electrolyte losses. The significant narrowing seen in the transverse colon suggests the possible progression to toxic megacolon, a rare complication in severe acute disease that carries a high mortality rate and requires emergency colectomy. Amebic colitis (choice A) is characterized by acute inflammation with multiple areas of enzymatic tissue necrosis leading to submucosal, flask-shaped abscesses throughout the colon. The mucosal surface shows multiple ulcers separated by healthy-appearing mucosa that is nevertheless undermined by the submucosal abscesses. Clinical features include bloody and mucoid diarrhea with low-grade fever. Collagenous colitis (choice B) is a more recently recognized form of colitis typically characterized clinically by episodic or chronic watery diarrhea that is not severe enough to cause dehydration, and pathologically by the presence of a distinct collagenous band beneath the colonic surface epithelium. Onset is almost always greater than 30 years of age (mean age 60), and affects women almost four times as often as men. Patients very often have a variety of autoimmune and other diseases. Cytomegalovirus enterocolitis (choice C) is a common GI infection in acquired immunodeficiency syndrome (AIDS) patients that infects the entire GI tract and produces severe, chronic diarrhea. Both mucosal epithelial and vascular endothelial cells are infected. Vasculitis may result in focal ischemic necrosis of the intestinal wall. Ulcers of the esophagus, stomach, small intestine, or colon may result in bleeding or perforation. Pseudomembranous colitis (choice D) is caused by a necrolytic enzyme produced by *Clostridium difficile* bacteria that most often proliferates in the bowel secondary to a variety of antibiotic therapies, although clindamycin is a frequent culprit. Diarrhea is most often watery and profuse. Sigmoidoscopy reveals patchy areas of mucosal inflammation with multiple, discrete yellowish plaques constituting the pseudomembrane, which is composed of fibrin, mucin, and necrotic debris.

548. (B) Myasthenia gravis is an autoimmune disease characterized by autoantibodies to acetylcholine receptors, and weakness of both facial and ocular muscles. Conjunctivitis (choice A) defines an inflammatory or infectious condition of the conjunctiva. Orbital inflammatory pseudotumor (choice C) is a benign mass lesion of the eye region not associated with muscle weakness and autoantibodies. Parkinson disease (choice D) is a neurologic movement disorder that does not demonstrate either weakness or acetylcholine autoantibodies. Polymyositis (choice E) is a rheumatic disease of skeletal muscle.

549. (C) Multiple sclerosis is a chronic demyelinating neurologic disorder of young adults. Pathologic abnormalities associated with the disease include the formation of fibrous plaques within the central nervous system and the presence of cerebrospinal fluid oligoclonal immunoglobulins. Amyotrophic lateral sclerosis (choice A) is a neurologic disease of unknown etiology characterized by degeneration of motor neurons and muscle wasting. Huntington disease (choice B) is an autosomal dominant neuropathy. Early dementia and generalized involuntary movements are characteristic. Pemphigus vulgaris (choice D) is an autoimmune blister-forming dermatologic condition with normal neurologic status. Spinocerebellar degeneration (choice E) is a rare degenerative neurologic condition that affects the cerebellum and spinal cord.

550. (A) The photograph displays a benign reactive plasmacytic and lymphocytic chronic inflammatory infiltrate. This inflammatory pattern is consistent with nonspecific chronic inflammation at various body sites. Chronic salpingitis is the only option listed that represents a chronic inflammatory disorder. Ectopic tubal pregnancy (choice B) would display chorionic villi and hemorrhage. The histology of endometriosis (choice C) features benign endometrial glands, benign endometrial stroma, and usually accompanying hemorrhage. Endosalpingosis (choice D) is not a chronic inflammatory condition. Benign

cervical glandular epithelium would be a necessary histologic attribute. The microanatomy of serous papillary carcinoma (choice E) is characterized by malignant glandular epithelium with a micropapillary architecture. Chronic inflammation, if present, is a minor secondary phenomenon.

551. (C) Following tissue injury (in this case caused by the insect sting), vasoactive inflammatory mediators originating from both cellular and humoral sources are released at the site of injury. These produce vasodilation of arterioles and increased blood flow producing the redness, and increased vascular permeability of venules allowing the formation of an exudate that produces swelling. All of the other choices can produce edema, but do not feature an increase in vascular permeability (they produce noninflammatory edema). Decreased plasma oncotic pressure (choice A) can result from either excessive loss (e.g., nephrotic syndrome) or decreased synthesis (e.g., cirrhosis, protein malnutrition) of plasma proteins, principally albumin. Increased hydrostatic pressure (choice B) occurs, for example, in heart failure where the pressure builds up behind the failing pump. Lymphatic obstruction (choice D) occurs where there is blockage to the normal lymphatic drainage. This could be due to the growth of an obstructing cancer or to inflammation and fibrosis (e.g., postsurgery, filariasis). Venous obstruction (choice E) leads to increased hydrostatic pressure as the blood backs up behind the obstruction.

552. (A) Achalasia is an esophageal disorder due to inadequate peristalsis. The most consistent feature is a decreased number of ganglion cells in the myenteric plexus. Clinically, there is regurgitation, chest pain, and odynophagia. Fibrous strictures (choice B) of the esophagus may be congenital or occur after damage to the submucosa. Diverticula formation (choice C) is not a consistent feature of achalasia. *Helicobacter pylori* infections (choice D) are unrelated to the development of achalasia. These infections are usually seen in the stomach and predispose to ulcer formation.

Hiatal hernia (choice E) is a herniation of the stomach through the diaphragm.

553. **(D)** Gout is caused by elevated uric acid levels. Symptoms may include joint pain, joint effusions, renal calculi, and subcutaneous collections of uric acid crystals. Examination of fluid aspirated from an inflamed joint may reveal diagnostic needle-shaped urate crystals that are negatively birefringent when observed under polarized light microscopy. Acute bacterial pyarthrosis (choice A) should display neutrophils, necrotic debris, and perhaps, bacteria. Crystals would not be seen. Calcium pyrophosphate deposition disease (choice B) is a nonspecific crystalline deposit found in joints damaged by various etiologies. Pyrophosphate crystals differ from urate crystals by their rhomboid shape and positive birefringence. A ganglion cyst (choice C) would reveal abundant mucoid debris and scant benign fibrous elements on aspiration. No crystals would be seen. Ochronosis (choice E) is a hereditary condition due to an inability to metabolize homogentisic acid. Clinically, there is pigmented arthritis, but joint crystals are not evident.

554. **(C)** The history and laboratory results strongly suggest systemic lupus erythematosus (SLE). The test for anti-nuclear antibodies is positive in nearly every patient with SLE, but is also positive in some other autoimmune diseases. In active cases, a more specific test is the demonstration of anti–double-stranded DNA antibodies, which are virtually diagnostic. A differential count on synovial fluid (choice A) is not diagnostic, even though the majority of patients with SLE have joint involvement. A renal biopsy (choice B) may at some time be necessary to assess renal status, but it would not be done at this time as a diagnostic procedure. A majority of patients with SLE have skin changes, but because these are not specific, a skin biopsy (choice D) is not diagnostic. Patients with porphyria also have skin lesions that are exacerbated by sun exposure. However, they do not have the other findings of this patient,

so a urine test for porphyrins (choice E) is not appropriate.

555. **(B)** A deficiency of thiamine classically produces beriberi marked by polyneuropathy, heart failure, and edema. However, in chronic alcoholism, this deficiency may produce Wernicke syndrome marked by the triad of ataxia, ophthalmoplegia, and dementia as seen in this patient. Vitamin A deficiency (choice A) is associated with night blindness, with or without keratomalacia and papular dermatitis. Vitamin B_{12} deficiency (choice C) produces a megaloblastic anemia and a subacute combined degeneration of the spinal cord. Vitamin C deficiency (choice D) produces scurvy in which there is impaired synthesis of collagen leading to hemorrhage, tooth loss, defective wound healing, and skeletal deformities in children. Vitamin D deficiency (choice E) produces osteomalacia in adults and rickets in children due to defective mineralization of bone. Vitamin K deficiency (choice F) can result in a bleeding diathesis because it is required for the activity of clotting factors II, VII, IX, and X.

556. **(D)** The sudden dyspnea and the V/Q mismatch point to a pulmonary embolism. Given the man's age and chronic illness, a likely sequence of events is inactivity, venous stasis, thrombophlebosis, and thromboembolism. Anemia (choice A) could produce a gradually evolving dyspnea, but not a V/Q mismatch. Cirrhosis of the liver (choice B) could produce portal hypertension, but this does not relate to the patient's condition. The pulmonary arteries are at a lower pressure than the systemic arteries so they do not develop arteriosclerosis unless there is chronic pulmonary hypertension. Therefore choice C is unlikely.

557. **(D)** Cretinism is due to a neonatal lack of thyroxine. Thyroid agenesis, iodine deficiency, ingestion of goitrogens, and hereditary enzymatic deficiencies may all result in a relative lack of biologically active thyroxine. Affected children may display lethargy, jaundice, hypothermia, muscular hypotonia, and mental

retardation. Medicinal replacement of thyroxine is therapeutic. The mental retardation may not be reversible, however, unless treated early. Antibiotics (choice A) have no effect in treating cretinism. Growth hormone (choice B) is an effective treatment for pituitary dwarfism. It has no benefit in cretinism. Treatment with thiamine (choice C) is the appropriate therapy for beriberi, not cretinism. A lack of vitamin D (choice E) causes rickets, not cretinism.

558. **(B)** Hepatitis C viral infections commonly cause necrosis of hepatocytes. One of the major products synthesized by hepatocytes is albumin. As liver cells are damaged, there is a concomitant reduction in the synthesis of albumin. Therefore, serum albumin levels are likely to decline during chronic hepatocellular injury. Alanine aminotransferase (choice A), aspartate aminotransferase (choice C), and lactate dehydrogenase (choice E) are all enzymes normally found in liver cells. As liver cells die these enzymes leak from the necrotic cells into the bloodstream. An increased serum content of these enzymes is a useful laboratory method to detect hepatocellular injury. Gamma globulin (choice D) is increased in most chronic inflammatory states, especially with chronic hepatitis.

559. **(D)** Figure 5–2 displays granulomatous inflammation characterized by multinucleate giant cell formation, lymphocytes, plasma cells, and monocytes. Of the listed choices, only Crohn disease characteristically invokes a granulomatous inflammatory response. Abetalipoproteinemia (choice A) is a genetic disorder. Malabsorption without granulomatous inflammation is the typical clinical picture. A biopsy of ileal adenocarcinoma (choice B) would demonstrate malignant gland-forming epithelium without granulomatous inflammation. Carcinoid tumor (choice C) should display islands or ribbons of cohesive neoplastic epithelial cells. Granulomatous inflammation is not evident. Ulcerative enterocolitis (choice E) is a type of idiopathic inflammatory bowel disease. Granulomatous inflammation is not present.

560. **(C)** Sjögren syndrome is an autoimmune disease in which there is immune-mediated destruction of lacrimal and salivary gland epithelium leading to diminished secretion by these organs. This disease may occur as a primary disorder or more commonly secondary to another autoimmune disorder such as rheumatoid arthritis as seen in this patient. One of the long-term risks for Sjögren syndrome is a 40-fold increase in malignant lymphoma. The development of esophageal carcinoma (choice A) is associated with alcohol use, smoking, Barrett metaplasia, and Epstein–Barr virus infections. Chronic Sjögren syndrome is not known to cause an increased incidence of leukemia (choice B). Melanoma (choice D) is a malignancy of melanocytes unrelated to Sjögren syndrome. Pleomorphic adenoma (choice E) is a benign salivary gland tumor composed of both neoplastic epithelium and stroma. Its occurrence is not associated with Sjögren syndrome.

561. **(E)** In a population of 100,000, 1000 people will have the disease and 99,000 will be disease free (the prevalence of the disease equals 1%). The sensitivity equals 90%, which indicates that in a population of people with the disease, 90% will have a positive test result (true positives) and 10% will have a negative test result (false negatives). The specificity also equals 90%, which indicates that in a population of people without the disease, 90% will have a negative test result (true negatives) and 10% will have a positive test result (false positives). Thus, looking at the negative test results, there were 100 false negatives (10% of the 1000 people with the disease) and 89,100 true negatives (90% of the 99,000 people without the disease). Therefore the chances of the test result being a true negative are (true negatives)/(true negatives + false negatives) = (89,100)/(89,100 + 100) = 99.9%. Mathematically, 1% (choice A), 10% (choice B), 50% (choice C), and 90% (choice D) can be eliminated.

562. **(C)** Ninety percent of individuals with chronic myelogenous leukemia have an acquired Philadelphia chromosome abnormal-

ity consisting of a translocation between chromosomes 22 and 9. The translocation places the proto-oncogene c-abl from chromosome 9 next to the breakpoint cluster region (bcr) on chromosome 22. The unique gene sequence bcr-abl confers a growth advantage with subsequent clonal expansion. Acute lymphoblastic leukemia (choice A) does not have a known reproducible gross chromosomal derangement. Burkitt lymphoma (choice B) is associated with a translocation of the c-myc oncogene from chromosome 8 to chromosome 14. Follicular lymphoma (choice D) is associated with a translocation between chromosomes 14 and 18. Hodgkin lymphoma (choice E) is characterized by the presence of Reed–Sternberg cells and has a number of subtypes.

563. **(E)** Rheumatoid arthritis (RA) occurs about four times more often in women than men and the majority of patients develop the disease between ages 35 and 50. Rheumatoid arthritis often develops slowly and insidiously with nonspecific symptoms such as malaise, fatigue, weight loss, and vague musculoskeletal discomfort. Later the joints become more obviously involved with a presentation similar to that found in this patient. About 80% of patients have rheumatoid factor (autoantibodies to the Fc portion of their own IgG). At this stage one would expect to see plasma cells and lymphocytes in a synovial biopsy. Caseous necrosis (choice A) is typically associated with tuberculosis. Fibrosis (choice B) is a late manifestation of RA. Macrophages and multinucleated giant cells (choice C) can be found later when the pannus forms. Necrotizing vasculitis (choice D) would not be seen in this patient. Rheumatoid vasculitis can occur in patients with long-standing RA and produce visceral infarction, skin lesions, and leg ulcers.

564. **(D)** Carcinomas in the head of the pancreas often obstruct the ampulla of Vater and the common bile duct, producing jaundice; carcinoma in the body and tail do not obstruct and remain clinically silent much longer. A dull, continuous abdominal pain is also a typical symptom and many patients report that the pain decreases when they lean forward. About 10% of patients with pancreatic carcinoma develop a migratory thrombophlebitis known as Trousseau syndrome. Alcoholic cirrhosis (choice A), cholecystitis (choice B), cholelithiasis (choice C), and viral hepatitis (choice E) may all be associated with abdominal pain and jaundice, but not the other findings in this case.

565. **(C)** The clinical and laboratory findings indicate that this man has nephrotic syndrome. In adults, the most common cause is membranous nephropathy and in a patient of this age may indicate an underlying malignancy. Although a small percentage of diabetic patients (choice A) can develop nephrotic syndrome, there are no other findings in this case that point to that disease. Goodpasture syndrome (choice B) is characterized by rapidly progressive (crescentic) glomerulonephritis and pulmonary hemorrhage. Minimal change disease (choice D) is the most common cause of nephrotic syndrome in children. Postinfectious glomerulonephritis (choice E) produces nephritic syndrome, not nephrotic syndrome.

566. **(E)** This patient manifested the classical pain of an acute myocardial infarction. The damaged and necrotic myocardial fibers leak enzymes and other proteins, which appear in the serum and serve as convenient markers of the tissue injury. Troponin I levels start to rise about 4 to 8 hours after a myocardial infarction and peak at 14 to 36 hours. Lactate dehydrogenase (choice C) is also released by damaged myocardial fibers, but does not begin to increase until about 8 to 12 hours after infarction. This patient was admitted 6 hours after the onset of his pain, so troponin I is more likely to yield a useful result. Bilirubin (choice A), glucose (choice B), and lipase (choice D) levels do not increase following a myocardial infarct.

567. **(C)** Mönckeberg (medial calcific) sclerosis is a degenerative aging change of medium-sized muscular arteries of the lower and upper extremities, and the genital tract. Calcium is de-

posited in the media of these vessels often as transverse rings, giving a "railroad track" appearance by x-ray. These changes usually do not have any clinical significance and are usually an incidental finding on x-ray. Dystrophic calcification (choice A) is the deposition of calcium in areas of necrosis or tissue injury and in some neoplasms. Serum calcium levels are normal. Mönckeberg sclerosis is an example of dystrophic calcification, but is a more specific diagnosis in this case and is therefore the best answer. Metastatic calcification (choice B) occurs in patients with hypercalcemia and results in deposition of calcium in otherwise normal tissues—typically lung, kidney, arteries, and stomach. The broken leg (choice D) could result in fat emboli being released into the circulation, but would not result in the x-ray findings described here.

568. **(E)** Figure 5–3 depicts a chronic peptic ulcer. There is a loss of mucosal continuity, an ulcer bed with necrotic tissue, and fibrosis of the submucosa. Peptic ulcers are associated with increased gastric acid secretion and *Helicobacter pylori* mucosal infestation. Hemorrhage, perforation, and penetration may complicate an ulcer. Adenocarcinoma (choice A) may form an ulcer. Within the ulcer, however, there would be diagnostic malignant glandular epithelium. Adenomatous polyps (choice B) are not associated with gross ulcer formation. Histologically, there is an increased number of benign glandular elements. Brunner gland adenoma (choice C) frequently presents as a duodenal mass. The microanatomy reveals hyperplasia of submucosal Brunner glands. A leiomyoma (choice D) is a benign smooth muscle tumor. Figure 5–3 does not display a neoplasm.

569. **(D)** This is a patient with multiple myeloma and one of the earliest symptoms of the disease is back pain. These patients have increased levels of Ig in the blood (which produces an increased erythrocyte sedimentation rate and will be seen as rouleaux formation on the blood smear) and light chains (Bence–Jones protein) in the urine. Multiple myeloma causes multifocal osteolytic lesions throughout the skeletal system and these are apparent on x-rays and are also responsible for the hypercalcemia as the ongoing bone destruction releases calcium. Fibrous dysplasia (choice A) is a disorder of bone in children with progressive replacement of a localized area of bone by an abnormal proliferation of benign fibrous tissue and bony trabeculae composed of haphazardly arranged woven bone. It occurs as a monostotic and polyostotic form, but neither could account for the findings in this case. Iron-deficiency anemia (choice B) does not produce any of the findings in this case. Metastatic prostatic carcinoma (choice C) can spread quite easily to the lumbar-sacral spine and this causes back pain. However, these bone lesions are osteoblastic rather than osteolytic. Osteosarcoma (choice E) is typically found in teenagers or young adults. When seen in older individuals, it usually occurs in association with Paget disease of the bone.

570. **(D)** The combination of diabetes, arthritis, congestive heart failure, cirrhosis, and golden-brown pigment in the organs indicate that this is an advanced case of hemochromatosis (the excessive accumulation of hemosiderin in the tissues). The best way to demonstrate this iron pigment is with Prussian blue. Congo red (choice A) demonstrates amyloid. Gomori methenamine silver (choice B) is commonly used to stain certain fungi. Periodic acid-Schiff (choice C) demonstrates glycogen, basement membranes, epithelial mucin, and most fungi. Trichrome (choice E) is a method for demonstrating collagen.

571. **(D)** The described lesion is a keloid. Keloids are an example of excessive scar formation due to a relative abundance of collagen matrix ground substance laid down in a disorganized manner. Keloids most frequently occur in blacks and may recur after excision. Brenner tumor (choice A) is a benign neoplasm of the ovary. A dermoid cyst (choice B) is a mature teratoma of the ovary. Excessive collagenization is not evident with this tumor. A hamartoma (choice C) is a collection of sev-

eral different types of adult tissue in an abnormal organization. The lung is the most frequent site. A teratoma (choice E) is a neoplasm derived from germ cells and usually displays several types of partially mature tissues. They usually occur in the ovary, testicles, or mediastinum.

572. **(E)** This is a patient who is inactive due to his age, myocardial infarct, and hospitalization. Such a patient is at risk for deep vein thrombosis and thromboembolism. In a patient with heart failure, this most likely produces an infarct of the lung. Microscopically, it appears as an area of coagulative necrosis and grossly as a hemorrhagic, wedge-shaped area. An infarct of the brain (choice A) is an area of liquefactive necrosis, not coagulative. An infarct of the heart (choice B) is irregular and pale (not wedge-shaped and hemorrhagic). An infarct of the kidney (choice C) is most likely to be pale and wedge-shaped. The liver (choice D) is an unusual site for infarction because of its dual circulation.

573. **(B)** Because both parents are phenotypically normal, this must be a recessive disease. In addition, knowing that the father is heterozygous and unaffected indicates that it is not sex-linked. Thus, it is autosomal recessive. This reasoning effectively rules out choices A, C, and D. Multifactorial (choice E) can also be eliminated because the disease occurrence in this family can be explained by simple mendelian genetics.

574. **(E)** Transudates are an ultrafiltrate of plasma that enter the extracellular space by either increased hydrostatic pressure or decreased colloid oncotic pressure. Transudates typically have a specific gravity < 1.012, < 1.5 g/dL protein, minimal fibrin, and minimal cells. Clinically, transudates are seen with heart failure, cirrhosis, kwashiorkor, and nephrotic syndrome. A collection of fat-rich fluid within the thoracic cavity is called a chylothorax (choice A). The fat stain would be positive. Trauma, tuberculosis, and lymphoid malignancies are associated with chylothorax formation. An empyema (choice B) is a col-

lection of pus within the thoracic cavity with many neutrophils. An exudate (choice C) is an extracellular fluid accumulation that has a specific gravity > 1.020, > 3 g/dL protein, a high content of fibrin, and many cells. Most exudates are inflammatory in nature. Hemothorax (choice D) is a collection of blood within the thoracic spaces. Analysis reveals many erythrocytes and a total protein > 3 g/dL.

575. **(E)** This is a case of typhoid fever. During the prodromal stage there is a gradual, step-like increase in fever with malaise, anorexia, myalgia, and headache. By the second week, the fever usually plateaus and the patient is very sick. There may be constipation or diarrhea with abdominal pain and distention, weakness, and a maculopapular rash (rose spots), particularly on the abdomen. If there are no complications, the patient may gradually improve over the next 2 weeks. One of the classic pathologic findings in typhoid is intestinal ulcerations over hyperplastic and necrotic Peyer patches. These may perforate and hemorrhage, as in this patient. Amebiasis (choice A) can produce a range of symptoms from being subclinical to producing a fulminant dysentery. However, it involves the large bowel rather than the small intestine and produces flask-shaped ulcers separated by areas of normal bowel. Cholera (choice B) does not actually invade the intestinal epithelium and therefore causes insignificant microscopic changes and no ulceration. Cryptosporidiosis (choice C) causes a severe, chronic diarrhea in AIDS patients. The protozoa attach to the brush border of the intestinal epithelial cells but do not cause ulceration. Giardia (choice D) attach to duodenal epithelial cells but do not invade those cells and do not cause ulceration.

576. **(E)** Figure 5–4 shows a large tumor mass originating in the kidney. Wilms tumor (or nephroblastoma) is the most common primary renal tumor of childhood and the second most common malignancy overall after lymphoma/leukemia. It typically presents as a large abdominal mass discovered by a parent. An ab-

scess (choice A) is a localized collection of pus that is not compatible with the solid mass shown here. A neuroblastoma (choice B) is most commonly primary in the adrenal and is unlikely to arise in the kidney. Renal cell carcinoma (choice C) is the most common primary renal tumor in adults, but is not expected in a child. Tuberculosis (choice D) would be identified by caseous necrosis, which has the appearance of amorphous crumbled cheese, not the solid appearance shown here.

577. **(B)** A 20-hour-old ischemic infarct of the myocardium should demonstrate coagulative necrosis without much of an inflammatory response. Abundant neutrophils and monocytes (choice A) typically are seen about 2 to 4 days after an infarction. Fibrosis and collagen deposition (choice C) are late healing phenomena that do not begin until at least 1 week after the infarct has occurred. Monocytic infiltration and neovascularization (choice D) usually occur about 3 to 6 days after an infarction. Plasma cells and caseous necrosis (choice E) are not seen with ischemic myocardial damage. This pattern occurs with the granulomatous inflammation of tuberculosis.

578. **(D)** The productive cough and leukocytosis with a high percentage of neutrophils and bands indicates that this is a bacterial infection and, of the choices given, is most likely an abscess. Bronchogenic carcinoma (choice A) can obstruct an airway and produce infection, but there is no evidence presented to support this. Interstitial pneumonia (choice B) is typically caused by mycoplasma or viruses and produces a mononuclear response rather than a neutrophilic response; the cough is usually nonproductive. Lobar pneumonia (choice C) fills the affected lobe with exudate, but does not typically result in necrosis or abscess formation. Pulmonary tuberculosis (choice E) can produce a cavitary lesion, typically at the apices, but also is marked by a mononuclear response.

579. **(A)** Hirschsprung disease is caused by the congenital absence of parasympathetic ganglion cells in the submucosal and myenteric plexus. This presents clinically soon after birth as an inability to pass stool and abdominal distention. The diagnosis is usually confirmed by a full-thickness colon biopsy showing disorganized, nonmyelinated nerve fibers replacing the missing ganglion cells. In Hirschsprung disease, the ganglion cells, not the nerve fibers (choice B), are missing. Muscular hypertrophy (choice D) or atrophy (choice C) are not specific diagnostic findings with Hirschsprung disease. Mucosal polyp development (choice E) is not associated with Hirschsprung disease.

580. **(B)** This clinical picture immediately following a difficult delivery makes amniotic fluid embolism a likely event. The amniotic fluid contains thromboplastic substances that initiate disseminated intravascular coagulation. Bilateral adrenal necrosis (Waterhouse–Friderichsen syndrome) (choice A) is typically associated with meningococcemia. This can also cause shock and disseminated intravascular coagulation, but there is no evidence for this in this patient. The three principal signs of preeclampsia (choice C) are hypertension, proteinuria, and generalized edema. Pulmonary thromboembolism (choice D) can occur in association with pregnancy and could cause dyspnea and cyanosis, but does not fit the rest of the clinical presentation. During pregnancy, the pituitary enlarges and this can, on occasion, lead to infarction of the pituitary, or Sheehan syndrome (choice E), but would not produce the constellation of clinical findings seen in this patient.

581. **(C)** Heat stroke is a life-threatening condition resulting from a failure of heat regulation. It is marked by high body core temperature and the failure of sweating. Heat cramps (choice A) are the result of the loss of fluid and electrolytes through sweating. Painful cramping of muscles can occur but core temperature remains normal. Heat exhaustion (choice B) results from excessive sweating and failure to replace the lost fluid. This results in hypovolemia, venous pooling, and reduced cardiac output. The skin is wet and the temperature is usually normal. Heat exhaustion is not life threatening, and there is

usually spontaneous recovery when the person is moved to a cool place. Malignant hyperthermia (choice D) is an inherited condition in which there is an increased temperature when the person is exposed to certain anesthetics. It has no relationship to environmental temperature. Pyrexia (choice E) is fever and is usually defined as a cytokine-mediated increase in body temperature as part of a response to disease. This results in the hypothalamus having a higher "set point" for the body's temperature.

582. **(D)** Lobar pneumonia may progress through four stages: congestion, red hepatization, gray hepatization, and resolution. The second stage, red hepatization, is characterized grossly by a liver-like firm consistency to the lung due to filling of the alveolar spaces by erythrocytes, fibrin, and leukocytes. Alcoholic toxic necrosis (choice A), tracheobronchial epithelial desquamation (choice B), fibroblastic proliferation (choice C), and pleural deposits (choice E) are not pathologic processes that usually cause red hepatization.

583. **(A)** Pancreatic fat necrosis is seen in acute pancreatitis and is commonly associated with dystrophic calcific deposits. Acute pancreatitis allows digestive enzymes to leak out of damaged acinar cells. Liberated lipases act on the adjacent fat to precipitate calcific deposits, which may be visualized by radiographic means. Lipofuscin (choice B) is a noncalcific degradation pigment that is not radiopaque. Liquefaction necrosis (choice C) is a form of cell death that is usually seen only in the brain and with abscesses. Calcification is not part of the process. Melanin (choice D) is a black pigment made by melanocytes that cannot be visualized radiographically. Viral infections (choice E) are rare in the pancreas, and none are associated with calcium deposition.

584. **(D)** The photomicrograph shows noncaseating granulomas. Given that similar lesions were found throughout her other organs, the most likely diagnosis is sarcoidosis. CREST syndrome (choice A) is a variant of progressive systemic sclerosis (choice C) in which there is calcinosis, Raynaud phenomenon, esophageal disease, sclerodactly, and telangectasia. Metastatic lung carcinoma (choice B) could have widespread involvement of the organs, but would demonstrate malignant cells, not granulomas. Progressive systemic sclerosis (choice C), also called scleroderma, is an uncommon connective tissue disorder in which there is vasculitis of small vessels and widespread collagen deposition. Tuberculosis (choice E) is an infectious granulomatous disease, but the granulomas usually have central caseous necrosis and do not usually involve all of the other organs as occurred in this case.

585. **(E)** Nearly all cases of mitral stenosis are the result of chronic rheumatic heart disease. Because of resistance to passage of blood through the stenotic valve, there is a compensatory left atrial hypertrophy and dilation. The decreased and altered flow in this enlarged chamber increases the likelihood of mural thrombus formation (with subsequent thromboembolism) as does the atrial fibrillation. Cardiac amyloidosis (choice A) can produce a restrictive cardiomyopathy, but there is no involvement of the valves. Dilated cardiomyopathy (choice C) also has no involvement of the valves. Hypertrophic cardiomyopathy (choice D) can mimic aortic stenosis, but the mitral valve is not involved. Chronic interstitial lung disease (choice B) (as well as other causes of pulmonary hypertension) would be expected to lead to right ventricular hypertrophy, not left atrial hypertrophy.

586. **(C)** The heart demonstrates left ventricular hypertrophy. Chronic essential hypertension is the most common etiology in the United States. Atrial septal defect (choice A) is an anomalous mural defect between the two atria. Chagas disease (choice B) is a protozoan infection of the heart that does not produce left ventricular hypertrophy. Congestive heart failure (choice D) is characterized by dilation of the cardiac chambers. Tricuspid valvular stenosis (choice E) is usually caused by rheumatic carditis and is not associated with left ventricular hypertrophy.

587. **(D)** The genetic lack of antiprotease (antitrypsin) activity predisposes an individual to the early development of panacinar emphysema. Alveolar proteinosis (choice A), chronic viral pneumonia (choice B), intralobular sequestration (choice C), and pulmonary hamartomas (choice E) are all pulmonary disorders that are not related to hereditary antiprotease deficiency.

588. **(D)** Epidemic rotavirus diarrhea is the correct choice. Other less likely etiologic agents that might fit this scenario would include Norwalk virus, adenovirus, calicivirus, and astrovirus infections. Cytomegalovirus (choice A) infection is usually subclinical except in immunocompromised individuals. Herpes simplex virus (choice B) is a DNA virus associated with oral or genital cutaneous vesicle formation. Parvovirus B19 (choice C) infection may result in erythema infectiosum (fifth disease), transient aplastic crisis, and fetal hydrops. Variola (choice E) virus causes smallpox. Skin lesions, not diarrhea, typify this disease.

589. **(A)** Galactosemia is an autosomal recessive disorder due (in this more common and more severe form of the disease) to a lack of galactose-1-phosphate uridyl transferase. This results in the formation and accumulation of galactose metabolites. If the infant's diet is not modified to exclude milk products, this will result in damage to the liver (fatty change, cholestasis, cirrhosis, liver failure), eyes (cataract formation), and brain (mental retardation). Hurler syndrome (choice B) is a severe form of mucopolysaccharidosis that typically becomes apparent between 6 months and 2 years of age. Prominent feature include coarse facies, dwarfism, organomegaly, cataracts, and mental retardation, not diarrhea, vomiting, and jaundice. Pyloric stenosis (choice C) can occur as a congenital condition, more frequently in baby boys (M:F = 4:1). It is marked by projectile vomiting in the first month of life but not the other findings in this case. Tay–Sachs (choice D) is a lipid storage disease due to a deficiency of hexosaminidase A. There is an inexorable deteri-

oration of mental and motor functions within a few months of birth culminating in a vegetative state and death within 3 or 4 years. Type I glycogen storage disease or von Gierke disease (choice E) is due to a deficiency of glucose-6-phosphatase and usually becomes apparent in the first year of life as hypoglycemia and/or hepatomegaly.

590. **(E)** Mallory–Weiss syndrome consists of a clinical history of prolonged vomiting or retching, hematemesis, and longitudinal mucosal tears in the lower esophagus. Blind loop syndrome (choice A) is associated with nonhemorrhagic malabsorption with bacterial overgrowth. Conn syndrome (choice B) is another term for primary hyperaldosteronism. Adrenal cortical hyperplasia or adenoma are the usual anatomic findings. Dubin–Johnson syndrome (choice C) describes a genetic disorder of intermittent jaundice and black hepatocytic pigmentation. Letterer–Siwe syndrome (choice D) is a malignant systemic disorder of Langerhans cells that usually affects infants and young children.

591. **(A)** Syphilitic saccular aneurysms of the thoracic aorta result from endarteritis obliterans of the vasa vasorum with subsequent mural ischemic necrosis. Hypersensitivity reactions, multinucleate giant cells, and fibrinoid necrosis (choice B) play no significant role in the development of syphilitic aortic aneurysms. Immune complex formation and complement activation (choice C) may be seen with tertiary syphilis, but involve only the small vessels, without aneurysm formation. Intimal fibroplasia and lipid deposition (choice D) are the early lesions of atherosclerosis. Cystic medial necrosis (choice E) is a noninfectious disorder characterized by abnormally weak connective tissue in the aortic media and deposits of myxoid substances.

592. **(C)** Figure 5–6 depicts macrophages filled with lipids from an infant with Gaucher disease. The disease is due to a genetic lack of the catabolic enzyme glucocerebrosidase, which fosters the abnormal accumulation of glucocerebroside within the reticuloendothelial cells and neurons. Gaucher disease is not caused by deficient cellular immunity (choice A), radiation (choice B), viral infection (choice D), or trauma (choice E).

593. **(E)** The clinical history, surgical findings, and described microscopic pattern all support the diagnosis of Warthin tumor, a benign neoplasm of the major salivary glands. Acute suppurative sialoadenitis (choice A) would have a more acute clinical history, pus may be observed at the time of surgery, and the histology would confirm an acute inflammatory process rather than neoplasm. Adenoid cystic carcinoma (choice B) and mucoepidermoid carcinoma (choice C) are both malignant neoplasms of the salivary gland. Neither displays the benign histology described for Warthin tumor. Pleomorphic adenoma (choice D) is also a common benign neoplasm of the salivary glands. However, it differs from Warthin tumor in several aspects. Pleomorphic adenoma is rarely cystic, usually lacks significant oncocytic epithelial elements, and the stroma is myxoid rather than lymphoid.

594. **(C)** A significant proportion of low-grade squamous intraepithelial lesions are the result of human papillomavirus infection. Viral subtypes 16 and 18 are more likely to progress to high-grade dysplasias. Koilocytosis is the usual morphologic marker of viral infection. It is unlikely that these changes would result from a hereditary disorder (choice A), hormonal imbalances (choice B), normal intermenstrual reactions (choice D), or a protozoan infection (choice E).

595. **(C)** Gynecomastia usually occurs in the setting of hyperestrinism. Puberty, cirrhosis, old age, certain pharmaceutical agents, and estrogen-secreting tumors may all induce gynecomastia. The hyperplasia of ducts and periductal stroma seen with gynecomastia are not clonal (choice A). Dietary deficiency states (choice B) are not known at present to be agents of gynecomastia. Ionizing radiation (choice D) and subacute inflammation (choice E) are not etiologic concerns in the formation of gynecomastia.

596. **(B)** Polyarteritis nodosa is a systemic vasculitis primarily seen in young adult males. Fibrinoid necrosis and acute inflammation are seen microscopically in the acute phase. Mucocutaneous lymph node syndrome (Kawasaki disease) (choice A) is a childhood disorder with coronary vasculitis, cervical lymphadenopathy, and acute onset. Takayasu disease (choice C) is characterized by fibrosis of the upper aorta. The classic patient is a Japanese woman with HLA-DR4. Temporal or giant cell arteritis (choice D) is a granulomatous arterial inflammation seen in the elderly. The superficial temporal and intercranial arteries are preferentially involved. Thromboangiitis obliterans (choice E) is an occlusive disease of small arteries strongly related to cigarette smoking.

597. **(B)** The majority of people who die in fires succumb to smoke inhalation with subsequent anoxia. Thermal burns (choice D) are the second most common cause of acute fire deaths. Hypovolemia (choice A) may be fatal in a minority of fire deaths because thermally damaged skin weeps protein-rich fluid, but death occurs in a subacute or chronic time frame rather than acutely. Stroke (choice C) and vascular thrombosis (choice E) are rarely seen as cause of death in fires unless there is concomitant severe thermal damage.

598. **(D)** Liposarcoma is a malignant tumor derived from nonepithelial lipomatous mesenchyme. A chondroma (choice A) is a benign neoplasm derived from chrondrocytes. Hemangioma (choice B) is a benign tumor composed of blood vessels. Hepatocellular carcinoma (choice C) is a malignant epithelial neoplasm of hepatocytic origin. Serous cystadenoma (choice E) is a benign epithelial tumor.

599. **(E)** Budd–Chiari syndrome is due to extensive occlusive fibrosis of the hepatic venous drainage. The clinical findings usually include ascites, hepatomegaly, and portal hypertension. Budd–Chiari syndrome is unlikely to be caused by agenesis of a hepatic lobe (choice A), congenital disorders of

bilirubin metabolism (choice B), a dietary deficiency (choice C), or malignant biliary transformation (choice D).

600. **(A)** Hyaline membranes are usually seen microscopically in lungs showing diffuse alveolar damage. Grossly, the lungs are heavy, wet, and meaty. The clinical course is termed adult respiratory distress syndrome and is characterized by relative unresponsiveness to oxygen therapy. Eosinophilic inflammatory infiltrates (choice B), hemorrhagic infarction (choice C), pleural effusions (choice D), and vascular microthrombi (choice E) are not typically seen with diffuse alveolar damage.

601. **(A)** Most of the amniotic fluid is derived from the urine of the fetus. In a fetus with bilateral cystic renal dysplasia, little or no urine is being produced, which leads to the oligohydramnios seen in this case. Bronchopulmonary dysplasia (choice B) may be seen in babies who have respiratory distress syndrome and are given oxygen therapy. Hypoplasia of the lungs (choice C) is a consequence of oligohydramnios because inhalation of amniotic fluid by the fetus is necessary for normal lung development. Klinefelter syndrome (choice D) occurs in males with XXY karyotype and does not explain the findings in this case. Placenta previa (choice E) occurs when there is abnormally low implantation of the fertilized ovum in the uterus such that is overlies the internal os.

602. **(A)** Opportunistic infections can occur in posttransplant patients on immunosuppressive therapy. Figure 5–7 shows greatly enlarged renal tubular cells containing both nuclear and multiple cytoplasmic inclusion bodies. These findings in combination are diagnostic of cytomegalovirus infection. Epstein–Barr virus (choice B) has been associated with a number of diseases, including infectious mononucleosis, Burkitt lymphoma, and nasopharyngeal carcinoma. However, even though this is also a herpes virus, it does not give the morphologic appearance described. Human immunodeficiency virus

(choice C) does not produce inclusion bodies in infected cells. *Pneumocystis carinii* (choice D) is an opportunistic fungus that can cause a pneumonia in immunocompromised individuals, particularly AIDS patients. It may be visualized with silver staining methods. *Staphylococcus epidermidis* (choice E) and *S. pyogenes* (choice F) are bacteria that one would not associate with this histologic appearance.

603. **(C)** One might see all of these microscopic findings in a malignant neoplasm, but invasion is the strongest indicator. Hyperchromatism (choice A) is a typical finding in malignant cells indicating their increased DNA content. However, it is not a reliable marker for malignancy. Increased nuclear/cytoplasmic ratio (choice B) can also be seen as part of the normal proliferative response. Mitoses (choice D) indicate an increased proliferative rate, but again the proliferation is not necessarily neoplastic. Necrosis (choice E) is often a feature of rapidly dividing tumors but is also found with infarction, infection, and other conditions. Pleomorphism (choice F) is another feature that is common in malignant tumors, but it can be seen in non-neoplastic conditions and there are some malignancies that are fairly monomorphic.

604. **(E)** Necrotic brain tissue tends to disintegrate very quickly, perhaps due to the inherent softness of the tissue and its high fat content, and produces a liquefactive necrosis. Caseous necrosis (choice A) is seen particularly in tuberculosis and also in some fungal infections. Coagulative necrosis (choice B) is seen following ischemic infarction of all organs, except in the CNS. Enzymatic fat necrosis (choice C) is associated with the release of enzymes from the damaged pancreas. Fibrinoid necrosis (choice D) is a microscopic vascular change seen in many autoimmune diseases as well as malignant hypertension.

605. **(A)** Pemphigus vulgaris is an autoimmune disorder. The autoantibodies are directed against keratinocyte antigens with subsequent dyshesion and fluid-filled blister for-

mation. Bacterial infections (choice B), dietary deficiencies (choice C), chemical toxins (choice D), and local ischemia (choice E) are not thought to be the causative agent of pemphigus vulgaris.

606. **(A)** Family history indicates that the disease must be autosomal recessive. Of this list of five diseases, only cystic fibrosis is both autosomal recessive and compatible with a diagnosis being made at the age of 5. Duchenne muscular dystrophy (choice B) is an X-linked disorder. Galactosemia (choice C) and Tay-Sachs disease (choice E) are both autosomal recessive, but would be apparent at a very early age and lethal before the age of 5. Klinefelter syndrome (choice D) occurs in males who have two (or more) X chromosomes (47, XXY).

607. **(E)** Pheochromocytoma is a neoplasm of the adrenal medulla. Episodic hypertension and elevated catecholamines usually accompany the clinical finding of an adrenal mass. Adrenal cortical carcinoma (choice A) and adrenal cortical hyperplasia (choice B) are not usually associated with elevations of catecholamines. Ganglioneuroma (choice C) is a rare neoplasm of young children composed of both differentiated and immature neural elements. Neuroblastoma (choice D) is a malignant childhood neoplasm composed of undifferentiated neuroblasts.

608. **(C)** Chronic lymphocytic leukemia is a disease of the elderly with mature lymphocytosis, B-cell markers, light chain restriction, and expression of CD5. Adult T-cell leukemia (choice A) would not demonstrate B-cell lymphocyte markers such as CD20. Castleman disease (choice B) usually is defined by a histologically unique pattern of lymphadenopathy without a peripheral lymphocytosis. Plasma cell leukemia (choice D) has different CD markers and appears morphologically as plasma cells rather than mature lymphocytes. It is a very rare entity. Reactive lymphocytosis (choice E) demonstrates a mixed κ and λ pattern and different CD markers.

609. **(C)** This is a neuroblastoma, and is one of a group of childhood tumors described as "small, round, blue-cell tumors," consisting as they do of monotonous small cells with dense, blue nuclei. The characteristic microscopic feature of a neuroblastoma is the pseudorosette, a ring of primitive neuroblasts surrounding a central space filled with fibrillar extensions from the cells. Many of these can be seen in Figure 5–8. These are called pseudorosettes because they do not have a central lumen as is found, for example, in the rosettes in retinoblastoma. Embryonal rhabdomyosarcoma (choice A) is a type of rhabdomyosarcoma typically found in children under the age of 10. It can arise in a number of locations and sarcoma botryoides is one form. It does not form rosettes. Malignant lymphomas (choice B) and leukemias are together the most common malignancies of childhood in the United States, but rosette formation is not a distinctive microscopic feature. Teratomas (choice D) in infants and young children are usually benign tumors found in the midline (e.g., sacrococcygeal, mediastinal). They are composed of tissues with a normal histologic appearance derived from all three germ layers. Wilms tumor (choice E) or nephroblastoma is derived from primitive blastema cells and sometimes displays aborted attempts to form glomeruli or renal tubules, but not rosettes.

610. **(E)** Tetralogy of Fallot includes right ventricular hyperplasia, pulmonary stenosis, ventricular septal defect, and dextroposition of the aorta. It is a cyanotic congenital heart disorder with a dismal prognosis unless surgically corrected. Anomalous pulmonary venous drainage (choice A) occurs when there is aberrant drainage of the pulmonary veins into the left atrium. Dextrocardia (choice B) is a mirror image inversion of the heart. Ebstein malformation (choice C) is a congenital abnormality of the tricuspid valve and right ventricle. Transposition of the great arteries (choice D) is a congenital heart disease defined as the aorta arising from the right ventricle and the pulmonary artery originating from the left ventricle.

611. **(E)** Osteogenesis imperfecta type I, is a genetic disorder characterized by synthesis of an abnormal type I collagen. Frequent childhood fractures, blue sclera, poor hearing, and misshapen teeth may all occur clinically because of the abnormal collagen synthesis. Abnormal intestinal receptors for calcium (choice A), inability to metabolize vitamin D (choice B), inadequate mineralization of bone matrix (choice C), and renal inability to conserve phosphorous (choice D) are not the primary pathologic alterations responsible for this disorder.

612. **(D)** Stein–Leventhal syndrome is seen as a constellation of polycystic ovaries, hirsutism, obesity, and amenorrhea. The pathogenesis probably relates to luteinizing hormone-dependent ovarian overproduction of androgens. Multiple endocrine neoplasia type 2A (choice A) may display pheochromocytoma, thyroid medullary carcinoma, gliomas, and parathyroid hyperplasia. It is a sporadic cause of female infertility in the United States. Multiple endocrine neoplasia type 2B (choice B) consists of a possible combination of pheochromocytoma, medullary thyroid carcinoma, and mucosal neuromas. Pseudomyxoma peritonei (choice C) is a peritoneal collection of mucinous debris due to rupture of appendiceal or ovarian mucinous tumors. A true hermaphrodite (choice E) has both testicular and ovarian gonads.

613. **(E)** The most common cause of pulmonary bone marrow emboli is trauma. Long bone fractures and resuscitative efforts that fracture the ribs are likely premortem events. Dislodged marrow elements gain access to the venous circulation during trauma and the circulating marrow is then subsequently trapped in the narrowing pulmonary vasculature. Acute leukemia (choice A), anomalous venous drainage (choice B), idiopathic thrombocytopenia (choice C), and pulmonary fibrosis (choice D) are not usually associated with pulmonary bone marrow emboli.

614. **(E)** Hookworms infect the human small bowel producing mucosal lacerations, blood loss, and subsequent anemia. In the United States the most common etiologic agent is *N. americanus*. *Ascaris lumbricoides* (choice A) is an intestinal nematode. Most infections with this roundworm are asymptomatic. *Dracunculis medinensis* (choice B) is a tissue nematode found in the Middle East that causes subcutaneous ulcers and allergic reactions along the lower extremities. *Entamoeba coli* (choice C) is nonpathogenic intestinal amoeba. *Enterobius vermicularis* (choice D) is the intestinal nematode responsible for pinworm infection.

615. **(A)** The finding of an enlarged left supraclavicular lymph node (Virchow or signal node) should raise the question of an underlying GI malignancy. This is confirmed in the above case by the microscopic findings. The pleomorphism of these cells and the fact that they are located in a lymph node indicate that these are malignant cells. Additionally, the glandular appearance identifies this as an adenocarcinoma metastatic to a lymph node. Carcinoid tumors (choice B) arise from neuroendocrine cells present in the mucosa throughout the GI tract. About 40% are found in the appendix where they are benign in 99% of cases. Another 25% are found in the ileum. Of these, about 60% are malignant. If they metastasize to the liver they can give rise to the carcinoid syndrome. Fibroadenoma (choice C) is the most common benign tumor of the female breast. Fibrosarcoma (choice D) and malignant fibrous histiocytoma (choice E) are both fibroblastic sarcomas; the photomicrograph clearly indicates a malignancy of epithelial (glandular) origin.

616. **(A)** Antibiotic-induced overgrowth of *C. difficile* is frequently associated with the occurrence of pseudomembranous colitis. The bacterial organism mediates these pathologic changes via a potent toxin. Rapid laboratory tests are available to detect the toxin in feces. *Helicobacter pylori* (choice B) is associated with gastric ulcers. *Shigella* (choice C) and *Salmonella* species (choice D) may both produce severe diarrhea. Neither, however, is commonly associated with pseudomembranous colitis. *Yersinia* species (choice E) are usually associated with ileal infections and mesenteric lymphadenitis.

617. **(D)** In postinfectious acute glomerulonephritis the major renal alterations are evident within the glomerulus. Hypercellularity and ultrastructural changes are morphologic correlates to the clinical observations of hematuria and hypertension. The other sites in the kidney such as afferent arteriole (choice A), calyx (choice B), the distal convoluted tubule (choice C), and proximal convoluted tubule (choice E) are not usually directly altered in acute postinfectious glomerulonephritis.

618. **(A)** Acute tubular necrosis due to ischemia is commonly caused by severe shock. Prolonged vasoconstriction of the kidney produces necrosis of renal tubular epithelial cells and the patient becomes oliguric. In patients who survive shock, renal function does not return until the tubular cells have time to regenerate (usually 2 to 3 weeks). Bone marrow embolization (choice B) does not result in oliguria and in a normal adult the long bones contain fat rather than bone marrow. Glomerulonephritis (choice C) has many different causes, but does not include shock. Interstitial nephritis (choice D) can be either acute, featuring interstitial edema, neutrophils, and focal tubular necrosis, or chronic, with mononuclear cells, tubular atrophy, and fibrosis, but neither apply to this patient. Pyelonephritis (choice E) typically has an infectious etiology.

619. **(E)** Pick disease has a clinical presentation very similar to that of Alzheimer disease. However, it principally affects the frontal and temporal lobes, often unilaterally. The resulting atrophy is often sufficiently severe to give the involved gyri a "knife-edge" appearance. Microscopically, surviving neurons may contain distinctive silver-positive inclusions. Alzheimer disease (choice A) may be clinically indistinguishable from Pick disease, but is quite different pathologically. There is cortical atrophy principally affecting the frontal, temporal, and parietal lobes. Microscopically

there are neurofibrillary tangles, senile plaques, and amyloid angiopathy. Creutzfeldt–Jacob disease (choice B) is a prion disease that presents clinically as a rapidly progressive dementia, usually resulting in death within 1 year of onset of symptoms. Huntington disease (choice C) is an autosomal dominant disorder. Clinically there are involuntary movements and deterioration of cognitive functions. There is a marked symmetric atrophy of the caudate nuclei and to a lesser extent the putamen. Microscopically, the neurons in these areas are seen to be greatly reduced. Krabbe disease (choice D) is an autosomal recessive leukodystrophy due to a deficiency of the enzyme galactocerebroside β-galactosidase. This is a rapidly progressive disease that becomes apparent in infancy and usually results in death by the age of 2 years.

620. **(B)** Overdoses of acetaminophen overwhelm the liver's glutathione reductase capacity. The toxic metabolites that accumulate predictably produce hepatic necrosis. Acute renal tubular necrosis (choice A), infarction of the spleen (choice C), meningeal inflammation (choice D), and pulmonary necrosis (choice E) are not associated with acetaminophen overdoses.

621. **(B)** Figure 5–10 shows areas of necrosis and cell nuclei containing Cowdry A inclusions, indicating that this is a disseminated herpes infection acquired during passage through the birth canal. Cytomegalovirus (choice A), rubella (choice C), syphilis (choice D) and toxoplasma (choice E) are the other members of the TORCHS complex, but are typically acquired transplacentally. Cytomegalovirus (choice A) has Cowdry A nuclear inclusions but, in addition, has multiple cytoplasmic inclusions and greatly increased cell size. The other agents do not generate Cowdry A inclusions.

622. **(A)** Amyloid is an acellular material that is eosinophilic. After Congo red staining, there is apple-green dichroism when examined under polarized light microscopy. Calcium salts

(choice B) tend to be deeply basophilic, not eosinophilic, with routine stains. Cholesterol deposits (choice C) tend to dissolve out of tissues with routine processing agents and only empty outlines of where the crystals once were are present. Myocyte fibrinoid necrosis (choice D) would be moderately cellular and eosinophilic. Congo-red dichroism is not evident. A postinfarctive cicatrix (choice E) also displays a relatively acellular eosinophilic morphology. Congo-red staining would not be dichromic, however.

623. **(C)** The asthma-like pulmonary disorder that develops after long-term inhalation of cotton fibers is byssinosis. Anthracosis (choice A) is commonly seen in human lungs. Coal miners have a particularly severe form of the disorder. City dwellers and smokers tend to have more moderate disease. Berylliosis (choice B) is a pneumoconiosis seen with beryllium inhalation. Occupational exposure is usually through the production of fluorescent lighting. Silicosis (choice D) is a pneumoconiosis resulting from the inhalation of silica. Occupational exposure can be seen with mining, sandblasting, stone masonry, pottery manufacture, and glass making. Inhalation of tin fumes or debris may result in pulmonary stannosis (choice E).

624. **(C)** Environmental exposure to vinyl chloride is associated with the later development of hepatic angiosarcoma. Focal nodular hyperplasia (choice A) and hepatic fibroma (choice D) do not at present have well-defined antecedent environmental exposure histories. Hepatic adenomas (choice B) occur sporadically in the setting of exogenous steroid hormone usage. Hepatocellular carcinoma (choice E) is associated with cirrhosis, chronic viral hepatitis, and aflatoxin exposure.

625. **(C)** Figure 5–11 displays viable benign chorionic villi that are diagnostic of an ectopic tubal pregnancy. The clinical history of acute lower abdominal pain and hypotension are expected findings with an ectopic pregnancy. Chorioadenoma destruens (choice A) is also referred to as invasive mole, and would display invasion of chorionic elements into the

uterine, not tubal, muscular layers. Choriocarcinoma (choice B) is a malignant neoplasm composed of gestational trophoblastic tissue. Figure 5–11 displays benign chorionic elements. Granular cell tumor (choice D) is a neoplasm of neural-type tissue. The photomicrograph is incompatible with this diagnostic consideration. Leiomyomas (choice E) rarely occur in the fallopian tube. They are most commonly seen in the wall of the uterus. Bundles of benign smooth muscle cells are seen microscopically.

626. **(E)** Cryptorchidism is associated with increased risk for infertility and the development of testicular neoplasms. Testicular germ cell neoplasms are most likely to develop in undescended testes. Cryptorchidism is not usually associated with an increased risk for testicular feminization syndrome (choice A), hemorrhage (choice B), infarction (choice C), or infection (choice D).

627. **(E)** Wilson disease is an autosomal recessive disorder of copper metabolism, probably due to defective biliary excretion of the metal. Cells of the liver and brain are particularly vulnerable to the toxic effects of excessive copper accumulation. Treatment with copper chelating agents, such as penicillamine or triethylene tetramine, have a dramatically beneficial effect. Congenital hepatic fibrosis (choice A) is a rare disorder of unknown etiology. It is most prevalent in India. Peliosis hepatis (choice B) demonstrates small, blood-filled spaces within the liver. Steroid hormone usage is associated with its development in some instances. Primary sclerosing cholangitis (choice C) is due to chronic fibrosis of bile ductules. The etiology is obscure. Most of those affected also have ulcerative colitis. Reye syndrome (choice D) is acute hepatic failure in infants following ingestion of aspirin.

628. **(E)** Liver cell adenomas may occur after several years of taking oral contraceptives but the actual mechanism of tumor formation is unknown. The clinical presentation is often acute abdominal pain due to necrosis of the tumor and hemorrhage. Given the patients'

history, liver cell adenoma is by far the most likely choice. Angiosarcomas of the liver (choice A) are very rare tumors associated with exposure to vinyl chloride (used in the manufacture of the plastic polyvinyl chloride), Thorotrast (formerly used in radiology as a contrast medium), and arsenic. They are not associated with oral contraceptives. Cholangiosarcomas (choice B) are rare tumors that arise in the intrahepatic bile ducts. However, they are more common in the Far East, where there is an association with the liver fluke, *Clonorchis sinensis*. Focal nodular hyperplasia (choice C) is a tumor-like lesion that occurs more frequently in women. It has a weak association with oral contraceptive use. On cut section, it typically has a central stellate scar. It is usually asymptomatic and is only resected in the symptomatic patient. Hepatocellular carcinoma (choice D) in the United States usually arises in a background of cirrhosis due either to alcoholism or hepatitis B virus infection. However, worldwide, hepatitis B is the major etiologic factor and up to 50% of patients with hepatocellular carcinoma may be noncirrhotic.

629. **(A)** Mesenteric adenitis with enterocolitis is associated with *Yersinia* species infections. Clinically, the disorder closely mimics acute appendicitis, presenting as acute right lower quadrant abdominal pain, fever, and leukocytosis. If the patient comes to surgery, the appendix usually appears fairly normal, and instead there is striking enlargement of the mesenteric lymph nodes. The nodes display an acute necrotizing granulomatous pattern if examined histologically. Mesenteric adenitis is unlikely to be caused by fungal infection (choice B), local vascular insufficiency (choice C), parasitic infection (choice D), or viral infection (choice E).

630. **(C)** Figure 5–12 displays interweaving bundles of smooth muscle cells, which, as a discrete myometrial nodule, define a leiomyoma. These are common tumors that may be asymptomatic or produce menorrhagia. Gross appearance is that of a solid white nodule. Adenomyosis (choice A) may clinically

and grossly mimic leiomyomas. Adenomyosis, however, has a triphasic microscopic appearance consisting of benign endometrial glands, benign endometrial stroma, and smooth muscle hypertrophy. A Krukenberg tumor (choice B) is replacement of the ovary by metastatic GI adenocarcinoma. The diagnosis of metastatic malignancy (choice D) is not supported by the photomicrograph of a benign process. Ovarian ectopia (choice E) is exceedingly rare and is incompatible with the histology of the photomicrograph.

631. **(E)** Primary sclerosing cholangitis is a chronic progressive periductal fibrosing biliary tract disease primarily affecting middle-aged men. It is associated with ulcerative colitis in about 70% of patients. Radiographic procedures are essential to show the diagnostic beading of the intrahepatic or extrahepatic bile ducts caused by the periductal fibrosis alternating with areas of ectasia. Ascending cholangitis (choice A) is caused by bacteria entering the biliary tract via the sphincter of Oddi, usually as a result of obstruction to bile flow. Choledochal cysts (choice B) are congenital dilations of the common bile duct. Polycystic liver disease (choice C) is an autosomal dominant condition in which multiple fluid-filled cysts appear throughout the liver. They appear in association with adult polycystic renal disease. Primary biliary cirrhosis (choice D) is a chronic progressive cholestatic disease primarily affecting middle-aged women. There is a strong association with autoimmune disorders and anti-mitochondrial antibodies are usually present.

632. **(D)** Sézary syndrome is the leukemic variant or phase of mycosis fungoides. Mycosis fungoides is a peripheral epidermotrophic T-cell lymphoma that afflicts middle-aged and elderly individuals. Most Sézary cells have a highly convoluted, cerebriform nucleus. Extranodal gastric B-cell lymphoma (choice B) does not define Sézary syndrome. Large B-cell lymphoma arising in the setting of chronic lymphocytic lymphoma (choice C) is termed Richter syndrome. Adult T-cell leukemia due to HTLV-1 infection (choice A) and lymphoma

that arises in HIV-positive patients (choice E) do not define Sézary syndrome.

633. **(E)** Paget disease of the nipple usually presents as an ulcerated crusted lesion of one nipple. Biopsy reveals intraepithelial adenocarcinoma. On further examination the underlying breast tissue may show an intraductal or infiltrating ductal adenocarcinoma. Bowen disease (choice A) is another term for cutaneous squamous cell carcinoma in situ. It frequently occurs on sun-exposed, aged skin. Dermatitis herpetiformis (choice B) is a gluten sensitivity-related cutaneous disorder characterized by pruritic plaque formation. Desmoid tumor (choice C) is a form of fibromatosis usually occurring in the ventral abdominal subcutis. Epidermolysis bullosa (choice D) is a benign dermatologic condition characterized by cutaneous blister formation with minor trauma.

634. **(D)** Peutz–Jeghers syndrome is an autosomal dominant condition in which large numbers of hamartomatous polyps are found throughout the GI tract, particularly in the small intestine. The hamartomatous polyps themselves are not premalignant, but these patients have an increased incidence of carcinomas at various sites, including the GI tract, breast, gonads, lung, and pancreas. Another characteristic finding in these patients is the appearance of pigmented macules in and around the mouth and over the genitalia and palmar surfaces of the hands. Familial polyposis coli (choice A) and Gardner syndrome (choice B) have the same genetic defect, are autosomal dominant, and are probably different expressions of the same disease process. Familial polyposis coli is associated with the occurrence of large numbers (hundreds to thousands) of adenomatous polyps throughout the large intestine and all of these patients eventually develop colon carcinoma unless a prophylactic colectomy is performed. Gardner syndrome in addition features extraintestinal lesions including osteomas of the skull, jaw, and long bones; epidermal cysts; fibromas of the skin; and fibromatosis of soft tissues. Juvenile retention

polyps (choice C) are a fairly common finding in children and young adults. These hamartomas of the mucosa, typically found in the rectum, have no malignant potential. Turcot syndrome (choice E) is a very rare autosomal recessive condition in which there are multiple colonic adenomas that carry a high potential for malignant transformation. This condition is also associated with malignant brain tumors, in particular glioblastoma multiforme.

635. **(D)** Pleomorphic adenoma is the most common tumor of the salivary glands, particularly of the parotids. It is benign, but often recurs due to incomplete surgical removal. It has a distinctive histologic appearance, being composed of sheets of myoepithelial cells containing ducts and tubules. Also apparent are chondroid, myxoid, and mucoid areas, presumably derived from the myoepithelial cells. This appearance gives rise to the earlier erroneous idea that this tumor was derived from both epithelial and mesenchymal elements and was thus called a "mixed tumor." Acinic cell carcinoma (choice A) is an uncommon (about 2% of all salivary gland tumors), low-grade tumor usually arising in the parotids. The microscopic appearance is variable, but often is composed of fairly uniform cells resembling the normal acinic cells of the salivary glands. Adenoid cystic carcinoma (choice B) is more common in the minor salivary glands, where it represents about 20% of the total. It has a great tendency to invade the perineural spaces and is, therefore, painful. Microscopically, it is composed of small cells with little cytoplasm surrounding cystic spaces containing hyaline. Mucoepidermoid carcinomas (choice C) account for about 10 to 15% of all salivary gland tumors with a greater incidence in the parotids. As the name suggests, microscopic examination reveals well-differentiated mucous cells lining glandular spaces with intervening sheets of epidermoid cells. Warthin tumor (choice E) is the second most common salivary tumor after pleomorphic adenoma and nearly always occurs in the parotids. It has a strong link with smoking and more commonly occurs in

males. Microscopically, it is composed of a double layer of epithelial cells composed of large cells with abundant cytoplasm (oncocytes), beneath which is dense lymphoid stroma.

636. **(D)** Malakoplakia is most frequent in middle-aged women with a clinical history of repeated bladder infections. Gross appearance is characterized by scattered, soft yellow plaques in the bladder mucosa. Chronic interstitial cystitis (choice A) is also called Hunner ulcer. The bladder mucosa is red, fibrotic, and may be ulcerated. Microcalcospherites are not part of the usual histology. Michaelis–Gutmann bodies are present microscopically. Endometriosis (choice B) is not associated with bladder infections, appears red on gross exam, and microscopically would display a mixture of benign endometrial glands and stroma. Exstrophy (choice C) of the bladder refers to a birth defect in which the bladder mucosa is everted through an abdominal wall defect. Polypoid cystitis (choice E) is associated with indwelling urinary catheters. The bladder lesion is usually single, polypoid, and red.

637. **(D)** Vitamin B_{12} deficiency is classically associated with the slow onset of fatigue, sore tongue, and peripheral neurologic changes, the latter due to myelin degeneration of the posterior and lateral columns of the spinal cord. This deficiency produces a macrocytic anemia (thus the increased MCV) and leukopenia with hypersegmented granulocytes. Hemolysis-induced hyperbilirubinemia may produce slight jaundice, as seen in this patient. Folic acid deficiency (choice A) produces an identical anemia but not the neurologic changes; the distinction between the two is very significant. Iron deficiency (choice B) produces microcytic, hypochromic anemia and does not produce the neurologic changes described. Vitamin B_1 deficiency (choice C) is associated with beriberi and Wernicke encephalopathy in alcoholics, but does not produce anemia. Vitamin K is required for the production of clotting factors VII, IX, and X and prothrombin; a deficiency (choice E) can lead to a bleeding diathesis, but has no direct neurologic consequences.

638. **(E)** This is a benign cystic teratoma of the ovary. It is a common tumor accounting for about 15% of ovarian tumors. Nearly all contain dermal elements and in most cases tissues derived from all three germ layers can be found. These tumors are typically benign, although about 1% do undergo malignant transformation. Choristoma (choice A) is a mass of maldeveloped tissue of a type not normally found at that site. Hamartoma (choice B) is a mass of maldeveloped tissue of a type that is normally found at that site. The lung is a more common location for these. Mixed tumor (choice C) is another name for pleomorphic adenoma, the most common benign tumor of salivary glands. Myxoma (choice D) is a benign neoplasm derived from connective tissue and is the most common primary tumor of the heart in adults. Most occur in the left atrium and they may become clinically significant by blocking the mitral valve or by embolization of fragments.

639. **(C)** Small-cell undifferentiated pulmonary carcinoma (oat cell carcinoma) is closely linked to cigarette smoking. This highly lethal malignancy is thought to arise from neuroendocrine cells of the bronchial mucosa. Clara cells (choice A) may give rise to certain pulmonary adenocarcinomas. Metaplastic bronchial epithelium (choice B) is the likely source of squamous cell carcinoma. The alveolar pneumocytes (choices D and E) rarely sustain malignant transformation.

640. **(C)** Figure 5–13 shows a clear cell adenocarcinoma, which is the most common histologic appearance for renal cell carcinoma. The patient's age, gender, and clinical presentation are typical for this malignant neoplasm. Angiomyolipoma (choice A) is a benign renal tumor that displays a mixture of blood vessels, smooth muscle, and mature fat on microscopic examination. Oncocytoma (choice B) is a benign renal neoplasm constructed by monomorphic cells with granular eosinophilic cytoplasm. Transitional cell carcinoma (choice

D) usually arises in the renal pelvis and histologically is composed of anaplastic transitional cells without a clear cell adenocarcinoma component. Xanthogranulomatous pyelonephritis (choice E) is a benign inflammatory condition of the kidney that may produce a mass effect. The gross appearance, but not the microscopic appearance, may be confused with renal cell carcinoma.

641. **(D)** The baby boy was born prematurely and had insufficient pulmonary surfactant to prevent the collapse of the alveoli during expiration. This led to the respiratory distress syndrome described in the history. Surfactant is made up of several polylipids, including lecithin and sphingomyelin. Its composition changes as the fetus matures; lecithin levels increase rapidly as the fetus approaches term. When the ratio of lecithin to sphingomyelin is above 2, this is an indication of sufficient lung activity for the baby to breathe normally without getting respiratory distress syndrome. Alpha-fetoprotein levels in the mother's blood (choice A), if increased, may indicate a neural tube defect in the fetus. For unknown reasons, a decrease is associated with the trisomies. Chromosomal analysis of fetal amniotic cells (choice B) could aid in the prenatal diagnosis of chromosomal abnormalities, but would not be useful in this case. Cytomegalovirus antibody levels in the mother's blood (choice C) is not of value because there is no indication that the baby has been infected with this virus. Toxicology screening of the mother's urine (choice E) would not be useful in the absence of any evidence for drug effects upon the infant.

642. **(A)** The inadequacy of surfactant leads to collapse of the lungs and expiration resulting in hypoventilation, hypoxemia, alveolar damage, and protein exudation. This exudate protein with necrotic cells forms a layer that lines the alveoli and respiratory bronchioles. It is referred to as a hyaline membrane. Foreign body granulomas and interstitial fibrosis (choice B) can be seen, for example, in the lungs of intravenous drug abusers as a response to some of the substances such as talc

used to "cut" or dilute the drug. Interstitial lymphocytes and plasma cells with early fibrosis (choice C) are found in a chronic inflammatory response rather than the acute process described. Intra-alveolar neutrophils and fibrin with hyperemia (choice D) are found in an acute inflammatory response that is not seen in respiratory distress syndrome. Intranuclear and intracytoplasmic inclusions (choice E) are an indication of a viral infection and in abnormally long cells are classic for cytomegalovirus.

643. **(B)** Treatment of babies with mechanical ventilation and high oxygen levels can result in bronchopulmonary dysplasia. This is marked by proliferation of type II pneumocytes, squamous metaplasia of bronchioles, and peribronchial and interstitial fibrosis. Asthma (choice A) is recognized microscopically by thickened basement membranes, hyperplasia of bronchial smooth muscle, goblet cell metaplasia, and eosinophils. Cystic fibrosis (choice C) is an autosomal recessive disease resulting in abnormally thick mucous secretions in the lungs and other organs. Panacinar emphysema (choice D) features a uniform involvement of the acinar involving alveoli, alveolar ducts, and respiratory bronchioles. It is the type of emphysema associated with alpha-fetoprotein deficiency. Sequestrated lung (choice D) is a congenital anomaly in which an area of the lung becomes isolated during development and is not connected to the bronchial tree.

644. **(C)** The manner of death refers to whether it is natural, an accident, a suicide, or a homicide. For a violent death, intent is considered. For example, a fatal gunshot wound could be either accidental, a suicide, or a homicide. In this case, even though the bank guard survived for a few days and then succumbed to pneumonia, the act that initiated the sequence of events was homicide. Accident (choice A) indicates an accidental discharge of the gun; because this occurred during a robbery attempt, this is clearly not the case. Gunshot wound to the head (choice B) and pneumonia (choice E) are causes, not man-

ners, of death. Natural death (choice D) refers to a nonviolent death that is usually the result of a disease process.

645. **(D)** The event that initiated the sequence of events resulting in death is the underlying cause. In this case it was the gunshot wound. If this event is prevented, none of the subsequent events will occur. Theoretically, the man could remain comatose for many years before dying and the underlying cause of death would still be gunshot wound (and the manner of death would still be homicide). Bronchopneumonia (choice A) is the immediate cause of death, not the initiating cause of death required for the death certificate. Cardiopulmonary arrest (choice B) is a meaningless term that should never appear on a death certificate. Cerebral edema with tonsillar herniation (choice C) and intracerebral hemorrhage (choice D) are probable consequences of the gunshot wound but, again, are not initiating events.

646. **(E)** Thrombotic thrombocytopenic purpura is an acute microangiopathic hemolytic anemia. The clinical picture usually includes mental alterations, anuria, mucosal bleeding, and purpura. An abnormal platelet aggregating substance is the likely initiating event. Acute idiopathic thrombocytopenia (choice A) does not have a hemolytic component, lacks renal failure, and does not display thrombi in the skin biopsy. Bernard–Soulier syndrome (choice B) and Glanzmann thrombasthenia (choice C) are hereditary disorders of platelet aggregation. Clinical symptoms of a coagulopathy usually occur in infancy. May–Hegglin anomaly (choice D) is an inherited condition with thrombocytopenia and morphologically abnormal white blood cells. Hemolysis, acute onset, and mental aberrations do not typify this disorder.

647. **(D)** Therapeutic apheresis is the currently recommended treatment for thrombotic thrombocytopenic purpura. Plasmapheresis is performed daily for about a week in most instances. The cure rate with this therapy approaches 90%. Antibiotics (choice A), antivi-

ral therapy (choice B), immunosuppressive agents (choice C), and renal transplant (choice E) are not the primary modalities used to treat thrombotic thrombocytopenic purpura.

648. **(E)** The recent use of therapeutic apheresis in the treatment of thrombotic thrombocytopenic purpura (TTP) is an encouraging development in medicine. Prior to the use of plasmapheresis, about 90% of patients with TTP died acutely. The statistics are now reversed, with about 90% of TTP patients surviving if given rapid and appropriate therapeutic apheresis. The other options of 10% (choice A), 25% (choice B), 40% (choice C), and 60% (choice D) are incorrect.

649. **(C)** Ichthyosis is a hereditary condition characterized clinically by coarse, fish-like, scaly skin. The microanatomy demonstrates marked thickening of the stratum corneum. Dermal fibrosis (choice A), basal hyperpigmentation (choice B), perivascular chronic inflammation (choice D), and subepidermal blister formation (choice E) are not the histologic hallmarks of ichthyosis.

650. **(B)** Ichthyosis is a hereditary condition. The most common form of the disorder in the United States is inherited in an X-linked fashion. The disease is not caused by bacterial infection (choice A), a hormonal imbalance (choice C), a hypersensitivity reaction (choice D), or viral infection (choice E).

651. **(A)** Figure 5–14 displays the histology of a basal cell carcinoma. These tumors are slow growing, appear as flesh- to pearl-colored cutaneous nodules, and arise principally on sun-exposed areas. The histologic pattern is one of infiltrating small dermal clusters of basophilic cells with peripheral basal orientation. Bowen disease (choice B) is another term for cutaneous intraepidermal squamous cell carcinoma. An epidermal cyst (choice C) is a benign dermal collection of central keratotic debris with a peripheral cyst wall formed by benign, mature, stratified squamous epithelium. Molluscum con-

tagiosum (choice D) is a viral disorder. Molluscum bodies are the critical histologic finding. Verruca vulgaris (choice E) is a cutaneous viral disorder with prominent papillomatosis.

652. **(A)** Basal cell carcinomas arise from actinically damaged skin. Areas of the body that are rarely exposed to ultraviolet light are unlikely to develop these tumors. Lumenal occlusion (choice B), fungal infection (choice C), papillomavirus infection (choice D), and poxvirus infection (choice E) are not significant etiologic factors in the development of basal cell carcinoma.

653. **(C)** Primary biliary cirrhosis is primarily a disease of middle-aged women (M:F = 1:6). Early in the course of the disease the clinical presentation is nonspecific, but the microscopic findings of a nonsuppurative, granulomatous distribution of medium-sized intrahepatic bile ducts is distinctive. Alcoholic hepatitis (choice A) features hepatocytic swelling and necrosis, neutrophilic infiltration, and Mallory bodies, but not granulomas. The microscopic appearance of hepatitis C (choice B) varies depending on the stage of the disease, but does not have a granulomatous response. Primary sclerosing cholangitis (choice D) has some similarities to primary biliary sclerosis, but now often occurs in men (M:F = 2:1) and does not feature granulomas. Schistosomiasis (choice E) can result in granulomas being formed in the liver in response to the parasite eggs. However, these are not centered on the bile ducts and is a much less likely possibility in this case.

654. **(C)** Primary biliary cirrhosis is an autoimmune disorder. Autoantibodies against mitochondria are usually present. Hyperbilirubinemia, steatorrhea, portal hypertension, and osteomalacia may be seen in the later stages of the disease. Vascular abnormalities (choice A), alcohol abuse (choice B), parasitic infections (choice D), and viral infections (choice E) all may mimic the clinical picture of primary biliary cirrhosis. They are not, however, the usual etiologic agents.

655. **(E)** In the later stages of primary biliary cirrhosis the serum chemistry studies usually display a striking elevation of alkaline phosphatase, bilirubin, and cholesterol. This pattern of chemical abnormality suggests that there is intrahepatic obstruction of the biliary tract. It is very unlikely that these three chemical studies would all be decreased (choice A) in the later stages of primary biliary cirrhosis. Usually these three tests are all elevated strikingly and in tandem with this disorder. An elevation of only one test (choices B and C), or of only two tests (choice D), is also very uncommon.

656. **(D)** Figure 5–15 reveals a poorly differentiated infiltrating ductal mammary adenocarcinoma. A family history of breast carcinoma puts other female relatives at increased statistical risk to develop breast cancer themselves. Asians (choice A) are less likely to develop breast cancer than are Caucasians or blacks. Both early age of first pregnancy and multiparity (choice B) decrease the risk of developing mammary carcinoma. Early menopause (choice C) decreases the relative risk of developing breast cancer. Late menarche (choice E) also decreases the relative risk of developing breast cancer.

657. **(C)** Overexpression of NEU oncogene in invasive breast carcinoma is an adverse prognostic indicator. Breast cancers that are estrogen-receptor positive (choice A), have a low S phase (choice B), are progesterone-receptor positive (choice D), and are well differentiated (choice E) are considered to have more favorable prognostic implications. Size of the primary breast carcinoma and the status of the axillary lymph nodes are also major factors that influence the prognosis of invasive ductal breast adenocarcinoma.

658. **(A)** Barrett esophagitis is a metaplastic alteration of the lower esophagus in response to chronic acid reflux. Figure 5–16 displays the specialized type of Barrett esophagitis, complete with numerous goblet mucous cells. *Candida* esophagitis (choice B) does not contain glandular epithelium. Squamous epithe-

lium, yeast, and pseudohyphae are expected instead. Granulomatous esophagitis (choice C) and viral esophagitis (choice E) are not characterized by metaplastic glandular epithelium. Giant cells or inclusion bodies may be seen, depending on the etiology. Plummer-Vinson syndrome (choice D) describes the formation of a lumenal web in the upper third of the esophagus. Microanatomy displays squamous epithelium, not metaplastic glandular epithelium.

659. **(A)** Long-standing Barrett metaplasia substantially increases the risk of developing adenocarcinoma in the lower esophagus. Most lesions pass through a dysplastic stage from which the carcinoma later arises. Frequent endoscopic monitoring of Barrett esophagus may identify these worrisome dysplastic changes early enough to allow prophylactic surgical therapy. The presence of Barrett metaplasia of the esophagus does not predispose an individual to an increased risk of esophageal varices (choice B), fungal septicemia (choice C), squamous cell carcinoma (choice D), or viral encephalitis (choice E).

660. **(E)** Nephroblastoma (Wilms tumor) is a childhood malignant neoplasm composed of primitive renal blastema. Microscopically, there is usually a mixture of immature tubular, stromal, and glomerular elements. Malignant adrenal neural crest cells (choice A) describe a neuroblastoma. An angiosarcoma is composed of malignant endothelial cells forming abortive vascular structures (choice B). Malignant gland-forming epithelium with glycogen-containing clear cytoplasm and abundant vascularity (choice C) is an accurate description of a renal cell carcinoma, which is an adult neoplasm. Malignant osteoid or cartilage (choice D) describe an osteosarcoma and a chondrosarcoma, respectively.

661. **(A)** Nephroblastoma usually harbors a partial deletion of chromosome 11. Down syndrome (trisomy 21) is an example of this type of chromosomal abnormality. Trisomy is not routinely seen with Wilms tumor. Inversion

(choice B) involves the reordering of gene sequences within the same chromosome. This alteration is not seen with nephroblastoma. Neither type is associated with nephroblastoma. Ring formation (choice C) describes the fusion of the telomeric portions of the chromosome into a ring-shaped structure. It is not usually seen with Wilms tumor. Translocations (choice D) may be reciprocal or Robertsonian. A third copy of a chromosome is termed trisomy (choice E).

662. **(E)** With appropriate combined therapy the 5-year survival rate for nephroblastoma is about 90%. Lack of therapy, inadequate therapy, and the anaplastic variant of this tumor may imply a negative outcome. The other choices 5% (choice A), 30% (choice B), 40% (choice C), and 60% (choice D) are incorrect.

663. **(B)** Hemophilia A is a genetic disorder characterized by very low levels of factor VIII, elevated partial thromboplastin time, normal prothrombin time, normal platelet aggregation with ristocetin, and spontaneous hemorrhages into joints, soft tissues, and mucosal surfaces. Christmas disease (choice A) is an alternative term for hemophilia B. Hemophilia B (choice C) is a hereditary coagulopathy due to a very low level of factor IX. Rosenthal syndrome (choice D) defines a deficiency of factor XI. Von Willebrand disease (choice E) is characterized by a mild hereditary bleeding diathesis and abnormal platelet aggregation with ristocetin.

664. **(E)** Hemophilia A is an X-linked recessive disorder. This mode of inheritance means that the disorder is only fully expressed in males and that females may be unaffected carriers of the trait. Hemophilia A is not usually inherited in an autosomal codominant (choice A), autosomal dominant (choice B), autosomal recessive (choice C), or X-linked dominant (choice D) manner.

665. **(E)** Multiple myeloma is a disease of the elderly classically characterized by numerous lytic bony areas containing atypical plasma cells. The neoplastic plasma cells may secrete

a monoclonal paraprotein that can be detected in the patient's serum or urine. The presence of a paraprotein usually results in elevated total protein and low serum albumin. Malignant lymphoma (choice A) demonstrates atypical lymphoid cells if examined by fine-needle aspiration. Total protein is usually decreased. Metastatic adenocarcinoma (choice B) displays atypical glandular epithelial cells on fine-needle biopsy. Total protein is usually low, not elevated. Metastatic melanoma (choice C) demonstrates atypical melanocytes on fine-needle biopsy, not plasma cells. Total protein is usually low, not elevated. Mononucleosis (choice D) is a viral disorder of young adults characterized by sore throat, lymphadenopathy, and fever. There are no bony lytic lesions with mononucleosis.

666. **(C)** The neoplastic clones of plasma cells usually secrete a monoclonal paraprotein that can be detected by laboratory methods in the serum, urine, or both. Bisalbuminemia (choice A) is a rare hereditary condition characterized by a biclonal albumin band on serum protein electrophoresis. It is a laboratory anomaly in an otherwise healthy individual. The presence of the myeloma paraprotein usually produces hypergammaglobulinemia, rather than hypogammaglobulinemia (choice D). The myeloma paraprotein results in a monoclonal hypergammaglobulinemia, rather than a polyclonal hypergammaglobulinemia (choice C). The alpha fractions (choice E) are usually normal or increased with multiple myeloma.

667. **(B)** Forty to 50 years ago diethylstilbestrol was actively used to prevent miscarriages. Surviving female fetuses exposed to this agent later demonstrated an increased incidence of vaginal adenosis. The development of vaginal adenosis is not known to be associated with aspirin ingestion (choice A), administration of methotrexate (choice C), radiation (choice D), or rubella virus (choice E).

668. **(A)** The most serious long-term consequence of vaginal adenosis is the increased risk of developing clear cell adenocarcinoma. Vaginal adenosis does not significantly predispose to the development of endometrial adenocarcinoma (choice B), serous papillary carcinoma (choice C), uterine leiomyomas (choice D), or vaginal sarcoma (choice E).

669. **(B)** The clinical scenario describes a classic example of Duchenne muscular dystrophy. The weakness is symmetric and most often begins at the pelvic girdle. Fatty pseudohypertrophy with alternating muscle fiber atrophy and hypertrophy typify the histologic changes. Many patients die before reaching their 20s. The other diagnostic options, cerebral palsy (choice A), myositis ossificans (choice C), poliomyelitis (choice D), and trichinosis (choice E), do not fit the clinical picture.

670. **(B)** Muscular dystrophy is a hereditary disorder. In most instances there is a deletion of a portion of the X chromosome that codes for the dystrophin muscle protein. Muscular dystrophy is not caused by *Trichinella spiralis* infestation (choice A), a neoplastic process (choice C), neonatal trauma (choice D), or viruses (choice E).

671. **(B)** Healthy skeletal muscle cells contain a number of enzymes that are required for routine physiologic functions. When these cells are damaged, enzymes may leak out into the blood and be used clinically as a marker for muscle cell death. Muscular dystrophy typically displays an elevation of creatine kinase, aldolase, and lactate dehydrogenase. Decreases in the muscular enzymes (choice A) would not be expected with muscular dystrophy. Other options (choices C and D) offer only one of the three enzymes as being elevated. Normally, dying skeletal muscle cells release all three diagnostic enzymes. The normal phenotype is present as choice E.

672. **(B)** Right-sided colon cancers typically produce a large ulcerative lesion. Blood loss from the tumor can be detected in the feces as a positive test for occult blood. If sufficient blood is lost, the patient becomes anemic. Serum CEA is usually elevated as a marker

of tumor dedifferentiation back toward a more primitive fetal antigen-synthesizing tissue. In choice A there is only one item (elevated CEA) of the three that is usually seen with right-sided colonic carcinomas. The elevated hemoglobin in choice C is highly unlikely in this clinical vignette. The other two items are normal. A normal CEA, negative occult blood, and normal hemoglobin (choice D) is a triplet of normal laboratory studies. In choice E there is only one item (positive occult blood) of the three that is usually seen with right-sided colon cancers.

673. **(D)** After metastasizing first to the pericolonic lymph nodes, colonic tumor cells usually are then drained by the mesenteric lymphatics into the blood vessels, the portal vein, and finally, into the liver. The liver is the most common distant site of metastatic right-sided colon carcinoma. The adrenal (choice A), appendix (choice B), brain (choice C), and lung (choice E) are all less likely sites of initial distant tumor spread.

REFERENCES

Chandrasoma P, Taylor CR. *Concise Pathology,* 3rd ed. Stamford, CT: Appleton & Lange; 1998.

Cotran RS, Kumar V, Collins T. *Pathologic Basis of Disease,* 6th ed. Philadelphia: Saunders; 1999.

Handbook of Diseases, 2nd ed. Springhouse, PA: Springhouse; 2000.

Rubin F, Farber JL. *Pathology,* 3rd ed. Philadelphia: Lippincott; 1999.

Subspecialty List: Pathology

Question Number and Subspecialty

547. Alimentary system
548. Immunopathology
549. Nervous system
550. Inflammation
551. Inflammation
552. Alimentary system
553. Genetic or metabolic syndromes
554. Immunopathology
555. Nongenetic syndromes
556. Respiratory system
557. Endocrine syndromes
558. Alimentary system
559. Alimentary system
560. Neoplasia
561. Laboratory medicine
562. Blood and lymphatic system
563. Immunopathology
564. Alimentary system
565. Kidney and urinary system
566. Cardiovascular system
567. Cardiovascular system
568. Alimentary system
569. Blood and lymphatic system
570. Genetic or metabolic syndromes
571. Abnormal growth and development
572. Cell injury and response
573. Genetic or metabolic syndromes
574. Inflammation
575. Infectious diseases
576. Neoplasia
577. Cardiovascular system
578. Respiratory system
579. Alimentary system
580. Blood and lymphatic system
581. Nongenetic syndromes
582. Respiratory system

583. Alimentary system
584. Inflammation
585. Cardiovascular system
586. Cardiovascular system
587. Respiratory system
588. Infectious diseases
589. Genetic or metabolic syndromes
590. Alimentary system
591. Cardiovascular system
592. Genetic or metabolic syndromes
593. Alimentary system
594. Genital system
595. Breast pathology
596. Cardiovascular pathology
597. Environmental pathology
598. Neoplasia
599. Alimentary system
600. Respiratory system
601. Abnormal growth and development
602. Infectious diseases
603. Neoplasia
604. Cell injury and response
605. Immunopathology
606. Genetic or metabolic syndromes
607. Endocrine system
608. Blood and lymphatic system
609. Endocrine system
610. Cardiovascular system
611. Genetic or metabolic syndromes
612. Genital system
613. Environmental pathology
614. Infectious diseases
615. Neoplasia
616. Infectious diseases
617. Kidney and urinary system
618. Kidney and urinary system
619. Nervous system
620. Environmental pathology

621. Infectious diseases
622. Cardiovascular system
623. Environmental pathology
624. Neoplasia
625. Genital system
626. Genital system
627. Genetic or metabolic syndromes
628. Neoplasia
629. Infectious diseases
630. Genital system
631. Alimentary system
632. Blood and lymphatic system
633. Breast pathology
634. Alimentary system
635. Neoplasia
636. Kidney and urinary system
637. Genetic or metabolic syndromes
638. Genital system
639. Respiratory system
640. Kidney or urinary system
641. Abnormal growth and development
642. Abnormal growth and development
643. Abnormal growth and development
644. Environmental pathology
645. Environmental pathology
646. Hemostasis and coagulation
647. Hemostasis and coagulation
648. Hemostasis and coagulation
649. Cutaneous pathology
650. Cutaneous pathology
651. Cutaneous pathology
652. Cutaneous pathology
653. Alimentary system
654. Alimentary system
655. Alimentary system
656. Breast pathology
657. Breast pathology
658. Alimentary system
659. Alimentary system
660. Kidney and urinary system
661. Kidney and urinary system
662. Kidney and urinary system
663. Genetic or metabolic syndromes
664. Genetic or metabolic syndromes
665. Blood and lymphatic system
666. Blood and lymphatic system
667. Abnormal growth and development
668. Abnormal growth and development
669. Muscular system
670. Muscular system
671. Muscular system
672. Neoplasia
673. Neoplasia

$$674$$
$$50$$
$$\overline{724}$$

$$674$$
$$63$$
$$\overline{737}$$

CHAPTER 6

Pharmacology
Questions

Bertram G. Katzung, MD, PhD

674. The following are pharmacokinetic data for the drug propranolol in a 70-kg person: clearance, 50 L/h; volume of distribution, 270 L; effective plasma concentration, 20 ng/mL; oral availability (percentage), 25%. Calculate the oral maintenance dosing rate for propranolol in a 70-kg person.

   (A) 10 µg/h
   (B) 200 µg/h
   (C) 1 mg/h
   (D) 4 mg/h
   (E) 54 mg/h

675. In the operating room, a patient is anesthetized with an inhalation anesthetic and given a single intravenous dose of pancuronium. Power is lost in the operating room, and the surgeon wishes to stop the procedure. What is the best pharmacologic treatment to reverse the actions of pancuronium?

   (A) Atracurium
   (B) Bethanechol
   (C) Neostigmine
   (D) Physostigmine
   (E) Pralidoxime

676. A teenage patient is brought to the emergency room in an agitated state. He must be restrained from leaving because he believes that he can fly and wants to jump off the roof.

His friend confides that the patient has consumed an extract made from some weeds. The patient has an elevated body temperature, but is not perspiring. His pupils are dilated, and his heart rate is markedly elevated. Although the diagnosis is necessarily tentative, the pharmacologic treatment of choice for the patient if his condition appears to be worsening is

   (A) carbachol
   (B) ipratropium
   (C) methscopolamine
   (D) neostigmine
   (E) physostigmine

677. Which of the following agents decreases the circulating levels of norepinephrine?

   (A) Amphetamine
   (B) Clonidine
   (C) Phentolamine
   (D) Phenoxybenzamine
   (E) Prazosin

Questions 678 through 680

A.W. is a 73-year-old woman complaining of difficulty sleeping, exercise fatigue, and shortness of breath. Examination reveals mental confusion, swollen ankles, pulmonary rales, and dyspnea upon reclining.

678. Chronic treatment of this patient with an angiotensin-converting enzyme (ACE) inhibitor such as captopril may be beneficial because ACE inhibitors

(A) decrease both ventricular preload and afterload

(B) increase coronary perfusion

(C) increase efficiency of oxygen extraction by skeletal and cardiac muscle

(D) produce a positive inotropic effect and negative chronotropic effect

(E) promote ventricular remodeling and compensatory enlargement

679. Immediate treatment may be needed if signs and symptoms, especially those of pulmonary congestion, worsen rapidly. Which of the following would be most beneficial in treating pulmonary edema?

(A) Amiloride

(B) Furosemide

(C) Hydrochlorothiazide

(D) Losartan

(E) Metoprolol

680. Use of a cardiac glycoside such as digoxin in addition to captopril may be warranted in the chronic treatment of this patient. Periodic monitoring of patients being treated with digoxin is necessary because of the serious hazard of

(A) digoxin-induced cardiac arrhythmias

(B) desensitization of cardiac β-adrenoreceptors produced by increased bradykinin levels

(C) hypokalemia produced by digoxin's effects on the kidney

(D) hypotension produced by an interaction of captopril with digoxin

(E) toxic accumulation of digoxin, produced by captopril's inhibition of renal excretion of the glycoside

681. Which of the following descriptions best describes the molecular mechanism underlying the therapeutic actions of the statins, such as simvastatin?

(A) Binding to peroxisome proliferator-activated receptor-α (PPAR-α) resulting in stimulation of lipoprotein lipase activity

(B) Increased fecal excretion of bile acid resulting in increased conversion of cholesterol to bile acid

(C) Inhibition of hepatic cholesterol synthesis resulting in increased expression of LDL receptors

(D) Inhibition of hepatic VLDL secretion resulting in reduced production of IDL and LDL

(E) Inhibition of lecithin:cholesterol acyl-transferase activity resulting in decreased conversion of IDL to LDL

682. Multidrug resistance is a major cause of treatment failure in cancer chemotherapy. A single mechanism for multidrug resistance (and therefore a target for pharmacologic intervention) to doxorubicin, vincristine, paclitaxel, and dactinomycin (actinomycin D) is produced when tumor cells have

(A) decreased doubling time so that a smaller percentage of cells are caught in S phase

(B) increased activity of dihydrofolate reductase

(C) increased activity of DNA repair pathways

(D) increased expression of an outward transport system that removes drug from cells

(E) reduced activity of deoxycytidine kinase

683. Additive and potentially dangerous hypertensive interactions may occur between cardiovascular stimulant drugs and which of the following herbal preparations?

(A) Echinacea

(B) Gingko biloba

(C) Ginseng

(D) Kava

(E) Ma-huang

684. A 37-year-old African-American man with a known allergy to sulfonamides is diagnosed with open-angle glaucoma. Several days after treatment is initiated with topical timolol, he experiences difficulty in breathing and goes to the emergency room. He is treated with inhaled albuterol and released with a referral to his ophthalmologist. What was the likely mechanism by which timolol caused this episode?

(A) Bronchoconstriction resulting from blockade of β-adrenoreceptors

(B) Drug allergy to timolol

(C) Hemolysis caused by hereditary glucose-6-phosphate dehydrogenase deficiency

(D) Idiosyncratic response to timolol

(E) Induction of erythrocyte sickling

685. A patient suffers from partial seizures that have been well controlled by treatment with a carbamazepine regimen. Which of the following new conditions is most likely to cause carbamazepine-induced diplopia and ataxia if the regular regimen is not altered?

(A) Coadministration of phenobarbital

(B) Gout treated with probenecid

(C) Hypertension treated with hydrochlorothiazide

(D) Initiation of smoking

(E) Peptic ulcer treated with cimetidine

Questions 686 through 688

Figure 6–1 shows plasma concentrations of drug W in a patient following IV injection of a single dose of 100 mg of the drug, an agent eliminated from the body by renal excretion. At hour 12, the patient is treated with sodium bicarbonate.

686. Using the data before hour 12, the calculated volume of distribution (V_d) for drug W is

(A) 1 L

(B) 10 L

(C) 25 L

(D) 50 L

(E) 100 L

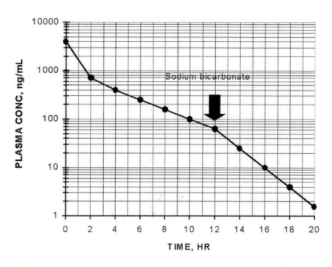

Figure 6–1

687. Using the data before hour 12, the half-life ($t_{1/2}$) for drug W is

(A) 0.5 h

(B) 1 h

(C) 3 h

(D) 7 h

(E) 10 h

688. The change in elimination rate after hour 12 when sodium bicarbonate was administered is expected if drug W is which of the following chemical types?

(A) Nonelectrolyte

(B) Strong acid

(C) Strong base

(D) Weak acid

(E) Weak base

Questions 689 and 690

T.W. calls 911 because of severe substernal crushing pain that has not responded to three nitroglycerin tablets taken sublingually. The paramedic team suspects that Mr. W. has suffered an acute myocardial infarction. His blood pressure is 110/70 and his heart rate is 70, with occasional premature extra beats.

689. What drug should be administered immediately, even before the patient reaches the hospital?

(A) Aspirin

(B) Dobutamine

(C) Lidocaine

(D) Metoprolol

(E) Streptokinase

690. After initial treatment in the hospital, Mr. W. is found to be suffering from more severe hypotension (his blood pressure is now 70/40) and reduction of cardiac function with an elevated left ventricular filling pressure. His urine output is low and he has mental clouding. The pharmacologic treatment of choice for this condition in this patient is

(A) atenolol

(B) digoxin

(C) dobutamine

(D) norepinephrine

(E) procainamide

691. H.M. is being treated for metastatic prostate cancer. Which of the following agents is used parenterally in prostate cancer to reduce luteinizing hormone (LH) release from the pituitary?

(A) Diethylstilbestrol

(B) Finasteride

(C) Flutamide

(D) Ketoconazole

(E) Leuprolide

692. A patient complains of severe itching of the eyes and a runny nose during the spring. He is responsible for operating dangerous farm machinery and does not want any drug that will make him sleepy. Which of the following agents would be most suitable?

(A) Chlorpheniramine

(B) Cimetidine

(C) Diphenhydramine

(D) Hydroxyzine

(E) Loratadine

693. A drug being developed as an antiarrhythmic agent was studied in the laboratory using microelectrode techniques for measuring the transmembrane potential. The results of this study are shown in Figure 6–2. Which of the following standard antiarrhythmic agents does the new drug most resemble?

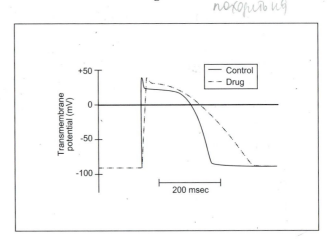

Figure 6–2

(A) Adenosine

(B) Lidocaine

(C) Procainamide

(D) Propranolol

(E) Sotalol

694. K.M. is admitted for acute coronary syndrome with signs of impending myocardial infarction. She undergoes emergency angioplasty with double coronary stenting to maintain the patency of her coronary vessels. Which of the following drugs will probably be administered to prevent clotting in the region of the wire mesh stents?

(A) Clopidogrel

(B) Low-molecular-weight heparin

(C) Regular heparin

(D) Tissue plasminogen activator (t-PA)

(E) Warfarin

695. A patient who underwent a liver transplant is found to be suffering from nephrotoxicity without any signs of bone marrow depression. This situation might arise from toxicity from which of the following agents?

(A) Azathioprine

(B) Cyclophosphamide

(C) Cyclosporine

(D) Muromonab-CD3 monoclonal antibody

(E) Prednisone

696. A patient became ill and vomited at a wedding reception where champagne was served. A week earlier, vaginal culture showed the presence of *Trichomonas vaginitis*. She was treated with an antiprotozoal agent. An interaction with alcohol best fits which antiprotozoal agent?

(A) Mebendazole

(B) Methimazole

(C) Metronidazole

(D) Primaquine

(E) Trimethoprim

697. Which of the following antiviral drugs is associated with the appropriate primary toxicity?

(A) Amantidine—neutropenia

(B) Didanosine—pancreatitis

(C) Ribavirin—hepatitis

(D) Ritonavir—hemolytic anemia

(E) Zidovudine—CNS stimulation, GI complaints

698. Because this anti-herpesvirus agent uses viral thymidine kinase as part of its activation pathway, resistance is associated with thymidine-kinase deficient strains of herpesvirus.

(A) Acyclovir

(B) Amantadine

(C) Foscarnet

(D) Saquinavir

(E) Zidovudine

699. Resistance to this agent used in *Escherichia coli* urinary tract infections can arise through bacterial expression of altered forms of dihydrofolate reductase acquired by spontaneous mutation or plasmid transfer.

(A) Amoxicillin

(B) Imipenem

(C) Methotrexate

(D) Sulfamethoxazole

(E) Trimethoprim

700. Because this antitubercular agent is an inducer of hepatic cytochrome P450, dosing regimens for oral anticoagulants must be adjusted when it is administered with them.

(A) Ethambutol

(B) Isoniazid

(C) Rifampin

(D) Streptomycin

(E) Sulfisoxazole

701. R.S. comes to migraine clinic with a complaint of poor control of her frequent migraine attacks. She would like a prophylactic drug that will reduce their frequency. Which of the following is most likely to be prescribed?

(A) Codeine

(B) Ergotamine

(C) Ibuprofen

(D) Propranolol

(E) Sumatriptan

702. A 47-year-old man being treated for moderately severe hypertension with this agent responded well with minimal adverse effects (tachycardia, which was treated with another agent). However, the patient now returns complaining of joint pains, fever, and a facial rash. The probable cause of these effects is

(A) captopril

(B) clonidine

(C) hydralazine

(D) hydrochlorothiazide

(E) methyldopa

703. A patient with type II (noninsulin-dependent) diabetes had been treated with an oral hypoglycemic agent for 2 years with good control of her blood sugar. After an attack of hepatitis, she develops severe lactic acidosis and dies. Which of the following agents is most likely to be involved in the lactic acidosis?

   (A) Glyburide
   (B) Metformin
   (C) Pioglitazone
   (D) Rosiglitazone
   (E) Tolbutamide

704. A 54-year-old flutist is treated for hypertension with this agent. Although his blood pressure was reduced, he complains that he is now unable to play his instrument because of a dry cough.

   (A) Captopril
   (B) Clonidine
   (C) Hydralazine
   (D) Prazosin
   (E) Propranolol

705. This cancer chemotherapeutic agent requires metabolism by cytochrome P450 for formation of the active alkylating species.

   (A) Bleomycin
   (B) Cisplatin
   (C) Cyclophosphamide
   (D) 5-Fluorouracil
   (E) Paclitaxel

706. This agent, used in treating testicular cancer, requires hydration and diuresis to prevent nephrotoxicity.

   (A) Bleomycin
   (B) Cisplatin
   (C) Cyclophosphamide
   (D) 5-Fluorouracil
   (E) Paclitaxel

707. This chemotherapeutic agent's mechanism of action involves inhibition of thymidylate synthase and incorporation into RNA.

   (A) Anastrozole
   (B) Cytarabine
   (C) Doxorubicin
   (D) 5-Fluorouracil
   (E) Methotrexate

708. This chemotherapeutic agent's mechanism of action involves inhibition of topoisomerase II and results in DNA strand breakage.

   (A) Dacarbazine
   (B) Etoposide
   (C) Lomustine
   (D) Prednisone
   (E) Vincristine

709. When a steady-state concentration of drug is present in the systemic circulation and equilibration between the systemic circulation and tissue compartments has been achieved, which of these fluid compartments has the largest total fluid–blood concentration ratio for the weak acid sulfadiazine ($pK_a = 6.5$)?

   (A) Alkalinized urine at pH 8.0
   (B) Acidified urine at pH 5.0
   (C) Breast milk at pH 6.4
   (D) Jejunum-ileum contents at pH 7.6
   (E) Stomach contents at pH 2.0

710. A 13-year-old boy with severe asthma has been treated for 6 months with good control of nocturnal wheezing. His parents now complain that he seems to be very fat around the face and shoulders, bruises easily, and has discolored streaks on his abdomen. Lab tests reveal moderate hyperglycemia. He has probably been receiving which of the following drugs?

   (A) Ipratropium
   (B) Prednisone
   (C) Salmeterol
   (D) Terbutaline
   (E) Theophylline

711. Which of the following is a correct statement regarding vasopressin (antidiuretic hormone [ADH]) and its actions?

(A) Ethanol stimulates vasopressin secretion.

(B) Hyperosmolality of the blood inhibits vasopressin secretion.

(C) The major site of action is the ascending limb of the loop of Henle.

(D) Thiazide diuretics are useful in treating nephrogenic (vasopressin-resistant) diabetes insipidus.

(E) Vasopressin relaxes vascular smooth muscle.

712. Which of the following statements combines a drug used clinically to prevent or relieve anginal pain with its correct mechanism of action?

(A) Isoproterenol—decreased myocardial contractile force

(B) Isosorbide dinitrate—increased extraction of oxygen from blood

(C) Nifedipine—selective venodilation and reduced cardiac size

(D) Nitroglycerin—increased diastolic cardiac filling

(E) Propranolol—decreased heart rate

713. Which of the following is (are) a possible adverse effect(s) of long-term chronic treatment of schizophrenia with a phenothiazine such as fluphenazine?

(A) Diarrhea, nausea, and vomiting

(B) Reduced secretion of prolactin

(C) Tardive dyskinesia

(D) Tourette syndrome

(E) Weight loss

714. Which of the following psychotropic drugs has the greatest sedative action?

(A) Buspirone

(B) Fluoxetine

(C) Haloperidol

(D) Lithium carbonate

(E) Mirtazapine

715. Which of the following is a predictable side effect of treatment with a monoamine oxidase inhibitor (MAOI) antidepressant?

(A) Chronic hypertension while taking the drug

(B) Hair loss

(C) Hypertensive reaction after eating foods containing serotonin

(D) Interaction with serotonin reuptake inhibitors

(E) Sedation

716. Which of the following is the drug of choice to reverse bronchoconstriction in an acute asthma attack?

(A) Albuterol

(B) Aminophylline

(C) Cromolyn

(D) Ipratropium

(E) Salmeterol

717. Which of the following drugs is useful in treatment of gouty arthritis because it inhibits the formation of uric acid?

(A) Allopurinol

(B) Colchicine

(C) Indomethacin

(D) Probenecid

(E) Sulfinpyrazone

718. Which of the following drugs can be used in rheumatoid arthritis with the lowest probable incidence of GI complications?

(A) Aspirin

(B) Ibuprofen

(C) Nabumetone

(D) Piroxicam

(E) Rofecoxib

719. Bromocriptine is used to treat which of the following conditions?

(A) Allergic rhinitis

(B) Bronchial asthma

(C) Diabetes insipidus

(D) Parkinsonism

(E) Peptic ulcer

Questions 720 and 721

In a study of cardiovascular drugs, normal volunteers were given drug X in a small bolus dose while blood pressure and heart rate were recorded. After recovery, a long-acting blocking agent, Y, was administered. The direct effects of Y were not recorded. After drug Y had equilibrated with the tissues of the body, drug X was repeated in the same dosage. The results are shown in Figure 6–3.

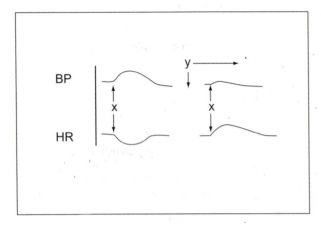

Figure 6–3

720. Drug X behaves most like

(A) bethanechol
(B) epinephrine
(C) isoproterenol
(D) norepinephrine
(E) phenylephrine

721. Drug Y behaves most like

(A) atropine
(B) pralidoxime
(C) prazosin
(D) reserpine
(E) timolol

722. The β-adrenoreceptor antagonist atenolol has a pA_2 value of 7.0 for cardiac muscle β-adrenoreceptors and a pA_2 value of 5.3 for lung β-adrenoreceptors. This suggests that atenolol

(A) has a greater efficacy in the heart than in the lung

(B) has greater efficacy in the lung than in the heart
(C) is equally potent in the heart and lung
(D) is more potent in blocking β-adrenoreceptors in the heart than in the lung
(E) is more potent in the lung than in the heart

723. In a functioning transplanted heart, which of the following agents would cause the greatest increase in heart rate?

(A) Amphetamine
(B) Cocaine
(C) Ephedrine
(D) Isoproterenol
(E) Phenylephrine

724. Which of the following agents produces vasodilation by increasing nitric oxide synthesis in endothelial cells?

(A) Diazoxide
(B) Histamine
(C) Minoxidil
(D) Nitroprusside
(E) Verapamil

725. A patient is scheduled for surgery that requires spinal anesthesia. This patient has documented allergy to ester-type local anesthetics. Which of the following local anesthetics should NOT be used?

(A) Etidocaine
(B) Lidocaine
(C) Mepivacaine
(D) Ropivacaine
(E) Tetracaine

726. A patient who previously suffered an allergic reaction to streptokinase when treated for acute myocardial infarction now returns to the hospital with a new coronary occlusion. Which of the following drugs is contraindicated?

(A) Abciximab
(B) Alteplase (t-PA)

(C) Anistreplase

(D) Clopidogrel

(E) Reteplase

727. Severe renal damage resulting from oxalate formation is characteristic of intoxication by

(A) ethanol

(B) ethylene glycol

(C) isopropanol

(D) methanol

(E) methylene chloride

728. Which of the following statements correctly associates a psychotherapeutic agent with a demonstrated effect on neurotransmitter mechanisms?

(A) Diazepam—facilitation of GABA-stimulated chloride channel opening

(B) Fluoxetine—selective inhibition of presynaptic norepinephrine uptake

(C) Pentobarbital—inhibition of NMDA receptors

(D) Tranylcypromine—inhibition of O-methylation of catecholamines

(E) Trifluoperazine—competitive antagonism of GABA$_A$ receptors

729. Which of the following agents is associated with numerous drug–drug interactions because of its inhibition of hepatic cytochrome P450 activity?

(A) Atracurium

(B) Cimetidine

(C) Cromolyn

(D) Diazepam

(E) Phenobarbital

730. Two members of the same family are admitted to the Emergency Department complaining of vomiting, abdominal cramps, and diarrhea. Examination reveals hypotension, tachycardia, possible difficulty swallowing, and upper extremity muscle weakness. Immediate liver function tests are within normal limits. During the next 24 hours their

condition improves and they ask to be discharged. However, 48 hours after admission some yellowing of their irises is noted and repeat liver function tests show significant elevation in serum alanine aminotransferase (ALT) and aspartate aminotransferase (AST) levels. What is the most probable cause of their illness?

(A) *Amanita muscaria* intoxication

(B) *Amanita virosa* intoxication

(C) Botulinum intoxication

(D) Scombroid fish intoxication

(E) Shellfish intoxication

731. Mr. K.L. has completed a course of cancer chemotherapy and now has severe anemia, neutropenia, and thrombocytopenia. If only one intervention is possible, which of the following is the most appropriate therapy?

(A) Epoetin-α (erythropoietin)

(B) Filgrastim (G-CSF)

(C) Growth hormone

(D) Sargramostim (GM-CSF)

(E) Testosterone

732. A single dose of propofol has a brief duration of action because it is

(A) eliminated by active tubular renal secretion

(B) metabolized rapidly in the blood

(C) metabolized rapidly in the brain

(D) rapidly redistributed

(E) very hydrophilic

733. Ketamine is characterized by which of the following pharmacologic properties?

(A) Association with disagreeable dreams during and after recovery

(B) Depression of blood pressure and heart rate in a dose-dependent fashion

(C) High minimum alveolar concentration (MAC) value

(D) Moderately high risk of bronchospasm

(E) Production of excellent skeletal muscle relaxation

734. The most rapid onset of action of inhaled general anesthetics correlates with the smallest value for the

   (A) blood-gas partition coefficient
   (B) MAC
   (C) oil–gas partition coefficient
   (D) onset of hepatic metabolism
   (E) rate of distribution from the blood

735. The MAC for which of the following inhaled general anesthetic agents exceeds normal atmospheric pressure?

   (A) Enflurane
   (B) Halothane
   (C) Isoflurane
   (D) Nitrous oxide
   (E) Sevoflurane

736. The agent of choice for chronic treatment of simple hypothyroidism (myxedema) is

   (A) desiccated thyroid
   (B) levothyroxine (T_4)
   (C) liothyronine (T_3)
   (D) potassium iodide
   (E) reverse T_3

737. K.R. is admitted to the hospital with signs of acute severe adrenal insufficiency (Addisonian crisis). Which of the following drug combinations is most appropriate?

   (A) Aldosterone and fludrocortisone
   (B) Cortisol and fludrocortisone
   (C) Dexamethasone and estrogen
   (D) Fludrocortisone and progesterone
   (E) Triamcinolone and betamethasone

738. A 24-year-old woman presents with hypertension and hypokalemic metabolic alkalosis. Although these symptoms are normally indicative of hyperaldosteronism, this patient's aldosterone levels are undetectable, and no other mineralocorticoid activity is found. A diagnosis of Liddle syndrome is made on the basis of the signs and symptoms and a family history. Liddle syndrome is caused by a genetic defect leading to excess expression of the apical sodium channel in the principal cells of the cortical collecting duct and excess sodium transport in this part of the nephron. Which of the following agents is the best choice for treatment of the hypertension and hypokalemic metabolic alkalosis in this patient?

   (A) Amiloride
   (B) Fludrocortisone
   (C) Hydrochlorothiazide
   (D) Lisinopril
   (E) Spironolactone

739. Which of the following correctly describes the mechanism of action of streptokinase?

   (A) Combines with plasminogen to form an enzymatically active complex
   (B) Competitively blocks binding of plasminogen to fibrin
   (C) Converts plasmin to plasminogen
   (D) Inhibits platelet cyclooxygenase activity
   (E) Provides a template for combination of thrombin and antithrombin III

740. T.R. is a 17-year-old patient who suffers from tonic–clonic seizures. This condition has been well controlled with a regimen of phenytoin. Which of the following signs or symptoms indicates phenytoin toxicity?

   (A) Diplopia and abnormal gait
   (B) Hyperprolactinemia
   (C) Polydipsia and polyuria
   (D) Postural hypotension
   (E) Rigidity and tremor

741. A substance that reduces the incidence of congenital neural tube defects is

   (A) β-carotene
   (B) folic acid
   (C) vitamin A
   (D) vitamin C (ascorbic acid)
   (E) vitamin E (α-tocopherol)

742. A 70-year-old man reports to the emergency room complaining of shortness of breath and a rapid, irregular heart beat. An ECG showed

the pattern shown in Figure 6–4, panel A. A diagnosis of atrial fibrillation, heart rate 140, is made. He is treated with an IV drug, which results in a change of the ECG to the pattern shown in panel B. This ECG was read as atrial fibrillation, heart rate 65. What drug was used?

A

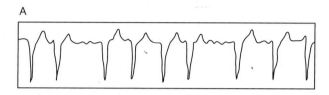

B

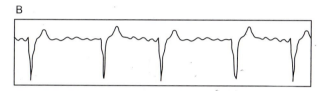

Figure 6–4

(A) Atropine
(B) Diltiazem
(C) Disopyramide
(D) Ibutilide
(E) Quinidine

743. Which of the following is a correct statement regarding the treatment of adverse effects of neuroleptic agents such as haloperidol?

(A) Acute dystonic reactions are best treated with clonidine.
(B) Akathisia is best treated by increasing the dosage of the neuroleptic.
(C) Neuroleptic malignant syndrome is first treated by administering a β-adrenoreceptor antagonist such as propranolol.
(D) Parkinsonian syndrome is best treated with anticholinergic agents such as benztropine.
(E) Tardive dyskinesia is best treated with levodopa.

744. A patient with AIDS has bacterial meningitis and is being treated with an antimicrobial agent cleared by both hepatic metabolism and renal excretion. The volume of distribu-

tion is 10 L and the half-life for elimination is 7 h in this patient. If the renal contribution to the plasma clearance of the drug is 8.3 mL/min, approximately what percentage of the drug's elimination can be attributed to hepatic metabolism?

(A) 10%
(B) 25%
(C) 50%
(D) 75%
(E) 90%

745. Patient W.W. has a bacterial infection that is to be treated with azithromycin. Which of the following mechanisms applies to azithromycin?

(A) Inhibition of peptide synthesis by binding to the 50S ribosome
(B) Inhibition of peptidoglycan chain elongation
(C) Inhibition of peptidoglycan cross-linking
(D) Inhibition of the formation of the ribosomal initiation complex
(E) Inhibition of topoisomerase II (DNA gyrase)

746. The target therapeutic plasma steady state concentration for drug Z is 500 μg/mL. When an IV loading dose of 30 mg is administered to a patient followed by the "standard" IV maintenance dosing rate of 30 mg/h, a plasma steady-state level of 300 μg/mL is obtained, too low to provide adequate therapy. Starting at the plasma concentration of 300 μg/mL, which of the following strategies will most safely achieve and maintain a plasma level of 500 μg/mL in this patient?

(A) Give 10 mg further loading dose as an IV bolus
(B) Give 20 mg further loading dose as an IV bolus
(C) Increase the maintenance infusion to 40 mg/h
(D) Increase the maintenance infusion to 45 mg/h
(E) Increase the maintenance infusion to 50 mg/h

747. A young boy was treated for 2 years with several antibacterial agents to eradicate tuberculosis. When entering school the following year, his teacher reports that he seems to be retarded. Upon investigation, he is found to have profound hearing loss. Which of the following agents may have been responsible for this hearing loss?

    (A) Ethambutol
    (B) Isoniazid
    (C) Pyrazinamide
    (D) Rifampin
    (E) Streptomycin

748. E.W. is a 40-pack-year ex-smoker with severe angina. In addition, he experiences periodic attacks of bronchospasm associated with chronic obstructive pulmonary disease. Which of the following regimens is most appropriate as treatment for his angina?

    (A) Atenolol and nitroglycerin
    (B) Diltiazem and isosorbide dinitrate
    (C) Isosorbide dinitrate and propranolol
    (D) Nitroglycerin and metoprolol
    (E) Verapamil and nifedipine

749. Regular (high-molecular-weight [HMW]) heparin differs from low-molecular-weight (LMW) heparin preparations in that

    (A) LMW heparin can be used by mouth; HMW heparin cannot
    (B) LMW heparin has a short half-life and must be given twice as often as HMW heparin
    (C) LMW heparin is indicated for use in acute coronary syndrome but not in deep venous thrombosis; HMW heparin is indicated in both
    (D) LMW heparin is not monitored by the activated partial thromboplastin time (aPPT) test; HMW heparin is
    (E) LMW heparin is safe in pregnancy; HMW heparin is teratogenic

750. Which of the following drugs exerts its effects through inhibition of cyclic GMP phosphodiesterase?

    (A) Hydralazine
    (B) Minoxidil
    (C) Nitroprusside
    (D) Prazosin
    (E) Sildenafil

Questions 751 through 753

P.D. is a 57-year-old obese woman with type II (noninsulin-dependent) diabetes mellitus of 15 years duration. Because her hyperglycemia is not well controlled with diet and oral hypoglycemic agents, she self-administers insulin injections. She comes to her physician's office with a fever and a draining external ear infection; *Pseudomonas aeruginosa* is cultured from the drainage.

751. Which of the following insulin regimens most closely mimics insulin release from a normally functioning pancreas?

    (A) Pre-breakfast and pre-dinner injections of lente insulin plus a pre-snack injection of regular insulin
    (B) Pre-meal injections of insulin lispro plus morning and evening injections of lente insulin
    (C) Pre-meal injections of NPH insulin plus an injection of insulin lispro at bedtime
    (D) Post-meal injection of lente insulin plus a pre-breakfast injection of regular insulin
    (E) Post-meal injections of insulin lispro

752. Which of the following drugs or drug combinations is appropriate treatment for the *P. aeruginosa* infection in this patient?

    (A) Chloramphenicol
    (B) Nafcillin plus kanamycin
    (C) Sulfamethoxazole plus trimethoprim
    (D) Tetracycline
    (E) Ticarcillin plus tobramycin

753. Two years after the infection described, the patient returns complaining of severe bloating after meals, which is sometimes followed by vomiting. A diagnosis of diabetic gastroparesis is made. Which of the following

agents is most useful in treating this patient's GI problem?

(A) Diphenhydramine
(B) Metoclopramide
(C) Omeprazole
(D) Ondansetron
(E) Scopolamine

754. A 20-year-old man suffers a broken arm in a bicycle accident. After a cast is applied he is to be discharged from the Emergency Department with a prescription for an analgesic to be used if over-the-counter acetaminophen or NSAIDs are not effective in providing pain relief. Which of the following is the best choice for prescription pain relief in this case?

(A) Codeine
(B) Diphenoxylate
(C) Meperidine
(D) Methadone
(E) Morphine

755. On the basis of their mechanisms of action, which of the following combinations of drugs produces a beneficial additive or synergistic effect in therapy when each agent is present at its effective concentration?

(A) Chlortetracycline plus amoxicillin
(B) Clomiphene plus chorionic gonadotropin
(C) Lovastatin plus cholestyramine
(D) Pentazocine plus morphine
(E) Succinylcholine plus atracurium

756. Figure 6–5 shows the quantal population dose–response curves for the therapeutic and toxic effects of drugs X and Y. Both drugs are agonists at the same receptor to produce the therapeutic response, and the maximum responses obtained with each agent are the same. The toxicity curve in the figure shows the superimposed toxic response curves for drugs X and Y; they are identical in terms of the concentration dependence. Which of the following statements is most correct?

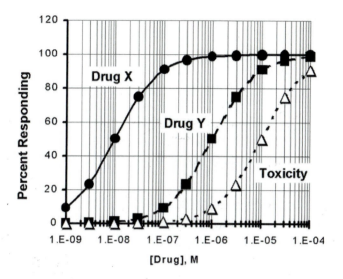

Figure 6–5

(A) At 1×10^{-5} M both drugs cause adverse effects in 90% to 100% of patients.
(B) Drug X has a larger therapeutic index than drug Y.
(C) Drug X is more efficacious than drug Y.
(D) Drug Y is more potent than drug X.
(E) Drug Y is safer than drug X.

757. A 78-year-old man has ankle edema, tachycardia, and shortness of breath on mild exercise. His blood pressure is 155/98. He has been diagnosed with hypertension and mild congestive heart failure. Which of the following regimens is most appropriate for starting therapy?

(A) Captopril plus dobutamine
(B) Captopril plus hydralazine
(C) Enalapril plus hydrochlorothiazide
(D) Furosemide plus spironolactone
(E) Losartan plus hydralazine

758. Figure 6–6 shows measurements of systolic blood pressure (top of bars), mean pressure (filled circle), and diastolic pressure (bottom of bars) in a normal subject. The solid bar at the top of the figure shows the duration for an IV infusion of a constant, low concentration of drug X. The arrow shows the point at which an IV bolus of drug X was administered. Drug X is

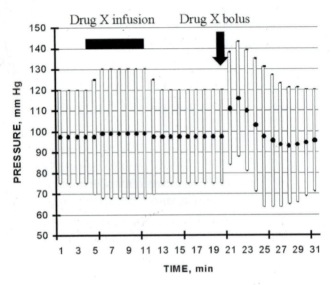

Figure 6–6

(A) acetylcholine
(B) amphetamine
(C) epinephrine
(D) norepinephrine
(E) phenylephrine

759. An asthmatic 63-year-old woman is admitted to the hospital suffering from palpitations and syncopal episodes (fainting spells). She is found to be hypotensive and her ECG shows a very rapid AV nodal reentrant tachycardia. Which of the following drugs provides appropriate acute treatment of this condition?

(A) Adenosine
(B) Bethanechol
(C) Isoproterenol
(D) Propranolol
(E) Quinidine

760. A 38-year-old man has been treated for myasthenia gravis with pyridostigmine and propantheline for 8 years. He has had the "flu" for 10 days and his wife calls reporting that he now has serious muscle weakness. What course of action should be followed after admitting this patient to the Emergency Department?

(A) Administer a test dose of edrophonium
(B) Administer a test dose of tubocurarine
(C) Administer atropine to reverse the effects of an overdose
(D) Administer pralidoxime on the assumption that he inadvertently overdosed
(E) Administer the daily dose of pyridostigmine on the assumption that he forgot to take his medication

761. A 75-year-old man has prostate cancer that has metastasized to bone. He is receiving hormonal therapy to slow progression of the neoplasm and codeine by mouth when it is absolutely required, but still complains of severe pain. What should be done about this symptom?

(A) He should be given additional codeine when he complains
(B) He should be given aspirin and told that additional narcotics cannot be used because he would become tolerant to their analgesic action
(C) He should be given a strong NSAID such as naproxen as needed to supplement his codeine therapy
(D) He should be given morphine in a long-acting oral preparation on a regular schedule and parenteral morphine when pain breaks through
(E) He should be given parenteral morphine when pain requires it

762. In a study of a new drug, the agent was administered to anesthetized animals while blood pressure, heart rate, and salivation were recorded. The results of a typical experiment are shown in Figure 6–7. What is the best characterization of this new agent?

(A) α-Adrenoreceptor agonist
(B) α-Adrenoreceptor antagonist
(C) Cholinesterase inhibitor

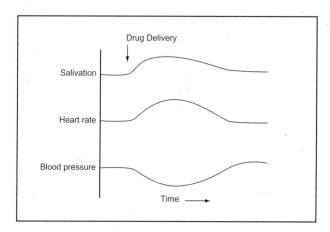

Drug Delivery

Salivation

Heart rate

Blood pressure

Time →

Figure 6–7

(D) Direct-acting muscarinic agonist
(E) Ganglionic nicotinic agonist

763. After administration of drug X, IV isoproterenol still causes tachycardia but no longer
causes a drop in blood pressure. What is the
site of drug X's action?

(A) α-Adrenoreceptors in blood vessels
(B) $β_1$-Adrenoreceptors in heart
(C) $β_2$-Adrenoreceptors in blood vessels
(D) M_2 muscarinic cholinoceptors in heart
(E) N_G nicotinic cholinoceptors in ganglia

764. Carbidopa is often used in patients with
Parkinson disease because it

(A) acts on D_2 receptors in the basal ganglia
(B) inhibits the metabolism of dopamine in
the blood and peripheral tissues
(C) inhibits the metabolism of dopamine in
the brain
(D) inhibits the metabolism of levodopa in
the brain
(E) inhibits the metabolism of levodopa in
peripheral tissues

765. B.L. is to receive chemotherapy for cancer.
The oncologist plans to use ondansetron to
reduce the nausea and vomiting associated
with the chemotherapeutic agents. What is
the mechanism of action of ondansetron?

(A) Cannabinoid receptor agonist
(B) Corticosteroid agonist
(C) Dopamine antagonist

(D) H_1 histamine antagonist
(E) Serotonin 5-HT_3 antagonist

766. Your new patient suffers from both rheumatoid
arthritis and gout. Which of the following analgesics provides appropriate coverage for moderately severe pain during acute flares of gout
and the chronic pain of rheumatoid arthritis?

(A) Aspirin
(B) Codeine
(C) Colchicine
(D) Ibuprofen
(E) Morphine

767. The neurotoxic actions of botulinum toxin are
associated with

(A) blockade of cholinergic nerve transmit-
ter exocytosis
(B) inhibition of smooth muscle myosin
light chain kinase
(C) irreversible inhibition of cholinesterase
(D) nicotinic receptor blockade
(E) reversal by infusion of large doses of
choline

768. H.R. has post-cataract surgery glaucoma, a
moderate elevation of intraocular pressure
that often follows replacement of the crystalline lens. Which of the following is a rational choice for treatment and the correct
mechanism for that drug?

(A) Atracurium—increased outflow of aqueous humor
(B) Dorzolamide—increased outflow of
aqueous humor
(C) Latanoprost—increased outflow of aqueous humor
(D) Pilocarpine—decreased synthesis of
aqueous humor
(E) Timolol—increased outflow of aqueous
humor

769. C.R. has started taking a medication for a psychiatric condition and has blood drawn weekly for complete blood counts. A psychotropic drug that causes agranulocytosis in up to 2% of patients is

    (A) amitriptylline
    (B) clozapine
    (C) haloperidol
    (D) lithium carbonate
    (E) thioridazine

770. Which of the following correctly describes the antiarrhythmic mechanism of action for ibutilide?

    (A) Blockade of cardiac β_1-adrenoreceptors
    (B) Blockade of delayed rectifier potassium channels
    (C) Blockade of voltage-dependent calcium channels
    (D) Blockade of voltage-dependent sodium channels
    (E) Opening of diastolic potassium channels

771. Oral anticoagulants such as warfarin exert their anticoagulant effects by

    (A) acting as a template for complexing thrombin and antithrombin III
    (B) breaking down thrombin
    (C) forming an active complex with plasminogen
    (D) inhibiting calcium binding to coagulation factors
    (E) inhibiting hepatic posttranslational carboxylation of coagulation factors

772. Potassium supplementation is often necessary for patients taking large doses of

    (A) amiloride
    (B) captopril
    (C) hydrochlorothiazide
    (D) losartan
    (E) spironolactone

773. Figure 6–8 illustrates a current concept of the control of gastric acid secretion. Which of the following drugs acts at the site labeled H_2?

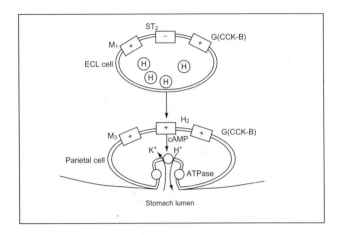

Figure 6–8

    (A) Aluminum hydroxide
    (B) Misoprostol
    (C) Omeprazole
    (D) Ranitidine
    (E) Sucralfate

774. Which of the following statements is correct regarding the use of ACE inhibitors?

    (A) ACE inhibitors are contraindicated in pregnancy.
    (B) ACE inhibitors are of little value in therapy of CHF.
    (C) Chronic therapy with ACE inhibitors impairs renal function in diabetics.
    (D) Rebound hypertension after abrupt cessation of therapy is a frequent problem.
    (E) The use of ACE inhibitors depresses renin activity.

775. Which of the following antidepressants is most selective in blocking reuptake of serotonin as compared with norepinephrine?

    (A) Amitriptyline
    (B) Citalopram
    (C) Desipramine
    (D) Imipramine
    (E) Trazodone

776. The most common problem associated with use of NSAIDs such as ibuprofen is

(A) bronchospasm
(B) drowsiness
(C) fluid retention
(D) GI complaints
(E) increased bleeding tendency

777. Megaloblastic anemia associated with gastrectomy is best treated with

(A) IM iron dextran
(B) IM vitamin B_{12}
(C) oral ferric chloride
(D) oral folic acid
(E) oral vitamin B_{12}

778. The actions of tamoxifen are best described by which of the following statements?

(A) Estrogen agonist in breast and bone
(B) Estrogen antagonist in breast; progesterone partial agonist in uterus
(C) Estrogen partial agonist in breast; agonist in bone
(D) Progesterone agonist in uterus
(E) Progesterone partial agonist in uterus

779. Which of the following items correctly associates the mechanism of action with the corresponding agent used in hyperlipidemia?

(A) Cholestyramine—increased activity of lipoprotein lipase
(B) Clofibrate—decreased activity of lipoprotein lipase
(C) Gemfibrozil—inhibition of microsomal triglyceride transfer protein
(D) Nicotinic acid—altered excretion of bile acids
(E) Simvastatin—inhibition of HMG-CoA reductase

780. Calcium disodium edetate is most effective as an antidote for poisoning with

(A) arsenic
(B) atropine
(C) iron

(D) lead
(E) mercury

781. The current drug of choice for treatment of roundworm (Ascaris) infections is

(A) diethylcarbamazine
(B) ivermectin
(C) mebendazole
(D) niclosamide
(E) praziquantel

782. G.W. is planning a trip to Africa. In the absence of contraindications, which of the following drugs should be prescribed as prophylaxis against falciparum malaria?

(A) Chloroquine
(B) Ciprofloxacin
(C) Doxycycline
(D) Mefloquine
(E) Pyrimethamine plus sulfadoxine

783. The leukotrienes LTC_4, LTD_4, and LTE_4

(A) are chemotactic agents for polymorphonuclear leukocytes
(B) are potent bronchoconstrictor substances
(C) are synthesized and stored in platelet granules
(D) have few cardiovascular effects
(E) have their biosynthesis greatly reduced by aspirin

784. Which of the following correctly matches an antiseizure agent with its mechanism of action?

(A) Carbamazepine—blockade of calcium channels
(B) Ethosuximide—activation of chloride channels
(C) Lamotrigine—activation of potassium channels
(D) Tiagabine—inhibition of the uptake of GABA
(E) Vigabatrin—competitive blockade of $GABA_A$ receptor

785. The mechanism of anesthetic action for local anesthetic agents involves

(A) blockade of axonal voltage-dependent calcium channels
(B) blockade of axonal voltage-dependent sodium channels
(C) hyperpolarization of axons via enhanced chloride influx
(D) hyperpolarization of axons via enhanced potassium efflux
(E) inhibition of nerve terminal pain receptors

786. Acute intoxication with antihistamines (H_1-receptor antagonists) in children is correctly described as

(A) causing severe respiratory depression early
(B) being characterized by hypothermia
(C) producing a state similar to atropine poisoning
(D) producing joint pain
(E) treatable with histamine therapy

787. Which of the following associates the correct mechanism of action with the drug used in type II (noninsulin-dependent) diabetes?

(A) Acarbose—reduction of insulin resistance
(B) Glipizide—inhibition of intestinal α-glucosidase
(C) Metformin—inhibition of ATP-sensitive potassium channels
(D) Repaglinide—modulation of pancreatic insulin release
(E) Rosiglitazone—reduction in circulating glucagon levels

788. Which of the following properties best correlates with the rate of recovery from anesthesia for a series of inhaled general anesthetic agents, each administered at its MAC partial pressure?

(A) Anesthetic potency
(B) Blood–gas partition coefficient
(C) Lipid solubility
(D) MAC for anesthesia
(E) Water solubility

789. Which of the following agents is used in thyroid storm because of its ability to inhibit both thyroid iodine organification and peripheral deiodination of thyroxine to tri-iodothyronine?

(A) Potassium perchlorate
(B) Propranolol
(C) Propylthiouracil
(D) Radioactive iodine (^{131}I)
(E) Reverse T_3

790. Which of the following drugs is used to promote ovulation through inhibitory actions in the hypothalamus?

(A) Cabergoline
(B) Clomiphene
(C) Ethinyl estradiol
(D) Norethindrone
(E) Progesterone

791. The table below provides several possible descriptions of the actions of nondepolarizing neuromuscular blockers such as tubocurarine. Which description is most accurate?

Choice	Train of Four Stimulation	Posttetanic Potentiation	Reversal by Neostigmine
(A)	Fade	No	No
(B)	Constant	Yes	No
(C)	Fade	No	Yes
(D)	Fade	Yes	Yes
(E)	Constant	Yes	Yes

792. A.H. has severe skeletal muscle spasms due to cerebral palsy. What is the site of action of dantrolene when used in the treatment of skeletal muscle spasticity?

(A) α_2-Adrenoreceptors in the spinal cord
(B) GABA receptors in the brain
(C) Glycine receptors in the spinal cord
(D) Neuromuscular junction of skeletal muscle
(E) Sarcoplasmic reticulum calcium channels

793. Which of the following agents is most effective as a cardiac stimulant in the treatment of severe β-blocker overdose?

(A) Atrial natriuretic peptide
(B) Epinephrine
(C) Glucagon
(D) Human growth hormone
(E) Insulin

794. At a blood alcohol level of 200 mg/dL (0.2%), which of the following correctly describes the systemic elimination process for ethanol?

(A) Constant clearance via liver, kidney, and lungs
(B) First-order elimination via pulmonary exhalation
(C) First-order elimination via renal excretion
(D) Second-order elimination via biliary secretion
(E) Zero-order elimination via hepatic metabolism

795. During the course of an ophthalmologic examination, W. H. was treated topically with eye drops. Two days later she complained that she was blinded by bright light the first day and is still unable to read. She had probably been given

(A) echothiophate
(B) edrophonium
(C) homatropine
(D) phenylephrine
(E) tropicamide

796. A patient is admitted to a drug detoxification program after a history of repeated bouts of increased motor activity, loss of appetite, and excitement. After very high-dose abuse of this drug, stereotyped and psychotic behavior was observed. Finally, significant tolerance developed. The drug used by this patient is

(A) amphetamine
(B) cocaine
(C) ethanol

(D) heroin
(E) tetrahydrocannabinol

797. The mechanism of action for the therapeutic effect of saquinavir involves

(A) incorporation into RNA
(B) inhibition of thymidylate synthase
(C) inhibition of viral DNA polymerase
(D) inhibition of viral protease
(E) inhibition of viral reverse transcriptase

798. B.T. is a tall, thin 58-year-old postmenopausal woman of northern European origin. She has been diagnosed with osteoporosis after measurements of bone density. She has a strong family history of breast cancer and is concerned about her high risk for this disease. Which of the following agents offers the best single treatment choice for osteoporosis in this patient?

(A) Alendronate
(B) Conjugated estrogen
(C) Dietary calcium supplementation
(D) Parathyroid hormone (PTH)
(E) Raloxifene

799. An unconscious 48-year-old man is brought to the Emergency Department following an industrial fire. He appears flushed but is not breathing spontaneously. His blood pressure on artificial ventilation is 100/60 and heart rate 120. A sample of venous blood is bright red. Coworkers report that he complained of headache before losing consciousness but was not coughing. What is the most likely cause of his inhalation toxicity?

(A) Carbon monoxide
(B) Carbon tetrachloride
(C) Nitrogen dioxide
(D) Ozone
(E) Sulfur dioxide

Answers and Explanations

674. (D) The maintenance dosing rate (D/T) is calculated using the formula D/T = target × CL/F, where D is the dose administered, T is the time interval between doses, target is the desired steady-state plasma concentration (for which the effective plasma concentration is used), CL is the systemic clearance, and F is the fractional absorption. After multiplying the clearance (50 L/h) times the effective plasma concentration (0.02 mg/L), the resulting product of 1 mg/h must be divided by the fractional absorption of 0.25, giving a dosing rate of 4 mg/h. Note that the units for clearance and target concentration must be consistent with respect to volume. The extensive first-pass metabolism of propranolol means that to achieve the same systemic concentration, an oral dose four times larger than the intravenous dose must be administered.

675. (C) The nondepolarizing blocking agent pancuronium acts as a nicotinic receptor antagonist at the neuromuscular junction and prevents depolarization. It has a prolonged action of 60 minutes or more, so rapid pharmacologic reversal is appropriate under the conditions described. A drug that increases (amplifies) the actions of physiologically released acetylcholine in the neuromuscular synapse is needed. Neostigmine is the best choice because it blocks acetylcholinesterase, amplifying the action of released acetylcholine and, unlike physostigmine, enters the CNS poorly. Atracurium (choice A) is a nicotinic receptor antagonist like pancuronium. Bethanechol (choice B) is a direct-acting muscarinic agonist with negligible action at nicotinic sites. The anticholinesterase physostig-

mine (choice D) increases acetylcholine concentrations, but is undesirable in this situation because it enters the CNS and may cause convulsions. Pralidoxime (choice E) is an important agent for reactivation of acetylcholinesterase that has been inhibited by organophosphates, but has no use in this case.

676. (E) The elevated body temperature without perspiration, but with dilated pupils and elevated heart rate, indicate parasympathetic blockade, such as might occur with atropine intoxication and blockage of muscarinic receptors. The delusional state indicates central nervous system (CNS) involvement. Scopolamine and similar antimuscarinic compounds are found in the seeds and leaves of plants such as Jimson weed (*Datura* species). Symptomatic management (temperature control, sedation, restraint) is often adequate in mild intoxications. If required, pharmacologic treatment consists of inhibition of acetylcholinesterase to increase concentrations of acetylcholine at muscarinic synapses in the CNS and peripheral tissues. Physostigmine will accomplish this. Carbachol (choice A) is a muscarinic agonist, but does not have CNS activity because, as a charged molecule, it does not cross the blood–brain barrier. Ipratropium (choice B) is a muscarinic antagonist administered by inhalation for the acute treatment of asthma. Methscopolamine (choice C) is a muscarinic antagonist like scopolamine that would exacerbate the toxicity. Neostigmine (choice D) is a cholinesterase inhibitor but, unlike physostigmine, does not enter the CNS because of its positive charge and low lipid solubility. This difference in distribution between physostigmine and neostigmine is the reason for using neostigmine, but not physostigmine, for treatment of myasthenia gravis, where central effects of the drug are undesirable.

677. **(B)** Clonidine, an α_2-adrenoreceptor agonist, acts at the level of the vasomotor centers in the brainstem to decrease sympathetic outflow, thus decreasing synaptic norepinephrine release and reducing its diffusion into the blood. Amphetamine (choice A) is an indirect-acting sympathomimetic agent that elevates plasma norepinephrine and blood pressure by causing nonexocytotic release of norepinephrine from sympathetic nerve endings. Phentolamine (choice C) is a nonselective α-adrenoreceptor antagonist that blocks arteriolar alpha receptors, lowers blood pressure, and causes a compensatory (reflex) increase in norepinephrine release. Phenoxybenzamine (choice D) is another α-adrenoreceptor antagonist that increases norepinephrine release by the same mechanism. Prazosin (choice E), an α_1-selective adrenoreceptor antagonist, also lowers blood pressure by blockade of arteriolar α_1 receptors and causes a reflex stimulation of the sympathetic nervous system and release of synaptic norepinephrine.

678. **(A)** The description of this patient is characteristic of the presentation of congestive heart failure (CHF). Goals in the treatment of CHF include decreasing the cardiac workload including preload and afterload, reducing sodium and fluid retention, and increasing myocardial contractility. ACE inhibitors decrease ventricular preload and afterload through the inhibition of ACE and the consequent decrease in production of the pressor peptide angiotensin II, along with prolongation of the actions of the vasodilator peptide bradykinin that is normally degraded by ACE. ACE inhibition also reduces angiotensin II–dependent augmentation of sympathetic nervous system activity. Decreased intrarenal levels of angiotensin II help correct CHF-induced salt and water retention by the kidney. Because aldosterone production in the adrenal cortex is also regulated by an-

giotensin II, the mineralocorticoid actions that promote sodium retention are also lessened. At the level of the heart, the use of ACE inhibitors decreases hypertrophy and ventricular remodeling associated with CHF. All of these factors support the use of ACE inhibitors as first-line drugs in the chronic treatment of CHF. Choice B is incorrect in that ACE inhibitors exert no direct effects on coronary perfusion. Choice C is incorrect because efficiency of oxygen extraction by muscle is unaffected by ACE inhibitors. Choice D is incorrect because ACE inhibitors exert no direct effects on cardiac force or rate. Choice E is incorrect. Use of ACE inhibitors *reduces* ventricular remodeling and compensatory enlargement, a very valuable effect in CHF.

679. **(B)** Rapid worsening of pulmonary congestion is suggestive of life-threatening acute cardiac decompensation. Rapid pulmonary vasodilation and reduction of preload through excretion of retained salt and water are very effective in the immediate treatment of this condition. Furosemide, a loop diuretic, is one of the most effective agents available because it has powerful diuretic action and also reduces pulmonary vascular pressures. Amiloride (choice A) is a much less efficacious diuretic with primary action in the collecting tubule of the nephron and little effect on pulmonary vessels. Hydrochlorothiazide (choice C) is a diuretic of intermediate efficacy that acts in the distal convoluted tubule. Losartan (choice D) is an angiotensin receptor blocker and is not effective in acute reduction of congestive symptoms. Metoprolol (choice E) is an α-adrenoreceptor blocker that is valuable in the long-term, chronic therapy of CHF, but not effective (and sometimes contraindicated) in acute decompensation. Morphine has also been used for acute pulmonary edema and is usually effective.

680. **(A)** Cardiac arrhythmias are the most common serious adverse effects of cardiac glycosides. These arrhythmias may affect any part of the heart and are particularly dangerous when they involve the ventricles. Other adverse effects of digoxin include GI upset

and neuroendocrine abnormalities. Although captopril is used in the treatment of hypertension, there is no significant hypotensive interaction between digoxin and captopril (choice D). Digoxin does not cause hypokalemia (choice C), although massive digoxin overdose may cause *hyper*kalemia by inhibiting the sodium pump in all tissues. ACE inhibitors such as captopril may cause renal insufficiency in patients with preexisting renal disease, but they do not interfere with the excretion of digoxin (choice E) unless renal damage is marked. Increased bradykinin levels, which may result from the action of captopril, do not result in β-adrenoreceptor desensitization (choice B).

681. **(C)** Hepatic intracellular cholesterol levels are tightly controlled through regulation of endocytotic uptake of cholesterol within LDL particles, de novo synthesis of cholesterol, incorporation into VLDL particles, and loss due to conversion to bile acids. Inhibition of cholesterol biosynthesis through statin inhibition of the enzyme 3-hydroxymethylglutaryl-CoA reductase (HMG-CoA reductase) lowers intracellular cholesterol levels. This lowering results in increased expression of the genes for the LDL receptor and HMG-CoA reductase. Increased expression of LDL receptors leads to increased endocytic uptake of LDL particles from the blood and consequent reduction of circulating levels of LDL cholesterol. This dependence on increased synthesis of LDL receptors explains why patients homozygous for defective LDL receptors (familial hypercholesterolemia) have extremely high levels of LDL cholesterol that do not respond to statin treatment. Choice D is incorrect because the statins do not affect hepatic VLDL secretion. Inhibition of VLDL secretion is probably the mechanism of action for nicotinic acid in lowering VLDL and LDL. Choice E is incorrect because the statins do not affect lecithin:cholesterol acyltransferase (LCAT) activity. Binding to PPAR-α and activation of lipoprotein lipase (choice A) appears to be the mechanism for lowering elevated VLDL levels by the fibric acids such as gemfibrozil. Bile acid–binding resins such as cholestyramine promote increased fecal excretion of bile acids (choice B) and ultimately lead to increased expression of hepatic LDL receptors.

682. **(D)** P-glycoprotein, the product of the MDR genes, is an ATP-dependent efflux protein that pumps a number of structurally dissimilar drugs out of cells. The chemotherapeutic agents named in this question have dissimilar mechanisms of action, but are all substrates for P-glycoprotein. Doxorubicin and dactinomycin are DNA-intercalating agents and are not cell-cycle–specific in their actions. Paclitaxel and vincristine are M-phase specific agents that promote and inhibit microtubule formation, respectively. Deletion of deoxycytidine kinase (choice E) is a mechanism for resistance to cytosine arabinoside. Increased activity of dihydrofolate reductase (choice B) is a mechanism for resistance to methotrexate. Decreased doubling time so that a smaller percentage of cells are caught in S phase (choice A) applies only to S phase-specific agents such as 5-fluorouracil. Increased activity of DNA repair (choice C) is a mechanism for resistance specific to DNA alkylating agents.

683. **(E)** Unregulated herbal preparations are in heavy use by the public and several have been documented to interact with regularly prescribed drugs. Ma-huang (choice E) contains the indirect-acting sympathomimetic ephedrine in varying concentrations and therefore can additively interact with other sympathomimetic stimulants such as amphetamine, cocaine, or phenylpropanolamine. Stroke, arrhythmias, or myocardial infarction may result. Echinacea (choice A) has no reported drug interactions to date but many preparations contain alcohol, which may add to alcohol-containing beverages. Gingko biloba (choice B) has antiplatelet activity and should not be used with aspirin or other antiplatelet drugs. Ginseng (choice C) may cause CNS stimulation and should not be used by patients taking psychoactive drugs. Kava (choice D) has sedative actions and interacts additively with sedative-hypnotics and sedative-antihistaminics.

684. (A) Open-angle glaucoma is treated either by increasing outflow of aqueous humor or by decreasing production of aqueous humor by the ciliary body. Miosis and cyclospasm, which can increase outflow, are produced by direct muscarinic stimulation with agonists such as pilocarpine or by inhibition of acetylcholinesterase with drugs such as physostigmine. The carbonic anhydrase inhibitors dorzolamide and acetazolamide decrease production of aqueous humor. β-Blockers inhibit production of aqueous humor. Topical timolol is a widely used agent for treatment of glaucoma. However, it can undergo systemic absorption from the nasolacrimal system. Use of β-blockers may precipitate an asthmatic attack, and their use is contraindicated in severely asthmatic patients. Drug allergy (choice B) might cause angioedema with breathing difficulties, but this condition would not be immediately resolved with inhaled albuterol. Hemolysis (choice C) may produce breathing difficulties, but this condition would not be immediately resolved with inhaled albuterol, a β-adrenoreceptor agonist used in asthma attacks. An idiosyncratic response to timolol (choice D) might also result in breathing difficulties, but the response to albuterol again points to β-blockade–induced bronchoconstriction. Induction of RBC sickling (choice E) may also cause breathing difficulties, but this condition would also not be resolved with inhaled albuterol.

685. (E) Carbamazepine is a drug of choice for treatment of partial seizures. Its pharmacokinetic profile is complex because a number of other drugs as well as the drug itself can induce carbamazepine metabolism and reduce its blood levels. However, diplopia and ataxia are indicative of carbamazepine toxicity (*increased* blood levels of the drug). Drugs inhibiting the hepatic P450 isoforms that metabolize the drug result in a rise in steady-state carbamazepine plasma concentrations if the dosing regimen is not adjusted. Cimetidine, often used for the treatment of peptic ulcer (choice E), is a potent inhibitor of hepatic P450. Phenobarbital (choice A) is an *inducer* of hepatic drug metabolism and its

coadministration is expected to *decrease* carbamazepine steady-state levels. Coadministration of probenecid, an inhibitor of active uric acid tubular reabsorption for gout (choice B), should have no effect because hepatic metabolism rather than renal excretion controls elimination of the drug. Hydrochlorothiazide for hypertension (choice C) should have no effect on carbamazepine steady-state levels because hepatic metabolism rather than renal excretion is responsible for its clearance. Smoking (choice D) induces hepatic drug metabolism and is expected to decrease carbamazepine levels.

686. (E) The apparent volume of distribution is calculated using the equation $V_d = X/C$, where V_d is the volume of distribution, X is the amount of drug present in the body, and C is the plasma (or blood) concentration. We must use time 0 for our calculations because this is the only time at which we know the amount of drug in the body; after administration it is immediately subjected to elimination. The curvature seen in the early data points results from distribution of the drug from blood into tissue compartments. The linear portion of the data reflects the elimination process and must be extrapolated back to time 0 to determine the plasma concentration that would have been obtained if distribution had been instantaneous. The administered dose of 100 mg divided by the extrapolated plasma concentration of 1 µg/mL (or 1 mg/L) yields an apparent V_d of 100 L. Volume of distribution is a useful parameter that describes the relationship between the administered dose and the resulting plasma concentration. It is used for calculating loading doses.

687. (C) Using the extrapolated linear portion of the data, the concentration at time 0 is 1 µg/mL. By definition, the elimination half-life is the time interval for a 50% reduction in concentration for single-dose drug disappearance under conditions when the drug disappearance is controlled by the elimination process. The plasma concentration of 0.5 µg/mL is achieved after 3 h. The elimination half-life provides information necessary for calculation of the dosing interval for maintenance dosing regimens that achieve and maintain the plasma concentration at a specified concentration without excessive swings in the concentration. Half-life can also be calculated if both volume of distribution and clearance are known from the equation $t_{1/2} = V_d \times 0.693 / CL$, where 0.693 is the natural logarithm of 2.

688. **(D)** By inspection of the graph, it is observed that administration of sodium bicarbonate increases the rate of elimination of the drug (the slope of the line increases and the half-life is shortened). Sodium bicarbonate causes alkalinization of urinary pH. Alkalinization causes increased ionization of weak acids and accelerates their urinary excretion; the ionized (charged) forms cannot be easily reabsorbed through the tubular epithelium, whereas the uncharged forms of many weak acids are readily reabsorbed. Urinary alkalinization is a strategy sometimes used to hasten the excretion of weak acids such as aspirin in overdose situations. Excretion of a nonelectrolyte (choice A) is unaffected by changes in urinary pH because the polarity of nonelectrolytes is insensitive to pH. A strong acid (choice B) is fully ionized (unprotonated) at all attainable urinary pH values so that alteration of urinary pH has no effect on its excretion. A strong base (choice C) is protonated and charged at all attainable urinary pH values so that alteration of urinary pH has no effect on its excretion. Excretion of a weak base (choice E) is slowed by alkalinization of urinary pH because the uncharged form of the base that is readily reabsorbed from the tubular urine predominates.

689. **(A)** Immediate administration of one aspirin tablet by mouth (choice A) has been shown to reduce morbidity and mortality from myocardial infarction. Because this dose is essentially free from adverse effects, this therapy is appropriate even before the diagnosis is confirmed by ECG or other means. Dobutamine (choice B) is a β_1-selective agonist that has positive inotropic action. It is not appropriate at this time because there is no evidence of contractile failure. Lidocaine (choice C), an antiarrhythmic, is not appropriate at this time because the patient is in sinus rhythm with only occasional arrhythmic beats. Metoprolol (choice D), a β-blocking drug, is often used after the acute period of a myocardial infarction, but is inappropriate until the patient's condition is stabilized. Streptokinase (choice E), a thrombolytic agent, is inappropriate because coronary thrombosis has not been confirmed and this IV drug is given in the hospital setting.

690. **(C)** The description of the patient's reduced cardiac function and elevated left ventricular filling pressure, with reduced peripheral perfusion (clouded mentation, reduced urine output) indicates cardiogenic shock. In cardiogenic shock, an agent is needed that increases myocardial contractility without increasing heart rate and peripheral resistance. Dobutamine (choice C), a selective β_1-adrenoreceptor agonist, increases myocardial contractility without producing an increase in peripheral resistance and may even lower resistance slightly. Atenolol (choice A), a β_1-selective blocker, is inappropriate in the setting of reduced cardiac function, although it may be quite appropriate later when the patient's condition is stabilized. Epidemiologic evidence shows that chronic therapy with β-blockers reduces mortality after recovery from an acute MI. Digoxin (choice B), a cardiac glycoside, may increase cardiac contractility but has a slow onset of action and may exacerbate arrhythmias. Norepinephrine (choice D) increases myocardial contractility but also greatly increases peripheral resistance. The latter effect increases the cardiac workload, a situation that must be avoided in cardiogenic shock. Procainamide (choice E), a group IA antiarrhythmic agent, is not indicated because the patient does not have an arrhythmia.

691. **(E)** Leuprolide is a GnRH agonist that when given in pulsatile fashion stimulates pituitary LH release, but when given continuously, or in a depot preparation, *suppresses* LH release and reduces plasma testosterone levels to the level of pharmacologic castration. Because it

is a peptide, it must be given parenterally. It is used extensively in the treatment of metastatic prostatic cancer. Diethylstilbestrol (choice A) is an oral nonsteroidal synthetic estrogen that is now rarely used in the treatment of prostatic cancer. Use of this agent produces undesirable feminization and is reserved for cases unresponsive to other agents. Finasteride (choice B) is an orally active inhibitor of the 5α-reductase that converts testosterone to dihydrotestosterone in the prostate. Because continuous conversion of testosterone to dihydrotestosterone is essential for the androgenic effects in the prostate, inhibition of the 5α-reductase decreases the stimulation of the prostate. Unfortunately, the drug is not effective in prostate malignancy. Finasteride is used for the treatment of benign prostatic hyperplasia because it produces a moderate decrease in prostatic size and improvement in urinary flow. It is also used for the treatment of androgenic hair loss. Flutamide (choice C) is a nonsteroidal antiandrogen occasionally used in the treatment of prostatic cancer that is unresponsive to leuprolide. It is active orally. Ketoconazole (choice D) is an oral antifungal agent that has the property of inhibiting the cytochrome P450 isoforms involved in steroid biosynthesis. It has been used in the treatment of prostatic cancer with mixed results.

692. **(E)** This patient's presentation is typical of seasonal rhinitis (hay fever). This condition is mediated largely by histamine release from sensitized mast cells. Loratadine is a second generation H_1-blocker that is almost completely lacking in sedative effects (probably because it enters the CNS poorly) and is the drug of choice. It should be noted that the efficacy of second-generation antihistamines at the manufacturers' recommended dosages has been questioned. At higher dosages, these newer drugs are more consistently efficacious but also somewhat sedating. Chlorpheniramine (choice A), diphenhydramine (choice C), and hydroxyzine (choice D) are all first-generation H_1-blocking antihistamines and possess varying degrees of sedative effect. Diphenhydramine and hydroxyzine are extremely sedating and are often used for that purpose, rather than for their antihistaminic properties. Cimetidine (choice B) is an H_2-blocking antihistamine and is of no value in this case.

693. **(C)** The recorded transmembrane potential indicates that the new drug slows the upstroke velocity and prolongs the action potential duration of the ventricular muscle fiber. These effects are characteristic of blocking sodium channels and delayed rectifier potassium (I_{Kr}) channels, actions shown by group IA antiarrhythmic drugs. Procainamide (choice C) is a group IA drug. Adenosine (choice A) hyperpolarizes AV nodal cells and blocks propagation of impulses through this part of the heart. It does not prolong the action potential. Lidocaine (choice B) is a group IB drug and slows upstroke velocity of the action potential in susceptible cells but shortens, rather than prolongs, the action potential duration. Propranolol (choice D), a β-blocker, is a group II drug and has little effect on ventricular cell action potentials at clinically relevant concentrations. Sotalol (choice E) is a group III drug and prolongs the action potential duration through its ability to block the delayed rectifier potassium channel. However, it does not significantly slow upstroke velocity (a sodium channel-blocking effect).

694. **(A)** Foreign material (such as a stent) in blood vessels invites clotting and the stented vessel will rapidly occlude if clotting is not prevented. The primary process in the formation of this *arterial* clot is platelet aggregation, so an antiplatelet drug is suitable (choice A). Abciximab and tirofiban are also sometimes used in this setting. Heparin (both forms, choices B and C) and warfarin (choice E) are useful in the prevention of *venous* thrombosis. t-PA (choice D) is useful in accelerating the dissolution of a fibrin clot (e.g., after myocardial infarction), but is not useful in this situation.

695. **(C)** Cyclosporine is a major agent used for immunosuppression in organ transplantation. Use of this agent and tacrolimus is

largely responsible for recent progress in the prevention and treatment of organ rejection. Cyclosporine acts by blocking the activation of T cells through formation of complexes with the cyclophilin family of proteins. These cyclosporine–cyclophilin complexes inhibit function of the protein complex calcineurin, preventing the transcriptional activation necessary for lymphokine expression. Cyclosporine produces nephrotoxicity in a majority of patients, but exhibits no bone marrow depression. Azathioprine (choice A) is a purine antimetabolite that prevents the clonal expansion of B and T lymphocytes, thus producing immunosuppressive actions. Because it is a cytotoxic agent, it produces bone marrow depression along with toxicity to GI cells. Cyclophosphamide (choice B) is an alkylating agent used in immunosuppression as well as in cancer chemotherapy. Toxicities include bone marrow depression along with hemorrhagic cystitis and cardiotoxicity. Muromonab-CD3 monoclonal antibody (choice D) is a mouse monoclonal antibody whose T-cell epitope is in close proximity to the antigen recognition complex. Binding to T cells prevents antigen binding to the antigen recognition complex and activates cytokine release. This ultimately results in the appearance of T cells with CD3 and antigen recognition complex being absent, resulting in the immunosuppressive actions. Toxicities include cytokine release syndrome, anaphylactoid reactions, and CNS effects, but do not include nephrotoxicity or bone marrow depression. Prednisone (choice E) is used in transplantation because it reduces circulating levels of lymphocytes and inhibits T-cell proliferation. Toxicity is that expected of glucocorticoids (ulcers, hyperglycemia, and osteoporosis) and includes neither nephrotoxicity nor bone marrow depression.

696. **(C)** Metronidazole is the agent of choice for the treatment of trichomoniasis. It produces a selective toxicity in anaerobic organisms by initiating redox cycling in these organisms. Because metronidazole produces a disulfiram-like action (inhibition of aldehyde dehydrogenase), it can result in the rapid accumulation of toxic levels of acetaldehyde after consumption of small amounts of ethanol. Therefore, patients must be cautioned to avoid alcohol consumption when taking the drug. Mebendazole (choice A) is an antihelmintic agent used to treat roundworm infections such as ascariasis, pinworms, or whipworm. Methimazole (choice B) is an antithyroid agent that inhibits formation of thyroid hormone. Primaquine (choice D) is used to treat relapsing malarias caused by *Plasmodium vivax* and *P. ovale.* Trimethoprim (choice E), in combination with sulfamethoxazole, is used prophylactically in antiparasitic treatments to prevent *Pneumocystis carinii* infections in immune-deficient patients, as well as being used to treat bacterial urinary tract infections.

697. **(B)** Didanosine causes pancreatitis in a significant number of patients treated for AIDS. Amantadine (choice A) is used in the prevention and treatment of influenza and causes CNS stimulation and light headedness. Ribavirin (choice C) is used for the treatment of respiratory syncytial virus in infants and causes dose-dependent hemolytic anemia in about 10% of patients. Ritonavir (choice D), a protease inhibitor used in AIDS, causes hepatitis. Zidovudine (choice E), another drug used in AIDS, causes neutropenia as its primary dose-limiting effect.

698. **(A)** Acyclovir is an acyclic guanine nucleoside analog that undergoes phosphorylation by herpesviral thymidine kinase to form the acyclovir triphosphate form and causes DNA chain termination. Resistance involves deletion or reduction, along with altered catalytic activity, of herpesvirus thymidine kinase. Amantadine (choice B) is a tricyclic amine that inhibits uncoating of influenza A virus. It is also used for the treatment of parkinsonism. Foscarnet (choice C) is a pyrophosphate analog that inhibits herpesvirus nucleic acid synthesis at the level of the viral DNA polymerase. Resistance involves point mutations in the viral DNA polymerase. Saquinavir (choice D) is an HIV protease inhibitor. Resistance involves point mutations in the protease. Zidovudine (choice E) is an antiretrovi-

ral thymidine analog. The triphosphate is a competitive inhibitor of reverse transcriptase and a DNA chain terminator. The monophosphate is a competitive inhibitor of thymidine kinase. Resistance involves point mutations in reverse transcriptase.

699. **(E)** Trimethoprim is an inhibitor of dihydrofolate reductase that exhibits great specificity for binding to the bacterial form as opposed to the human form (10^5 higher concentrations are required for inhibition of host dihydrofolate reductase). Trimethoprim is combined with sulfamethoxazole to provide inhibition of sequential steps in bacterial tetrahydrofolate synthesis. Resistance may arise by mutation of bacterial dihydrofolate reductase, although acquisition of a plasmid encoding altered dihydrofolate reductase is more common for gram-negative bacteria. Amoxicillin (choice A) is a β-lactamase–sensitive penicillin whose spectrum of activity includes the gram-negative bacteria. Because amoxicillin achieves high concentrations in the urine, it is useful for *E. coli* urinary tract infections, although resistance is increasingly a problem. Its mechanism of action involves inhibition of cell wall synthesis. Imipenem (choice B) is a β-lactam antibiotic whose structure is distinct from the penicillins and cephalosporins. It exhibits good activity against a wide variety of bacteria. It is resistant to hydrolysis by bacterial β-lactamases and kills susceptible organisms by inhibiting cell wall synthesis. Methotrexate (choice C) is an inhibitor of dihydrofolate reductase but this drug, unlike trimethoprim, shows no specificity for bacterial forms as opposed to host cell forms. This lack of specificity makes it unsuitable for antibacterial therapy. Methotrexate and similar antifolates such as trimetrexate and 5,10-dideazatetrahydrofolate are used in cancer chemotherapy. Methotrexate is also used in rheumatoid arthritis. Sulfamethoxazole (choice D) is a sulfonamide that shares the property of inhibiting incorporation of p-aminobenzoic acid into folate in bacteria. It is often combined with trimethoprim to provide sequential inhibition of reduced folate synthesis as indicated above.

700. **(C)** Rifampin selectively inhibits bacterial DNA-dependent RNA polymerase. It is highly useful in treating mycobacterial infections since it can penetrate cells and kill intracellular mycobacteria. It is a potent inducer of cytochrome P450, leading to increased hepatic clearance of many other drugs including the oral anticoagulants, cyclosporine, propranolol, digitoxin, corticosteroids, and oral contraceptives. Ethambutol (choice A) is often combined with isoniazid in antitubercular regimens. Clearance is primarily via renal excretion. Isoniazid (choice B) is the most widely used antitubercular agent worldwide. It functions by inhibiting mycolic acid biosynthesis. Isoniazid is cleared by metabolism via N-acetylase and hydrolytic activity. Streptomycin (choice D) was the first effective drug for the treatment of tuberculosis, but, because of its ototoxicity and nephrotoxicity and the development of less toxic agents, use of streptomycin is limited to more severe forms of the disease. Sulfisoxazole (choice E) may rarely be used in antitubercular regimens in combination with other drugs. Clearance is primarily via glomerular filtration.

701. **(D)** Prophylaxis of migraine is poorly understood; drugs from several groups have partial activity and must be tried to find which is effective in a particular patient. Propranolol is effective in reducing the frequency of migraine attacks in a significant percentage of patients. The mechanism of action is unknown. Codeine (choice A), a moderate opioid analgesic, would not be tried; it has no prophylactic effect and might cause constipation and habituation. Ergotamine (choice B), an ergot derivative useful in the treatment of acute attacks, is not prescribed for prophylaxis. It has powerful and long-lasting vasoconstrictor effects that can cause ischemia and even gangrene when given chronically. Ibuprofen (choice C), an NSAID analgesic, is useful in control of acute headache but has no prophylactic efficacy. Sumatriptan (choice E) is a synthetic 5-HT$_{1D}$ agonist useful in the treatment of acute migraine attacks. It is not usually used for prophylaxis.

702. **(C)** The patient's drug-induced condition resembles lupus erythematosus and can be caused by several drugs. Unlike naturally occurring lupus, drug-induced lupus is reversible upon discontinuing the causative drug and does not involve the kidneys. Hydralazine causes the reversible type of lupus described. Captopril (choice A) does not cause lupus. This ACE inhibitor causes cough, renal damage in the fetus, and renal impairment in renovascular disease. Clonidine (choice B) causes some sedation and rebound hypertension when stopped suddenly, but does not cause lupus. Hydrochlorothiazide (choice D) may cause hypokalemia, dilutional hyponatremia, elevated lipids, hyperuricemia, and glucose intolerance, but not lupus. Methyldopa (choice E) causes sedation and formation of red blood cell antibodies, but does not cause lupus. It may cause hemolytic anemia.

703. **(B)** Metformin, a biguanide, causes lactic acidosis (although less often than earlier biguanides, such as phenformin). Patients with renal or liver disease are at higher risk. The sulfonylurea hypoglycemic drugs (choices A and E) are rarely associated with lactic acidosis. Their major toxicity is excessive hypoglycemia, especially with high-potency agents such as glyburide. The new glitazone agents (choices C and D) are not associated with a high incidence of lactic acidosis, although an earlier glitazone (troglitazone) was withdrawn because of a high incidence of liver damage.

704. **(A)** Captopril and other ACE inhibitors cause a dry cough in 5% to 20% of patients. This may be due to accumulation of bradykinin in the lungs as a result of ACE inhibition; ACE also metabolizes bradykinin. The cough disappears with cessation of ACE inhibitor treatment. Pretreatment with aspirin reduces its frequency and severity in some patients. Clonidine (choice B), the centrally acting α_2-receptor agonist, produces sedation and xerostomia but not cough. The arteriolar smooth muscle relaxing agent hydralazine (choice C) produces troublesome tachycardia along with a lupus-like syndrome, but does not cause cough. The α_1-receptor antagonist prazosin (choice D) produces postural hypotension but not cough. The β-blocker propranolol (choice E) may produce a variety of side effects including precipitating heart failure and asthma in susceptible patients. It does not cause cough. Propranolol has been used by musicians to control palpitations associated with stage fright.

705. **(C)** Cyclophosphamide is metabolized by the cytochrome P450 CYP2A isoform to species that eventually lead to phosphoramide mustard, an alkylating agent, and acrolein, a chemical irritant that causes hemorrhagic cystitis. The natural product bleomycin (choice A) binds to DNA and forms an iron complex capable of generating active oxygen species in the presence of a reducing agent. The reactive oxygen species then generate single- and double-strand breaks, leading to cytotoxicity. Cisplatin (choice B), an inorganic platinum-containing complex, binds to DNA where it forms intra- and interstrand cross-links. The pyrimidine analog 5-fluorouracil (choice D) is metabolized by ribosylation and phosphorylation to the nucleotide level. See answer 707 for further details. Paclitaxel (choice E) is a natural product isolated from the bark of the Western yew tree. Paclitaxel is a mitotic inhibitor that prevents microtubule disassembly.

706. **(B)** As described, cisplatin binds to DNA where it forms intra- and interstrand cross-links. Cisplatin is particularly effective in testicular and ovarian cancers in combination with other antitumor agents. Cisplatin exerts a renal toxicity that may be prevented by the infusion of saline to maintain a high urine flow. Ototoxicity involving high-frequency hearing loss is an effect that is not prevented by hydration. The natural product bleomycin (choice A) binds to DNA and causes single- and double-strand breaks, leading to cytotoxicity. The drug is particularly useful against Hodgkin lymphoma and testicular tumors. Bleomycin has the serious toxicity of pul-

monary fibrosis. Cyclophosphamide (choice C) is widely used in combination regimens. Nausea and vomiting are the most common toxicities. Hemorrhagic cystitis attributable to the acrolein also produced from cyclophosphamide may be minimized by hydration and use of the drug mesna. Note that this toxicity is not at the level of the kidney. The pyrimidine analog 5-fluorouracil (5-FU) (choice D) is used to treat a wide variety of carcinomas. Toxicity from 5-FU is expressed as GI disturbances (anorexia, nausea, stomatitis, and diarrhea) and myelosuppression. Paclitaxel (choice E) is a natural product isolated from the bark of the Western yew tree. Paclitaxel is particularly useful in treating metastatic breast and ovarian cancer. The primary toxicity of paclitaxel is bone marrow suppression.

707. **(D)** The pyrimidine analog 5-fluorouracil (5-FU) is metabolized by ribosylation and phosphorylation to the nucleotide level (F-UMP). F-UMP is further metabolized to F-dUMP, an inhibitor of thymidylate synthase. Cells then become starved for TTP and incorporate F-dUTP and dUTP in its place in DNA. 5-FU also becomes incorporated in RNA, leading to inhibition of RNA processing. Anastrozole (choice A) is a nonsteroidal inhibitor of aromatase, an enzyme required for synthesis of estrogens. This drug is useful against advanced estrogen- or progesterone-receptor–positive breast cancer. Cytarabine (cytosine arabinoside, ara-C, choice B), is an S phase-specific antimetabolite that is metabolized to the triphosphate form, which blocks DNA synthesis. It is used exclusively in acute myelogenous leukemia. Doxorubicin (choice C) is an anthracycline antibiotic that intercalates into DNA causing strand breakage and blockage of both DNA and RNA synthesis. This agent is widely used in combination regimens for breast, endometrial, ovarian, testicular, and thyroid carcinomas, and several sarcomas and lymphomas. Methotrexate (choice E) is a folic acid antagonist that blocks dihydrofolate reductase and interferes with the synthesis of purines and pyrimidines necessary for cell proliferation. It is a key drug in

the treatment of acute lymphocytic leukemia and choriocarcinoma.

708. **(B)** Etoposide is a semisynthetic derivative of podophyllotoxin, a constituent of the mandrake plant. Etoposide is an inhibitor of topoisomerase II, an enzyme that relaxes supercoiled DNA by breaking one strand and passing the second strand through the break before closing the break. Etoposide inhibits the closure step and results in an accumulation of DNA strand breaks, leading to cell death. Etoposide is used to treat testicular tumors and small cell carcinoma of the lung in combination with cisplatin. Leukopenia is the dose-limiting toxicity seen with this drug. Dacarbazine (choice A) is a synthetic prodrug activated in the liver to a metabolite that alkylates DNA leading to cytotoxicity. The drug is useful against melanoma and Hodgkin lymphoma. Lomustine (CCNU, choice C) is a lipid-soluble nitrosourea agent that acts as an alkylating agent. The nitrosoureas are unusual in having relatively good access to the CNS and are therefore useful in treating brain tumors. Prednisone (choice D) is a potent, orally active corticosteroid with good lymphotoxic potency. Its mechanism is not fully understood but may involve activation of apoptotic pathways in lymphocytes. Vincristine (choice E) is a natural product isolated from the vinca plant. It is classified as a spindle poison and inhibits mitosis by inhibiting microtubule assembly. This drug is particularly useful in treating acute leukemias in children and Hodgkin lymphoma.

709. **(A)** Sulfadiazine is stated to be a weak acid with a pKa value of 6.5. The protonated form is uncharged and is the permeant species that crosses biological membranes. At equilibrium, concentration of the permeant species is the same on both sides of the membrane, but the total amount (protonated form + anion) present in each compartment depends on the pH of the compartment. For a weak acid, the total amount is highest in the most alkaline compartment. This is because higher pH values cause dissociation of the acid to

the anion, which becomes trapped in the compartment because the charged anion cannot cross the membrane. The higher the pH value for the compartment, the greater the total amount present. Alkalinized urine at pH 8.0 has the highest pH value. The value for the protonated and unprotonated forms may be calculated using the Henderson–Hasselbalch equation [log (protonated form/unprotonated form) = pKa – pH].

710. **(B)** This patient's presentation is typical of glucocorticosteroid toxicity (iatrogenic Cushing syndrome). Prednisone is an effective corticosteroid frequently used by mouth to control severe asthma that is not responsive to inhaled corticosteroids. High doses of prednisone given chronically very predictably cause signs and symptoms of hypercorticism. Ipratropium (choice A) is an antimuscarinic agent used in asthma by inhalation. Salmeterol (choice C) is a long-acting β_2-selective agonist used by inhalation. Terbutaline (choice D) is a short-acting β_2-selective agonist, also used by inhalation. Theophylline (choice E) is a long-acting oral drug that causes CNS stimulation (including convulsions in toxic overdosage), but not hypercorticism.

711. **(D)** Vasopressin is a peptide hormone synthesized in the hypothalamus and transported to the posterior lobe of the pituitary gland. As explained below, thiazides are used in the treatment of nephrogenic diabetes insipidus. Ethanol (choice A) inhibits vasopressin secretion, resulting in the well-known alcohol-induced diuresis; thus, choice A is incorrect. Osmoreceptors in the hypothalamus, close to the nuclei that synthesize and secrete ADH, are stimulated to cause release of vasopressin by an increase in plasma osmolality. Thus, choice B is incorrect. Vasopressin acts through G protein-linked receptors on vascular smooth muscle (V_1 receptors) to mediate vasoconstriction (thus, choice E is incorrect) and on V_2 receptors in the collecting ducts (thus choice C is incorrect) to increase permeability to water, thus aiding in the formation of hypertonic urine. Diabetes insipidus is characterized by

formation of large quantities of dilute urine due to either inadequate vasopressin secretion (pituitary diabetes insipidus) or inadequate renal response to vasopressin (nephrogenic, or vasopressin-resistant, diabetes insipidus). Vasopressin-resistant diabetes insipidus can be treated with thiazide diuretics. These drugs act by decreasing plasma volume, which increases proximal tubular reabsorption, and thus decreases fluid delivery to the collecting ducts and the bladder. Choice D is correct. Desmopressin, a longer-acting analog of vasopressin, is used as an intranasal spray for the treatment of pituitary diabetes insipidus.

712. **(E)** Propranolol is used to prevent the onset of anginal attacks because of its β-blocking action, which decreases heart rate and prevents increases in heart rate with exertion. This effect decreases myocardial oxygen demand and prevents the ischemic episodes that trigger anginal pain. The drug also decreases cardiac force and blood pressure, two additional factors that contribute to its efficacy in angina prophylaxis. It is not useful in treatment of an acute attack because it has a slow onset of action. Isoproterenol (choice A) is a β-receptor agonist that increases heart rate and contractile force, and may *precipitate* an anginal attack or even myocardial infarction in a patient with compromised coronary blood flow. Isosorbide dinitrate (choice B) is another organic nitrate drug, like nitroglycerine. No anti-anginal drug has significant effects on myocardial oxygen extraction. Nifedipine (choice C) is a dihydropyridine calcium channel blocker that can be beneficially combined with nitrate drugs to treat angina. Nifedipine selectively dilates arterial resistance vessels with much less effect on veins. The decreased peripheral resistance causes a decrease in cardiac workload and oxygen demand. The slow-release formulation of nifedipine should be used in patients with coronary artery disease. Nitroglycerin (choice D) is used to prevent or terminate anginal attacks. Its venodilating action causes venous pooling of blood and decreased cardiac filling in diastole. This results in a

diminution of cardiac fiber tension and a consequent decrease in myocardial oxygen demand.

713. **(C)** Long-term treatment of schizophrenia with potent dopamine D_2 receptor antagonists is associated with a high incidence of the irreversible extrapyramidal dystonias called tardive dyskinesia. The phenothiazines (and haloperidol) are D_2 receptor antagonists in the CNS; their success in the treatment of schizophrenia resulted in the hypothesis that the antipsychotic effect requires D_2 blockade. Data from newer, atypical antipsychotic agents casts some doubt on this hypothesis because drugs such as clozapine and risperidone have a low affinity for D_2 receptors. Older drugs in the phenothiazine class (e.g., chlorpromazine) have both antimuscarinic and antiemetic action; thus diarrhea, nausea, and vomiting (choice A) are very unlikely. Because prolactin secretion (choice B) from the anterior pituitary is inhibited by dopamine, blockade of D_2 receptors by fluphenazine increases prolactin secretion. This may result in breast engorgement and galactorrhea in women. Tourette syndrome (choice D) involves tics and other involuntary movements and obscene vocalizations. The neuroleptic agent haloperidol is the current drug of choice for the treatment of this disease. Weight loss (choice E) is associated with the use of selective serotonin reuptake inhibitors (SSRIs), not phenothiazines. In fact, the phenothiazines are often associated with weight gain.

714. **(E)** Mirtazapine is a third-generation antidepressant related to antihistaminics and has significant sedative action. Buspirone (choice A) is an antianxiety agent with minimal sedative action. Fluoxetine (choice B) is the prototype SSRI antidepressant. Sedation does not occur but sexual dysfunction is often reported. Haloperidol (choice C) is an older, highly potent antipsychotic drug used in schizophrenia. Lithium carbonate (choice D) is an important antimanic drug. It apparently acts by interfering with inositol phosphate cycling and second messenger synthesis in neurons.

715. **(D)** A very important serotonin syndrome may occur in patients taking MAOIs if they also ingest an SSRI drug such as fluoxetine. This syndrome is characterized by hyperthermia, muscle spasms, and autonomic instability and may be fatal. MAOIs do not cause an increase in blood pressure (choice A); at one time they were promoted for the treatment of hypertension. They do not cause hair loss (choice B). Tyramine in the diet, not serotonin (choice C), may result in a hypertensive crisis in patients taking MAOIs. MAOIs often cause some stimulation or alerting, so choice E is incorrect. Tricyclic antidepressants may cause sedation.

716. **(A)** Inhaled albuterol (or other β_2-selective receptor agonists including bitolterol, metaproterenol, pirbuterol, and terbutaline) are the usual agents of choice for treating bronchoconstriction in an acute asthma attack. These β_2-selective agonists produce bronchial relaxation by stimulating cyclic AMP (cAMP) formation in bronchiolar smooth muscle and cause less tachycardia than nonselective β-agonists. Unfortunately, they do cause some tachycardia and skeletal muscle tremor. Aminophylline (choice B) and other methylxanthines are rarely used to terminate acute episodes of asthma because they must be administered parenterally for rapid onset of effect. Cromolyn sodium (choice C) must be used prophylactically to prevent acute episodes. It is not a smooth muscle relaxing agent and probably acts by stabilizing mast cells. Inhaled ipratropium (choice D) is prophylactic in preventing asthmatic episodes but has less general efficacy in acute attacks than β-agonists. Salmeterol (choice E) is an effective β_2-selective agonist but has a slow onset and long duration of action. Therefore, it is used for prophylaxis, not treatment of acute attacks.

717. **(A)** All of the drugs listed are used in the treatment of gout. Allopurinol and its metabolite alloxanthine inhibit xanthine oxidase, thus preventing conversion of xanthine and hypoxanthine to uric acid. Although xanthine and hypoxanthine then accumulate, these compounds are more soluble than uric

acid and less likely to deposit in joints. Allopurinol is not useful in an acute gout attack; it must be used prophylactically. Colchicine (choice B) is an inhibitor of microtubule function that brings relief in an acute gout attack by inhibiting the motility of granulocytes and preventing the formation of mediators of inflammation by leukocytes. Because of its toxicity at higher doses, it is now used chiefly at low doses to prevent acute attacks. Indomethacin (choice C) is a nonsteroidal anti-inflammatory drug (NSAID) that inhibits cyclooxygenase (COX) and reduces formation of prostaglandins and eicosanoids involved in gouty arthritis. It has no effect on the formation of uric acid. Probenecid (choice D) and sulfinpyrazone (choice E) are uricosuric agents—they increase the excretion of uric acid by the kidney. Renal uric acid excretion is determined by the balance between the amount filtered plus that actively secreted and the amount undergoing passive and active reabsorption. At very low doses, these agents inhibit active secretion and thus promote retention of uric acid. At higher (clinical) doses, both active secretion and active reabsorption are inhibited, with the result that excretion is enhanced.

718. **(E)** All of the drugs listed are NSAIDs. NSAIDs have long been drugs of first choice in arthritis treatment. Their primary mechanism of action in arthritis appears to be inhibition of COX, an enzyme required for the synthesis of inflammatory and other prostaglandins. Two forms of COX are present in the body: COX-1, which is required for synthesis of useful prostaglandins (e.g., PGE_1, a cytoprotective agent in the stomach), and COX-2, the isoform responsible for synthesis of most of the damaging prostaglandins. The older NSAIDs (choices A through D) inhibit both COX-1 and COX-2 with little or no selectivity and thus reduce protective prostaglandins, resulting in a high incidence of GI disorders. Rofecoxib (choice E) and celecoxib are newer NSAIDs that are much more selective for COX-2 and thus have a lower incidence of adverse GI effects.

719. **(D)** Bromocriptine is a synthetic ergot derivative with potent dopamine agonist effects in the CNS. It is most useful in the treatment of parkinsonism and amenorrhea/galactorrhea syndrome. Adverse effects include GI disturbance, hallucinations, dyskinesias, orthostatic hypotension, and erythromelalgia, a painful swelling and reddening of the feet and hands. Allergic rhinitis (choice A) is treated with H_1-blocking antihistamines such as chlorpheniramine and with nasal corticosteroids such as fluticasone. Bronchial asthma (choice B) is treated with β_2-selective adrenoreceptor agonists (e.g., metaproterenol) and corticosteroids by inhalation. Diabetes insipidus (choice C) is treated with vasopressin or desmopressin (if pituitary deficiency is the cause), or with thiazide diuretics (if vasopressin resistance is the cause; see 711). Peptic ulcer (choice E) is treated with H_2-blocking antihistamines such as cimetidine, or with proton pump inhibitors such as omeprazole.

720. **(D)** Elevated blood pressure typically evokes a compensatory baroreceptor reflex with slowing of heart rate. Thus, the decrease in heart rate shown in the initial data can be interpreted as a reflex bradycardia. Bethanechol (choice A) is a muscarinic agonist and typically causes vasodilation, with a drop in blood pressure and a compensatory tachycardia. Epinephrine (choice B), an α_1-, α_2-, β_1-, and β_2-agonist, causes hypertension at high doses, but usually also causes tachycardia. Isoproterenol (choice C) is a β_1-, β_2-agonist, and does not cause hypertension or bradycardia. Norepinephrine (choice D) and phenylephrine (choice E) can both cause hypertension and reflex bradycardia. However, norepinephrine has β_1-agonist action, whereas phenylephrine has only α effects. Thus, in the presence of an α-blocking agent, norepinephrine causes a β_1-mediated tachycardia; phenylephrine has no effect on heart rate.

721. **(C)** As noted in the answer to question 720, the agonist drug in the data presented is the α-agonist norepinephrine. Prazosin (choice C) is an α-blocker that prevents the pressor effects of α-agonists such as norepinephrine and phenylephrine. If norepinephrine's α-agonist effects on the vessels are blocked, its β-agonist action on the heart becomes evident, causing tachycardia. Phenylephrine, on the other hand, has no β-agonist effects, and tachycardia does not result. Atropine (choice A) is a muscarinic blocker and does not prevent hypertension due to α-agonists. Pralidoxime (choice B) is a cholinesterase regenerator used in the treatment of organophosphate insecticide toxicity. Reserpine (choice D) is a blocker of postganglionic sympathetic nerve function (it prevents storage of norepinephrine in transmitter vesicles and depletes the nerve ending of its transmitter stores); it has no effect in the experiment described. Timolol (choice E), a β-blocker, does not prevent the pressor effects of α-agonists.

722. **(D)** The pA_2 value is the negative logarithm of the concentration of a competitive antagonist required to cause a doubling of the apparent effective concentration at 50% response (EC_{50}) for the receptor agonist. This method is used for determining the affinity of the antagonist for the receptor. Assuming a 1:1 relationship between receptor occupancy and the response (i.e., no spare receptors), the pA_2 value should be equivalent to the negative logarithm of the dissociation constant for the inhibitor-receptor complex. In the situation described, cardiac β-adrenoreceptors require 10^{-7} M atenolol to double the agonist EC_{50} whereas lung β-adrenoreceptors require 50 times more (5×10^{-6} M). This indicates that atenolol is considerably more potent in blocking cardiac β-adrenoreceptors than lung β-adrenoreceptors. Choices C and E are incorrect as indicated above. Choices A and B are incorrect because they refer to efficacy. Efficacy (or maximal efficacy) is a property of agonists and the system they act upon, not of antagonists. Ordinary antagonists do not have efficacies because they do not produce a response by themselves. They only alter the response to an agonist.

723. **(D)** The transplanted heart lacks functional innervation for at least 2 years, and possibly longer, after surgery. Because the nerves are cut in the procedure, nerve endings degenerate (Wallerian degeneration) and transmitter stores are lost. Adrenoreceptors on the myocardial cells are normal or even increased in sensitivity, so responses to direct-acting β-adrenoreceptor agonists such as isoproterenol are retained. Indirectly acting sympathomimetics, on the other hand, are relatively ineffective (choices A, B, and C) because they act through the release or amplification of endogenous norepinephrine. Phenylephrine (choice E), a direct-acting α-agonist, has no significant β-agonist activity and in the intact, innervated heart causes only reflex bradycardia. It has no effect on the rate of the denervated heart.

724. **(B)** Histamine activates nitric oxide synthase by binding to H_1 receptors in the endothelium. Nitric acid synthesis is increased, and this molecule rapidly diffuses into the adjoining smooth muscle, where it causes vasodilation. Diazoxide (choice A) is a powerful vasodilator used in hypertensive emergencies. It acts by opening potassium channels in vascular smooth muscle and hyperpolarizing these cells. Minoxidil (choice C), another vasodilator used in severe hypertension, is converted to the sulfate metabolite, which similarly opens potassium channels and hyperpolarizes vascular smooth muscle. Nitroprusside (choice D) contains nitric oxide that is spontaneously released in the blood. Stimulation of endothelial synthesis is not involved. Verapamil (choice E) blocks calcium channels in vascular smooth muscle and thereby causes relaxation.

725. **(E)** Patients with documented allergy to ester-type local anesthetics are rare, but can suffer severe reactions if such agents are used. At present, it is easy to distinguish between ester and amide local anesthetics because the amide members of this drug group have two *i*s in their names. Thus choices A through D are all amide local anesthetics and could be used in this patient. Tetracaine, on the other hand, is an ester and is contraindicated. Note that with the introduction of new local anesthetics, this simple mnemonic may become invalid.

726. **(C)** Any drug containing streptococcal antigens is contraindicated in this allergic patient. (Some patients are sensitized by prior administration of streptokinase, others by a previous streptococcal infection.) The only drug in this list that contains streptococcal protein is anistreplase, a complex of streptokinase and recombinant human plasminogen. This patient would probably be treated with t-PA (choice B), a purified recombinant human protein. Although much more expensive than streptokinase, clinical studies show that t-PA is at least as effective as the bacterial protein in dissolving coronary thrombi in patients with myocardial infarction. Reteplase (choice E) is another, newer human thrombolytic enzyme that could be used safely. Abciximab (choice A), a chimeric human-mouse monoclonal antibody, and clopidogrel (choice D), a synthetic nonprotein agent, are not thrombolytics but have antiplatelet activity and are indicated in patients who have angioplasty and insertion of stents.

727. **(B)** Ethylene glycol, commonly used as antifreeze in cars, is metabolized via several enzymatic steps to acidic intermediates and finally to oxalic acid. Ethylene glycol is sometimes used as an ethanol substitute by alcoholics. Its low molecular weight means that ingestion of relatively small amounts generate high concentrations of metabolites, thus producing a profound metabolic acidosis. Oxalic acid precipitates in the renal tubules, causing severe renal damage. Treatment consists of sodium bicarbonate for the metabolic acidosis and measures to inhibit further metabolism, which may include ethanol as a competitive substrate for alcohol dehydrogenase or 4-methylpyrazole as an inhibitor. Hemodialysis may be useful. Ethanol (choice A) is metabolized to acetaldehyde and acetic acid. Isopropanol (choice C) is slowly metabolized to acetone. Methanol (choice D) follows the same path of metabolism as ethanol, with the toxic metabolites being formaldehyde and formic acid. Formic acid causes

retinal damage. Methylene chloride (choice E) is metabolized by cytochrome P450 to carbon monoxide.

728. **(A)** The benzodiazepine anxiolytic agents, including diazepam, potentiate the actions of the inhibitory neurotransmitter GABA, which acts on $GABA_A$ receptors to open chloride ion channels. Fluoxetine (choice B) is a selective inhibitor of serotonin uptake. Pentobarbital (choice C) is a modulator of the same GABA-sensitive chloride channel affected by benzodiazepines, although its mechanism of action is slightly different. Tranylcypromine (choice D) is an inhibitor of MAO rather than catechol-O-methyltransferase (COMT). Trifluoperazine (choice E) is a phenothiazine that blocks dopamine receptors.

729. **(B)** The H_2-receptor antagonist cimetidine has been shown to cause many drug-drug interactions. Alone among the H_2-blocking agents, it is a potent inhibitor of cytochrome P450 inhibition by cimetidine and therefore increases the plasma concentrations of other P450 substrate drugs. Because other H_2-receptor antagonists (ranitidine, nizatidine, and famotidine) cause little or no inhibition of P450, use of cimetidine has declined. Development of the proton pump inhibitors such as omeprazole, and antibiotic regimens to eradicate *Helicobacter pylori*, a causative agent for peptic ulcers, have also contributed to a decline in use of H_2-blockers. Atracurium (choice A) is a competitive antagonist for nicotinic receptors at the neuromuscular junction. It is used to produce skeletal muscle relaxation during surgery. Atracurium is eliminated by a spontaneous chemical reaction and by plasma cholinesterases, and is not a substrate or inhibitor of cytochrome P450. Cromolyn sodium (choice C) is used in prophylaxis of asthma because of its ability to inhibit the release of histamine and other mediators of inflammation from mast cells. It is not a substrate or inhibitor of cytochrome P450. The drug is excreted unchanged in the urine and bile. Diazepam (choice D) is used to treat anxiety and muscle spastic states by virtue of its ability to facilitate inhibitory ac-

tions exerted by the GABA$_A$ receptor at chloride channels. It is eliminated by cytochrome P450 metabolism, but is not an inducer of activity. Although it may compete with other P450 substrates for metabolism, diazepam and other benzodiazepines do not inhibit the metabolism of other drugs. Phenobarbital (choice E) produces many drug interactions because of its ability to induce (rather than inhibit) cytochrome P450 activity. Phenobarbital was widely used as a sedative-hypnotic and antiepileptic agent, but its use today is limited because of respiratory depression and drug interaction properties.

730. **(B)** The presentation of these patients is typical of mushroom intoxication of the *A. phalloides* type. *Amanita virosa* (choice B) is a member of this group and is common in many temperate climates. Initial symptoms resemble excessive muscarinic stimulation (GI upset) and may be difficult to distinguish from *A. muscaria* consumption (choice A). (The neuromuscular symptoms reported in these patients were nonspecific.) However, *A. muscaria* symptoms are usually self-limited, disappearing after 6 to 12 hours. No liver damage is involved. Amanitin and phalloidin, the toxins in *A. phalloides* and *virosa*, on the other hand, are irreversible inhibitors of RNA polymerase in the liver and kidney, and produce progressive cellular damage that becomes evident after a delay of 36 to 48 hours. Liver failure is common and may require a liver transplant. Botulinum intoxication (choice C) results in block of cholinergic transmission, with respiratory weakness as the most dangerous effect. Scombroid fish intoxication (choice D) results from consumption of spoiled fish, especially bluefin, tuna, skipjack, mackerel, and marlin. The tissues of these fish release significant amounts of histamine if bacterial action is not prevented by adequate refrigeration. The histamine causes marked hypotension, flushing, urticaria, and paresthesias. Shellfish intoxication (choice E) can take two forms: diarrheic (GI symptoms are dominant, neuromuscular function is not affected) and paralytic (neuromuscular weakness, paresthesias, and anesthesia are domi-

nant). The latter form involves the toxin saxitoxin, which is produced by algae and stored and concentrated by shellfish. Saxitoxin, like tetrodotoxin, blocks sodium channels and inhibits axonal action potential propagation.

731. **(D)** A patient who is anemic, neutropenic, and thrombocytopenic requires stimulation of all three major cell lines in the bone marrow. The only drug currently available that accomplishes this broad-spectrum stimulant effect is sargramostim (granulocyte–macrophage colony stimulating factor [GM-CSF]). Epoetin-α (choice A) is a more selective stimulant of erythrocyte production and is very useful in isolated anemia. Filgrastim (choice B) is a somewhat selective stimulant of leukocyte production and has much less effect on erythrocytes and platelet production than sargramostim. Growth hormone (choice C) and testosterone (choice E) have both been tried in the treatment of anemia with negligible success.

732. **(D)** The IV anesthetic propofol shares the property of rapid induction of anesthesia with thiopental because both agents are highly lipid soluble and are rapidly distributed to the brain via the relatively large percentage of cardiac output the brain receives. The drugs are then rapidly redistributed from the brain to skeletal muscle and eventually to adipose tissue in proportion to the relative rates of perfusion for these tissues, resulting in a brief duration of action. Although propofol is rapidly metabolized in the liver by glucuronide conjugation, the controlling factor for the duration of action is the redistribution from brain to other tissues. Propofol is widely used for induction of anesthesia because of its rapidity of onset and rate of recovery, which is more rapid than that from thiopental. Propofol is devoid of major side effects and may be used by infusion for maintenance of anesthesia as well. Propofol does not undergo active tubular secretion (choice A). Propofol is not metabolized in the blood (choice B) or brain (choice C). Propofol is very hydrophobic as opposed to being hydrophilic (choice E).

733. **(A)** Use of the dissociative anesthetic agent ketamine is associated with disagreeable dreams during and after recovery. The frequency of these effects is lower in children. Coadministration of midazolam or another benzodiazepine lessens this phenomenon. Ketamine is unusual among anesthetic agents in that it stimulates sympathetic nervous system activity rather than depressing it (choice B). Heart rate may increase by 25%. This property is considered useful for patients in shock. Ketamine is an IV anesthetic and does not have a minimum alveolar anesthetic concentration (MAC) value (choice C). Its use is associated with increased muscle tone, making it a poor agent for production of skeletal muscle relaxation (choice E). Ketamine reduces bronchospasm rather than causing it (choice D). Ketamine is related chemically to the veterinary anesthetic phencyclidine (PCP), a drug officially discontinued for human use because of the high frequency of hallucinations and psychological problems. PCP is still widely abused for its hallucinogenic effects.

734. **(A)** The blood-gas partition coefficient is a measure of the solubility of the inhalation anesthetic in the blood relative to its solubility in the inspired air. Blood provides the means of delivery to the brain. The solubility of an agent in blood determines how rapidly the partial pressure rises in the blood. Agents with high solubility (large blood-gas partition coefficients) require large amounts of the anesthetic to dissolve in the blood before the partial pressure in the blood increases enough to effectively deliver them to the brain. Thus, agents with lower blood solubilities (small blood-gas partition coefficients) have more rapid rates of onset of anesthesia. Desirable properties for inhalation anesthetic agents include high potency and low blood solubility. The halogenated hydrocarbons such as desflurane and sevoflurane fit these criteria and are used extensively. The MAC value required for anesthesia (choice B) is a measure of the potency of the agent, but does not give an indication of the rate of onset of anesthesia. The oil–gas partition coefficient

(choice C) is a measure of the lipid solubility of the anesthetic agent. This correlates with the potency as measured by the MAC. Hepatic metabolism (choice D) plays no role in onset of action, but may be important in terms of possible liver and kidney damage resulting from the production of toxic metabolites from some of the halogenated inhaled anesthetic agents. The organ system distribution from the blood (choice E) does not play a role in the rate of onset for inhaled general anesthetic agents, unlike the situation with thiopental and propofol, where high lipid solubility and relative tissue perfusion rates cause distribution and redistribution to be primary determinants of rates of onset and recovery.

735. **(D)** The MAC value for nitrous oxide is 105% (i.e., 5% greater than atmospheric pressure), meaning that for nitrous oxide to be used as the sole anesthetic agent, hyperbaric conditions would have to be used to deliver both the nitrous oxide for anesthesia and oxygen needed for life. The other commonly used inhaled agents, including the halogenated hydrocarbons enflurane, isoflurane, halothane, and sevoflurane (choices A, B, C, and E) have MAC values of 6% or less. Although these data might be interpreted to imply that nitrous oxide is not useful in anesthesia, it is highly valued because of its very low toxicity and additive effects with more potent (but more toxic) agents. It is therefore very commonly combined with other inhaled agents, especially the halogenated hydrocarbons. For example, 0.5% MAC of nitrous oxide plus 0.5% MAC of isoflurane delivers a full anesthetic concentration of gases to the lungs but requires less than 60% of the inspired air partial pressure, so oxygen can utilize the other 40%.

736. **(B)** The agent of choice in treating simple hypothyroidism is levothyroxine (T_4). Administered thyroxine is bound in plasma in the same way and metabolized to tri-iodothyronine in the same manner as native thyroxine. Although liothyronine (tri-iodothyronine [T_3] choice C) is more active than T_4 as an agonist at thyroid hormone receptors, its shorter half-life of 1 day as compared with the 6- to 7-day half-life of T_4 means that thyroxine has a longer duration of action and provides smoother control. The use of desiccated thyroid (choice A) has been abandoned in the United States because of variations in potency. T_4 (3,5,3′,5′-tetraiodothyronine) is converted by deiodinases to the active T_3 (3,5,3′-triiodothyronine) and the inactive reverse T_3 (3,3′,5′-triiodothyronine [choice E]) in equal amounts. T_3 is used in therapy under special circumstances when immediate actions of thyroid hormone are desired, but it is not generally used to treat hypothyroidism because of its higher cost and shorter duration of action. At high concentrations, iodide in the form of potassium (choice D) or other salts is an inhibitor of thyroid gland function and is used in hyperthyroidism. Iodide inhibits its own uptake into thyroid cells and inhibits the release of thyroxine and T_3 from the gland. Iodide treatment is useful in preparation for surgical thyroidectomy because the gland becomes firmer and vascularity is reduced.

737. **(B)** Addisonian crisis is a life-threatening emergency and must be treated with both glucocorticoids and mineralocorticoids. Aldosterone (choice A) is a pure mineralocorticoid and fludrocortisone is primarily mineralocorticoid. Cortisol and fludrocortisone (choice B) provide an appropriate balance of effects. Dexamethasone (choice C) is a potent glucocorticoid and is devoid of mineralocorticoid effects; estrogen adds nothing to the therapy. Fludrocortisone (choice D) has some glucocorticoid effect in addition to its primary mineralocorticoid action and is sometimes used as sole therapy in stable adrenal insufficiency. However, in Addisonian crisis its glucocorticoid action is insufficient and progesterone does not provide the needed glucocorticoid effect. Triamcinolone and betamethasone (choice E) are both potent, selective glucocorticoids devoid of mineralocorticoid action.

738. **(A)** Liddle syndrome is an autosomal dominant disease in which there is unregulated, excess activity of the apical sodium channel in the principal cells in the cortical collecting duct

due to mutations in its structure. Treatment consists of direct inhibition of the sodium channel by either amiloride (choice A) or triamterene, both of which are classified as potassium-sparing diuretics. Triamterene is less useful than amiloride because of its low potency and low solubility, which may lead to the formation of stones. Fludrocortisone (choice B) is a synthetic mineralocorticoid used for replacement therapy in hypoaldosteronism. Although aldosterone levels are reduced in this patient, administration of a mineralocorticoid will exacerbate rather than relieve the hypertension and hypokalemic metabolic alkalosis. Hydrochlorothiazide (choice C), a thiazide diuretic, will exacerbate the problem because inhibition of the Na^+/Cl^--symporter in the distal convoluted tubule results in delivery of more sodium to the cortical collecting duct, where the hyperactivity of the sodium channel and resulting potassium extrusion along with increased proton exchange from type A intercalated cells results in greater hypokalemia and alkalosis. Lisinopril (choice D) is an ACE inhibitor used in the treatment of essential hypertension. Because the problem in Liddle disease is specific to sodium channel hyperactivity within the principal cells in the cortical collecting duct, use of an ACE inhibitor would not correct the pathophysiology underlying the hypokalemia and metabolic alkalosis. Spironolactone (choice E) is a synthetic steroid that acts as a selective antagonist at the aldosterone receptor. It is used as a potassium-sparing diuretic. In the case of Liddle disease, spironolactone has no utility; aldosterone does not play a causative role and its levels are already depressed.

739. **(A)** Streptokinase is a protein produced by β-hemolytic streptococci. It has no intrinsic enzymatic activity, but instead forms a stable complex with the patient's plasminogen making it enzymatically active in cleaving free plasminogen to plasmin. The streptokinase–plasminogen complex is not inhibited by antiplasmin. Anistreplase is a preformed complex of streptokinase and recombinant human plasminogen, a complex that becomes enzymatically active spontaneously. The other thrombolytic

agents—t-PA, reteplase, and urokinase—activate plasminogen directly. Competitive blocking of binding of plasminogen to fibrin (choice B) is a property of aminocaproic acid (AMICAR), a lysine analog used to inhibit fibrinolysis. Conversion of plasmin to plasminogen (choice C) is incorrect; it is plasminogen that is converted to plasmin in the thrombolytic action. Inhibition of cyclo-oxygenase activity (choice D) is a property of the NSAIDs that contributes to prevention of platelet aggregation and thrombosis. Heparin exerts its anticoagulant actions by providing a template for the combination of thrombin and antithrombin III (choice E).

740. **(A)** Diplopia, abnormal gait, and other signs of cerebellar dysfunction are important symptoms of phenytoin toxicity. Other manifestations of toxicity include gingival hyperplasia, nystagmus, and vertigo. Metabolic effects of phenytoin include hyperglycemia (by inhibiting insulin release from the pancreas) and osteomalacia (by altering vitamin D metabolism and increasing the metabolism of vitamin K, a factor necessary for production of bone proteins). Hyperprolactinemia (choice B) is an adverse effect of antipsychotic agents such as the phenothiazines, which are antagonists at dopamine receptors; dopamine exerts negative control of prolactin secretion at the anterior pituitary. It is not an effect of phenytoin toxicity. Polydipsia and polyuria (choice C) are symptoms of diabetes insipidus. These symptoms may be produced by lithium toxicity during treatment of bipolar depression, and are not associated with phenytoin toxicity. Postural hypotension (choice D) is not an adverse effect of phenytoin. Postural hypotension can be produced by antihypertensive agents that work peripherally rather than centrally, as well as antipsychotic agents such as the phenothiazines that have α_1-adrenoreceptor–blocking actions. Rigidity and tremor (choice E) are symptoms of parkinsonism. These symptoms may also be produced by dopamine antagonists such as antipsychotic agents, but are not associated with phenytoin toxicity.

741. **(B)** Folic acid has been found to be important in the prevention of neural tube defects during fetal development. It is now added to flour and other foodstuffs in the United States. In vitro studies of β-carotene (choice A) have demonstrated antioxidant properties for this precursor of vitamin A, but it does not affect neural tube development. High doses of β-carotene have been implicated in increasing the risk of lung cancer. Although vitamin A (choice C) is lipid soluble and has antioxidant properties, its most important physiologic role seems to be in the control of cell differentiation and proliferation (retinoic acid) and vision (retinal). High doses of vitamin A are teratogenic and analogs such as isotretinoin are absolutely contraindicated in pregnancy. Vitamin C (ascorbic acid, choice D) is water soluble and functions as an antioxidant in the aqueous phase of cells, and as a cofactor for many hydroxylation biosynthetic reactions. α-Tocopherol (choice E) becomes associated with lipoprotein particles after dietary absorption. It is under study for a possible role in the prevention of atherosclerosis.

742. **(B)** The initial atrial fibrillation ECG shows a very rapid ventricular rate, which decreases cardiac output and explains the patient's shortness of breath. After administration of the drug, the ventricular rate markedly slowed, but QRS duration and QT interval were not altered. This pattern of effects is observed with drugs that selectively slow AV conduction (i.e., β-blockers [antiarrhythmic group II] and calcium channel blockers [group IV]). Atropine (choice A) accelerates AV conduction through its antimuscarinic action. Disopyramide (choice C) and quinidine (choice E) are group IA antiarrhythmic drugs and prolong the QRS and QT intervals. Ibutilide (choice D) is a group III drug and prolongs the QT interval. Cardiac glycosides such as digoxin also slow AV conduction (through their parasympathomimetic action), but have a slower onset of action than parenteral calcium or β-blockers.

743. **(D)** Parkinsonian syndrome is a common adverse effect whose occurrence is predictable from the dopamine-blocking actions of the neuroleptics. This syndrome, which is charac-

terized by akinesia and rigidity, can be treated with a centrally acting muscarinic antagonist such as benztropine. Dopamine agonists cannot be used in this iatrogenic Parkinson syndrome because the dopamine receptors are blocked. Acute dystonic reactions (choice A) are the earliest occurring adverse effects of neuroleptic treatment. They are characterized by spasms of the muscles of the face, tongue, neck, and back. The dystonia may be treated with a centrally acting antihistamine such as diphenhydramine. Akathisia (choice B) or motor restlessness is an early occurring adverse effect treated by dose reduction or changing the neuroleptic. It must be differentiated from agitation, because the latter is treated by increasing the neuroleptic dose. Neuroleptic malignant syndrome (choice C) is a rare medical emergency that carries a 10% fatality rate. Propranolol, a β-adrenoreceptor antagonist, has no role in its treatment. Neuroleptic malignant syndrome is characterized by catatonia and fluctuations in blood pressure and heart rate. The first step in treatment is to stop administration of the neuroleptic. Muscle relaxants such as benzodiazepines or dantrolene are helpful. Tardive dyskinesia (choice E) is a late-occurring syndrome that is most frequently seen in elderly female patients after chronic treatment. The syndrome is characterized by choreoathetoid movements that appear to arise as a consequence of dopamine supersensitivity in the basal ganglia. Because there is no satisfactory treatment of the condition, prevention is crucial.

744. **(C)** The total plasma clearance of the drug can be calculated from the relationship $CL = 0.693 \times V_d/t_{1/2}$. The total clearance is therefore 6.93×10 L/7 h or 0.99 L/h (which is equal to 16.5 mL/min). Because we know that the renal clearance is 8.3 mL/min, hepatic metabolism must account for the remaining 8.2 mL/min. Thus, hepatic metabolism accounts for about 50% of the total drug elimination.

745. **(A)** Macrolides such as erythromycin, azithromycin, and clarithromycin inhibit bacterial peptide synthesis at the 50S ribosome.

Rather minor mutations of the binding site render organisms resistant to these drugs. Chloramphenicol and the lincomycins (e.g., clindamycin) also act on the 50S ribosome but not at the same binding site. Inhibition of peptidoglycan chain elongation (choice B) is the mechanism of action of vancomycin. Peptidoglycan cross-linking (choice C) is inhibited by β-lactams such as penicillins and cephalosporins. Aminoglycosides (e.g., gentamicin) inhibit the formation of the initiation complex of ribosomes on messenger RNA (choice D). These agents also cause miscoding of synthesized proteins and block the translocation of the ribosome on mRNA. Inhibition of topoisomerase (choice E) is the mechanism of action of fluoroquinolones.

746. **(E)** The plasma level (C_p) is already at 60% of the target concentration. To achieve and maintain 100% of the target of 500 mg/mL, the infusion needs to be increased by two-thirds (40% is two-thirds of 60%). Administering an additional loading dose (choices A and B) produces only a transient increase in concentration. The present infusion rate is 30 mg/h, so an increase of two-thirds (20 mg/h) requires an infusion rate of 50 mg/h (choice E). Another way of reaching this answer is to calculate a corrected clearance based on the known initial infusion rate and the present steady state C_p; then compute the new infusion rate on the basis of the corrected clearance. Thus, $CL_{(corrected)} = $ infusion rate$/C_p = 30$ mg/h/0.3 mg/mL $= 100$ mL/h. Then infusion rate$_{(corrected)} = CL_{(corrected)} \times C_{p(target)} = 100$ mL/h $\times 0.5$ mg/mL $= 50$ mg/h.

747. **(E)** The agents listed are the primary drugs used in the treatment of tuberculosis. Isoniazid and rifampin are the most efficacious and least toxic, but even when used together are insufficient in many cases to prevent the development of resistance. Therefore, most cases of tuberculosis are treated with three or even four agents in an effort to eradicate the infection before resistance develops. Because each drug has distinctive toxicities, it is sometimes possible to achieve a cure without severe toxicity. Ethambutol (choice A) causes visual dysfunction and possible retinal damage, not hearing loss. Isoniazid (choice B) causes peripheral neuropathies and hepatic damage. Fortunately, hepatitis is uncommon in children treated with this drug. Pyrazinamide (choice C) causes joint pains and swelling, GI upset, and rash. Rifampin (choice D) causes proteinuria, rash, and thrombocytopenia. Streptomycin (choice E) and other aminoglycosides cause eighth nerve damage, which is often irreversible and may take the form of auditory or vestibular dysfunction.

748. **(B)** The combination of diltiazem, a calcium channel blocker (for prophylaxis) and isosorbide dinitrate (for treatment of acute angina attacks) is effective and safe. Patients with bronchial hyperreactivity should never be treated with β-blocking drugs if other drug groups are sufficient to control symptoms. Atenolol (choice A), propranolol (choice C), and metoprolol (choice D) are all β-blockers and place the patient at risk for severe asthmatic attacks. Verapamil and nifedipine (choice E) are both calcium channel blockers and the combination does not provide significant advantages over monotherapy.

749. **(D)** LMW heparin does not significantly alter the aPPT test so its effect cannot be readily monitored. Fortunately, these drugs are relatively reliable in use, so that regular monitoring is not needed. The aPPT test is the standard test for HMW heparin effect and because of the irregular and unpredictable response to HMW heparin in many patients, the test should be performed regularly. No form of heparin is active orally (choice A). LMW heparin has a somewhat longer half-life than HMW heparin and does not have to be given as often (choice B). Both LMW and HMW heparins are indicated in coronary syndromes and deep venous thrombosis (choice C). HMW heparin has been shown to be safe in pregnancy; the safety of LMW heparin has not been demonstrated (choice E).

750. **(E)** Vasodilators act by one of three mechanisms: increase cyclic GMP (cGMP) levels in

vascular smooth muscle cells; open potassium channels; or block calcium channels. The organic nitrates and nitroprusside (nitrovasodilators) increase cGMP synthesis by generating nitric oxide (NO) that subsequently activates a soluble form of guanylyl cyclase. Activation of muscarinic receptors on vascular endothelial cells results in formation of NO (earlier identified as endothelial-derived relaxing factor) that diffuses to smooth muscle cells and relaxes them through increased cGMP levels. Erection of the penis involves neuronally regulated formation of NO, increased cGMP levels in the corpus cavernosum, and relaxation of corporal and vascular smooth muscle in erectile tissue. Rather than stimulating guanylyl cyclase, sildenafil (Viagra) acts as a selective inhibitor of cGMP phosphodiesterase type 5 to increase the half-life of cGMP in the tissues. The fact that sildenafil acts downstream of NO stimulation of guanylyl cyclase accounts for the toxic interactions between nitrovasodilators and sildenafil. The mechanism for relaxation of vascular smooth muscle by hydralazine (choice A) is unknown, but may involve NO. Minoxidil (choice B) is metabolized to minoxidil sulfate, which activates an ATP-sensitive potassium channel in smooth muscle. The outflow of potassium produces hyperpolarization and subsequent relaxation of smooth muscle cells. Nitroprusside (choice C) is a nitrovasodilator as described. It spontaneously releases NO by a mechanism distinct from that of the organic nitrates. Prazosin (choice D) produces vasodilation by inhibiting α$_1$-adrenoreceptors on arteriolar smooth muscle to block norepinephrine-induced vasoconstriction.

751. **(B)** A normally functioning endocrine pancreas provides a low basal level of circulating insulin and spikes of insulin release in response to the ingestion of food and subsequent elevation of blood sugar. In a diabetic, use of morning and evening injections of a slowly released form such as lente insulin provides a low basal level of circulating insulin. The pre-meal injections of rapid-acting insulin provide the spikes of circulating in-

sulin needed to deal with the dietary glucose load. Regular insulin or insulin lispro is needed here because the release kinetics from the intermediate (NPH) and slow (lente) formulations do not provide a sufficiently rapid increase in circulating levels of insulin to control blood glucose level after a meal.

752. **(E)** *Pseudomonas aeruginosa* is an aerobic gramnegative bacterium that is frequently the causative agent in diabetic malignant external otitis. Increased susceptibility to infection in diabetics with poor glycemic control probably arises through impairment of leukocyte function. Such serious *P. aeruginosa* infections are best treated parenterally with a broad-spectrum β-lactam cell wall synthesis inhibitor such as ticarcillin in combination with an aminoglycoside such as tobramycin. Chloramphenicol (choice A) is a protein synthesis inhibitor. *Pseudomonas aeruginosa* is resistant to chloramphenicol. Nafcillin plus kanamycin (choice B) is a combination of a penicillinase-resistant penicillin plus a limited spectrum aminoglycoside. Nafcillin is useful in treating penicillinaseproducing staphylococcal infections, but does not possess a broad enough antibacterial spectrum to treat *P. aeruginosa*. Kanamycin is ineffective against *P. aeruginosa* and is used orally or topically, not parenterally as needed here. Sulfamethoxazole plus trimethoprim (choice C) is a combination of a folate synthesis inhibitor and a dihydrofolate reductase inhibitor that is effective in treating urinary tract infections. *Pseudomonas aeruginosa* is resistant to this combination. Tetracycline (choice D) is a bacteriostatic protein synthesis inhibitor. When first introduced, tetracycline was effective in treating *Pseudomonas*, but now all strains are resistant.

753. **(B)** Diabetic gastroparesis is a late complication of diabetes that involves loss of normal motility of the stomach and small intestine. Gastric retention occurs after meals and if the stomach does not empty within several hours, vomiting often results. Prokinetic drugs increase GI motility and promote gastric emptying. Metoclopramide has dopamine receptor antagonistic properties in the CNS and the GI tract. Its CNS actions include inhibition of

vomiting induced by chemotherapy. In this patient, metoclopramide can increase the motility of smooth muscle from the esophagus to small bowel and is therefore effective in promoting gastric emptying. Diphenhydramine (choice A) is an antihistamine (H₁ blocker) with antimuscarinic activity that is useful in treating extrapyramidal dystonias and emesis due to chemotherapy. In the GI tract, diphenhydramine produces hypomotility because of its antimuscarinic activity. Omeprazole (choice C) is a proton pump inhibitor that is very useful in the treatment of peptic disease such as gastroesophageal reflux and peptic ulcer. It is of no value in gastroparesis. Ondansetron (choice D) is a very effective antiemetic for chemotherapy-induced and postsurgical vomiting. It is not effective in gastroparesis. Scopolamine (choice E) is a muscarinic receptor antagonist with good anti-motion sickness properties. It produces hypomotility of the GI tract and is contraindicated in this patient.

754. **(A)** Excellent analgesia and significant addictive properties are associated with drugs that act at mu-type (μ-type) opioid receptors. Of the analgesics listed, codeine is a weak agonist at μ-receptors, whereas the other opioid analgesics listed (choices C, D, and E) are full agonists. Therefore codeine (choice A) is less efficacious but also has the lowest addiction and abuse liability; it is therefore the agent of choice within this list. Diphenoxylate (choice B) is a congener of meperidine (and the primary component of Lomotil) that is used to control GI motility in diarrhea. At its therapeutic dose levels, neither analgesia nor addiction are observed. Meperidine (choice C) is a synthetic μ-opioid receptor agonist with high addiction liability. Methadone (choice D) is a μ-opioid receptor agonist with good oral efficacy and a long plasma half-life (15 to 40 h). It is used in the treatment of opioid addiction. Morphine (choice E) is the prototype μ-opioid receptor agonist and possesses high addiction liability.

755. **(C)** The hydroxymethylglutaryl-CoA (HMG-CoA) reductase inhibitor lovastatin and the bile acid-binding resin cholestyramine (choice

C) both exert hepatic effects through lowering the intracellular concentration of cholesterol. Because they act by different mechanisms, combination therapy is at least additive. The combination of chlortetracycline and amoxicillin (choice A) results in antagonism of amoxicillin's antibacterial action. The β-lactam cell wall synthesis inhibitors such as the penicillins and cephalosporins are bactericidal, but are effective primarily when the bacteria proliferate rapidly. Tetracyclines are bacteriostatic agents that slow or inhibit the growth of bacterial cells by inhibiting protein synthesis. The combination of clomiphene and chorionic gonadotropin (choice B) does not produce any beneficial additive action. Both agents are used to treat female infertility. Clomiphene is an estrogen-receptor antagonist that functions at the level of the hypothalamus to stimulate release of gonadotropin-releasing hormone (GnRH). The increased release of GnRH results in increased release of the gonadotropins LH and FSH from the anterior pituitary. This results in stimulation of ovulation. Administration of chorionic gonadotropin also stimulates ovulation. Because both preparations function through increases in gonadotropin levels and both are present at their effective concentrations, a beneficial additive effect is unlikely. The combination of pentazocine and morphine (choice D) does not produce a beneficial interaction. Pentazocine exerts its pain-relieving activity by a weak (partial) agonist action at μ-opioid receptors. Morphine is a full agonist at the same receptors. When the two analgesic agents are combined, pentazocine acts as an antagonist for morphine at μ-receptors. The result is precipitation of withdrawal in addicted patients, and dysphoria and loss of morphine analgesia in nonaddicted patients. Succinylcholine and atracurium (choice E) are both skeletal muscle-relaxing agents that block muscle contraction by actions at the neuromuscular junction. Succinylcholine is a depolarizing blocker that acts as a long-lasting agonist at the nicotinic receptor. Atracurium is a competitive antagonist at the same receptor. Because they both act at the same receptor and are present at their effective concentrations, atracurium interferes with the action of succinylcholine.

756. (B) Drug X has a larger therapeutic index (calculated as TD_{50}/EC_{50}) than drug Y. At a concentration of 1 E-05 M (1×10^{-5} M, choice A), both drugs produce adverse effects in about 50%, not 90% to 100% of patients. Drug X is not necessarily more efficacious than drug Y (choice C); quantal dose–response data provide no information about maximum efficacy. Drug Y is not more potent than drug X (choice D); it is less potent (it has a higher EC_{50}). Drug Y is not safer than drug X (choice E) from the data presented; if anything, more adverse effects are produced by drug Y at its EC_{50} than by drug X at its EC_{50}.

757. (C) Long-standing hypertension is often complicated by congestive heart failure. Angiotensin antagonists of the ACE inhibitor or angiotensin receptor-blocking type are first-line therapy for both congestive heart failure and hypertension. Diuretics are similarly appropriate for both conditions. Enalapril (an ACE inhibitor) and hydrochlorothiazide (a diuretic) are complementary in their actions and are most appropriate for this case. Dobutamine (choice A) must be given parenterally and is suitable only for treating acute congestive heart failure. A vasodilator such as hydralazine (choices B and E) should be accompanied by a sympathoplegic agent such as a β-blocker to control reflex tachycardia. Hydralazine is not a first-line drug for treating congestive heart failure. Furosemide and spironolactone (choice D) are both diuretics and act at different sites in the nephron; furosemide is a short-acting agent (2 to 4 h duration) and spironolactone is much longer acting (24 to 48 h). The combination should be reserved for severe edema associated with cardiac failure.

758. (C) With a constant infusion of drug X, there is an increase in pulse pressure, which indicates an increase in stroke volume. Increased stroke volume indicates an increase in cardiac force of contraction that might result from an agent with positive inotropic action. Epinephrine acts on cardiac β_1-adrenoreceptors to stimulate contractile force. The decrease in diastolic pressure indicates that peripheral resistance has decreased. Epinephrine acts on β_2-adrenoreceptors in skeletal muscle blood vessels to reduce vascular resistance. Because skeletal muscle contains a large vascular bed, total peripheral resistance decreases even though epinephrine can also act on α_1-adrenoreceptors in arterioles in the skin and splanchnic vascular beds to produce vasoconstriction. This reduction of total peripheral resistance depends on the concentration of epinephrine. β-Adrenoreceptors are somewhat more sensitive and respond at lower concentrations than α-adrenoreceptors. At higher epinephrine concentrations, more α-adrenoreceptors are activated, and an increase in total peripheral resistance is usually observed. The large pulse pressure (the difference between systolic and diastolic) and small effect on mean pressure are characteristic of small and intermediate doses of epinephrine. With the bolus injection, epinephrine initially produces increases in both systolic and diastolic pressures. As the plasma epinephrine concentration declines with time, the systolic pressure rapidly decreases toward the baseline value, and diastolic pressure remains depressed for a longer period due to the higher affinity of the β_2-adrenoreceptors for epinephrine. Acetylcholine (choice A) decreases total peripheral resistance through activation of vascular muscarinic receptors (present in spite of the lack of cholinergic innervation), and causes relaxation of vascular smooth muscle. Amphetamine (choice B), because it displaces norepinephrine from adrenergic nerve terminals, produces responses similar to those of norepinephrine (i.e., α-agonist effects with increased peripheral resistance and weaker β_1 effects on the heart). Amphetamine does not exhibit any direct β actions. Isoproterenol (choice D), a strong β_1- and β_2-agonist, causes a large decrease in total peripheral resistance, thereby reducing diastolic pressure. The drug also stimulates the heart, causing an increase in pulse pressure, but the systolic pressure does not rise as much as shown in the figure and diastolic pressure falls regardless of

the mode of administration. Phenylephrine (choice E) is an α-adrenoreceptor agonist. It increases diastolic pressure by increasing total peripheral resistance. It has little direct effect on the heart, but the increase in blood pressure causes a reflex bradycardia.

759. **(A)** The current drug of choice for acute AV node reentrant tachycardia (a supraventricular tachycardia [SVT]) is the nucleoside adenosine. This agent, when given as a bolus, causes marked hyperpolarization of AV node tissue and transiently blocks conduction of AV node action potentials. This abolishes the reentrant impulse and allows normal sinus rhythm to be reestablished. The half-life of adenosine is about 3 seconds and the duration of action of the dose used is about 15 seconds, so toxicities from this therapy are minimal. Calcium channel blockers such as verapamil and diltiazem are also effective in SVT. Bethanechol (choice B) is a muscarinic agonist and produces hypotension and other muscarinic effects. It is ineffective in SVT. Isoproterenol (choice C) is a β-selective adrenoreceptor agonist that causes hypotension and reflex sympathetic discharge to the heart, along with direct stimulation. It is more likely to cause than to abolish arrhythmias. Propranolol (choice D) slows AV conduction and might abolish the AV reentrant rhythm, but because this patient has asthma, β-blockers are contraindicated. Furthermore, β-blockers are not very effective in converting preexisting SVT. Similarly, quinidine (choice E) and related group IA antiarrhythmic drugs are not as effective as adenosine in converting SVT to normal sinus rhythm.

760. **(A)** Myasthenia gravis is an autoimmune disease attributable to an impairment of nicotinic receptor function at the neuromuscular junction by antireceptor antibodies. Severe, progressive skeletal muscle weakness is the major manifestation. Treatment consists of increasing the junctional concentration of acetylcholine with a carbamate anticholinesterase such as pyridostigmine. Because anticholinesterase treatment causes excess muscarinic effects in some patients, an antimuscarinic drug such as

propantheline is often also used. Infections such as influenza may change the anticholinesterase dose requirement in myasthenia either up or down. In this patient, the problem is to distinguish whether the muscle weakness is attributable to myasthenic crisis (too little medication) or cholinergic crisis (too much medication); both conditions cause muscle weakness. The safest definitive method is to administer a small dose of the short-acting anticholinesterase edrophonium. If the patient is in myasthenic crisis, an immediate improvement in muscle function should be evident. If the patient is in cholinergic crisis, the patient's condition may worsen, but because the duration of action for edrophonium is just 5 to 10 minutes, this test provides less risk than other alternatives. Parenteral atropine should be available to treat excess parasympathetic activity. Administration of a test dose of a long-acting agent such as tubocurarine (choice B) to elicit muscle weakness is a provocative test that is dangerous and does not provide definitive evidence for diagnosis. Symptoms of parasympathetic hyperactivity (choice C) are normally evident in cholinergic crisis, except that this patient is being treated with the muscarinic antagonist propantheline. Administration of pralidoxime (choice D) is incorrect because pralidoxime is useful for reactivation of cholinesterase only in the case of recent organophosphate intoxication. Administration of pyridostigmine (choice E) is unwise because a patient in cholinergic crisis is put at risk of exacerbation and extension of the toxic episode for a significant period of time.

761. **(D)** Pain of malignancy is still a badly undertreated condition, due to misunderstanding of the nature of opioid tolerance and addiction and an unwillingness to deal with the complications of prescribing controlled substances. Codeine has limited maximum efficacy, so additional doses of this drug (choice A) are unlikely to control this patient's pain. It was previously thought that regular use of strong opioids for any purpose inevitably led to tolerance and a loss of analgesic effect, as well as addiction (choice B). However, excellent clinical studies have shown that this is not the case. Regular use (as opposed to as-needed use) of small to moderate doses of opioids effectively controls pain in most cases without causing tolerance or addiction. In fact, restricting opioids to use only when absolutely needed results in larger total analgesia requirements and greater toxicity. Use of NSAIDs (choice C) should be started early, when pain is mild and supplemented with oral opioids such as codeine as soon as it becomes necessary. NSAIDs are not adequate at this stage of this patient's disease. Parenteral morphine given when necessary (choice E) is as not as effective as regularly scheduled morphine and leads to greater drug toxicity.

762. **(D)** Salivation is under parasympathetic control; salivary glands contain muscarinic receptors, primarily of the M_3 subtype. Agonists such as bethanechol and indirect agents such as neostigmine mimic parasympathetic nerve stimulation. Blood vessel endothelial cells contain M_3 receptors that are not innervated, but respond to circulating direct-acting muscarinic agonists. When these endothelial receptors are activated, nitric oxide synthesis is stimulated and smooth muscle relaxation occurs promptly with vasodilation and a drop in blood pressure. Because no nerve endings are present, indirect-acting cholinomimetics such as cholinesterase inhibitors do not have this vasodilating effect. In the presence of hypotension induced by a direct-acting muscarinic agonist, a strong compensatory reflex originates in the baroreceptors and results in increased sympathetic outflow to the heart. Tachycardia results. In the case of cholinesterase inhibitors, the normal slowing effect of the vagus is amplified and at normal doses, bradycardia results. The effect of the new drug illustrated in Figure 6–7 is most consistent with a direct-acting muscarinic agonist (choice D). Alpha receptor ligands (choices A and B) have little effect on salivation, although indirectly acting agents like ephedrine can cause a sensation of dry mouth. However, ephedrine causes increased blood pressure. A ganglionic stimulant drug (choice E) causes increased salivation but also increases sympathetic discharge

to the blood vessels and results in increased, not decreased, blood pressure.

763. **(C)** Isoproterenol acts directly on β_2-adrenoreceptors in blood vessels to cause vasodilation and a drop in blood pressure. It also directly activates β_1- and β_2-receptors in the heart to cause tachycardia. Finally, the reduced blood pressure that results from vasodilation evokes a compensatory reflex tachycardia that is transmitted through the sympathetic ganglia. Prevention of isoproterenol's tachycardia would require that both β_1- and β_2-receptors in the heart be blocked. On the other hand, prevention of isoproterenol's vasodilation requires only that β_2-receptors be blocked. Selective β_2-blockers prevent vasodilation without blocking the direct β_1-mediated tachycardia. β_2-Selective blockers are not used clinically, but the research drug butoxamine has this property. A drug acting at vascular α-receptors (choice A) has no effect on the β actions of isoproterenol. A β_1-blocker (choice B) might reduce the tachycardia but not prevent it, and does not prevent the hypotensive action of the drug. Muscarinic agonists or antagonists (choice D) do not influence the action of isoproterenol. A ganglion blocker (choice E) might reduce the reflex tachycardia induced by isoproterenol, but does not affect the direct vasodilation or the direct cardiac effects of the drug.

764. **(E)** Carbidopa is a peripheral inhibitor of dopa decarboxylase. Dopa decarboxylase is an enzyme present in large amounts in the GI tract and peripheral tissues, and in smaller amounts in the nerve terminals of dopaminergic neurons in the basal ganglia. It is required for the conversion of DOPA to dopamine in the biosynthesis of dopamine and norepinephrine. However, when the prodrug levodopa is used for parkinsonism, over 90% is metabolized in the periphery by the enzyme to dopamine and inactive products and only about 3% of the administered dose enters the brain. Unfortunately, dopamine does not cross the blood–brain barrier, so dopamine formed outside the brain is of no value in treating parkinsonism. When carbidopa is given with levodopa, less levodopa is metabolized in the gut and other peripheral tissues, so more (about 10%) is available to enter the CNS. Carbidopa does not cross the blood–brain barrier, so it does not prevent conversion of levodopa to active dopamine in the basal ganglia. Combination therapy thus reduces the peripheral effects of levodopa–dopamine and allows patients to receive more benefit from levodopa. Choices A through D are incorrect.

765. **(E)** All of the mechanisms listed are valid mechanisms of antiemetic therapy that are used in cancer chemotherapy. Dronabinol is a cannabinoid agonist (choice A). Dexamethasone is a corticosteroid (choice B). Metoclopramide is a dopamine antagonist (choice C). Diphenhydramine is a histamine antagonist (choice D). Ondansetron is a 5-HT$_3$ antagonist. In the prevention of nausea and vomiting caused by chemotherapeutic agents, a cocktail of three, four, or more of these agents is often used. Ondansetron is also effective in reducing postsurgical vomiting.

766. **(D)** Ibuprofen, an NSAID, is appropriate for both rheumatoid and gouty arthritis. Aspirin (choice A) provides both analgesic and anti-inflammatory action in rheumatoid arthritis, but is a poor choice in a patient with gout. Although it can be uricosuric at very high dosages, it may actually increase uric acid retention at lower doses. Codeine (choice B) provides analgesia but no anti-inflammatory action. Colchicine (choice C) has high efficacy in reducing the pain of acute gout and in preventing attacks, but is of no value in rheumatoid arthritis. It is used mostly in low doses as a prophylactic against acute gout. Morphine (choice E), like codeine, has no anti-inflammatory action. Its analgesic efficacy is probably greater than that needed for the case described.

767. **(A)** Botulinum toxin is an enzyme that enters presynaptic cholinergic nerve terminals by endocytosis and cleaves proteins involved in neurotransmitter exocytosis. The resulting impairment of acetylcholine release causes autonomic blockade and somatic motor weakness.

The major hazard of botulinum poisoning is paralysis of skeletal muscle and respiratory failure. Therapeutic preparations of the toxin (Botox) are used by injection for severe muscle spasm in multiple sclerosis and cerebral palsy. It is also used cosmetically to reduce or obliterate facial frown lines. Inhibition of smooth muscle myosin light chain kinase (choice B) produces smooth muscle relaxation. Irreversible inhibition of cholinesterase (choice C) as seen in organophosphate intoxication results in excessive muscarinic actions and muscle paralysis attributable to depolarizing blockade at the neuromuscular junction. Nicotinic receptor blockade (choice D) is the mechanism for skeletal muscle relaxation by curare-like agents. Because the problem in botulism toxicity is at the level of loss of transmitter release, choline administration (choice E) to increase acetylcholine synthesis has no effect.

768. **(C)** Latanoprost is a $PGF_{2\alpha}$ analog used topically to increase aqueous outflow. Atracurium (choice A) is a nondepolarizing neuromuscular blocking agent that is of no value in glaucoma. Dorzolamide (choice B) is a topically active carbonic anhydrase inhibitor that inhibits the synthesis of aqueous humor. Pilocarpine is a muscarinic cholinomimetic that increases aqueous outflow. Timolol (choice E) is a β-adrenoreceptor blocker that reduces aqueous synthesis.

769. **(B)** Clozapine is an atypical antipsychotic that is more selective for D_4 than D_2 receptors and causes agranulocytosis in a small but significant fraction of patients. Amitriptyline (choice A) is a tricyclic antidepressant with a major toxicity of atropine-like antimuscarinic effects. Sedative effects and α-adrenoreceptor blockade may also be troublesome. Haloperidol (choice C) is an older, highly potent antipsychotic agent with major extrapyramidal toxicity. Lithium carbonate (choice D) is an antimanic drug that causes tremor, nephrogenic diabetes insipidus, and hypothyroidism. Thioridazine (choice E) is a phenothiazine antipsychotic agent that causes retinitis pigmentosa and cardiac arrhythmias in overdose.

770. **(B)** Ibutilide is a group III antiarrhythmic drug. Blockade of delayed rectifier potassium channels, which are important for repolarization of the cardiac action potential, is the mechanism of group III drugs such as ibutilide and dofetilide. These agents prolong the action potential duration, the QT interval, and the refractory period. Amiodarone, sotalol, and all group IA drugs (e.g., quinidine) also have these group III effects. Note that most antiarrhythmic drugs have actions of more than one group; for example, amiodarone has actions typical of groups IA, II, III, and IV. Blockade of cardiac β-adrenoreceptors (choice A) is the mechanism of action of group II antiarrhythmic drugs such as esmolol and propranolol. Blockade of voltage-dependent calcium channels (choice C) is the mechanism of action of group IV drugs such as verapamil and diltiazem. Blockade of voltage-dependent sodium channels (choice D) is the mechanism of action of all group I drugs such as lidocaine, flecainide, amiodarone, and quinidine. Opening of diastolic potassium channels appears to be the major mechanism of action of adenosine, a drug that is extremely effective in abolishing AV nodal reentrant arrhythmias.

771. **(E)** The oral anticoagulants such as warfarin block the vitamin K–dependent step in the synthesis of coagulation factors VII, IX, X, and prothrombin. Carboxylation of descarboxyprothrombin to form prothrombin containing γ-carboxyglutamate residues requires the reduced form of vitamin K as a cofactor. Vitamin K epoxide is formed as a product. KH_2 must be regenerated by an NADH-dependent epoxide reductase for the next round of carboxylation. It is the epoxide reductase step that is blocked by oral anticoagulants. Heparin exerts its anticoagulant actions by acting as a template for combining thrombin and antithrombin III (choice A). Warfarin has no degradative effect (choice B) on the thrombin molecule. The thrombolytic agent streptokinase becomes active in fibrinolysis by forming an active complex with plasminogen (choice C). The oral anticoagulants do not inhibit calcium binding to coagu-

lation factors (choice D), but calcium binding is reduced because of the absence of γ-carboxyglutamate residues within the sequences of the coagulation factors VII, IX, X, and prothrombin.

772. **(C)** Hydrochlorothiazide causes potassium wasting and may lead to hypokalemia requiring dietary potassium. Potassium wasting is characteristic of diuretics that present more sodium to the collecting tubule, where sodium is conserved in exchange for potassium under the control of aldosterone. Therefore, diuretics that act in the proximal convoluted tubule (carbonic anhydrase inhibitors), ascending limb of the loop of Henle (loop diuretics), and distal convoluted tubule (thiazides) cause potassium wasting and may lead to dangerous hypokalemia. Angiotensin antagonists (because they interfere with aldosterone secretion) and aldosterone inhibitors have the opposite effect. Amiloride (choice A) and spironolactone (choice E) are aldosterone antagonists; captopril (choice B) and losartan (choice D) are angiotensin antagonists. All of these agents cause potassium retention and may cause hyperkalemia, not hypokalemia.

773. **(D)** Ranitidine is an H_2-receptor antagonist. H_2-receptors have been identified in numerous sites, including the stomach, heart, uterus, ileum, and bronchial musculature. Gastric acid secretion involves activation of H_2-receptors, and peptic disorders such as duodenal ulcer often respond to treatment with H_2-receptor antagonists. Unless the ulcer is the result of NSAID therapy, treatment also calls for eradication of *Helicobacter pylori* because this bacterium is the causative agent for most duodenal ulcers. Aluminum hydroxide (choice A) is an antacid that may reduce symptoms of peptic disease, but is inconvenient to use and constipating. Misoprostol (choice B) is an orally active PGE_1 analog that is used in the treatment or prevention of NSAID-induced ulcers. Omeprazole (choice C) is a proton pump (H^+/K^+-ATPase) inhibitor that is extremely effective in the treatment of peptic disease, including ulcers, gastroesophageal reflux disorder, and gastrinoma. Lansoprazole and rabeprazole are similar. Sucralfate (choice E) is a sucrose–aluminum–sulfate compound that polymerizes in an acid environment and is able to form a protective coating over an ulcer bed. It must be taken four times a day, so it is less convenient than H_2-blockers or proton pump inhibitors.

774. **(A)** ACE inhibitors such as captopril and enalapril are effective agents for systemic hypertension in many patients. However, ACE inhibitors are contraindicated in pregnancy. Apparently, the action of angiotensin is needed for normal development of the fetal kidney. By inhibiting ACE, these drugs impair conversion of angiotensin I to angiotensin II and prolong the half-life of bradykinin, a vasodilator that ACE normally degrades. ACE inhibitors are highly useful in the treatment of CHF (choice B). The drugs decrease cardiac preload and afterload and prevent ventricular remodeling. ACE inhibition has a protective effect on renal function in diabetics (choice C). Unlike centrally acting sympathoplegic agents such as clonidine, there is no increase of rebound hypertension after abrupt cessation of therapy (choice D). Renin levels (choice E) rise as feedback inhibition via production of angiotensin II is removed.

775. **(B)** Citalopram is one of the newer, highly SSRIs. Most older, tricyclic/heterocyclic antidepressants block—to varying degrees—reuptake of both norepinephrine and serotonin amine neurotransmitters into the presynaptic nerve terminals. Different agents are relatively selective for one or the other amine. Amitriptyline (choice A), desipramine (choice C), imipramine (choice D), and trazodone (choice E) are members of the tricyclic/heterocyclic group and all have mixed effects on both norepinephrine and serotonin reuptake. Desipramine (choice C) is the most selective agent for blocking uptake of norepinephrine. The selective serotonin uptake inhibitors offer the advantage that they do not produce autonomic side effects, in contrast to the tricyclic/heterocyclic antidepressants.

776. (D) The most common adverse effects of NSAIDs are GI complaints including gastric upset, gastritis, and peptic ulcer. Prostaglandins PGI_2 and especially PGE_1 are cytoprotective agents important in inhibiting acid secretion by the stomach and promoting formation of mucus in the intestine. Nonselective inhibition of both COX-1 and COX-2 by NSAIDs prevents synthesis of these protective prostaglandins as well as the synthesis of the prostaglandins involved in inflammation. COX-2–selective NSAIDs such as rofecoxib and celecoxib cause less GI upset. Bronchospasm (choice A) may rarely be produced by NSAIDs in intolerant patients. The mechanism may involve shunting of arachidonic acid to the lipoxygenase pathway with subsequent formation of bronchoconstrictor leukotrienes. Drowsiness (choice B) is not a common adverse effect of NSAIDs. Fluid retention (choice C) is produced rarely by loss of prostaglandin function in the kidney. This is not a problem in normal individuals, but may become evident in patients with CHF, hepatic cirrhosis, or renal disease. Damage to the kidneys can occur with high or prolonged dosage, and the action of loop and other diuretics is reduced in patients taking NSAIDs. Prolongation of bleeding time (choice E) is attributable to inhibition of COX in platelets. This leads to reduced production of thromboxane A_2, a platelet-aggregating agent. This platelet function in coagulation is inhibited. Although easily demonstrated in the laboratory, NSAIDs other than aspirin have little effect on bleeding tendency because their inhibition of COX is reversible.

777. (B) Megaloblastic anemia is an indication of impaired maturation of erythrocytic precursors and erythrocytes. It usually results from either folic acid or vitamin B_{12} deficiency. Pernicious anemia involves vitamin B_{12} deficiency, with both the hematologic abnormality and impairment of myelination of nerves. The defect in myelination can result in permanent neurologic damage. Maturation of erythrocytes requires the synthesis of large amounts of RNA and DNA. Such synthesis requires a ready supply of tetrahydrofolate. This cofactor requires a source of folic acid in the diet and vitamin B_{12}. Folic acid is present in large quantities in a normal, "enriched" diet and is easily absorbed even in patients with abnormal GI function. Vitamin B_{12}, on the other hand, is present in small quantities and must be complexed with an endogenous protein, intrinsic factor, for absorption. Intrinsic factor is synthesized in the stomach; thus, gastrectomized individuals are unable to absorb ingested vitamin B_{12}. Folic acid supplements can reverse the hematologic abnormality in pernicious anemia but not the neuropathology. Therefore, folic acid supplements (choice D) should not be used in this disease. Because intrinsic factor is not available, oral vitamin B_{12} (choice E) is ineffective unless administered in large quantities. IM administration is the usual route and a single injection can be given monthly. Iron-deficiency anemias (but not megaloblastic anemias) can be treated with iron preparations. Ferric salts such as ferric chloride (choice C) show poorer absorption than the ferrous forms of iron. Parenteral administration of iron, in the form of iron dextran (choice A), is much more toxic than oral administration and is used only when oral iron cannot be given in adequate amounts.

778. (C) Tamoxifen and a newer related drug, raloxifene, are nonsteroidal estrogen analogs that slow the progression of breast cancer; thus, they act as antagonists or partial agonists in breast tissue. At the same time, these selective estrogen receptor-modulating agents have estrogenic agonist effects in bone; both drugs reduce the progression of postmenopausal osteoporosis in the same way as estrogen itself. Tamoxifen definitely does not act as an agonist in breast cancer (choice A); such action would promote tumor development. Neither drug has significant progestin activity (choices B, D, E).

779. (E) Simvastatin is one of the statin inhibitors of HMG-CoA reductase, the rate-limiting enzyme in cholesterol biosynthesis within the liver. The statins are the most efficacious agents in the treatment of elevated LDL cholesterol levels. Inhibition of HMG-CoA reductase prevents hepatocytes from synthesizing cholesterol from HMG-CoA. Lowering intracellular cholesterol levels results in increased transcription of the genes for LDL receptor and HMG-CoA reductase. The increased LDL receptors lower circulating LDL cholesterol levels through increased endocytosis of the lipoprotein particles. Bile acid-binding resins, including cholestyramine (choice A) and colestipol, sequester bile acids in the intestinal lumen, reducing their reabsorption and decreasing cholesterol levels within the liver cell. Clofibrate (choice B) and other fibric acid derivatives including gemfibrozil reduce plasma triglyceride levels by increasing lipoprotein lipase activity, allowing more rapid catabolism of VLDL particles in skeletal muscle and adipose tissue vascular beds. Gemfibrozil (choice C) causes a beneficial increase in HDL cholesterol levels through unknown mechanisms. Niacin (nicotinic acid, choice D), through unknown mechanisms, decreases the production of VLDL particles, which in turn leads to less conversion to LDL particles.

780. **(D)** Chronic lead poisoning results in multiple toxicities including headache, hypertension, infertility, anemia, and renal insufficiency. Mental and growth retardation occur in children. Acute lead intoxication usually presents as encephalopathy or severe abdominal colic, sometimes masquerading as pancreatitis. When blood lead levels exceed 50 µg/dL, chelation treatment is indicated. The calcium ion in calcium disodium edetate is readily displaced by lead, forming a lead chelate that is excreted in the urine. Arsenic poisoning (choice A) is treated with chelation therapy using dimercaprol, succimer, or penicillamine. Atropine (choice B) is a lipophilic muscarinic receptor antagonist that blocks parasympathetic function and at toxic levels produces hallucinations and psychosis. Treatment of atropine intoxication consists of symptomatic management or administration of the lipid-soluble anticholinesterase physostigmine. Toxicity from iron (choice C) may arise from ingestion of iron supplements (as with children swallowing adult preparations) or hemolytic

diseases such as thalassemia. Treatment consists of the use of the iron-chelating agent deferoxamine. EDTA does not chelate mercury (choice E). Inorganic mercury poisoning is treated by using chelation therapy with dimercaprol, succimer, or penicillamine. Organic mercury poisoning is more difficult to treat because of the lipophilic nature of organomercury compounds.

781. **(C)** Mebendazole is a broad-spectrum antihelmintic that is effective against a variety of nematodes including ascarids, hookworm *(Necator, Ancylostoma)*, whipworm *(Trichuris)*, threadworm *(Stronglyloides)*, and pinworm *(Enterobius)*. Adverse effects are rare. Diethylcarbamazine (choice A) was developed as a treatment for filariasis. Because of adverse effects that include nausea, vomiting, headache, leukocytosis, and proteinuria, it has been largely supplanted by other antifilarial agents, except in the case of *Loa loa*, where it remains the drug of choice. Ivermectin (choice B) is used to treat *Onchocerca volvulus*, the agent responsible for river blindness in west and central Africa. Niclosamide (choice D) and praziquantel (choice E) are agents with primary efficacy against flukes and tapeworms. In the case of *Fasciola hepatica* (sheep liver fluke), however, bithionol or triclabendazole (a veterinary drug) are drugs of choice; in cysticercosis, albendazole is the drug of choice.

782. **(D)** Mefloquine (choice D) has been a prophylactic antimalarial of choice for most parts of the world because of convenience, good efficacy, and relatively low toxicity. In most parts of the world, chloroquine (choice A) resistance is too great to safely use this agent for prophylaxis. Ciprofloxacin and other fluoroquinolones have been studied, but their efficacy is low. Doxycycline (choice C) is an effective prophylactic agent and must be used in areas where mefloquine and chloroquine resistance is widespread (e.g., Southeast Asia). However, it must be taken daily, whereas mefloquine is taken weekly. Pyrimethamine plus sulfadoxine (choice E), a mixture known as Fansidar, was widely used

in the past but resistance by *P. falciparum* is now widespread and toxicity associated with the sulfa component may be significant.

783. **(B)** The leukotrienes LTC_4, LTD_4, and LTE_4 are 5'-lipoxygenase metabolites of arachidonic acid. When lung tissue is challenged with antigen in sensitive individuals, LTC_4 is formed and subsequently metabolized to LTD_4 and LTE_4. These leukotrienes produce bronchoconstriction, increased capillary permeability, and increased mucus formation for an extended time because of their slow tissue clearance. Because the first enzyme in synthesis of leukotrienes from arachidonic acid is 5'-lipoxygenase rather than COX, aspirin (choice E) does not inhibit their biosynthesis. An increased formation of leukotrienes with COX inhibition and shunting of arachidonate to the lipoxygenase pathway by aspirin and other NSAIDs has been postulated. The leukotrienes possess significant cardiovascular effects (choice D); they produce hypotension by decreasing intravascular volume and reducing cardiac contractility by constricting coronary vessels, thus reducing coronary blood flow. Platelets do not contain 5'-lipoxygenase (although they do contain 12'-lipoxygenase), and leukotrienes are not stored in platelet granules (choice C). The COX product of arachidonic acid, TXA_2, is critical in platelet physiology, and acetylation of COX by aspirin accounts for the effect of this drug in inhibiting platelet function. Another leukotriene, LTB_4, is a potent chemotactic agent for polymorphonuclear leukocytes (choice A), but the cysteine-linked leukotrienes LTC_4, LTD_4, and LTE_4 do not share this property.

784. **(D)** The mechanisms of action for the agents that are effective in treating partial and generalized tonic–clonic seizures (e.g., grand mal) fall into two primary areas: promoting the inactive state of voltage-dependent sodium channels, which inhibits sustained repetitive neuronal firing; and enhancing GABA inhibition of synaptic transmission. The mechanisms of action for agents effective against absence seizures involve GABA enhancement and limiting the activation of T-type voltage-dependent calcium channels. GABA is the most abundant inhibitory neurotransmitter in the brain. Tiagabine was designed as an inhibitor of neuronal reuptake of GABA, thereby enhancing its inhibitory synaptic actions. It is effective against both partial and generalized tonic–clonic seizures. Its adverse effects include dizziness, tremor, and nervousness. Carbamazepine (choice A) slows the rate of recovery of inactivated sodium channels. It is a primary drug for the treatment of partial and tonic–clonic seizures. Carbamazepine is cleared by hepatic metabolism and induces its own metabolism. Adverse effects include drowsiness, vertigo, ataxia, and double vision. Ethosuximide (choice B) inhibits T-type calcium channels that are involved in the thalamic 3-Hz spike rhythm of absence seizures. Adverse effects include nausea, vomiting, drowsiness, dizziness, and headache. Lamotrigine (choice C), like phenytoin and carbamazepine, inhibits sodium channel function by promoting voltage- and use-dependent inactivation. Lamotrigine is effective alone against partial seizures as well as absence and generalized seizures. Adverse effects include dizziness, ataxia, double vision, and serious dermatitis. Vigabatrin (choice E) is an irreversible inhibitor of GABA aminotransferase, the enzyme responsible for metabolic inactivation of GABA. It is effective against partial seizures. Adverse effects include drowsiness, dizziness, and weight gain.

785. **(B)** Local anesthetic agents inhibit nerve conduction through state- and use-dependent blockade of voltage-dependent fast sodium channels. As a result, the threshold of excitability of the nerve is increased, and the ability of the nerve to propagate an action potential is decreased. Ultimately, transmission of sensory stimuli to the CNS is suppressed, and motor function involving small fibers in the vicinity of the injection is also lost. Inhibition of nerve conduction via blockade of calcium channels (choice A) is not a mechanism for local anesthetic agents. Inhibition of T-type calcium channels to inhibit synaptic transmission in the thalamus is the mechanism for the antiepileptic agent ethosux-imide. Hyperpolarization of neurons via en-hanced chloride influx (choice C) is not a mechanism for local anesthetic agents, but is the mechanism for inhibition of repetitive neuronal firing by the benzodiazepines, bar-biturates, and other GABA-mimetic and -enhancing agents that act on the GABA$_A$ recep-tor-chloride channel of neurons. Enhanced potassium efflux (choice D) does not occur. Inhibition of pain receptors (choice E) is not a current mechanism for analgesic agents, al-though antagonists at the neurokinin recep-tors involved in nociception (pain percep-tion) are an area of intense research.

786. **(C)** In an individual severely intoxicated by an antihistamine, the combination of initial central excitatory and the later depressant ef-fects is potentially lethal. In children, the dominant effect is excitation; hallucinations, ataxia, incoordination, and convulsions may occur. Symptoms such as fixed and dilated pupils, and a flushed face are common, and resemble those of atropine intoxication. There is no specific therapy for antihistamine in-toxication; treatment is usually supportive. Deepening coma and cardiorespiratory col-lapse (choice A) characterize the late or ter-minal phases of antihistamine intoxication (and many other intoxications). Hypothermia is not a common effect (choice B) and the at-ropine-like toxicity in children may include hyperthermia. Joint pain (choice D) is not as-sociated with antihistamine intoxication. His-tamine administration (choice E), in addition to being dangerous because of the potential for bronchospasm and hypotensive reactions, is not useful because major antihistamine toxicities involve the CNS, and histamine does not gain access.

787. **(D)** Pancreatic (β) cells are electrically polar-ized. Depolarization causes entry of calcium and activation of insulin exocytosis. In hy-poglycemia, the negative resting potential is maintained by the activity of an ATP-sensitive hyperpolarizing potassium channel and insulin secretion is inhibited. When ex-tracellular glucose levels are high, glucose enters the β cells via the GLUT-2 transporter and is metabolized to yield ATP. The in-creased ATP (or other unknown compound) levels cause closure of the potassium channel, allowing the cell to depolarize and secrete in-sulin. Acarbose (choice A) is an inhibitor of intestinal α-glucosidase and thus reduces ab-sorption of glucose. Sulfonylureas such as glipizide (choice B) bind to a cell-surface pro-tein to cause inhibition of the hyperpolarizing potassium channel, thereby allowing the β cell to depolarize and secrete insulin. Met-formin (choice C) and other biguanides are poorly understood, but do not inhibit the potassium channel that is the target of sul-fonylureas. Modulation of insulin release (choice D) is the mechanism of action of the meglitinides such as repaglinide. Although the details are not fully understood, these drugs share one binding site with sulfonyl-ureas and have a second, independent bind-ing site. Rosiglitazone (choice E) and pioglita-zone do not act by reduction of circulating glucagon; this is one proposed mechanism for the biguanides. These thiazolidinediones or "glitazones" appear to act by a peripheral mechanism that reduces insulin resistance, probably mediated by the peroxisome prolif-erator-activated receptor-γ nuclear receptor.

788. **(B)** Anesthetic gases behave as gases in the body and their partial pressure in the blood and tissue, rather than their concentration, is the determining factor in distribution to and from the brain. The blood–gas partition coef-ficient determines the rate of onset of, and re-covery from, anesthesia. The blood solubility of the agent determines how rapidly the par-tial pressure rises or falls in the blood. Agents with high solubility (large blood–gas parti-tion coefficients, such as methoxyflurane) re-quire large amounts of the anesthetic to be put into or removed from the blood before the partial pressure in the blood changes enough to effectively deliver the agent to or remove it from the brain. Such drugs have a very slow onset and offset of action. The MAC value (choice D) and the other proper-ties listed (anesthetic potency [choice A], lipid solubility [choice C], and water solubil-

ity [choice E]) are all direct or inverse measures of the potency, which determines the amount or partial pressure of the agent needed in the brain to produce anesthesia, not the rate of onset or offset. Potency and rate of onset or offset are independent properties of anesthetic agents. Desirable properties for inhalation anesthetic agents include high potency and low blood solubility. The halogenated hydrocarbons such as desflurane and isoflurane fit these criteria and are extensively used.

789.   **(C)** Thyroid storm, a malignant manifestation of thyrotoxicosis, involves an exaggeration of the features of thyrotoxicosis including fever, tachycardia, vomiting, and agitation. The thioamide propylthiouracil exerts its primary antithyroid actions by inhibiting the thyroid peroxidase, which carries out iodine organification and coupling of iodotyrosines. The ability of propylthiouracil to block the peripheral deiodination of thyroxine to tri-iodothyronine adds to the treatment of thyroid storm. Potassium perchlorate (choice A) is an agent that inhibits the uptake of iodide by the thyroid gland. It is rarely used because it can cause fatal aplastic anemia. Propranolol (choice B) is a nonselective β-adrenoreceptor antagonist used to treat the tachycardia of thyrotoxicosis and thyroid storm. Radioactive iodine (^{131}I) (choice D) is used in ablation of hyperactive thyroid tissue in Graves disease. The preparation is administered orally and rapidly accumulates in the thyroid gland where the ionizing radiation destroys the tissue. Reverse T_3 (3,3′,5′-tri-iodothyronine, choice E) is formed from thyroxine in almost equimolar amounts with normal tri-iodothyronine (3,5,3′-tri-iodothyronine). Reverse T_3 is metabolically inactive.

790.   **(B)** Clomiphene is a weak partial agonist at estrogen receptors. When clomiphene binds to these receptors in the hypothalamus and the pituitary, it acts as a competitive antagonist of endogenous estrogen. Clomiphene thus blocks estrogen feedback inhibition of gonadotropin-releasing hormone secretion from the hypothalamus. This allows levels of gonadotropin-releasing hormone and gonadotropins to increase, stimulating ovulation. Cabergoline (choice A) is an ergot derivative that acts as a dopamine agonist in the pituitary to reduce prolactin release. Ethinyl estradiol (choice C), a synthetic estrogen, and norethindrone (choice D), a synthetic progestin, are commonly used separately for replacement therapy in postmenopausal women or combined for oral contraception. Progesterone (choice E) is the most important endogenous human progestin, but is subject to a very high first-pass effect when administered orally. It does not promote ovulation.

791.   **(D)** Nondepolarizing neuromuscular blockers are heavily used in anesthesia because they produce full surgical relaxation without causing significant cardiovascular depression. They act as nicotinic cholinoceptor blockers at the neuromuscular nicotinic receptor with little or no ganglionic blockade. They have some effect on presynaptic cholinoceptors of motor nerves and it is believed that this site of action is the cause of alterations in the response of the motor nerve–muscle system to rapid stimulation. The train of four stimulation pattern is used by anesthesiologists to monitor the level of neuromuscular block in the anesthetized patient and consists of a brief period of stimulation that simulates slow tetanic stimulation. In the absence of drugs, and in the presence of a depolarizing blocker, the twitches during train of four are well maintained in strength. However, after a nondepolarizing blocker the contraction strength fades during the sequence (choices A, C, or D). In the absence of drugs, rapid tetanic stimulation results in moderate increase in contraction during the tetanus and a marked increase in strength of the muscle twitch following the end of the train due, at least in part, to a buildup of calcium in the motor nerve terminal. This post-tetanic potentiation is enhanced by nondepolarizing blockers (choices B, D, or E). Finally, nondepolarizing blockade results from competitive blockade of cholinoceptors, so increasing the amount of acetylcholine in the synapse by means of a drug like neostigmine

can reverse the blockade (choices C, D, or E). Thus, only choice D meets all three requirements.

792. **(E)** Skeletal muscle spasticity results from a loss of inhibitory signals from the brain to primary motor neurons in the spinal cord. These spasms can be very painful and often limit mobility and other functions. Therapies in use include facilitation of GABA action in the CNS (choice B) by benzodiazepines such as diazepam (at $GABA_A$ receptors) and by baclofen (at $GABA_B$ receptors); activation of cord α_2-receptors (choice A) by clonidine or tizanidine; activation of cord glycine receptors (choice C) by glycine itself; interference with neuromuscular transmission (choice D) with botulinum toxin; and interference with calcium release from the sarcoplasmic reticulum of skeletal muscle (choice E) by drugs such as dantrolene.

793. **(C)** The cardiac manifestations of β-blocker intoxication may be very severe, resulting in bradycardia, AV blockade, and markedly reduced force of contraction and cardiac output. Hypotension is common. However, the heart has glucagon receptors that are linked to stimulation of adenylyl cyclase independent of β-adrenoreceptors, which mediate marked increases in rate and force and substitute for the blocked β response. (Glucagon also plays a primary role in raising blood glucose levels through activation of glycogenolysis and gluconeogenesis.) Atrial natriuretic peptide (choice A) is released from the cardiac atria and causes vasodilation through activation of membrane-bound guanylyl cyclase in arteriolar smooth muscle, and sodium excretion in the urine through an increase in glomerular filtration rate and consequent increase in filtration fraction. It is of no value in β-blocker overdose. If the β-blocker overdose is sufficient, administration of β-agonists such as epinephrine (choice B) is inadequate to overcome the blockade. Human growth hormone (choice D) is a peptide hormone produced by the anterior pituitary. It stimulates growth at open epiphyses through production of the insulin-like growth factors.

It has no direct effect on cardiac function. Insulin (choice E) activates entry of glucose into most tissues and promotes glycogen and triglyceride storage. It has no direct effects on cardiac function.

794. **(E)** At a blood alcohol level of 200 mg/dL, most individuals are grossly inebriated; a level of 80 to 100 mg/dL (0.08% to 0.1%) is considered the legal threshold for intoxication in most states. Ethanol is metabolized by alcohol dehydrogenase (and to a lesser extent by the microsomal ethanol oxidizing system) to acetaldehyde, primarily in the liver. At most ethanol concentrations, the metabolizing system is saturated. As a result, zero-order kinetics are observed. A typical adult shows a constant elimination rate manifested as a decline in blood level of 16 to 22 mg/dL/h. As blood alcohol levels drop below about 100 mg/dL, elimination has characteristics intermediate between zero and first order. Only at concentrations below 1 mg/dL is the elimination truly first order. Constant clearance (choice A) requires first-order elimination. Pulmonary excretion (choice B) of ethanol accounts for only a minor component of elimination. Breath analyzers are used to estimate the blood alcohol level in drivers suspected of driving under the influence of alcohol. Renal excretion (choice C) also accounts for only a minor component of systemic elimination of alcohol. Because of the small size of the ethanol molecule, most of the alcohol undergoing filtration at the glomerulus is reabsorbed. Biliary secretion (choice D) is generally important only for large molecules. This route is not significant in ethanol elimination. At a concentration of 200 mg/dL, blood alcohol is eliminated at zero-order kinetics via hepatic alcoholic dehydrogenase.

795. **(C)** For a complete eye examination, both mydriasis (pupillary dilation) and cycloplegia (paralysis of accommodation) are useful. Muscarinic cholinoceptor antagonists produce both of these effects. The description of this patient best fits homatropine (choice C) because it produces mydriasis and cycloplegia

lasting 1 to 3 days. Echothiophate (choice A) is a stable organophosphate anticholinesterase that is occasionally used topically for glaucoma. It causes miosis and cyclospasm and has a very long duration of action. Edrophonium (choice B) is a short-acting anticholinesterase used to diagnose myasthenia gravis. It is very polar and therefore not well absorbed from the conjunctival sac. Anticholinesterase action in the eye produces miosis and contraction of the ciliary body, thus facilitating outflow of aqueous humor and reducing intraocular pressure in glaucoma. Phenylephrine (choice D), an α-adrenoreceptor agonist, produces mydriasis without cycloplegia. Tropicamide (choice E), a muscarinic receptor antagonist, is similar to homatropine but has a much shorter duration of action (6 h) as compared with 2 to 3 days for homatropine and 1 week for atropine.

796. **(A)** The description of this drug indicates a CNS stimulant such as amphetamine. The loss of CNS activity with frequent repeated use is common with amphetamine because tolerance develops rapidly. This may arise in part from depletion of cytoplasmic biogenic amine stores. Cocaine (choice B), by virtue of its actions in inhibiting synaptic reuptake of biogenic amines, is also a stimulant. Cocaine exhibits a shorter duration of action and has a lesser tendency to produce stereotyped behavior than does amphetamine. Tolerance to the stimulating actions is not seen with cocaine, probably because its duration of action is so short. Ethanol (choice C) is categorized as a CNS depressant rather than a stimulant, although certain behaviors may appear to be excitatory as a result of loss of inhibitory influences. Tachyphylaxis is not seen with ethanol, although a modified form of tolerance is common with chronic alcoholism. Heroin (diacetylmorphine, choice D), along with its metabolite monoacetylmorphine, gain rapid access to the CNS because of their high lipid solubility. Abuse of opioids causes sedation and decreased activity, and no evidence of psychotic behavior. Tolerance is observed with heroin and other opioids. Tetrahydrocannabinol (the active ingredient in marijuana, choice E) produces an effect that is different from that produced by the stimulants. Motor activity is usually decreased. Appetite is usually stimulated and although psychotic behavior may occur, it is very uncommon.

797. **(D)** Saquinavir is an HIV protease inhibitor. Viral protease cleavage of a polyprotein is necessary for production of the viral coat protein. The HIV protease inhibitors were designed as specific inhibitors of this activity. This group includes ritonavir, indinavir, nelfinavir, and amprenavir in addition to saquinavir. The current HIV protease inhibitors are not sufficient for monotherapy because of the rapid emergence of resistance due to mutations in the viral protease. Combination therapy using saquinavir with two reverse transcriptase inhibitors such as zidovudine, lamivudine, abacavir, or didanosine is currently effective in reducing viral load. Incorporation into RNA (choice A) is part of the mechanism of action for the antitumor agent 5-fluorouracil (5-FU). 5-FU may be converted to 5-fluorouridine and incorporated into RNA, where it affects both processing and function of RNA. Inhibition of thymidylate synthase (choice B) is another part of the mechanism of action for the antitumor agent 5-FU. 5-FU is converted to 5-FdUMP, a potent inhibitor of thymidylate synthase. Inhibition of viral DNA polymerase (choice C) is a mechanism of action for the anti-herpesvirus nucleosides acyclovir, valacyclovir, famciclovir, and ganciclovir. These agents are metabolized to their nucleotide triphosphate forms, which competitively inhibit the herpesvirus polymerase. Acyclovir and valacyclovir also cause DNA chain termination. Inhibition of viral reverse transcriptase (choice E) is a property of the nucleosides zidovudine (AZT), didanosine (ddI), lamivudine (3TC), stavudine (d4T), and zalcitabine (ddC). These nucleosides are metabolized to the triphosphate forms that competitively inhibit reverse transcriptase. Non-nucleoside reverse transcriptase inhibitors include nevirapine, delavirdine, and efavirenz. Combinations of agents are used because resistance, through mutations in the reverse transcriptase sequence, frequently arises during monotherapy.

798.   **(E)** Osteoporosis is one of the leading causes of morbidity in postmenopausal women. Loss of estrogen after menopause increases the rate of bone resorption and is a major factor in this process. Other risk factors for osteoporosis include being of Asian or Caucasian descent, slender body build, smoking, alcohol consumption, a low-calcium diet, sedentary life style, and a family history of the disease. Postmenopausal estrogen replacement therapy (choice B) is satisfactory for treatment of osteoporosis in many women. It is not recommended in women with a high risk of breast cancer because of the potential for carcinogenesis and stimulation of tumor growth. Raloxifene (choice E), a selective estrogen-receptor modulator (a partial agonist with different effects in different tissues), offers the best choice in this patient because it produces an estrogen-like effect in decreasing bone resorption, while giving anti-estrogenic activity in breast tissue to provide chemoprotection against breast cancer. Alendronate (choice A) is a bisphosphonate inhibitor of bone resorption. The bisphosphonates are analogs of pyrophosphate and appear to be incorporated into bone matrix, where they inhibit osteoclast function. Alendronate is useful in treating osteoporosis and Paget disease. It and other second-generation bisphosphonates do not inhibit bone mineralization, an adverse effect of the first-generation bisphosphonate etidronate. Although effective in treating osteoporosis alone, alendronate does not offer protection against breast cancer in this patient. Conjugated estrogen (choice B) and other estrogen preparations reduce or prevent osteoporosis, but are contraindicated in this patient because of her family history of breast cancer. Dietary calcium supplementation (choice C) slows bone loss and helps to increase bone mass in patients taking estrogen or bisphosphonates, but is minimally effective alone. This treatment does not offer protection against breast cancer. Parathyroid hormone (PTH, choice D) appears to work at the level of bone to stimulate bone resorption through inhibition of osteoblasts and recruitment of osteoclast precursor cells into bone remodeling units. Intermittent administration of PTH in combination with estrogen has shown efficacy in increasing bone mineralization. This combination is experimental and, because of the estrogen component, is inadvisable in this patient.

799.   **(A)** Carbon monoxide is a colorless, tasteless, odorless gas that combines avidly with hemoglobin, thus preventing normal carriage of oxygen. Carboxyhemoglobin is bright red, so that the blood looks oxygenated and because the carbon monoxide is not removed by the tissues, even venous blood appears fully oxygenated. Early symptoms include headache, tachycardia, mental confusion, and loss of visual acuity. Late effects include cardiovascular and respiratory failure. Treatment includes general supportive measures plus 100% or hyperbaric oxygen. Carbon tetrachloride (choice B) is a chemical used in dry cleaning and other processes. It is not usually produced in fires; intoxication, when it occurs, is usually chronic. Chronic exposure to carbon tetrachloride results in liver and kidney damage. Acute exposure may cause CNS depression. Nitrogen dioxide (choice C) is a brownish irritant gas that may be produced in fires or in silage (stored hay). It causes eye and nose irritation and inflammation, and severe deep lung irritation. The latter results in coughing, sputum production, dyspnea, pulmonary edema, and chest pain. Treatment is symptomatic and directed at reducing inflammation. Ozone (choice D) is a bluish irritant gas that occurs around electrical equipment and as an air pollutant in large cities. It is not commonly produced in fires. Exposure results in irritation of mucous membranes of the eyes, nose, and throat followed by bronchospasm and deep lung irritation. Treatment is symptomatic and directed at reducing inflammation. Sulfur dioxide (choice E) may be produced in fires, but is quite irritating and causes coughing and watering of the eyes. It causes marked bronchospasm. Treatment is again symptomatic and directed at reducing inflammation.

REFERENCES

Fauci AS, Braunwald E, Isselbacher KJ, et al. *Harrison's Principles of Internal Medicine,* 14th ed. New York: McGraw-Hill; 1998.

Hardman JG, Limbird LE, Molinoff PB, et al. *Goodman & Gilman's The Pharmacological Basis of Therapeutics,* 9th ed. New York: McGraw-Hill; 1996.

Jellin JM, Gregory P, Batz F, et al. *Pharmacist's Letter/Prescriber's Letter Natural Medicines Comprehensive Database,* 3rd ed. Stockton, CA: Therapeutic Research Faculty; 2000.

Katzung BG. *Basic & Clinical Pharmacology,* 8th ed. New York: McGraw-Hill; 2001.

Subspecialty List: Pharmacology

747. Antibacterial (TB) adverse effects
748. Cardiovascular adverse effects of β-blockers
749. Anticoagulants—heparins
750. Sexual dysfunction—sildenafil
751. Endocrine pancreas
752. Antibacterials for *Pseudomonas*
753. GI prokinetic agents
754. Analgesics—codeine
755. Lipid-lowering agents—statin mechanism
756. General principles—quantal dose–response curves
757. Antihypertensives—ACE + diuretics
758. Autonomic nervous system—effects of epinephrine on blood pressure
759. Cardiovascular antiarrhythmics—adenosine
760. Autonomic nervous system—myasthenia gravis
761. Analgesics—opioids
762. Autonomic nervous system—cholinomimetics
763. Autonomic nervous system—β-agonist
764. CNS—parkinsonism/carbidopa
765. CNS—antiemetics
766. Analgesics—NSAIDs/gout
767. Autonomic nervous system—botulism
768. Eye—glaucoma
769. Antipsychotics—adverse effects
770. Cardiovascular—antiarrhythmics
771. Anticoagulants—oral anticoagulants
772. Potassium-wasting diuretics
773. GI drugs
774. Antihypertensives—ACE inhibitors
775. Antidepressants—SSRIs
776. Analgesics—NSAID adverse effects
777. Blood anemia—B_{12}
778. Endocrine estrogens
779. Lipid-lowering agents—mechanism of action
780. Toxicology—chelators
781. Antiparasitics—worms
782. Antiparasitics—malaria
783. Eicosanoids—leukotrienes, prostaglandins
784. Anticonvulsants—mechanism of action
785. Local anesthetics—mechanism of action
786. Autacoids antihistamine—adverse effects
787. Endocrine pancreas—oral antidiabetics
788. General anesthetics
789. Endocrine—thyroid
790. Endocrine hypothalamus—clomiphene
791. Neuromuscular junction blocking agents
792. Neuromuscular junction blocking agents—spasticity
793. Toxicology—antidotes
794. Alcohols—metabolism of ethanol
795. Autonomic nervous system—cholinolytics
796. CNS drug abuse—amphetamines
797. Antivirals—mechanism of action
798. Endocrine bone—mineral
799. Toxicology—gases

CHAPTER 7

Behavioral Sciences
Questions

Hoyle Leigh, MD

66 %

DIRECTIONS: (Questions 800 through 899): Each of the numbered items or incomplete statements in this section is followed by answers or by completions of the statement. Select the ONE lettered answer or completion that is BEST in each case.

100

800. A patient who had a painful bee sting is now afraid of flies and birds. This is an example of

    (A) classical conditioning
    (B) flooding
    (C) operant conditioning
    (D) shaping
    (E) stimulus generalization

801. Which of the following is an id function?

    (A) Cognition
    (B) Conscience
    (C) Libido
    (D) Perception
    (E) Psychological defense mechanisms

802. The multiaxial diagnostic system in psychiatric disorders implies that

    (A) all medical diseases have psychiatric symptoms
    (B) all psychiatric disorders are personality disorders
    (C) psychiatric disorders and other diseases can coexist
    (D) psychiatric disorders are complex

803. A most characteristic element of managed care is

    (A) capitated payment
    (B) that it emphasizes prevention and health promotion
    (C) that it is a fee-for-service system
    (D) that it provides specialized care
    (E) that physicians may be salaried

804. The average age for puberty is

    (A) 11 for boys and 13 for girls
    (B) 11 for girls and 13 for boys
    (C) 14 for boys and 16 for girls
    (D) 14 for girls and 16 for boys
    (E) 15 for both girls and boys

805. Which of the following statements is true concerning infant mortality in the United States?

    (A) Infant mortality in the United States is high compared to other developed nations.
    (B) Prenatal care, disappointingly, has not been shown to reduce infant mortality.
    (C) The leading cause of infant mortality in the United States is acquired immunodeficiency syndrome (AIDS).
    (D) The mortality rate for white infants is greater than that of black infants.
    (E) Very few Asian-Americans receive prenatal care as compared to African-Americans or Hispanic-Americans.

806. If a person drinks to deal with discomfort, and has never lost control, but has experienced unpleasant social consequences of drinking, which type of alcoholism might that person have?

    (A) Alpha
    (B) Blackouts
    (C) Crash
    (D) Epsilon
    (E) Gamma

807. The most significant contraindication to electroconvulsive therapy (ECT) is

    (A) advanced age
    (B) benign meningioma
    (C) cachexia
    (D) history of fracture
    (E) history of seizure disorder

808. A patient is convinced that an IV injection she received has made her immortal. This is an example of

    (A) delirium
    (B) delusion
    (C) hallucination
    (D) illusion
    (E) reality testing

809. The latest developmental phase according to Piaget is

    (A) concrete operations
    (B) formal operations
    (C) Oedipus complex
    (D) preoperational phase
    (E) sensorimotor period

810. A 32-year-old man presents to a sex therapy clinic with the chief complaint of premature ejaculation. Which of the following procedures is (are) appropriate?

    (A) CBC
    (B) Physical examination
    (C) Psychotherapy
    (D) Squeeze technique
    (E) All of the above

811. Which of the following is a normal sexual function?

    (A) Anorgasmia
    (B) Dyspareunia
    (C) Masturbation
    (D) Premature ejaculation

812. A 45-year-old woman comes to a sexual dysfunction clinic because of an inability to achieve orgasm. The patient was able to have orgasm in the past, but, of late, she has lost interest in sex. She comes to the clinic at her husband's insistence. She looks rather sluggish and unkempt. A likely diagnosis is

    (A) depressive disorder
    (B) dyspareunia
    (C) primary orgasmic dysfunction
    (D) Turner syndrome
    (E) vaginismus

813. A 57-year-old man complains of erectile dysfunction of a few months' duration. He is an executive at an HMO with a very stressful life style. He has a history of myocardial infarction, essential hypertension, and angina pectoris, which are controlled with medication. He is moderately obese. Which of the following is contraindicated?

    (A) Exercise training
    (B) Psychotherapy
    (C) Relaxation training
    (D) Sex therapy
    (E) Sidenafil (Viagra)

814. Which of the following is the most treatable dementing disease of the elderly?

    (A) Alzheimer disease
    (B) Creutzfeld–Jakob disease
    (C) Multi-infarct dementia
    (D) Pick disease
    (E) Secondary dementia

815. A 76-year-old man is brought to the clinic because of increasing confusion and episodes of dizziness. Upon examination, the patient shows upgoing toes on the left side, and his

blood pressure is found to be 178/115 mm Hg. The most likely diagnosis is

(A) Alzheimer disease
(B) Creutzfeld–Jakob disease
(C) multi-infarct dementia
(D) Pick disease
(E) secondary dementia

816. All patients who have trisomy of autosome 21 who survive to adulthood develop what condition?

(A) Creutzfeld–Jakob disease
(B) Down syndrome
(C) Multi-infarct dementia
(D) Pick disease
(E) Secondary dementia

817. Which form of dementia is often reversible with treatment with tricyclics such as imipramine or serotonin reuptake inhibitors such as fluoxetine?

(A) Alzheimer disease
(B) Creutzfeld–Jakob disease
(C) Multi-infarct dementia
(D) Pick disease
(E) Pseudodementia

818. The most common type of substance dependency in the United States is

(A) alcohol
(B) barbiturates
(C) cannabis
(D) heroin
(E) tobacco

819. The likelihood for physicians to become addicted to narcotics during their careers is estimated to be

(A) 1 in 10
(B) 1 in 100
(C) 1 in 1000
(D) 1 in 10,000
(E) 1 in 100,000

820. The abstinence syndrome to this drug is triphasic. During the second phase, protracted dysphoria occurs with decreased activity, amotivation, and intense boredom and anhedonia.

(A) Alcohol
(B) Barbiturates
(C) Cannabis
(D) Cocaine
(E) Opiates

821. One sensitive laboratory indicator of heavy use of alcohol is

(A) decreased mean corpuscular volume (MCV)
(B) decreased serum alkaline phosphatase
(C) elevated serum creatinine
(D) elevated serum gamma-glutamyl transpeptidase (GGT)
(E) elevated serum indirect bilirubin

822. The activity of which structure in the pons is suppressed by opioids, clonidine, and gamma-aminobutyric acid (GABA), and produces most of the noradrenergic input to the brain?

(A) Locus ceruleus
(B) Mammillary bodies
(C) Nucleus pulposus
(D) Nucleus solitarius
(E) Substantia nigra

823. Myelinated A-delta fibers are thought to carry which types of pain sensation?

(A) Aching
(B) Burning
(C) Dull
(D) Gnawing
(E) Pricking

824. Which theory concerning pain postulates that non-pain sensations such as vibration or pressure may affect the transmission and perception of pain sensation?

(A) Chemical transmission theory
(B) Electrical transmission theory
(C) Gate control theory
(D) Pattern theory
(E) Specificity theory

Questions 825 through 827

A man complaining of severe back pain is given an injection of saline. The pain seems to have subsided considerably.

825. The most likely reason for the pain relief is

(A) hypnotic suggestion
(B) that secondary gain was achieved
(C) that the pain of injection caused counterirritation
(D) that the saline injection induced endorphins
(E) that the saline injection induced GABA

826. This phenomenon indicates that placebos can be effectively used as a (an)

(A) differential diagnostic tool to distinguish between psychogenic and organic pain
(B) muscle relaxant
(C) opiate substitute
(D) research tool

827. If an injection of naloxone had preceded the injection of saline, the pain would be

(A) better, but the patient would be drowsy
(B) better, but the patient would be more anxious
(C) even more alleviated
(D) more localized
(E) worse

828. Anal-phase fixation may result in

(A) dependency
(B) fierce competitiveness

(C) parsimony
(D) schizophrenia

829. Harry Harlow's experiments with young monkeys separated from their mothers demonstrated that they

(A) all died of dehydration
(B) became docile and domesticated
(C) chose a terrycloth as a mother substitute
(D) had normal sexual development
(E) tended to adjust to stress rapidly

830. Susan was tending the goose eggs when they hatched. The young goslings started following Susan, even when the mother was calling them. This is an example of

(A) classical conditioning
(B) imprinting
(C) instinctual behavior
(D) maternal bonding
(E) operant conditioning

831. "Executive monkeys" as described by Brady tended to develop bleeding ulcers. They were

(A) alpha monkeys that have the highest level of testosterone in the colony
(B) humans with weak egos and many decisions to make
(C) male monkeys that had too many available females
(D) monkeys that had to keep pressing bars to avoid shock
(E) monkeys that had to press a bar to get a pellet of food

832. James is 3 years old and he will not part with his filthy terrycloth blanket. Whenever it is taken away from him, he throws a temper tantrum to get it back. He holds it, sucks on it, and seems content when he has it. This is an example of

(A) castration anxiety
(B) childhood fetishism
(C) codependence

(D) displacement

(E) transitional object

Questions 833 through 835

Sara is 15 years old.

833. Usually at this age, one expects her to spend a lot of time with

(A) a mixed group of peers

(B) adults

(C) animals

(D) furry toys

(E) guns

834. According to Piaget, children of this age typically engage in

(A) abstract thinking

(B) circular reactions

(C) concrete operations

(D) preoperational activities

(E) repetitive learning

835. During this period, according to Erikson, a major developmental task for the child is

(A) developing a clear identity

(B) developing a sense of integrity

(C) developing intimate relationships

(D) learning basic skills such as reading and arithmetic

(E) learning to be independent

836. According to psychoanalytic theory, which of the following is a function of the superego?

(A) Curiosity

(B) Guilt

(C) Music appreciation

(D) Perception

(E) Sexual urge

Questions 837 through 841

A 72-year-old woman is brought to the clinic by her family because she is exhibiting confusion.

837. Upon mental status examination, the patient demonstrates fluctuating levels of awareness. For example, she seems lucid one minute, then becomes somnolent or stuporous the next. The patient most likely has

(A) coma

(B) delirium

(C) dementia

(D) factitious illness

(E) stupor

838. The family informs you that the patient was found walking aimlessly in the fields in hot weather for several hours before being brought to the clinic. The most useful lab test would be a (an)

(A) electrocardiogram

(B) electroencephalogram

(C) HIV test

(D) serum electrolyte levels

(E) urinalysis

839. The serum electrolytes revealed Na$^+$ 150 mEq/L, K$^+$ 5.2 mEq/L. The most likely diagnosis is

(A) Alzheimer disease

(B) delirium

(C) Pick disease

(D) secondary dementia

(E) seizure disorder

840. Upon further inquiry, the family reports that the patient's mental status has been deteriorating for the past several years, during which time the patient had episodes of transient weaknesses of the arms and legs. The most likely diagnosis is

(A) Alzheimer disease

(B) Korsakoff syndrome

(C) multi-infarct dementia

(D) old age

(E) vitamin deficiency

841. If, upon further observation, this patient shows urinary incontinence and ataxia, a therapeutic procedure that may be considered is

   (A) benzodiazepines
   (B) electroconvulsive therapy
   (C) megavitamin therapy
   (D) urocholine
   (E) ventriculoperitoneal shunt

Questions 842 through 844

A 23-year-old woman complains of depression and anxiety. While describing her symptoms, she looks dazed. A minute later, she looks around the room slowly, and says, in a heavily accented voice with a different tone, "Where am I?"

842. This presentation is suggestive of
   (A) adjustment disorder
   (B) catatonia
   (C) dissociative identity disorder
   (D) major depression
   (E) schizophrenia

843. A careful history is likely to reveal

   (A) an excellent school record
   (B) a history of criminal behavior during childhood
   (C) physical or sexual abuse in childhood
   (D) setting of fires in childhood

844. An essential feature of this disorder, according to DSM-IV, is

   (A) amnesia
   (B) dependent personality traits
   (C) depersonalization
   (D) derealization
   (E) substance abuse

Questions 845 through 849

A 50-year-old man is brought to the emergency room by the police because he was on the street screaming that the water supply was poisoned.

845. The man is very agitated, and requires restraint by the attendants. As you, the on-call physician, try to interview him, he tries to hit you and screams at you. A reasonable first approach would be to

   (A) administer amobarbital by mouth
   (B) give him an injection of haloperidol
   (C) give him an injection of naloxone
   (D) perform a physical examination
   (E) reason with him that the water is not poisoned

846. Naloxone would be contraindicated if you find that the patient

   (A) had a psilocybin-induced psychosis
   (B) has hypertension
   (C) has just suffered a fracture
   (D) is a placebo responder
   (E) is an alcohol abuser

847. The mechanism of action of haloperidol seems to be

   (A) blockade of serotonin reuptake
   (B) facilitation of cholinergic transmission
   (C) generalized CNS depressant effect
   (D) postsynaptic blockade of dopamine receptors
   (E) presynaptic blockade of norepinephrine receptors

848. It is learned that the patient suddenly developed the idea that the water supply in the city was poisoned about 1 week ago. In considering the diagnosis of schizophrenia, a crucial piece of information would be that the patient

   (A) does not smoke
   (B) has a history of similar psychotic episodes in the past
   (C) has a history of substance abuse
   (D) is a toxicologist
   (E) is single

849. If, on further evaluation, you find that one of the patient's brothers was schizophrenic, the probability that this patient is schizophrenic is

(A) 1%
(B) 13%
(C) 18%
(D) 25%
(E) 50%

Questions 850 through 852

A 25-year-old man is admitted to the hospital after coming to the doctor carrying a bottle containing bloody urine. All tests were negative, and he was observed stealing a test tube of blood from the lab technician's cart.

850. Which of the following is a likely diagnosis?

(A) Antisocial personality disorder
(B) Conversion disorder
(C) Factitious disorder
(D) Malingering
(E) Schizophrenia

851. This condition can be considered a (an)

(A) form of psychosis
(B) integral part of borderline personality
(C) intentional antisocial act
(D) sick-role addiction

852. If the physician learns that the patient would have been incarcerated for a criminal offense if he had not been hospitalized, which of the following diagnoses becomes most likely?

(A) Antisocial personality disorder
(B) Borderline personality disorder
(C) Malingering
(D) Munchausen syndrome
(E) Sick-role addiction

Questions 853 and 854

Concerning "sick-role" as described by Talcott Parsons

853. One of the rights of the sick individual is to

(A) be hospitalized
(B) be exempted from income tax during the period of illness
(C) be provided low-cost medical care
(D) be provided outpatient care
(E) not be blamed for being sick

854. One of the obligations of the sick individual is to

(A) attempt to get better by "pulling oneself together"
(B) have a consultation with a physician
(C) participate in health-promotion activities
(D) pay for medical care received
(E) want to get well

Questions 855 through 859

A 48-year-old woman comes to the doctor complaining of vague pains in the abdomen, legs, and thighs.

855. On physical examination, the only positive findings are varicose veins of 20 years' duration. The patient, upon being told of this, insists on being operated on for the varicose veins immediately. Underlying this wish for immediate surgery is likely to be

(A) anxiety
(B) depression
(C) drug dependence
(D) psychosis

856. If the patient, instead of requesting surgery, told the doctor, "In spite of what you say, doctor, I know that I have a serious illness, probably cancer," the next step should be to

(A) ask why she thinks she has cancer
(B) tell her that she does not have cancer
(C) tell her that she has anxiety
(D) tell her that she has depression
(E) tell her to see a psychiatrist

857. The patient further confides in you that she has been losing weight with loss of appetite, has been unable to concentrate, and has had difficulty sleeping through the night. She has been, in fact, thinking of the means of killing herself. You should suspect

(A) borderline personality disorder
(B) factitious disorder
(C) generalized anxiety disorder
(D) hypochondriasis
(E) major depression

858. In obtaining further history, you find that the patient has become increasingly anxious, with a sense of impending doom, and vague abdominal discomfort. You decide to do further medical workup to rule out cancer. Which malignancy is most likely in this patient?

(A) Astrocytoma
(B) Carcinoma of the pancreas
(C) Carcinoma of the stomach
(D) Kaposi sarcoma
(E) Pancoast tumor

859. If cancer is ruled out in this patient, you are likely to use which of the following drugs to treat this patient?

(A) Diazepam
(B) Methylphenidate
(C) Olanzapine
(D) Paroxetine
(E) Valproic acid

860. Which of the following statements is true concerning medical care of persons of lower socioeconomic status?

(A) There is a problem of language that results from their unfamiliarity with physicians.
(B) They feel socially distant from physicians.
(C) They often regard physicians with a sense of awe.
(D) They sense that doctors do not expect them to ask questions.
(E) All of the above.

861. One advantage of technical language is

(A) ease of communication
(B) ease of visualization
(C) familiarity
(D) specificity

862. One of the social expectations of the doctor is that the doctor will

(A) be competent in what he or she does
(B) share all information
(C) treat all pathology he or she discovers
(D) treat the patient without the cost in mind

863. Affective neutrality expected of a doctor means

(A) countertransference should be analyzed
(B) the doctor should always have a stone face
(C) the doctor should not belong to any political organizations
(D) the doctor should suppress all feelings about patients
(E) the doctor should treat patients equally, whether or not he or she likes the patient

Questions 864 through 868

A young woman presents to the physician with the chief complaint of palpitations.

864. She also complains of feelings that she is going to die, with feelings of dizziness. A very useful question is:

(A) Are you anxious?
(B) Do you have a heart disease?
(C) Has anything like this happened before?
(D) What drugs do you use?
(E) Why do you think you will die?

865. If further evaluation reveals that the patient has used a substance heavily, but stopped about 3 days prior to experiencing symptoms, the most likely substance used is

(A) alprazolam

(B) cannabis

(C) cocaine

(D) dextroamphetamine

(E) heroin

866. If further evaluation reveals that the patient has not used any substances recently, but that she has been curtailing going outside, especially in open spaces, because she is afraid that she might have one of those attacks and become immobilized, which of the following diagnoses becomes more likely?

(A) Acute anxiety attack

(B) Agoraphobia with panic attack

(C) Agoraphobia without panic attack

(D) Anxiety secondary to a medical condition

(E) Cocaine withdrawal

867. If the patient turns out to have a panic disorder, a useful drug for treatment is

(A) bupropion

(B) olanzapine

(C) phenobarbital

(D) sertraline

(E) valproic acid

868. If laboratory tests determine that the patient has a general medical condition that underlies the symptoms, it is likely to be

(A) Addison disease

(B) cancer of the pancreas

(C) hyperparathyroidism

(D) hyperthyroidism

(E) hypothyroidism

869. Emotion

(A) is a conditioned reflex

(B) is a purely psychological phenomenon

(C) is a uniquely primate experience

(D) may be dysregulated

Questions 870 through 874

A 21-year-old female college student came to the doctor complaining of lightheadedness, palpitation, and tingling of the fingers and toes. She was terrified by this experience and is afraid that she may have a serious disease.

870. As her physician, your first approach is to

(A) ask about any stressors

(B) perform a physical examination

(C) prescribe a small dose of diazepam

(D) reassure her that she does not have a serious medical disease

871. Upon further evaluation, there is no evidence of a serious medical condition. The patient, however, has major stress related to her boyfriend. A likely diagnosis is

(A) agoraphobia

(B) generalized anxiety disorder

(C) hyperventilation syndrome

(D) panic disorder

(E) psychogenic syncope

872. Blood lab work on this patient is likely to reveal

(A) decreased hemoglobin

(B) increased hemoglobin

(C) increased MCV

(D) increased P_{CO_2}

(E) reduced P_{CO_2}

873. The tingling of fingers and toes may be due to

(A) hypocalcemia

(B) hypoxia

(C) niacin deficiency

(D) peripheral neuropathy

(E) thiamine deficiency

874. An effective treatment for the acute symptoms of this patient is

(A) ice packs
(B) IV injection of benztropine
(C) paper bag rebreathing
(D) rotating tourniquets
(E) Trendelenburg position

Questions 875 through 879

A 65-year-old man develops confusion and difficulty with memory and concentration over a period of several months. He also develops visual hallucinations and delusions that he has a secret identity.

875. This presentation is atypical for Alzheimer disease because

(A) confusion is not likely in Alzheimer disease
(B) difficulty in concentration indicates delirium rather than dementia
(C) the gender of the patient is atypical
(D) visual hallucinations and delusions are atypical

876. On physical examination, you are likely to find

(A) choreo-athetoid movement
(B) cog wheeling and tremor
(C) enlarged liver
(D) hemiparesis
(E) Kayser–Fleischer ring

877. If you decide to treat the hallucinations and delusions, your drug of choice is

(A) chlorpromazine
(B) fluphenazine
(C) haloperidol
(D) lorazepam
(E) risperidone

878. If further evaluation reveals that the patient also has myoclonus, ataxia, and seizures, the most likely diagnosis is

(A) Alzheimer disease
(B) Creutzfeldt–Jakob disease
(C) dementia secondary to a general medical condition
(D) Pick disease
(E) vascular dementia

879. If this patient has Creutzfeld–Jakob disease, a characteristic finding on autopsy is

(A) aluminum deposits in the brain
(B) multiple ischemic degeneration
(C) punctate hemorrhage in the hippocampus
(D) senile plaques
(E) spongiform encephalopathy

Questions 880 through 884

Sean is 8 years old. He is referred by his school because he is habitually disruptive in class.

880. A useful area to explore at this point would be

(A) his attention span
(B) his criminal record
(C) his relationship with his mother
(D) history of cruelty to animals
(E) history of enuresis

881. If further evaluation reveals that Sean has been unable to sleep at night for at least 3 months out of fear that his parents may divorce, an important diagnostic possibility is

(A) anaclitic depression
(B) attention deficit hyperactivity disorder
(C) conduct disorder
(D) generalized anxiety disorder
(E) separation anxiety disorder

882. If further evaluation reveals that Sean has had inattention, hyperactivity, and impulsivity since the age of 5, the likely diagnosis is

(A) anaclitic depression
(B) attention deficit hyperactivity disorder
(C) conduct disorder
(D) generalized anxiety disorder
(E) separation anxiety disorder

883. For the most likely diagnosis in question 882, the drug of choice is

(A) buspirone

(B) clomipramine

(C) dextroamphetamine

(D) nefazodone

(E) paroxetine

884. If further evaluation shows that Sean has had marked impairment in social interaction, and developed restricted, repetitive patterns of behavior and activities, including mannerisms, then the diagnosis that should be considered is

(A) Asperger disorder

(B) attention deficit hyperactivity disorder

(C) Munchausen syndrome

(D) Rett disorder

(E) schizophrenia

Questions 885 through 889

A 30-year-old woman complains of insomnia.

885. The differential diagnosis should include

(A) alcohol withdrawal

(B) depression

(C) hypothyroidism

(D) mania

(E) all of the above

886. Which of the following neurotransmitters is considered to be most involved in slow-wave sleep?

(A) Dopamine

(B) Endorphin

(C) Norepinephrine

(D) Phenylalanine

(E) Serotonin

887. If the patient states that one of the reasons she wakes up from sleep is that she has very vivid nightmares, which of the following drugs might provide most effective temporary relief?

(A) Aspirin

(B) Chloral hydrate

(C) Tranylcypromine

(D) Trazodone

(E) Zolpidem

888. If she states that in addition to the vivid nightmares, she has attacks of intense anxiety during sleep, such as feeling crushed, and wakes up with a blood-curdling scream, but cannot remember any specific dream, this is most likely a case of

(A) factitious disorder

(B) flashback

(C) hysteria

(D) night terror

(E) non-REM dream

889. For the condition defined in question 888, an effective treatment likely to show short-term results is

(A) behavioral therapy

(B) benzodiazepines

(C) hypnosis

(D) psychoanalysis

(E) tranylcypromine

890. The hospital system is characterized by

(A) democracy

(B) ease of mobility

(C) extreme division of labor

(D) lack of hierarchy

Questions 891 and 892

Concerning intensive or coronary care units (ICUs and CCUs)

891. The environment is often characterized by

(A) chaotic activity

(B) loud noise

(C) rigid and predictable schedule

(D) sensory deprivation and overload

(E) structured activity

892. This environment may lead to

   (A) delusional disorder
   (B) ICU psychosis
   (C) major depression
   (D) obsessive-compulsive disorder
   (E) panic disorder

Questions 893 through 895

A 53-year-old male executive undergoes an emergency appendectomy. Three days after surgery, he becomes tremulous and diaphoretic, and starts having frightening visual hallucinations.

893. At this point, the most likely diagnosis is

   (A) alcohol withdrawal
   (B) bipolar disorder
   (C) ICU psychosis
   (D) panic disorder
   (E) schizophrenia

894. If the patient turns out to have none of the disorders put forth in question 893, the most likely diagnosis is

   (A) Capgras syndrome
   (B) Cushing syndrome
   (C) drug-induced psychosis
   (D) schizoaffective disorder
   (E) thyrotoxicosis

895. If the patient turns out to have had a recent psychiatric procedure, it is likely to have been

   (A) electroconvulsive therapy (ECT)
   (B) hypnosis
   (C) psychoanalysis
   (D) psychosurgery
   (E) sodium amytal interview

896. During the course of an interview, a patient says that he is very happy to see you again. You know that this is the first time you are seeing him. Nevertheless, he tells you that he enjoyed the dinner he had with you and your family. The most likely diagnosis is

   (A) acute mania
   (B) delusional disorder
   (C) Ganser syndrome
   (D) Korsakoff syndrome
   (E) schizophrenia

897. If a patient has an amnestic syndrome due to thiamine deficiency, the lesions are most likely to be in the

   (A) cerebellum
   (B) frontal lobe
   (C) limbic system
   (D) occipital lobe
   (E) parietal lobe

898. Further history reveals that a patient has been hospitalized recently because of confusion, difficulty with walking, and inability to move his eyeballs. The diagnosis at that time was probably

   (A) cerebral hemorrhage
   (B) cerebral ischemia
   (C) pellagra
   (D) Wernicke syndrome
   (E) vitamin B_6 deficiency

899. Hypnosis

   (A) can cure warts
   (B) can recover memories that are tantamount to facts
   (C) causes the subject to be completely under the power of the hypnotist
   (D) utilizes animal magnetism

Answers and Explanations

800. **(E)** Stimulus generalization is a process through which a conditioned response is transferred from one stimulus to another stimulus that, in some sense, resembles the conditioned stimulus. In this case, the patient generalized the conditioned stimulus from bees to other flying objects—flies and birds. Classical conditioning (choice A), flooding (choice B), operant conditioning (choice C), and shaping (choice D) refer to other aspects of learning.

801. **(C)** The id is the collection of psychological functions having to do with basic instincts, such as sex and survival. Libido, as the energy arising from instincts, is an id function. The ego functions to mediate between the personality system on one hand and the demands of external reality and the superego on the other hand. Thus, psychological defense mechanisms (choice E), perception (choice D), and cognition (choice A) are all ego functions. Superego is the part of the personality system that encompasses conscience (choice B).

802. **(C)** Axis I of the multiaxial system is for clinical psychiatric disorders such as schizophrenia and mood disorders. Axis II is for personality disorders and mental retardation. Axis III is for general medical conditions (such as myocardial infarction). Axis IV is for psychosocial and environmental problems, and Axis V is for global assessment of functioning. This classificatory system clearly indicates that psychiatric disorders (Axis I) and general medical disorders (Axis III) often do coexist and may influence each other. Choices A, B, and D are not part of the multiaxial system.

803. **(A)** Managed care involves an entity (company, state, organization) managing health care through a capitated (head count) payment system. Within the managed care system, there are various models including specialized care and fee for service in addition to capitation.

804. **(B)** The onset of puberty varies, but girls usually enter puberty 12 to 18 months earlier than boys. The average age is 11 (range, 8 to 13) for girls and 13 (range, 10 to 14) for boys. Choices A, C, E are incorrect because they do not distinguish between girls and boys. Choice D is above the upper limit for both girls and boys.

805. **(A)** The infant mortality rate in the United States is 8.9 deaths per 1000 live births as of 1989, which ranks the United States behind 11 other developed countries. The leading causes of infant death are congenital anomalies, respiratory distress syndrome, and sudden infant death syndrome; therefore, choice C is incorrect. Choices B, D, and E are incorrect because prenatal care does reduce infant mortality, but only 80% of Caucasian women receive prenatal care, followed by 75% of Asian-American women, 65% of African-American women, and 60% of Native American women. The infant mortality rate for black infants is greater than that of white infants (choice D).

806. **(A)** Jellinek labeled the types of alcoholism as alpha through epsilon. Alpha alcoholics drink to deal with discomfort, and have not yet lost control. Blackouts (choice B) are common in this category, but not in epsilon alcoholics. Crash (choice C) is the first phase of cocaine abstinence, characterized by a crash of mood and energy immediately following the cessation of a binge. Epsilon alcoholics (choice D) are characterized by periodic or binge drinking. Gamma alcoholics (choice E) conform closely to the popular notion of alcoholism, with loss of control, tolerance, physical dependence, and withdrawal symptoms.

807. **(B)** Electroconvulsive therapy is a safe and painless procedure performed with muscle relaxation and general anesthesia (choices A, C, D, and E are not significant contraindications). The only serious contraindication is increased intracranial pressure, as in cases of recent cerebrovascular accident or a known space-occupying lesion such as meningioma, because of the danger of herniation due to transient further increase in intracranial pressure during the procedure.

808. **(B)** Delusion is a fixed idea or belief that does not correspond to reality. Delirium (choice A) involves an alteration of the sensorium, with confusion and disorientation. Hallucination (choice C) and illusion (choice D) are examples of impaired reality testing. Hallucination is perception without stimulus. In illusion, a stimulus is misperceived. Reality testing (choice E) refers to a person's ability to determine what percepts are real.

809. **(B)** Piaget described the development of intelligent thinking in stages where the last occurs from adolescence through adulthood and is referred to as the period of formal operations. Piaget described the other developmental stages as the sensorimotor period: 18 months to 2 years (choice E); preoperational phase, 2 to 7 years (choice D); and the phase of concrete operations, 7 to 11 years (choice A). Oedipus complex (choice C) is not a Piagetian stage, but is characteristic of ages 3 to 5.

810. **(E)** In evaluating sexual dysfunction, it is appropriate to perform a complete physical examination (choice B) and laboratory tests (choice A) to rule out a medical condition that may underlie the condition. Psychotherapy (choice C) is often indicated if there is major anxiety or conflict associated with the dysfunction. Squeeze technique (choice D) is a specific behavioral technique used to treat premature ejaculation. During manual stimulation of the penis by the partner, as soon as the patient feels a premonitory urge to ejaculate, he signals his partner, who then squeezes the coronal ridge of the glans. The urge then disappears, and stimulation is begun again.

811. **(C)** Masturbation is virtually universal among men and women of all cultures. It is common among married as well as single people. Many sex therapists recommend self-stimulation as an auxiliary treatment technique for a variety of sexual dysfunctions. Choices A, B, and D are sexual dysfunctions.

812. **(A)** Orgasmic phase dysfunctions include anorgasmia (frigidity), premature ejaculation, and erectile dysfunction (impotence), as well as delayed ejaculation. In this case, because the patient has experienced orgasm in the past, primary orgasmic dysfunction (choice C) is incorrect. Dyspareunia (choice B) is pain on intercourse, and vaginismus (choice E) is contraction of the muscles surrounding the vagina. Although Turner syndrome (choice D) may underlie some sexual dysfunctions, there is no evidence at this point of that disorder. The recent loss of interest in sex and her appearance indicate that depression is a likely diagnosis.

813. **(E)** Although sidenafil (Viagra) is an excellent drug for erectile dysfunction, it is contraindicated in patients who are receiving nitrates for angina pectoris because severe hypotension and death have occurred. Because the patient is receiving medications for his heart condition, angina, and hypertension, sidenafil is contraindicated until the medications are clarified. All other treatments listed may be helpful.

814. **(E)** Secondary dementia accounts for less than 10% of dementia cases in the elderly, but is important because the treatment of the un-

derlying disease may reverse or retard the progression of dementia. Alzheimer disease (choice A) is the most common primary dementia in the elderly. About 50% of brains of demented patients show evidence of Alzheimer disease. Creutzfeldt–Jakob (choice B) disease and kuru are slow virus infections that show clinical and histologic features similar to Alzheimer disease. Multi-infarct dementia (choice C) is secondary to repeated cerebrovascular accidents (CVAs) in patients with underlying atherosclerosis or hypertension. It is more common among men than women. Pick disease (choice D) is a rare cause of cortical dementia. The presence of unilateral cortical atrophy in Pick disease contrasts with the bilateral atrophy evident in Alzheimer disease. Microscopically, Pick bodies composed of densely packed neurofilaments are seen within diseased neurons.

815. **(C)** Because the patient shows signs of an old CVA (upgoing toes) and possible transient episodes of cerebral ischemia (episodes of dizziness) with hypertension, the most likely diagnosis is multi-infarct dementia. Multi-infarct dementia is a result of repeated CVAs, and successful treatment of the cardiovascular condition, including hypertension, may retard the progression of the dementia. Choices A, B, D, and E are therefore less likely.

816. **(B)** Down syndrome is a congenital mental retardation associated with trisomy of autosome 21. All patients with Down syndrome who survive into adulthood develop the brain pathologies of Alzheimer disease, rendering support to the notion that at least one form of Alzheimer disease may be associated with an autosome 21 abnormality. Choices A, C, D, and E are not associated with trisomy of autosome 21.

817. **(E)** Major depression may cause difficulty with concentration, memory, and mental acuity that are indistinguishable from dementia. Careful examination, however, usually reveals symptoms and signs of depression, such as depressed mood, anhedonia, loss of appetite, and sleep disturbance. Antidepressants are often effective for this type of syndrome called pseudodementia. Choices A, B, C, and D are not reversible with antidepressants.

818. **(E)** Tobacco addiction is the most common type of drug dependency in the United States. Nicotine is extremely addictive. Since the Surgeon General's report in 1964 that identified the health risks of tobacco smoking, there has been an encouraging trend in the United States. Approximately 42% of the U.S. adult population smoked cigarettes in 1965. The rate was 37% in 1975 and 30% in 1985. The reduction rate of smoking has been more pronounced in males than in females. Choices A, B, C, and D are incorrect.

819. **(B)** Because of easy drug availability and their high-stress occupation, physicians are at high risk for narcotic drug addiction; the incidence is estimated to be 1 in 100, which is 30 to 100 times greater than that of the general population. Choices A, C, D, and E are incorrect.

820. **(D)** The abstinence syndrome to cocaine is triphasic. Phase 1 is called "crash," phase 2 is a withdrawal phase with protracted dysphoria, and phase 3 is an "extinction" phase that follows the resolution of withdrawal anhedonia. Choices A, B, C, and E do not show this type of triphasic syndrome.

821. **(D)** An elevated GGT level may be the only laboratory abnormality in a patient who abuses alcohol. At least 70% of persons with a high GGT (over 30 U) are persistent heavy drinkers. Heavy drinkers may also have increased mean corpuscular volume (MCV), but this is not as sensitive as GGT. Choices A, B, C, and E are incorrect.

822. **(A)** The locus ceruleus, located in the pons, produces most of the noradrenergic input to the brain, and has receptors for opioids and autoreceptors for norepinephrine (α-2) as well as GABA. The locus ceruleus seems to be involved in alertness and anxiety re-

sponse. Choices B, C, D, and E refer to structures elsewhere.

823. **(B)** It is now believed that specific pain receptors (free nerve endings) are stimulated mainly by chemicals such as bradykinin, and that two types of pain sensations ("pricking" and "burning") are transmitted by different types of nerves. The burning pain sensation is transmitted by small C-fibers, and the pricking pain sensation is transmitted by larger, myelinated A-delta fibers. The pain fibers eventually terminate in the thalamus in a somatotopical fashion. Choices A, C, D, and E are incorrect.

824. **(C)** The theories involving pain perception are: (1) the specificity theory (choice E), postulating that there are specific pain receptors transmitting specific pain signals through specific neurons to specific areas of the brain; (2) the pattern theory (choice D), postulating the existence of "reverberating circuits" to explain phantom pain; and (3) the gate control theory (choice C), postulating an interaction between pain sensation and other sensations competing for transmission at the spinal cord level. Choices A and B do not postulate the interaction with non-pain sensations.

825. **(D)** Placebo-induced analgesia has been shown to be reversed with naloxone, indicating an endorphinergic mechanism. Therefore, choices A, B, C, and E are incorrect.

826. **(D)** Placebos are inconsistently effective, but they are far from being inert. Placebos should never be used as a differential diagnostic tool to distinguish between psychogenic and organic pain (choice A), because they may be equally effective in both. The best current use of placebo is as a research tool in double-blind, placebo-controlled studies. Therefore, choices A, B, and C are incorrect.

827. **(E)** Because placebo-induced analgesia is blocked by naloxone, the pain would be likely to worsen, because the naloxone would also block whatever endorphin there was alleviating pain before the saline injection. Fur-

ther, if the patient were habituated to opiates, there could be withdrawal symptoms, including heightened anxiety. Choices A, B, C, and D are incorrect.

828. **(C)** The anal phase of development occurs around age 2, around the type of toilet training. Developmental difficulty around this time may result in "anal-phase fixation," in which some characteristics of this phase may unduly influence the adult personality. Such characteristics include struggles over the issue of control. Excessive cleanliness and orderliness, or the opposite, as well as parsimony and hoarding may occur. Dependency (choice A) is characteristic of oral phase, and fierce competitiveness (choice B) may be characteristic of the Oedipal phase. Schizophrenia (choice D) is sometimes reminiscent of the autism in early oral phase, but is generally not considered to be a result of developmental arrest.

829. **(C)** During infancy, the presence of a mothering figure and close contact with her (or even a suitable substitute, such as a "terrycloth mother") provides a basic sense of security. Choices B, C, and E are incorrect; if anything, the opposite effects were observed. Death from dehydration (choice A) did not occur.

830. **(B)** Imprinting is an ethologic term that indicates a critical period in a newborn animal's life. For example, if goslings are exposed to humans rather than geese shortly after hatching, they will follow humans rather than their own mother.

831. **(D)** Monkeys that were placed in a highly complex operant conditioning program to avoid electric shock developed bleeding gastric ulcers, while yoked controls who received the same amount of shock, but did not have to perform the complex task, did not. The lack of a confirmatory feedback (such as a safe light or food to indicate a shock-free interval) seems to be especially ulcerogenic in Brady's "executive monkeys." Choices A, B, C, and E are incorrect.

832. **(E)** Transitional objects are "mother substitutes" such as a blanket or a soft toy, to which a child may become attached and that she or he may carry around all the time. This is a normal developmental phenomenon and not a sign of pathology. Choices A, B, C, and D do not refer to this phenomenon.

833. **(A)** An adolescent veers away from childish toys and develops an interest in the opposite sex. Peer relationships include members of the opposite as well as the same sex.

834. **(A)** According to Piaget, at about the time of puberty (which is on the average about age 11 in girls), the final stage of maturation in cognitive functioning, the period of formal operations, occurs. The individual's thought processes become more flexible, and transcends the here and now. Propositional thinking and hypothesis testing are prominent features of this stage.

835. **(A)** Erikson describes adolescence as the period of identity formation. In this period, a person develops a sense of inner sameness and continuity, a sense of direction and self. Career choices are also made during this phase. Failure of identify formation in this period results in "role confusion." The other choices refer to other developmental periods.

836. **(B)** The superego is the collection of functions having to do with conscience, social expectations, and guilt, which arises from failing to meet the demands of conscience. Id is the reservoir of basic instinctual drives, where sexual urge belongs (E). Ego is the collection of functions that mediate relations between the demands of the id and the constraints of social reality and conscience, as well as some innate, nonconflictual spheres of existence such as perception and movement. Choices A, C, and D are ego functions.

837. **(B)** Fluctuating levels of awareness are characteristic of delirium, which is indicative of an encephalopathy due to metabolic derangement of the brain, such as anoxia, electrolyte imbalance, or hypoglycemia. Although delirium may be superimposed on dementia, at this point there is no evidence that the patient has the more stable cognitive deficits characteristic of dementia (choice C). Coma (choice A) and stupor (choice E) refer to more severe disturbance of sensorium. Factitious illness (choice D) is unlikely unless there is evidence of self-induced metabolic derangement.

838. **(D)** An elderly woman exposed to hot sunlight for hours may be dehydrated, and testing serum electrolyte levels may confirm this suspicion. Although the other tests (choices A, B, C, and E) may be indicated at some point, they are not the most urgent tests in this case.

839. **(B)** The hypernatremia and hyperkalemia are indicative dehydration, which is a common cause of delirium. Choices A, C, D, and E do not explain this phenomenon.

840. **(C)** Multi-infarct dementia is caused by repeated cerebrovascular ischemia, indicated in this case by periods of transient paralysis. Alzheimer disease (choice A) is the most common primary dementia in the elderly. Old age (choice D) alone is no cause for dementia. Korsakoff syndrome (choice B), which is characterized by confabulation, is associated with alcohol withdrawal and thiamine deficiency (choice E). There is no evidence of either in this case.

841. **(E)** Normal pressure hydrocephalus is associated with the symptoms of dementia, ataxia, and urinary incontinence. On brain imaging, the ventricles are often enlarged, but cerebrospinal fluid (CSF) pressure is normal. A ventriculoperitoneal shunt is often therapeutic for this condition. Choices A, B, C, and D are inappropriate.

842. **(C)** Dissociative identity disorder (multiple personality disorder) is often associated with memory disturbance and an alternate personality who may have a different speech tone, accent, or voice. Schizophrenia (choice E) is unlikely; there is no sign of psychosis.

Major depression (choice D) is unlikely; there is no sign of depression. Catatonia (choice B) refers to muscle rigidity and mutism, and adjustment disorder (choice A) is a broad diagnostic category that does not include this presentation.

843. **(C)** Dissociative identity disorder (multiple personality disorder) is often associated with a history of severe emotional, physical, or sexual abuse in childhood. The dissociation may serve an adaptive function that enables the patient to tolerate an intolerable situation. The patient's school record is often poor due to memory disturbance associated with the disorder. Choices B and D are associated with antisocial personality, and choice A is unlikely because dissociation often causes inattention and poor school grades.

844. **(A)** DSM-IV diagnostic criteria for dissociative identity disorder include the presence of two or more distinctive identities or personality states, at least two or more of these identities or personality states recurrently taking control of the person's behavior, and an inability to recall important personal information. All the other choices may or may not be exhibited by a patient with dissociative identity disorder, but none is an essential diagnostic criterion.

845. **(B)** The management of acute psychosis involves use of parenteral antipsychotic drugs, such as haloperidol. Reasoning with a delusional patient (choice E) is usually futile, and an agitated and uncooperative patient is unlikely to permit a physical examination (choice D) or take an oral medication (choice A). Unless you know that the patient is intoxicated with opiates, naloxone (choice C) is unlikely to be of benefit.

846. **(C)** Naloxone is an opiate antagonist, and would be contraindicated in a patient with fracture who would require rapid pain relief. The placebo analgesic effect seems to be endorphin mediated, and naloxone would block it. The other choices do not deal with naloxone's specific anti-opioid activity.

847. **(D)** The mechanism of action of haloperidol is believed to be the blockade of dopaminergic receptors, particularly in the mesolimbic system. Many of the more recently marketed antidepressants are serotonin reuptake blockers. Choices A, B, C, and E are incorrect.

848. **(B)** Although all the other items (choices A, C, D, and E) may be significant, schizophrenia cannot be diagnosed if the patient has never had an episode of psychotic symptoms lasting for at least 6 months.

849. **(B)** The risk of developing schizophrenia in the general population is about 1%, and the prevalence for parents of children who are schizophrenic is 12%. The morbidity risk for schizophrenia for full siblings of schizophrenic patients is 13% to 14%. The risk for children of one schizophrenic parent is about 8% to 18%. The risk for children with both parents who are schizophrenic is about 50%.

850. **(C)** The essential feature of factitious disorder is the intentional production of physical signs or symptoms in the absence of an external incentive as a motivation. If there is an external incentive for fabricating an illness, then malingering is diagnosed (choice D). Antisocial personality disorder (choice A) requires a pattern of antisocial behavior. Conversion disorder (choice B) is incorrect because it involves symptoms or deficits involving voluntary motor or sensory function as a result of a psychological conflict. Schizophrenia (choice E) is incorrect because there is no evidence of psychotic symptoms even though the behavior may be bizarre.

851. **(D)** The caring environment of hospitalization and exemption from normal responsibilities accompanying the sick-role may be the unconscious motivation for many patients with factitious disorders to undergo very uncomfortable and often painful procedures or self-inflicted injuries to become a patient. There is no clear-cut learning, psychosis, or personality disorder that accompanies this condition; choices A, B, and C are incorrect.

852. **(C)** When there is an external incentive for causing the symptom or injury, malingering is more likely than factitious disorder (Munchausen syndrome), the motivation for which is often quite unclear. Although there may be concomitant personality disorders, malingering is not diagnostic of any specific personality disorder. Choices A, B, D, and E are less likely because there seems to be an obvious and conscious motivation in this case.

853. **(E)** According to Parsons, a sick person has a right not to be held responsible for being sick, and to be exempted from normal role expectations, such as going to school or work. A sick person is expected to be cared for, but this does not include any specific rights such as medical care, hospitalization, outpatient care, or legal obligations such as paying taxes (choices A, B, C, and D).

854. **(E)** With the obligation to consider being ill an undesirable state comes the obligation to want to get well, to seek competent help, but the help need not be by consultation with a physician (choice B). The sick role expectation also involves the notion that being ill is not one's own fault, and that the patient cannot be expected to get better alone (choice A) without help. Although participating in health-promotion activities (choice C) is laudable, it is not part of the original sick-role expectations formulated by Parsons, and neither is paying for medical care (choice D).

855. **(A)** Anxiety or concomitant stress is a common trigger for help-seeking behavior, especially if the symptom or sign is of long duration. Although depression (choice B) can cause vague discomfort and precipitate help seeking, insisting on an operation immediately seems to indicate anxiety rather than depression, which is more likely to cause indecision or inaction. A drug-dependent person (choice C) is more likely to insist on drugs. There is no evidence of psychosis (choice D).

856. **(A)** When a patient presents with a conviction that she has a serious illness, it is important to find out more about why the patient has the notion, because in the process the doctor may be able to diagnose emotional distress in the form of anxiety, depression, or simple misperception, as well as hypochondriasis. All the other choices (B, C, D, and E) bring about a premature closure.

857. **(E)** Depression is often accompanied by vague physical symptoms. When a depressed patient presents to a primary physician, it is important that the presence of depression be ascertained by careful history; depressed patients are often suicidal, and about 70% of successful suicides have seen their physician in the previous month. Choices A, B, C, and D are not supported by the signs presented.

858. **(B)** Carcinoma of the tail of the pancreas often presents with symptoms of depression. Although other carcinomas and neoplasms (choices A, C, D, and E) may also cause depression, pancreatic cancer has to be ruled out first in a patient with severe depression.

859. **(D)** Paroxetine is a selective serotonin reuptake inhibitor (SSRI), an antidepressant, and is the drug of choice for treating this patient's depression. Diazepam (choice A) is an antianxiety agent; methylphenidate (choice B) is a CNS stimulant; olanzapine (choice C) is an atypical antipsychotic; and valproic acid (choice E) is an anticonvulsant used to treat bipolar disorder.

860. **(E)** In spite of all the barriers listed, the general desire for medical knowledge, regardless of social status of the individual, is the same. Therefore, the seeming lack of interest should not deter the physician from providing appropriate information to all patients.

861. **(D)** Technical language can be quite specific and precise. It suffers, however, from being unfamiliar to lay persons, and often impedes rather than facilitates communication between physician and patient (choice A). For choices A, B, and C, the opposite is true, especially when technical language is spoken to a lay person.

862. **(A)** In addition to technical competence, Talcott Parsons listed universalism, functional specificity, affective neutrality, and collectivity orientation as being part of doctor role expectations. Although it may be desirable for doctors to share all information (choice B) and treat patients without cost in mind (choice D), these are not general social expectations of the doctor. Requiring a doctor to treat all pathology (choice C) is counter to the functional specificity expectation that the doctor will treat only conditions for which he or she has competence.

863. **(E)** Affective neutrality implies that the physician will not become emotionally involved with patients or act on emotions generated by the patient. This includes not becoming intimate with a patient or becoming emotionally aroused (either erotically or aggressively). Choices A, B, C, and D are incorrect and impractical.

864. **(C)** The patient presents with acute anxiety symptoms that might be due to panic or other acute situation. Panic disorder usually is recurrent and history of previous episodes would be extremely helpful. Choice A is inappropriate; the patient is obviously anxious. Choices B, D, and E may be useful but not yield as much information.

865. **(A)** Benzodiazepine withdrawal is often associated with anxiety symptoms. Cocaine (choice C) may cause a "crash" with anxiety soon after cessation of use, but by day 3 there is more likely to be dysphoria than anxiety. Although withdrawal from other substances (choices B, D, and E) can cause similar anxiety, benzodiazepine withdrawal is the most common cause of this type of symptomatology.

866. **(B)** The symptoms of panic associated with fear and avoidance of being in places where escape may be difficult or embarrassing call for the consideration of agoraphobia with panic attack. Choices A, C, D, and E are not associated with the phenomenon described here.

867. **(D)** In addition to SSRIs such as sertraline, paroxetine and fluoxetine, tricyclic antidepressants, MAOIs, and high-potency benzodiazepines such as alprazolam and clonazepam may be effective in panic disorder. Olanzapine (choice B) is an atypical antipsychotic and has not been shown to be effective in panic disorder. Bupropion, an antidepressant (choice A), phenobarbital, a CNS depressant (choice C), and valproic acid, an anticonvulsant and antimanic drug (choice E) are also ineffective in panic disorder.

868. **(D)** Hyperthyroidism is often associated with anxiety and panic symptoms. Although these symptoms may also occur with any of the other medical conditions (choices A, B, C, and E), depression and slowed mentation are more common in hypothyroidism, hyperparathyroidism, and Addison disease; cancer of the pancreas is often associated with severe depression.

869. **(D)** Emotions, or affects, include three main components—a subjective feeling tone, a neurophysiologic discharge, and perception of the bodily sensations caused by the motor discharge (e.g., palpitation). Dysregulation of emotion results in anxiety or mood disorders. It is certainly observable in animals other than primates. Certain aspects of emotions may be conditioned (choice A), but not the totality of it.

870. **(A)** Although the known symptoms are indicative of an anxiety disorder, more information is needed to proceed. Because stressors are important in anxiety symptoms, asking about them is the first approach. Choices B, C, and D bring about premature closure.

871. **(C)** Lightheadedness, palpitation, and tingling in the fingers and toes are characteristic of hyperventilation syndrome. Choice E is incorrect because there is no syncope, and choices A, B, and D need further evidence and are not supported by known symptoms.

872. **(E)** In hyperventilation syndrome, there is respiratory alkalosis due to CO_2 loss. This

may in turn lead to decreased ionization of calcium. Choices A, B, C, and D are incorrect; there is no reason for such changes.

873. **(A)** In hyperventilation syndrome, there is often hypocalcemia associated with respiratory alkalosis. Choices B, C, D, and E are not supported by the evidence presented.

874. **(C)** Paper bag rebreathing restores P_{CO_2} and normalizes blood pH and calcium. This technique, and education about hyperventilation and appropriate coping skills, can prevent and control hyperventilation syndrome. Choices A, B, D, and E may be appropriate for other conditions.

875. **(D)** Although hallucinations and delusions do occur in Alzheimer disease, they are less typical than in delirium or in Lewy body disease. Confusion and difficulty with concentration are quite common in Alzheimer, which affects both sexes, although females may be at slightly higher risk. Therefore, choices A, B, and C are less appropriate than D.

876. **(B)** Lewy body disease is characterized by Alzheimer-like dementia with visual hallucinations, delusions, and Parkinsonian features including cog wheeling and tremor, which this patient's presentation closely resembles. Kayser–Fleischer ring (choice E) is seen in Wilson disease. Other choices are possible but not appropriate with the symptoms presented.

877. **(D)** Lewy body dementia frequently manifests psychosis, but the patients are exquisitely sensitive to the extrapyramidal side effects of typical antipsychotic drugs such as chlorpromazine (choice A), fluphenazine (choice B), and haloperidol (choice C). Lorazepam is a benzodiazepine that may exacerbate the confusion. Atypical antipsychotics, such as risperidone (choice E), may be used carefully to treat the psychotic symptoms.

878. **(B)** Creutzfeldt–Jakob disease, caused by protein fragments called "prions," is characterized by relatively rapid onset of dementia,

myoclonus, seizures, and ataxia. Choices A, C, D, and E are not associated with these severe neurologic signs.

879. **(E)** Creutzfeldt–Jakob disease is a spongiform encephalopathy similar to kuru and mad cow disease. Unlike Alzheimer disease, senile plaques (choice D) or neurofibrillary tangles are usually absent in the brains of patients with Creutzfeld–Jakob disease. Punctate hemorrhage (choice C) in the hippocampus is seen in Wernicke disease, and multiple ischemic degeneration (choice B) is more likely in vascular dementia. Aluminum deposits (choice A) were suspected in Alzheimer, but not in Creutzfeld–Jakob disease.

880. **(A)** A common cause of disruptiveness is attention deficit hyperactivity disorder (ADHD), which is characterized by inattention and hyperactivity. Enuresis (choice E), cruelty to animals (choice D), and trouble with the law (choice B) are often found in the childhoods of those who are eventually diagnosed as having an antisocial personality, but disruptiveness in class is more indicative of hyperactivity. Exploring Sean's relationship to his mother (choice C) may be useful, but not as much as assessing his attention span.

881. **(E)** Separation anxiety disorder involves excessive anxiety concerning separation from the home or someone to whom the child is attached. The disturbance must continue for more than 4 weeks, with onset before age 18. Choices A, B, C, and D are not particularly indicated by the new information provided.

882. **(B)** The diagnostic criteria for ADHD include inattention, hyperactivity, and impulsivity in various areas, and the symptoms must have been present before the age of 7. The specific history of inattention and hyperactivity tend to rule out choices A, C, D, and E, although there may be some elements of conduct disorder.

883. **(C)** Dextroamphetamine and methylphenidate are effective in treating ADHD. Paroxe-

tine (choice E) and nefazodone (choice D) are antidepressants, clomipramine (choice B) is a tricyclic that has special use in obsessive-compulsive disorders, and buspirone (choice A) is an anti-anxiety agent.

884. **(A)** Asperger disorder and Rett disorder are forms of pervasive developmental disorder. In Rett disorder (choice D), there is the development of multiple, specific deficits following a period of normal functioning after birth. In Asperger disorder, there is severe and sustained impairment in social interaction and restricted, repetitive patterns of behavior, interests, and activities. There is no evidence of schizophrenia (choice E) or factitious disorder (choice C). If symptoms of ADHD exist (choice B) in addition to symptoms of pervasive developmental disorder, the latter is diagnosed.

885. **(E)** Insomnia is seen in depression, sedative withdrawal including alcohol, hypothyroidism, and mania, although in mania the patient may not feel the need to sleep or complain about the lack of sleep.

886. **(E)** Non-REM or slow-wave sleep is an active phenomenon probably brought about by the activation of the serotonergic neurons of the pontine raphe system. Noradrenergic (choice C) and possibly cholinergic systems are involved in REM sleep, and dopamine (choice A) seems more involved in attention and reward mechanisms. Phenylalanine (choice D) is an amino acid, and endorphins (choice B) are neuromodulators that may contribute to modulation of sleep.

887. **(C)** Vivid dreams usually occur during REM sleep. Many drugs suppress REM, but MAOIs such as tranylcypromine, are most potent in this effect. The other drugs listed (choices A, B, D, and E) have little effect on REM sleep.

888. **(D)** This is a typical description of night terrors, which, unlike nightmares, occur during NREM delta-wave sleep. Flashback (choice B) and hysteria (choice C) are not sleep disorders, and non-REM dreams (choice E) are usually not terrifying. Although in factitious disorder (choice A), the patient may give a manufactured account of what happened, the case fits the description of night terror the best.

889. **(B)** Because night terror is an NREM, particularly stage 4, sleep phenomenon, benzodiazepines (e.g., diazepam) that suppress stage 4 sleep can be effective. There is no evidence that psychotherapy, including psychoanalysis, hypnosis, or behavioral therapy (choices A, C, and D) are effective in the short term for this condition. Tranylcypromine (choice E), an MAOI, suppresses REM but not NREM sleep.

890. **(C)** The professional, administrative, and nonprofessional staffs in a hospital have clearly distinguishable and separate tasks, orientations, and loyalties. The clerk does not operate, and the doctor does not collect bills. A hospital is a hierarchy, and there is often blocked mobility—a nurse cannot be a doctor without first changing his or her career, and vice versa. Therefore, choices A, B, and C are incorrect.

891. **(D)** Various activities occur simultaneously in the ICU and CCU, and structured activity is often impossible due to the urgent nature of medical care needed. Noise is usually suppressed, and although there are a variety of activities, they are not chaotic, but instead are medically ordered. Sensory deprivation and overload both may occur due to the suppression of sound and lighting, contrasted with the constant beep of the monitors and the clamor of cardiac resuscitation. Therefore, choices A, B, C, and E are incorrect.

892. **(B)** Sensory deprivation and overload superimposed on physiologic aberrations such as electrolyte imbalance or narcotic analgesics may cause a psychotic syndrome characterized by hallucinations and delusions called ICU psychosis. Although panic disorder (choice E) is possible, all the other disorders listed (choices A, C, and D) are primary psy-

chiatric disorders that can be diagnosed only after ruling out ICU psychosis.

893. **(A)** Emergency surgery results in unexpected withdrawal from habituated drugs, including alcohol. The symptoms are characteristic of delirium tremens. Schizophrenia (choice E) is unlikely because the psychosis is sudden, and the hallucinations are primarily visual (in schizophrenia, they are more likely to be auditory). ICU psychosis (choice C) is not impossible, but most likely by the third postsurgical day, the patient is out of the ICU. Being tremulous and diaphoretic are not typical features of bipolar disorder (choice B), and hallucinations do not occur in panic disorder (choice D).

894. **(C)** Next to sedative drug withdrawal, visual hallucinations during the postoperative period should raise the index of suspicion for drug-induced psychosis, especially due to narcotic analgesics. Although all the other listed disorders (choices A, B, D, and E) could produce a psychotic syndrome, the acute course in this patient suggests delirium.

895. **(A)** ECT often causes memory disturbance, especially of short-term memory. Hypnosis (choice B), psychoanalysis (choice C), and amytal interview (choice E) may be used to attempt to recover certain types of memory, but are unlikely to be causes of this disturbance. Modern psychosurgery (choice D) is often very localized and unlikely to involve memory loss.

896. **(D)** Korsakoff syndrome, caused by thiamine deficiency in alcoholics, is characterized by confabulation, as in this case. Ganser syndrome (choice C) is associated with approximate but inaccurate answers, and schizophrenia (choice E) and acute mania (choice A) are usually associated with their characteristic symptoms, although confabulation may occasionally occur. Delusional disorder (choice B) is possible, but the patient presented with memory problems, which are a component of delusional disorder.

897. **(C)** Amnestic syndrome is associated with lesions in the limbic system, including the hippocampus, fornix, and mammillary bodies. Therefore, choices A, B, D, and E are incorrect.

898. **(D)** Wernicke syndrome is characterized by ophthalmoplegia, ataxia, and delirium. Wernicke syndrome may progress to Wernicke–Korsakoff syndrome, with amnesia, nystagmus, and ataxia. Peripheral neuropathy is usually present. Although all the other disorders (choices A, B, C, and E) could produce neurologic symptoms and confusion, the presenting symptoms are characteristic of Wernicke encephalopathy. Furthermore, the patient's current condition (Korsakoff syndrome) must be a progression of the recent Wernicke syndrome.

899. **(A)** Hypnotic suggestion can make warts disappear by reducing blood flow to their base. Hypnosis, however, is not an all-powerful tool to control others (choice C), but rather a method of enhancing the concentration and attention of the subject. Historically, Anton Mesmer proposed that the hypnotic phenomenon was based on animal magnetism (choice D), but the association between hypnosis and magnetism was disproved by the famous French Royal Commission Report. Memory retrieved under hypnosis (choice B) is no more accurate than nonhypnotic recall (in fact, it is less reliable).

REFERENCES

Elkin GD. *Introduction to Clinical Psychiatry.* Stamford, CT: Appleton & Lange; 1998.

Kaplan HI, Sadock BJ. *Comprehensive Textbook of Psychiatry/VI CD-ROM.* Jackson, WY: Teton Data Systems; and Baltimore: Williams & Wilkins; 1998.

Kaplan HI, Sadock BJ. *Kaplan and Sadock's Synopsis of Psychiatry,* 8th ed. Baltimore: Williams & Wilkins; 1998.

Leigh H, Reiser MF. *The Patient: Biological, Psychological, and Social Dimensions of Medical Practice,* 3rd ed. New York: Plenum; 1992.

Subspecialty List: Behavioral Sciences

874. Anxiety disorders
875. Organic dementia
876. Organic dementia
877. Organic dementia
878. Organic dementia
879. Organic dementia
880. Attention deficit hyperactivity disorder
881. Separation anxiety disorder
882. Attention deficit hyperactivity disorder
883. Attention deficit hyperactivity disorder
884. Developmental disorder
885. Sleep
886. Sleep
887. Sleep
888. Sleep
889. Sleep
890. Medical ethics
891. Psychological and social factors
892. Psychological and social factors
893. Substance abuse
894. Psychotic disorders
895. Organic correlates
896. Organic correlates
897. Organic correlates
898. Organic correlates
899. Hypnosis

Practice Tests

Carefully read the following instructions before taking the Practice Tests.

1. This examination consists of questions divided into three testing periods. Each test contains 100 questions. You are allowed 2 hours to complete each batch of 100 questions. At this pace you need to answer a question about every 50 seconds.
2. The tests simulate the USMLE. You should not carry any extra time from one test over to the other. Any remaining time from either test should be used to review your answers in that test only. You should take a break of 1 or 2 hours between each of the tests.
3. Be sure you have an adequate number of pencils and erasers, a clock, a comfortable setting, and an adequate amount of undisturbed, distraction-free time to complete each test.
4. After you have completed a test, check your responses against the answers that appear on the pages directly following each exam.
5. Good luck on these Practice Tests and on the USMLE.

CHAPTER 8

Practice Test I
Questions

75%

DIRECTIONS: Questions 1 through 100: Each of the numbered items or incomplete statements in this section is followed by answers or by completions of the statement. Select the ONE lettered answer or completion that is BEST in each case.

1. A deficiency in the urea cycle enzyme argininosuccinate synthetase will result in urinary, serum, and cerebrospinal fluid accumulation of

   (A) arginine
   (B) argininosuccinate
   (C) carbamoyl phosphate
   (D) citrulline
   (E) ornithine

2. You determine that your young patient has an enlarged right side of the heart due to significant shunting of blood from the left to the right atrium. You suspect that this interatrial septal defect is due to an abnormally large foramen ovale resulting from incomplete development of the

   (A) muscular interventricular septum
   (B) ostium primum
   (C) ostium secundum
   (D) septum primum
   (E) septum secundum

Refer to Figure 8–1 for questions 3 and 4.

3. Drug L, when administered as a single-bolus IV dose of 30 mg to a 70-kg (154-lb) patient, yields the plasma values shown in Figure 8–1

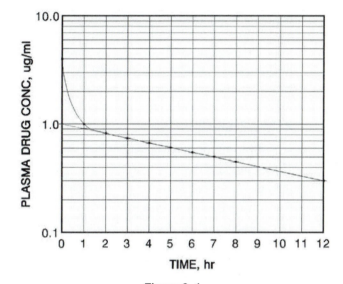

Figure 8–1

as a function of time after injection. The apparent volume of distribution is

   (A) 0.25 L
   (B) 4.0 L
   (C) 14.0 L
   (D) 30.0 L
   (E) 100.0 L

4. In Figure 8–1, the elimination half-life for drug L is

   (A) 0.25 h
   (B) 1.0 h
   (C) 7.0 h
   (D) 12.0 h
   (E) 28.0 h

5. When a person thinks about biting into a sour apple, he or she may experience increased salivation. This phenomenon is probably an example of

   (A) classical conditioning
   (B) cognitive learning
   (C) imprinting
   (D) operant conditioning
   (E) shaping

6. A 42-year-old woman presents with an acute onset of fever, jaundice, tender liver enlargement, and ascites combined with the histologic features of scattered foci of hepatocytes undergoing swelling and necrosis, with neutrophilic infiltration around the affected cells, and sinusoidal and perivenular fibrosis. This is most suggestive of

   (A) acetaminophen overdose
   (B) acute fatty liver of pregnancy
   (C) alcoholic hepatitis
   (D) Budd–Chiari syndrome
   (E) pyogenic liver abscess

7. Which of the following symptoms is attributable to the vitamin deficiency most commonly observed in chronic alcoholics?

   (A) Corneal vascularization
   (B) Dark, scaling skin lesions of the mouth
   (C) Periosteal hemorrhaging
   (D) Severe eye itch and burning
   (E) Weakening of the rectus muscles of the eye

Questions 8 and 9

A 24-year-old male model has a mononucleosis-like illness, characterized by apathy, slow responsiveness, fever, generalized enlargement of lymph nodes, leukopenia, and a maculopapular rash. Cultivation of lymphocytes obtained from this patient resulted in the isolation of the virus that was responsible for the illness of the 24-year-old model. The virus had an envelope, two molecules of single-stranded, positive-polarity RNA, and a reverse transcriptase.

8. The most likely diagnosis is

   (A) acquired immunodeficiency syndrome (AIDS)
   (B) infectious hepatitis
   (C) lymphocyte choriomeningitis
   (D) mumps
   (E) pleurodynia

9. The most notable opportunistic neoplasia associated with the illness found in the 24-year-old male model is

   (A) Burkitt lymphoma
   (B) herpes simplex type 1 lymphoma
   (C) herpes simplex type 2 carcinoma
   (D) Kaposi sarcoma
   (E) Rous sarcoma

10. A 36-year-old teacher has been treated with a β-lactam antibiotic. This antibiotic MOST likely will

    (A) bind to bacterial capsule
    (B) bind to bacterial nuclear membrane
    (C) inhibit synthesis of cell wall proteins
    (D) inhibit the transpeptidation reaction
    (E) neutralize bacterial autolytic hydrolases

11. In Figure 8–2, a patient receives a continuous infusion of gastrin. The production of gastric acid and pancreatic bicarbonate secretion is monitored before and after administration of peptide X (at arrow). Which of the following hormones is most likely to produce the changes observed?

    (A) Angiotensin II
    (B) Cholecystokinin (CCK)
    (C) Motilin
    (D) Secretin
    (E) Somatostatin

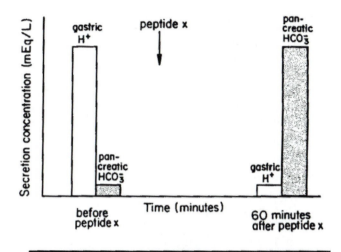

Figure 8–2

12. A 12-year-old boy is diagnosed with congenital coarctation (constriction) of the aorta. A posterior-to-anterior chest film reveals a characteristic notch in the aortic knob in the superior aspect of the left border of the cardiovascular shadow. This points to a constriction just past the origin of the left subclavian artery. Radiographic examination also reveals characteristic notching of the lower border of the upper ribs, most pronounced along the posterior segments. Upon simultaneous examination of the radial and posterior tibial pulses on the 12-year-old boy, you observe that the posterior tibial pulse is

(A) delayed and of greater volume than the radial pulse

(B) delayed and of lesser volume than the radial pulse

(C) in sequence with and equal in volume with the radial pulse

(D) in sequence with, but of greater volume than, the radial pulse

(E) in sequence with, but of lesser volume than, the radial pulse

13. Which of the following is true concerning tobacco?

(A) It is the most common type of drug dependency in the United States.

(B) Nicotine is associated with psychological dependence but no physical withdrawal symptoms.

(C) Physical complications of chronic tobacco use usually begin to appear in 40 pack-years.

(D) The relapse rate of most smoking cessation programs is 30%.

(E) Tobacco dependence usually begins in childhood.

14. The second law of thermodynamics states that

(A) energy cannot change form

(B) reactions that are spontaneous proceed as written because the products of the reaction possess a minimal energy content

(C) the natural tendency of molecules is to increase their state of disorder

(D) the total energy of a molecule is equal to the sum of all internal energies of all the bonds within that molecule

(E) the total energy of the universe cannot increase or decrease

15. Which of the following is a mechanism for resistance to trimethoprim by *E. coli*?

(A) Acquisition of altered forms of dihydrofolate reductase through plasmid transfer

(B) Expression of altered forms of the transpeptidase involved in cell wall synthesis

(C) Expression of β-lactamase activity

(D) Mutating ribosomal subunits to reduce drug binding

(E) Thickening of the bacterial cell wall

16. A 27-year-old recent Asian immigrant is hospitalized because of cyclic severe fevers occurring about every 72 hours due to infection by *Plasmodium malariae*. What is the pathogenic mechanism responsible for the recurrent quartan fever?

    (A) Cell-mediated cytokines invoke pyrogen production
    (B) Central hypothalamic fever due to cerebral malaria
    (C) Hepatocyte infestation with cyclic lysis
    (D) Immune mediated destruction of organisms by cytotoxic antimalarial antibodies
    (E) Red cell lysis upon release of proliferating merozoites

17. A 71-year-old man is admitted for thromboendarterectomy (TEA) because of an 85% stenosis of his left common carotid artery documented by Doppler echography. As part of this procedure, a brief occlusion of the carotid artery is unavoidable. During this occlusion the anesthesiologist would expect

    (A) a decrease in heart rate
    (B) an increase in arterial pressure
    (C) an increase in the number of impulses from the carotid sinus nerve
    (D) an increase in venous capacity
    (E) vasodilatation throughout the peripheral circulation

18. Binding of O_2 to hemoglobin

    (A) causes a large shift of the surrounding secondary structures leading to decreased affinity of the deoxy subunits for CO_2
    (B) is cooperative, meaning that after the first O_2 binds, the other subunits are more readily oxygenated
    (C) occurs with equal affinity at all four subunits
    (D) results in a release of heme from the interior to the exterior of the α-subunits leading to an increase in O_2 affinity of the β-subunits

    (E) results in a release of the heme from the interior to the exterior of the β-subunits leading to an increase in O_2 affinity of the α-subunits

19. You are about to remove a small lesion from the mucosa of the laryngeal vestibule and want to anesthetize the nerve that supplies general sensation to the mucous membrane of that area. The nerve you are interested in is the

    (A) external laryngeal
    (B) glossopharyngeal
    (C) inferior laryngeal
    (D) internal laryngeal
    (E) pharyngeal plexus

20. On routine examination, a 35-year-old man is found to have a blood pressure of 145/89 mm Hg. Thorough workup excludes an immediate cause of his hypertension. A diagnosis of essential hypertension is made. Long-term regulation of arterial blood pressure in this patient is primarily a function of

    (A) peripheral baroreceptors
    (B) the autonomic nervous system
    (C) the central nervous system (CNS)
    (D) total peripheral vascular resistance
    (E) urine output and fluid intake

21. A 37-year-old man has recurrent skin lesions that first appeared over his elbows and knees as well-defined pink papules covered by a micaceous silvery scale. A skin biopsy microphotograph is displayed from one of his lesions in Figure 8–3. The diagnosis is

    (A) basal cell carcinoma
    (B) malignant melanoma
    (C) pemphigus vulgaris
    (D) psoriasis
    (E) squamous cell carcinoma

22. Which of the following drugs is most likely to produce tachycardia as an adverse effect?

    (A) Clonidine
    (B) Digoxin
    (C) Nifedipine

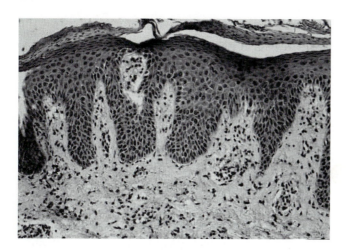

Figure 8–3

(D) Propranolol

(E) Pyridostigmine

23. Which of the following is associated with the use of benzodiazepines?

(A) Addictive effects

(B) Agitation in the elderly

(C) Muscle relaxant effects

(D) Nonimpairment of conditioned avoidance learning

24. The major amino acid precursor for gluconeogenesis is

(A) alanine

(B) aspartate

(C) cysteine

(D) glutamate

(E) serine

25. During the course of a neurologic exam you notice that your patient exhibits a loss of all somatosensation on the right side of the body, accompanied by obvious weakness and hyperreflexia in the arm and leg on that side. When protruded, the patient's tongue also deviates to the right. Occlusion of which of the following vessels accounts for these deficits?

(A) Anterior spinal artery on left

(B) Lenticulostriate arteries on left

(C) Lenticulostriate arteries on right

(D) Paramedian branches of basilar bifurcation on right

(E) Posterior spinal artery on right

26. A 48-year-old woman moved to a new area and is being seen for a routine physical examination as a new patient in a general medicine clinic. Her present medical history is significant for a 30-lb weight excess and an 8-year history of noninsulin-dependent diabetes mellitus, which she reports has been fairly well controlled with oral agents and a strict diet regimen. However, she is now anxious about her condition and admits to recently developing poor and irregular eating habits, and occasionally missing a medication dosage due to the high stress level surrounding her recent move. The most accurate estimation of this patient's recent glucose control would be

(A) fasting insulin and C peptide levels

(B) glucose tolerance test

(C) glycated hemoglobin level

(D) random serum glucose

(E) urine ketone body level

27. A 23-year-old quadriplegic patient has a complete spinal transection between the cervical and thoracic levels. If you were to test this patient you would most likely find that

(A) functional residual capacity equals residual volume

(B) the inspiratory reserve volume is greatly reduced (< 10% of normal)

(C) the maximal inspiratory pressures are more compromised than the expiratory ones

(D) the ventilatory response to limb exercise is characterized by an increase in tidal volume contributed by the expiratory reserve volume

(E) vital capacity is only slightly compromised

28. A 6-year-old child presents with diarrhea, malabsorption, and steatorrhea. A photomicrograph from a small intestinal mucosal biopsy is displayed in Figure 8–4. An appropriate treatment would be

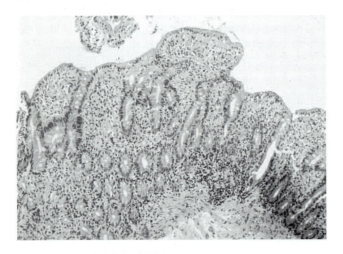

Figure 8–4

(A) a referral to hospice for supportive care
(B) a gluten-free diet
(C) antineoplastic drugs
(D) β-interferon therapy
(E) surgical resection of a segment of small bowel

29. A drug is administered to a patient with an arrhythmia. In the laboratory this drug has been observed to increase action potential duration. The ECG recorded before and after drug administration is shown in Figure 8–5. Which of the following drugs was administered?

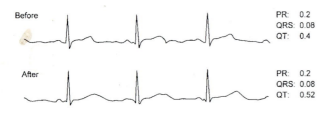

Figure 8–5

(A) Flecainide
(B) Ibutilide
(C) Lidocaine
(D) Propranolol
(E) Verapamil

30. Glutamate dehydrogenase is an extremely important enzyme involved in nitrogen homeostasis. This enzyme catalyzes a reversible reaction (Figure 8–6) that either incorporates or liberates ammonium ion. When catalyzing the reaction in the direction of ammonium ion liberation the enzyme is allosterically activated by

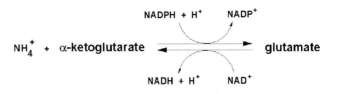

Figure 8–6

(A) ADP
(B) ATP
(C) citrate
(D) glutamine
(E) GTP

31. Your patient has a pituitary tumor that has encroached on the cavernous sinus, compressing the internal carotid artery and the adjacent abducens nerve. Interruption of the abducens nerve in the cavernous sinus is most likely to result in

(A) a loss of visual accommodation
(B) dilatation of the pupil
(C) lateral deviation of the pupil (external strabismus)
(D) medial deviation of the pupil (internal strabismus)
(E) ptosis of the upper eyelid

32. Which of the following statements concerning typical neuroleptic antipsychotic drugs is true?

(A) Combined use with anticholinergic agents is contraindicated.

(B) Most are dopamine receptor blockers.

(C) Most are effective against negative symptoms of schizophrenia.

(D) Most decrease serum prolactin levels.

(E) Most of them are nonsedating.

33. A 52-year-old man with a history of fainting episodes is admitted for cardiac monitoring. A representative section of his ECG is shown in Figure 8–7. Which of the following statements best describes the pathophysiologic condition of this patient?

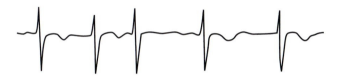

Figure 8–7

(A) A drug such as quinidine, which acts in part by prolonging the effective refractory period of conducting tissue, is useful therapy.

(B) Because the atria contribute little to ventricular function, this patient's pulse is expected to be extremely regular in spite of the abnormality.

(C) The interval between QRS complexes remains constant in this patient.

(D) The P waves on the ECG recordings are normal in this patient.

(E) This patient's ECG shows a life-threatening condition and requires immediate application of strong electric current to place the entire myocardium in refractory period.

34. The chance of successful transplantation is minimal when the donor and recipient have

(A) different class II molecules

(B) different MHC class I and class II molecules

(C) different MHC class I molecules

(D) similar MHC class I and class II molecules

(E) similar MHC class II molecules

35. In the titration of a weak acid, such as an amino acid, the point of dissociation at which the concentration of the acid (HA) is equal to that of the conjugate base (A⁻) is defined as

(A) K_a

(B) log[A⁻]

(C) log[HA]

(D) pH

36. A temporary increase in the number of circulating reticulocytes most predictably results when an individual

(A) experiences an allergic reaction to ragweed pollen

(B) has a bacterial infection

(C) has a viral infection

(D) moves from sea level to a high altitude

(E) receives a vaccination against measles

37. A 58-year-old woman who has previously been diagnosed with Graves disease undergoes an esophagogastroduodenoscopy (EGD) after complaining of weakness, tingling, and numbness of the extremities. Biopsy results reveal atrophic mucosa, intestinal metaplasia, lymphoplasmacytic infiltration, and endocrine cell hyperplasia. What is the most effective intervention for this patient?

(A) Cessation of alcohol use

(B) Chemotherapy

(C) Replacement of NSAID use with acetaminophen

(D) Triple antibiotic therapy

(E) Vitamin B_{12}

38. A 66-year-old woman has complained of hip pain for about 3 years. A prosthetic hip replacement is recommended. A photograph of her diseased femoral head is displayed in Figure 8–8. What is the likely cause of this abnormality?

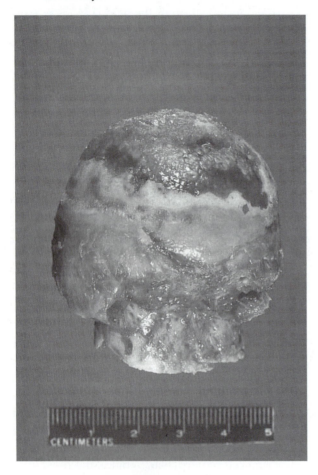

Figure 8–8

(A) Benign neoplastic process
(B) Coagulopathy
(C) Degenerative process
(D) Infection
(E) Malignant neoplastic process

39. An 8-year-old boy has chronic granulomatous disease. He most likely will be often infected with

(A) *Staphylococcus aureus*
(B) *Streptococcus agalactiae*
(C) *Streptococcus mitis*

(D) *Streptococcus pneumoniae*
(E) *Streptococcus pyogenes*

40. Which of the following is a pharmacologic effect commonly associated with opioid use, even in tolerant individuals?

(A) Intestinal hypermotility
(B) Pupillary constriction
(C) Relaxation of the lower end of the common bile duct
(D) Respiratory depression
(E) Stimulation of the cough reflex

41. Phosphofructokinase-2 can best be characterized as

(A) a bifunctional enzyme that can function as a kinase or as a phosphatase
(B) an allosteric activator of phosphofructokinase-1
(C) an enzyme regulated by phosphorylation, an event that increases the rate at which the enzyme phosphorylates its substrate
(D) an enzyme whose substrate is fructose 1,6-bisphosphate
(E) one of the enzymes whose activity is required in the TCA cycle

42. The protruded tongue tests the competence of the innervation to the muscles of the tongue. A deviation of the protruded tongue to the right indicates damage to the

(A) left hypoglossal nerve
(B) left lingual nerve
(C) right glossopharyngeal nerve
(D) right hypoglossal nerve
(E) right lingual nerve

43. Which of the following cancers is most likely to cause depression?

(A) Cervical
(B) Lung
(C) Pancreatic
(D) Skin
(E) Stomach

44. A 56-year-old man is slowly losing vision in his right eye. The ophthalmologist notes that the conjunctiva, sclera, and lens are normal on examination. The intraocular pressure, however, is markedly elevated and there is pressure atrophy of the optic disk. The most likely diagnosis is

(A) arcus senilis
(B) cataract
(C) glaucoma
(D) pinguecula
(E) retrolental fibroplasia

45. During a snowboarding accident a 19-year-old man suffers a complete transection of the upper lumbar spinal cord. During the first 12 h after this accident you would expect a (an)

(A) diminished bladder reflex
(B) exaggerated knee stretch reflex
(C) normal bladder reflex
(D) normal knee stretch reflex
(E) normal sense of vibration in the legs

46. A 33-year-old man employed in a nuclear power plant is exposed to 17 cGy. What acute clinical symptoms are likely to be observed?

(A) Acute radiation syndrome
(B) Cerebral syndrome
(C) GI syndrome
(D) Hematopoietic syndrome
(E) None

47. The conversion of fibrinogen to fibrin is catalyzed by

(A) antithrombin III
(B) heparin
(C) plasmin
(D) prothrombin
(E) thrombin

48. A 13-year-old girl has leukemia and needs a bone marrow transplant. Using this girl's leukocytes and irradiated leukocytes from her relatives in mixed leukocyte cultures, the following results were obtained.

SOURCE OF LEUKOCYTES	COUNTS/MIN OF TRITIATED THYMIDINE INCORPORATED
Sister	540
Brother	2000
Mother	280
Grandmother	650
Grandfather	980

The best bone marrow donor for this 13-year-old girl is her

(A) brother
(B) grandfather
(C) grandmother
(D) mother
(E) sister

49. A 5-year-old boy presents with bowing of the lower legs. There is a depression of the sternum leaving a sharp elevation at each of the rib margins. You also notice that movement of his limbs is painful and that he has numerous purpura and ecchymoses of the skin. These findings lead you to suspect that this child suffers from a dietary deficiency of vitamin

(A) A
(B) B_1 (thiamine)
(C) B_{12} (cyanocobalamin)
(D) C (ascorbate)
(E) D (calciferol)
(F) K

50. The thrombolytic mechanism of action of alteplase (tissue plasminogen activator [t-PA]) involves

(A) activation of antithrombin III
(B) direct conversion of plasminogen to plasmin
(C) formation of an active complex with plasminogen
(D) inhibition of activated factor X
(E) proteolytic activation of fibrinogen

51. A 61-year-old administrative assistant is a long-term smoker and has a sedentary life style. He has a chronic cough, which has worsened in the past 2 years. He has also developed a bulge in the groin area. Upon examination, you observe that the elongated swelling is located at the medial end of the inguinal ligament, superior and medial to the pubic tubercle. You can also detect the pulse of the inferior epigastric artery lateral to this bulge. This patient suffers from

    (A) a direct inguinal hernia
    (B) a femoral hernia
    (C) a sliding hiatal hernia
    (D) an indirect inguinal hernia
    (E) an umbilical hernia

52. HIV-affected individuals

    (A) can engage in kissing
    (B) may manifest a cortical but not subcortical dementia
    (C) may not safely masturbate
    (D) should not donate blood unless under triple therapy
    (E) should not engage in vaginal or anal intercourse under any circumstances

53. Phosphofructokinase-1 can best be characterized by which of the following statements?

    (A) The enzyme is activated as the concentration of AMP rises.
    (B) The enzyme is activated when the concentration of NADH is rising.
    (C) The enzyme is negatively regulated by fructose 1,6-bisphosphate.
    (D) The enzyme is positively regulated by fructose 1,6-bisphosphatase.
    (E) The enzyme uses AMP in a substrate level phosphorylation to yield ATP.

54. Insulin resistance is a major contributor to the difficulty in management of patients with diabetes mellitus. Which of the following tends to decrease insulin resistance?

    (A) Cortisol
    (B) Exercise
    (C) Growth hormone
    (D) Obesity
    (E) Pregnancy

55. A 30-year-old man has a viral infection characterized by fever, myalgia, headache, and a dry, nonproductive cough that lasts for 3 days. The virus responsible for this infection is an orthomyxovirus and undergoes frequent antigenic changes. It is reasonable to assume that this virus

    (A) has a segmented RNA genome
    (B) is a bullet-shaped virus
    (C) is a nonenveloped virus
    (D) lacks H antigen
    (E) lacks N antigen

56. A 24-year-old pregnant woman is infected with the rubella virus. Her embryo or fetus is at greatest risk for the development of a malformation if transplacental transmission occurs during

    (A) days 1 to 15
    (B) days 15 to 60
    (C) delivery
    (D) the second trimester
    (E) the third trimester

57. The section shown in the photomicrograph in Figure 8–9 is typical of the mucosa from the

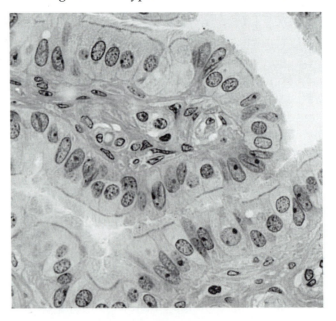

Figure 8–9

(A) epididymal duct

(B) oropharynx

(C) oviduct

(D) small intestine

(E) trachea

58. Which one of the following pairs of drugs with a description or mechanism of action is correct?

(A) Edrophonium—short-acting cholinesterase inhibitor

(B) Metrifonate—used in treatment of myasthenia gravis

(C) Neostigmine—cholinesterase inhibitor-specific for muscarinic synapses

(D) Physostigmine—irreversible cholinesterase inhibitor

(E) Pralidoxime—reversible cholinesterase inhibitor

59. A 25-year-old smoker reports a 3-week history of a productive cough with occasional blood streaking, low-grade fevers, night sweats, and a 6-lb weight loss over the past month. The most likely finding on chest radiography would be

(A) a single mass lesion

(B) an apical cavitary lesion

(C) bilateral hilar lymphadenopathy

(D) lobar consolidation

(E) patchy diffuse interstitial infiltrates

60. The graph in Figure 8–10 shows loss of vision (shaded areas) in the visual field of a patient. This patient most likely has a lesion in the

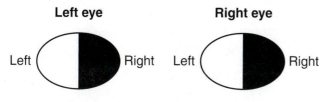

Figure 8–10

(A) left optical nerve

(B) left optical tract

(C) optic chiasm

(D) right optical nerve

(E) right optical tract

61. Ethanol consumption inhibits the delivery of glucose to the blood primarily as a consequence of the activity of alcohol dehydrogenase. The effect of this reaction is to reduce the level of NAD⁺, which in turn

(A) activates glycolysis by increasing the rate of ATP utilization, signaling a need to oxidize more carbohydrate within hepatocytes

(B) activates the glycolytic reaction catalyzed by glyceraldehyde-3-phosphate dehydrogenase, thereby inhibiting the rate of gluconeogenesis

(C) inhibits the ability of the cell to deliver gluconeogenic substrates in the form of phosphoenol pyruvate as a result of a shift in the equilibrium of the malate dehydrogenase catalyzed reaction

(D) inhibits the gluconeogenic reaction catalyzed by glyceraldehyde-3-phosphate dehydrogenase which requires NAD⁺ as a substrate

(E) signals a reduced level of hepatocyte ATP that results in activation of phosphofructokinase-1

62. Degeneration of the substantia nigra results in

(A) athetosis

(B) chorea

(C) "cog wheel" rigidity

(D) hyperkinesia

(E) intention tremor

63. The structure indicated by arrow #3 in Figure 8–11 is the

(A) ascending aorta

(B) descending aorta

(C) esophagus

(D) superior vena cava

(E) trachea

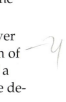

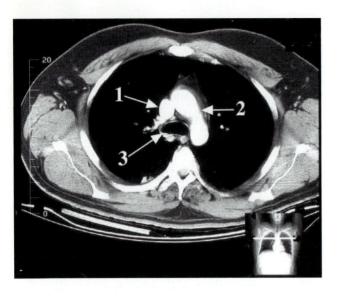

Figure 8–11

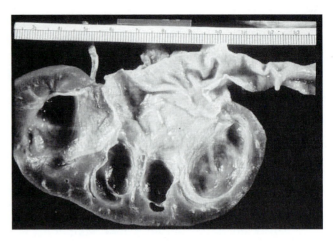

Figure 8–12

64. An antihyperlipidemic therapy whose efficacy in lowering LDL cholesterol depends on the expression of functional LDL receptors in the liver is

   (A) colestipol
   (B) diet
   (C) etretinate
   (D) gemfibrozil
   (E) niacin

65. The antibody residues that predominantly make up the antigen-combining site as the "contact" amino acids are located within the

   (A) constant domains
   (B) disulfide bonds
   (C) framework regions
   (D) heavy chains
   (E) hypervariable regions

66. The changes seen in the kidney shown in Figure 8–12 were an incidental finding in the autopsy of a 39-year-old woman. The most likely cause is

   (A) abuse of analgesics
   (B) hypertension
   (C) postrenal obstruction
   (D) renal cell carcinoma
   (E) renal infarct

67. The presence of villi are an important structural and functional specialization of the GI tract lumen. The villi of the small intestine are notable in part because they greatly increase the absorptive surface area. However the Crypts of Lieberkuhn, between the villi, also play a crucial role, including which of the following?

   (A) As a site of bile secretion
   (B) As a site of iron secretion
   (C) As the site of cellular proliferation of enterocytes
   (D) As the site of sloughing of dead and damaged cells
   (E) Location of membrane-bound enzymes of the brush border

68. Herniation of the uncal region of the temporal lobe over the free edge of the tentorium and through the tentorial notch compresses the ipsilateral crus cerebri and nearby structures such as the oculomotor nerve. Which of the following combination of signs might be seen in such a case?

   (A) Contralateral hemiplegia—contralateral upper facial expression paralysis
   (B) Contralateral hemiplegia—paralysis of ipsilateral lower facial expression
   (C) Contralateral hemiplegia—paralysis of the ipsilateral medial rectus muscle

(D) Ipsilateral hemiplegia—deviation of the tongue toward the side opposite the lesion

(E) Ipsilateral hemiplegia—paralysis of the ipsilateral medial rectus muscle

69. Which of the following is present only in the intrinsic pathway of clotting?

(A) Factor I (fibrinogen)
(B) Factor II (prothrombin)
(C) Factor V
(D) Factor VIII (antihemophilic factor)
(E) Factor X (Stuart factor)

Questions 70 through 75

A 30-year-old woman complains of fatigue, insomnia, and depression.

70. If the patient had a recent weight gain and has been feeling cold much of the time, which of the following tests would be most useful?

(A) Dexamethasone suppression test
(B) Rorschach test
(C) Serum calcium level
(D) Thyroid function test
(E) Trail-making test

71. If the patient seems very sluggish in movement and speech, and takes an inordinate amount of time to answer a question, this phenomenon is called

(A) hysteria
(B) pseudobulbar palsy
(C) psychomotor agitation
(D) psychomotor retardation
(E) restless leg syndrome

72. If the patient says that she intends to kill herself by taking an overdose, you should

(A) hospitalize her
(B) prescribe amitriptyline 50 mg at night for 30 days
(C) prescribe fluoxetine 20 mg every day for 14 days

(D) provide explorative psychotherapy
(E) provide supportive psychotherapy

73. If further history reveals that she had attempted suicide several times in the past, which of the following statements would be most correct?

(A) The patient is not a serious suicide risk.
(B) The patient probably has antisocial personality disorder.
(C) The patient should be evaluated for a psychotic disorder.
(D) The risk of successful suicide is decreased.
(E) The risk of successful suicide is increased.

74. Which additional information would be most useful in treating this patient at this point?

(A) Family history of bipolar disorder
(B) Family history of dysthymia
(C) Family history of schizophrenia
(D) Family history of somatization disorder
(E) Family history of suicide

75. If this patient turns out to have bipolar disorder, the pharmacologic agent most likely to help the patient's mood swings is

(A) buspirone
(B) fluoxetine
(C) nefazodone
(D) tranylcypromine
(E) valproic acid

76. The structure indicated by arrow #4 in Figure 8–13 is the

(A) left atrium
(B) left ventricle
(C) right atrium
(D) right ventricle

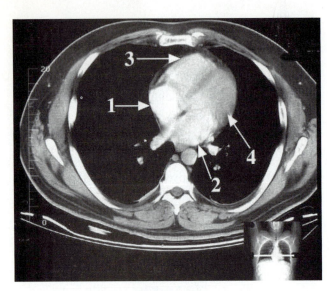

Figure 8–13

77. The blood protein thrombin is known to

(A) be an oligomeric protein

(B) contain γ-carboxyglutamate residues

(C) form clots by complexing with fibrin

(D) have an enzymatic specificity similar to trypsin

(E) require vitamin K in its activated form

78. Which of these agents is used in the acute treatment of cardiogenic shock because of its ability to increase cardiac contractility without producing large increases in heart rate?

(A) Albuterol

(B) Digoxin

(C) Dobutamine

(D) Epinephrine

(E) Phenylephrine

79. A patient's laboratory analysis of arterial plasma showed a pH of 7.44, bicarbonate 15 mEq/L, P_{O_2} = 80 mm Hg, and P_{CO_2} = 25 mm Hg. This patient probably

(A) has severe chronic lung disease

(B) is a lowlander who has been vacationing at high altitude for 2 weeks

(C) is a subject in a clinical research experiment who has been breathing a gas mixture of 10% oxygen and 90% nitrogen for a few minutes

(D) is an adult psychiatric patient who swallowed an overdose of aspirin

(E) is an emergency room patient with severely depressed respiration as a result of a heroin overdose

80. In a case of referred pain over the shoulder, you discover that the patient has irritation of the subdiaphragmatic parietal peritoneum due to inflammation of the gallbladder. The innervation of this area of the parietal peritoneum is by the

(A) least splanchnic nerve

(B) oligohypogastric nerve

(C) phrenic nerve

(D) subcostal nerve

(E) vagus nerve

81. A baseball player has pain in his stomach that is relieved by food intake. If gastritis due to *H. pylori* is suspected, the most useful and rapid diagnostic test is

(A) carbohydrate utilization tests

(B) culture of gastric contents on blood agar containing metronidazole and bismuth salts

(C) determination of IgE

(D) Gram stain of the gastric contents

(E) *in vivo* or *in vitro* tests for urease

82. On a routine physical examination of a 63-year-old woman, cardiac auscultation reveals the presence of a diastolic murmur, a loud S1 followed by a normal S2, and a subsequent clicking sound. These findings are most closely associated with

(A) aortic regurgitation

(B) aortic stenosis

(C) mitral regurgitation

(D) mitral stenosis

(E) pulmonic regurgitation

(F) pulmonic stenosis

(G) tricuspid regurgitation

(H) tricuspid stenosis

83. Neonatal urea cycle defects are usually misdiagnosed because of a failure to

    (A) assess the level of ammonia in the blood
    (B) assess the level of argininosuccinate in the blood
    (C) assess the level of citrulline in the blood
    (D) assess the level of orotic acid in the urine
    (E) recognize the odor of acetone on the breath

84. Figure 8–14 represents filtration through the glomerular membrane and shows the locations of the Starling forces. In which of the following is there a positive ultrafiltration pressure ($P_{uf} > 0$) for formation of glomerular filtrate? (Numbers in mm Hg.)

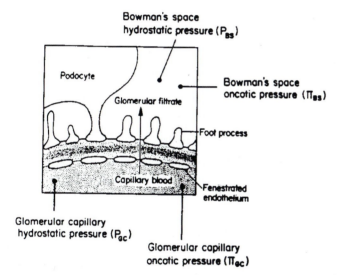

Figure 8–14

	P_{GC}	P_{BS}	Π_{GC}	Π_{BS}
(A)	40	10	20	0
(B)	40	15	25	0
(C)	40	20	30	10
(D)	50	20	30	0
(E)	55	25	40	5

85. A 3-year-old child has a temperature of 101°F. On examination, discrete vesiculoulcerative lesions (Koplik spots) are noted on the mucous membranes of the mouth. The most probable diagnosis is

    (A) herpangina
    (B) measles
    (C) rubella
    (D) scarlet fever
    (E) thrush

86. Which of the following statements about neuromuscular blocking drugs is most correct?

    (A) Atracurium is eliminated primarily by the kidneys.
    (B) Mivacurium has the longest duration of action.
    (C) Pancuronium can be reversed with neostigmine.
    (D) Succinylcholine is longer acting than vecuronium.
    (E) Tubocurarine has antihistaminic effects in addition to neuromuscular blockade.

87. Histologic examination of a lymph node reveals the presence of germinal centers but an absence of the deep cortical (paracortical) zone. This finding is consistent with

    (A) agammaglobulinemia
    (B) an acute bacterial infection
    (C) combined immunodeficiency
    (D) thrombocytopenia
    (E) thymic hypoplasia

88. A 35-year-old woman noticed a slowly growing mass in her left breast over the past 4 months. At surgery, the mass is found to be predominantly solid, tan-white, rubbery, well circumscribed, and measuring about $3 \times 3 \times 3$ cm. A representative photomicrograph of the lesion is displayed in Figure 8–15. What is the diagnosis?

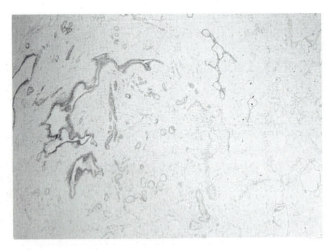

Figure 8–15

(A) Fibroadenoma
(B) Intraductal carcinoma
(C) Medullary carcinoma
(D) Paget disease of the breast
(E) Scirrhous carcinoma

89. Most blood vessels dilate under ischemic conditions. In which arterial region does hypoxia cause vasoconstriction?

(A) Coronary arteries
(B) GI arteries
(C) Pulmonary arteries
(D) Renal arteries
(E) Skeletal muscle arteries

90. Figure 8–16 depicts an important type of biological reaction necessary for metabolic homeostasis. The freely reversible reaction is catalyzed by the class of enzymes known as

(A) aminotransferases
(B) dehydrogenases
(C) hydrolases
(D) nitrogenases

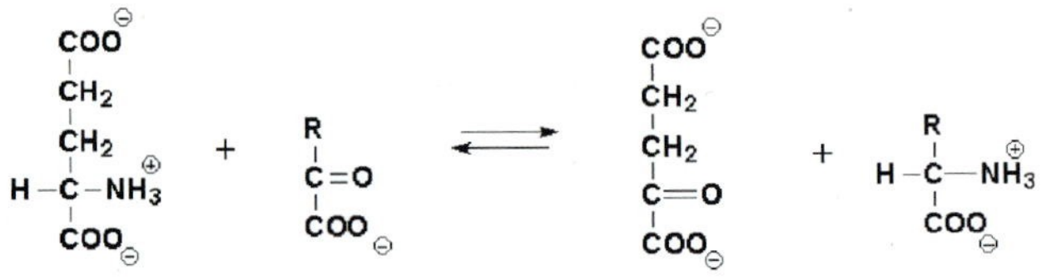

Figure 8–16

91. Irrigation of the seated patient's right ear with warm water should produce

(A) fast conjugate horizontal eye movement to the left
(B) no horizontal eye movements
(C) slow conjugate horizontal eye movement to the left
(D) slow conjugate horizontal eye movement to the right
(E) slow horizontal movement of right eye and fast movement of left eye

92. Concerning HIV infection, which of the following statements is correct?

(A) Most women acquire HIV infection through IV drug use.
(B) The number of infected men is growing at a higher rate than infected women.
(C) The percentage of heterosexual men with HIV is decreasing.
(D) The percentage of total cases among gay and bisexual men has declined in the United States.
(E) The sex ratio between infected males and females is about the same.

93. L.G. has severe cirrhosis and has developed marked peripheral pitting edema and ascites (edema fluid in the peritoneal cavity). Which of the following drugs is most likely to cause an effective diuresis?

(A) Captopril
(B) Digoxin
(C) Hydrochlorothiazide
(D) Spironolactone
(E) Triamterene

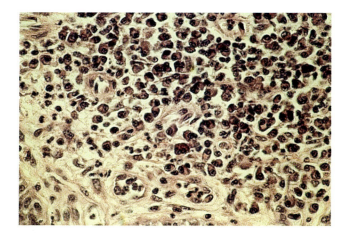

Figure 5–1 (Question 550)

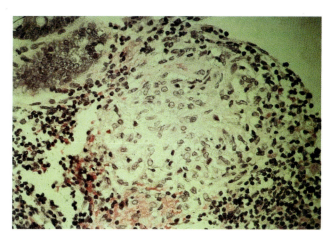

Figure 5–2 (Question 559)

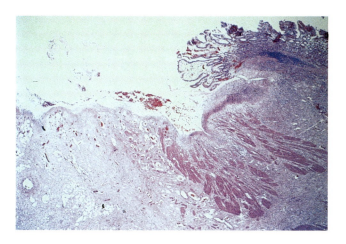

Figure 5–3 (Question 568)

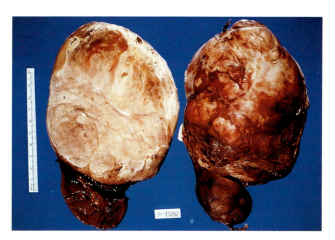

Figure 5–4 (Question 576)

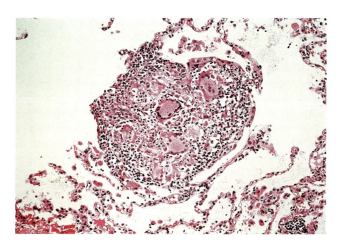

Figure 5–5 (Question 584)

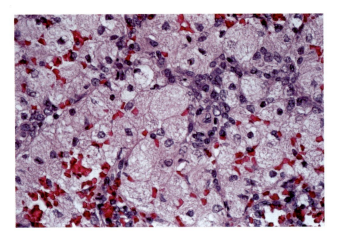

Figure 5–6 (Question 592)

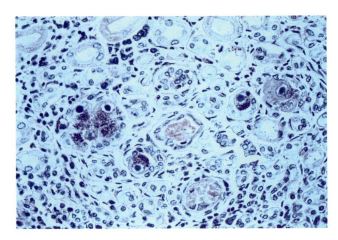

Figure 5–7 (Question 602)

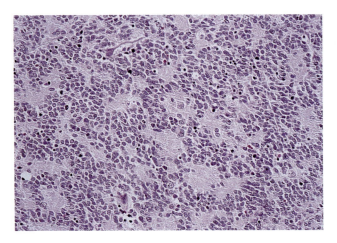

Figure 5–8 (Question 609)

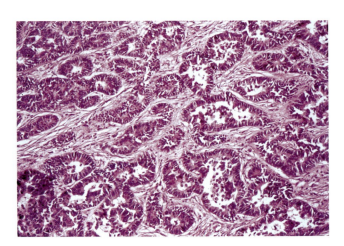

Figure 5–9 (Question 615)

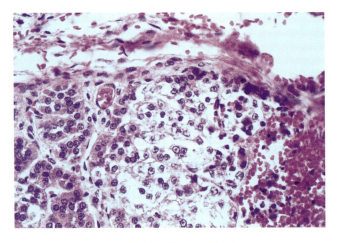

Figure 5–10 (Question 621)

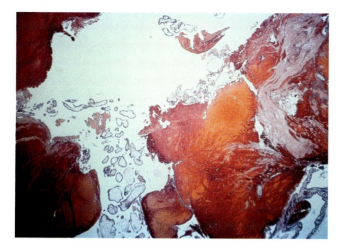

Figure 5–11 (Question 625)

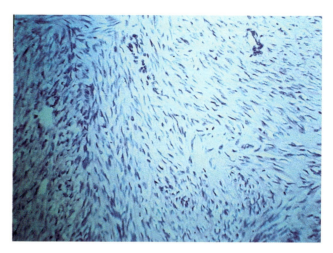

Figure 5–12 (Question 630)

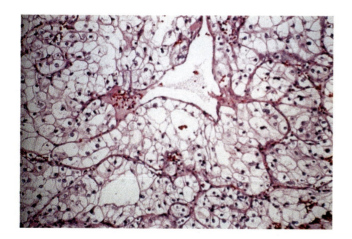

Figure 5–13 (Question 640)

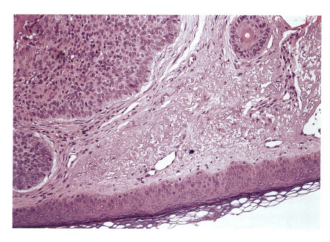

Figure 5–14 (Questions 651 and 652)

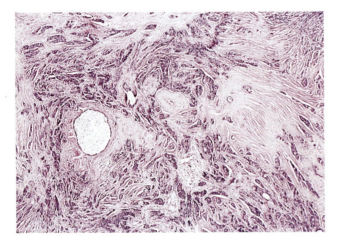

Figure 5–15 (Question 656 and 657)

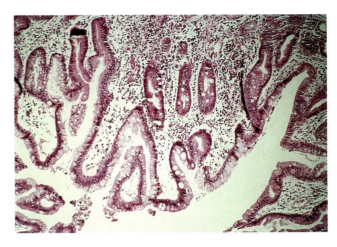

Figure 5–16 (Questions 658 and 659)

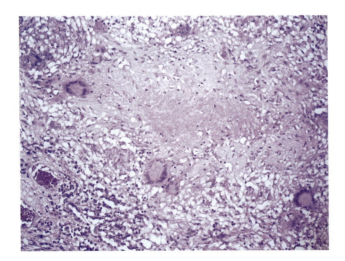

Figure 9–14 (Question 98)

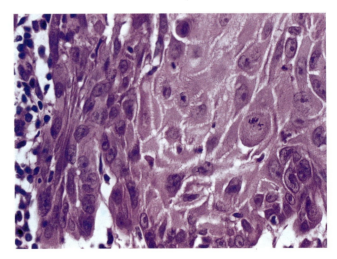

Figure 10–12 (Question 99)

94. DiGeorge syndrome is characterized by

(A) a defect in neutrophil chemotaxis

(B) a depletion of B-dependent areas in lymph nodes

(C) a depletion of lymph node lymphocytes in both T- and B-dependent areas

(D) an absence of isohemagglutinins

(E) defective development of the third and fourth pharyngeal pouches

Questions 95 and 96

A 12-year-old African-American boy develops a large facial tumor. The histology of the lesion obtained from a fine-needle biopsy is displayed in Figure 8–17.

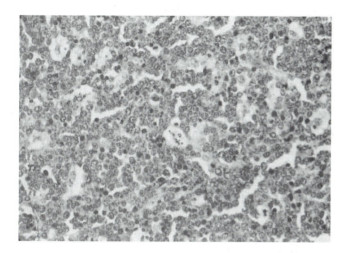

Figure 8–17

95. The most likely diagnosis is

(A) adenocarcinoma

(B) Burkitt lymphoma

(C) chronic lymphocytic leukemia-lymphoma

(D) parasitic lymphadenitis

(E) salivary gland lymphoepithelioma

96. The development of this lesion is associated with

(A) aflatoxin exposure

(B) deficiency of an essential dietary nutrient

(C) infection with Epstein–Barr virus

(D) infection with *Wuchereria bancrofti*

(E) Sjögren syndrome

97. When lactate is used as a source of carbon atoms for gluconeogenesis, the NADH required for the glyceraldehyde-3-phosphate dehydrogenase reaction comes from the action of which enzyme?

(A) Glucose-6-phosphate dehydrogenase

(B) Glycerol-3-phosphate dehydrogenase

(C) Lactate dehydrogenase

(D) Malate dehydrogenase

(E) Phosphoenol pyruvate carboxykinase

98. A 32-year-old man presents with diarrhea and symptoms of peptic ulcer disease. Endoscopy reveals two ulcers, one in the first portion of the duodenum and one in the mid-duodenum. However, they do not respond to the usual peptic ulcer treatment programs. The most likely explanation for the findings in this patient is

(A) antibodies to intrinsic factor

(B) ectopic hypersecretion of gastrin

(C) gastric mucosal atrophy

(D) pressure ulceration from bezoars

(E) vascular abnormality

99. A boil in the facial area bordered by the nose, eye, and upper lip can cause thrombosis of the facial vein, which may spread to a bony sinus within the skull. The resulting thrombosis in the sinus may be fatal unless treated with antibiotics. The sinus in question is the

(A) cavernous sinus

(B) ethmoidal sinus

(C) frontal sinus

(D) maxillary sinus

(E) sphenoidal sinus

100. Which of the following agents has good antipyretic activity but poor anti-inflammatory activity?

(A) Acetaminophen

(B) Aspirin

(C) Indomethacin

(D) Nabumetone

(E) Tolmetin

Answers and Explanations

1. **(D)** Argininosuccinate synthetase catalyzes the ATP-dependent synthesis of argininosuccinate from citrulline and aspartate. Therefore, deficiencies in this enzyme lead to accumulation of citrulline in the urine, plasma, and cerebrospinal fluid. Defects in argininosuccinate synthetase are also referred to as citrullinemias. The other urea cycle intermediates (choices A, B, C, and E) are either upstream or downstream of argininosuccinate synthetase and, therefore, do not accumulate to a significant degree as a result of deficiencies in this enzyme.

2. **(E)** The septum secundum is a crescent-shaped wedge of tissue that incompletely partitions the developing atria leaving a defect called the foramen ovale near the floor of the right atrium. The muscular interventricular septum (choice A) arises from the inferior part of the bulboventricular sulcus to incompletely partition the developing ventricles. The defect in the interventricular septum is closed by growth of the endocardial cushions creating the membranous interventricular septum. The ostium primum (choice B) is the opening between the right and left sides of the developing atrium that is gradually closed by the developing septum primum. The ostium secundum (choice C) is formed by the resorption of the superior part of the septum primum before it completely partitions the ventricles. The septum primum (choice D) is the first partition of the atria and results in complete partitioning except for the timely development of the ostium secundum.

3. **(D)** The apparent volume of distribution is a primary pharmacokinetic parameter and is calculated from the formula $V_d = X/C$, where V_d is the apparent volume of distribution, X is the amount of drug present in the body, and C is the plasma (or blood) concentration. We know the amount of drug administered. Because the drug is subject to elimination immediately after administration, we must use the concentration at time 0 for our calculations. The curvature seen in the early data points results from slow distribution of the drug from blood into the tissue compartments that comprise the volume of distribution. Therefore, we cannot use these data points directly. However, the linear portion of the data can be extrapolated back to time 0 to determine the plasma concentration that would have been obtained if distribution had been instantaneous. The administered amount X (30 mg) divided by the extrapolated plasma concentration (1 μg/mL or 1 mg/L) yields an apparent V_d of 30.0 L.

4. **(C)** Using the linear portion of the data (including the dashed extrapolation), the concentration at time 0 is 1 mg/mL. By definition, the half-life is the time interval for 50% reduction in concentration for single-dose drug disappearance. The plasma concentration of 0.5 mg/mL is reached after 7 h. The half-life predicts the approach to plateau for any situation in which first-order kinetics apply. Single-dose disappearance kinetics can be thought of as the approach to a plateau of zero.

5. **(A)** By repeated exposure to the pairing of a stimulus (thinking of an apple) to another stimulus (sour taste) that produces a response (salivation), simply thinking of a sour apple

produces salivation. This type of learning is called classical or Pavlovian conditioning. Choice B is incorrect because it refers to learning by thinking. The person in this case probably learned the association between sourness and salivation through experience first, not by thinking about it. Imprinting (choice C) involves learning during a critical period, as in the case of goslings that follow a human if exposed to a human just after birth. Operant conditioning (choice D) refers to learning by rewarding desired behavior. It is unlikely that salivation was rewarded. Shaping (choice E) is a form of operant conditioning.

6. **(C)** Alcoholic hepatitis (also called acute sclerosing hyaline necrosis of the liver) usually occurs acutely following an alcohol binge superimposed on steatosis (fatty liver) or cirrhosis. Variable degrees of liver cell necrosis are present with corresponding clusters of neutrophils and frequent accompaniment of pericellular and perivenular fibrosis. Intracellular Mallory bodies are common. Alcoholic hepatitis may range from asymptomatic to fulminant hepatic failure. Symptoms, which may persist for weeks or months, include upper abdominal pain, anorexia, fever, tender hepatomegaly, and jaundice. Severe disease may cause encephalopathy and death. Acetaminophen overdose (choice A) causes massive, dose-related centrilobular liver cell necrosis secondary to glutathione depletion. Toxicity begins with nausea, vomiting, diarrhea, abdominal pain, and sometimes shock, followed in a few days by jaundice. Liver injury occurs 24 to 48 hours following ingestion. Acute fatty liver of pregnancy (choice B) occurs in late pregnancy and is characterized by increased microvesicular fat in the hepatocytes and fibrin deposits in the sinusoids. Budd–Chiari syndrome (choice D) refers to acute or chronic hepatic vein thromboses that may occur as a result of a number of predisposing thrombotic conditions (e.g., pregnancy, neoplasms, polycythemia vera). Liver changes are those of severe venous congestion including sinusoidal and centrilobular space of Disse erythrocytic infiltration. Chronic disease is associated with fibrosis

and nodular regeneration. Clinical presentation includes hepatomegaly, portal hypertension, and very commonly ascites. Pyogenic liver abscesses (choice E) may be caused by many bacteria, most commonly *Escherichia coli*, or by *Entamoeba hisolytica* in regions where the parasite is endemic. Lesions are walled-off, focal collections of necrotic liver cells and accumulated neutrophils (pus). Clinical presentation is with upper right abdominal pain, high fever, and hepatomegaly.

7. **(E)** Chronic alcoholics are prone to many physiologic problems due to their poor dietary patterns and the effects of alcohol itself on the GI tract that lead to impaired nutrient absorption. The most common problems of chronic alcoholics are neurologic in nature, including mental confusion and depression, ataxia, and uncoordinated eye movements. The most severe symptoms are related to those seen in Wernicke–Korsakoff syndrome. Although thiamine deficiency is only one of many nutritional deficiencies seen in chronic alcoholics, administration of thiamine has a dramatic effect on reversing the course of these severe symptoms. None of the other choices (A, B, C, and D) reflect symptoms associated with thiamine deficiency, or to deficiencies in other vitamins.

8. **(A)** At an early stage of AIDS, the patient displays a mononucleosis-like illness, with lethargy, apathy, fever, generalized lymphadenopathy, leukopenia, and maculopapular rashes. All these symptoms are caused by human immunodeficiency virus (HIV), which is an enveloped, single-stranded, positive-polarity RNA virus. The RNA genome of HIV is composed of two identical molecules. The virus also contains in its nucleocapsid reverse transcriptase, protease, and an integrase. The mumps virus (choice D) is an enveloped virus with neuraminidase and hemagglutinin spikes; it has a nonsegmented single-stranded RNA of negative polarity. Infectious hepatitis (choice B) is caused by a single-stranded, positive polarity RNA, nonenveloped virus. The disease is characterized by fever, vomiting, and jaun-

dice. Lymphocytic choriomeningitis (choice C) is caused by a single-stranded, circular, segmented RNA, enveloped virus. It is characterized by vomiting, stiff neck, and changes in mental state. Mumps (choice D) is associated with tender swelling of the parotid glands. Pleurodynia (choice E) is caused by group B coxsackieviruses. These are nonenveloped viruses, and have a single-stranded, positive polarity RNA genome.

9. **(D)** The most notable opportunistic neoplasia associated with AIDS is Kaposi sarcoma. It has been recently published that human herpesvirus 8 may be the etiologic agent of Kaposi sarcoma. Burkitt lymphoma (choice A) is caused by the Epstein–Barr virus, not AIDS. Herpes simplex type 1 (choice B) is the causative agent of oral lesions, not lymphoma. Herpes simplex type 2 (choice C) is the causative agent of genital herpetic lesions. Both type 1 and type 2 herpes viruses may produce either local vesicular lesions or severe generalized disease in neonates infected during passage through an infected birth canal. Rous sarcoma (choice E) is caused by the Rous sarcoma virus, a retrovirus isolated by Peyton Rous who produced tumors in chickens with this virus.

10. **(D)** The mechanism of action of β-lactam antibiotics is inhibition of transpeptidases, which cross-link the amino group on the end of the pentaglycine and the terminal carboxyl group of D-alanine. β-Lactam antibiotics adhere primarily to the penicillin-binding proteins of the bacterial cytoplasmic membrane and cell wall. β-Lactam antibiotics do not bind to the bacterial capsules (choice A); they do not inhibit synthesis of cell wall proteins (choice C); and they may activate bacterial autolytic hydrolases (choice E). Bacteria lack nuclear membranes (choice B).

11. **(D)** Gastrin infusion stimulates gastric acid secretion. Thus, initially, before peptide X was given, there was high gastric acid concentration. Secretin, sometimes called "nature's antacid," must have been peptide X because it is known to inhibit gastric acid secretion and to stimulate pancreatic bicarbonate production. Peptide X could not have been angiotensin II (choice A), which has several functions (e.g., stimulation of aldosterone secretion), none of which is inhibition of gastric acid secretion or stimulation of pancreatic bicarbonate secretion. Nor could it have been CCK (choice B), which mainly stimulates pancreatic enzyme secretion and gallbladder contraction. Nor could it have been motilin (choice C), which has mainly to do with motility. Somatostatin (choice E) has many inhibitory effects and does not stimulate pancreatic bicarbonate production.

12. **(B)** In congenital coarctation of the aorta, the thoracic aorta is usually obstructed just past the origin of the left subclavian artery. If the constriction reduces the diameter of the aorta by more than 50%, then the patient develops symptoms such as decreased tolerance to exercise and greater fatigability. Because the radial artery arises from branches proximal to the coarctation and the posterior tibial artery from branches distal to the coarctation, simultaneous palpation of their pulses typically reveals posterior tibial pulses to be delayed and of lesser volume than the radial pulses.

13. **(A)** Tobacco dependence is the most common and most difficult to control drug dependence in the United States. Choice B is incorrect because nicotine is an extremely physically addicting substance, and sudden cessation of its use results in both physical and psychological withdrawal symptoms. Choice C grossly underestimates the harmfulness of tobacco because physical complications of chronic tobacco use begin to appear in 20 pack-years. Choice D is incorrect because the relapse rate of smoking cessation programs is 60% to 70%. Choice E is incorrect because tobacco dependence usually begins in adolescence.

14. **(C)** The second law of thermodynamics states that for a reaction to proceed spontaneously, the total entropy of the system must increase. Entropy is a measure of the disorder

of a system; therefore, the natural thermodynamically driven tendency is for systems (and the molecules of a system) to tend toward maximum disorder. Total energy must remain constant, but it can change form (choice A), such as heat energy into work energy. Some, but not many, reactions proceed spontaneously (choice B); however, the majority require a catalyst. In biological systems, the catalysts are enzymes. The total energy of a molecule (choice D) does not impact the second law, but the various entropies of a molecule do. Choice E reflects the first law of thermodynamics, stating that the total energy of a system plus that of its environment must remain constant.

15. **(A)** Trimethoprim is an inhibitor of dihydrofolate reductase that exhibits great specificity for binding to the bacterial form as opposed to the human form (10^5 higher concentrations are required for inhibition of human dihydrofolate reductase). Trimethoprim is usually combined with sulfamethoxazole, an inhibitor of dihydropteroate synthase, to provide inhibition of sequential steps in bacterial tetrahydrofolate synthesis. Resistance to trimethoprim may arise by mutation of bacterial dihydrofolate reductase, although acquisition of a plasmid-encoding, altered dihydrofolate reductase is more common for gram-negative bacteria. Expression of altered forms of transpeptidase (choice B) is a mechanism for resistance to the inhibitors of cell wall synthesis, such as the β-lactam penicillins and cephalosporins. Expression of β-lactamase activity (choice C) is a mechanism for resistance to the β-lactam antibacterial agents such as the penicillins and cephalosporins. Mutation of ribosomal subunits (choice D) is a mechanism for resistance to the protein synthesis inhibitors, such as the tetracyclines and aminoglycosides, including streptomycin. Thickening of the bacterial cell wall (choice E), as well as decreasing activity of pore-forming proteins such as porins, are mechanisms of resistance to the protein synthesis inhibitors for gram-negative bacteria; these agents must gain access to the protein synthetic machinery through the cell wall and cell membrane.

16. **(E)** The quartan fever that accompanies infection with *P. malariae* is secondary to cyclic release of proliferating merozoites from erythrocytes. The circulating ruptured red cell stroma and free hemoglobin are naturally occurring pyrogens capable of invoking an abrupt febrile episode. Cell-mediated cytokines (choice A) are minimally active in *Plasmodium* infections. They do not engender sufficient pyrogenic activity to account for the severe cyclic fevers seen with *P. malariae* infections. Cerebral malaria is a grave prognostic finding. It does not cause cyclic central hypothalamic fever (choice B). Hepatocytes (choice C) serve as a nonlytic reservoir for *P. malariae* infection. Immune-mediated destruction of the organism (choice D) is a minor feature of malaria infection. It does not produce quartan fever.

17. **(B)** Temporary occlusion of the common carotid arteries decreases vascular pressure within the carotid sinus area. This peripheral baroreceptor responds to changes in pressure and is an important reflex in maintaining relatively constant arterial pressure on a short-term basis. A decrease in pressure depresses the number of impulses that travel from the carotid sinus nerve. Because these impulses normally inhibit the central vasoconstrictor area and excite the vagal center, a decrease in impulses reflexively causes arterial pressure to rise and heart rate and contractility to increase. The entire circulation is stimulated to constrict, and thus there is a reduction in venous capacitance. Increased firing rate of the carotid sinus nerve (choice C) and subsequent vasodilatation (choice E) and decreased heart rate (choice A) result from an increase in vascular pressure within the carotid sinus area. The venous capacity (choice D) also increases with decreased sympathetic tone as a result of an increased firing rate of the carotid sinus nerve.

18. **(B)** The deoxygenated subunits of the hemoglobin tetramer exist in the T ("tense") conformational state. As erythrocytes enter the capillaries of the lung alveoli, the partial pressure of O_2 increases sufficiently to allow

binding to hemoglobin. When 1 mole of O_2 binds, it causes a shift in the overall conformation of the other subunits to a more R ("relaxed") conformational state. This change in conformation leads to higher affinity of the remaining monomers for O_2. Each deoxygenated monomer has a progressively increased affinity for O_2 as more oxygen binds. This cooperative binding is observed as a sigmoidal saturation curve when plotting the partial pressure of oxygen versus moles of O_2 bound. Oxygen binding impacts the secondary structure of hemoglobin, but only to a minor degree, and this has no impact on its affinity for CO_2 (choice A). As indicated, oxygen binds cooperatively to hemoglobin, not with equal affinity to each deoxy subunit (choice C). Oxygen binding shifts the position of the heme group, but not sufficiently to place it on the exterior of any hemoglobin subunit (choices D and E).

19. **(D)** The internal laryngeal nerve supplies the laryngeal mucosa above the level of the vocal fold as well as the mucosa of the piriform recess and the epiglottic valleculae. The external laryngeal nerve (choice A) is motor to the cricothyroid muscle and the lowest part of the inferior pharyngeal constrictor muscle. The glossopharyngeal nerve (choice B) carries afferent fibers from the mucosa of the middle ear, auditory tube, pharynx, palatine tonsils, and posterior one-third of the tongue, but does not supply the laryngeal mucosa. The inferior laryngeal nerve (choice C) is motor to the intrinsic muscles of the larynx, except the cricothyroid muscle, and is sensory to the mucosa of the larynx below the level of the vocal fold. The pharyngeal plexus (choice E) supplies most of the innervation to the pharynx, including general visceral afferent fibers from the pharyngeal mucosa that are carried in the glossopharyngeal nerve.

20. **(E)** Although short-term regulation of arterial blood pressure is primarily affected by the integrated responses of peripheral baroreceptors and the central and sympathetic nervous systems, the primary determinant of regulation of blood pressure in the long run is the relationship of urine output to fluid intake. This system is normally capable of returning blood pressure to normal levels, which is different from the short-term nervous regulation. By adjusting extracellular fluid and blood volumes, renal–body fluid mechanisms alter the venous return. Individual beds then adjust their resistance because of the interplay of local and neuronal factors, and thus arterial pressure is slowly readjusted to control levels. The baroreceptor reflex pathway (choice A) involves the autonomic nervous system (choice B) and vital centers in the brainstem portion of the CNS (choice C), but plays little role in long-term regulation of blood pressure. The total peripheral vascular resistance (choice D) is thus altered by those mechanisms rather than being the variable that directly determines blood pressure.

21. **(D)** Hyperkeratosis, parakeratosis, acanthosis, club-shaped dermal papillae, and clusters of neutrophils in the upper epidermis (Munro microabscesses) are the defining microscopic features of psoriasis. Clinically, the disease displays erythematous scaly plaques, which preferentially occur over the extensor cutaneous surfaces. Basal cell carcinoma (choice A) is a low-grade cutaneous malignancy and is characterized by dermal infiltration of small, basally oriented tumor cells. The histology of primary malignant melanoma (choice B) displays collections of atypical melanocytes within the epidermis and possibly invading into the dermis. Neither basal cell carcinoma nor melanoma present with recurrent multiple lesions that come and go. Pemphigus vulgaris (choice C) is a cutaneous blistering disease. Epidermal bleb formation is the critical histologic observation. Squamous cell carcinoma (choice E) is defined microscopically by collections of malignant cells with focal squamous differentiation.

22. **(C)** By inhibiting entry of calcium into vascular smooth muscle, the calcium channel blockers produce vasodilation with hypotension as an adverse effect in overdose situations. The hypotension may result in a reflex

increase in sympathetic stimulation to the heart and compensatory tachycardia, especially with dihydropyridine calcium blockers. This effect, along with systemic hypotension and decreased coronary flow, may exacerbate myocardial ischemia in patients being treated with fast-onset calcium channel blockers such as regular nifedipine. Bradycardia has been reported as an adverse effect of nifedipine with IV administration combined with concurrent β-blocker administration. Clonidine (choice A), an α_2-adrenoreceptor agonist, acts at the level of the vasomotor centers in the brainstem to decrease sympathetic outflow. Cardiac adverse effects, when seen, involve bradycardia. The cardiac glycosides such as digoxin (choice B) inhibit Na^+/K^+ ATPase. The glycosides increase vagal tone and decrease sympathetic nervous system activity. These effects also result in bradycardia. The nonselective β-blocker propranolol (choice D) produces bradycardia as a normal aspect of its actions. The anticholinesterase pyridostigmine (choice E) is used in the treatment of myasthenia gravis to increase the concentration of acetylcholine at the neuromuscular junction. Increased acetylcholine levels cause a decrease in heart rate.

23. **(B)** Benzodiazepines are antianxiety agents. They are also muscle relaxants and anticonvulsants as well as sedatives. Because of the sedative action, an elderly patient may develop paradoxical agitation due to the disinhibition of higher cortical function.

24. **(A)** The primary precursors for gluconeogenesis in the liver are lactate and alanine, which are produced in muscle during intense activity. Alanine is formed from pyruvate by transamination in a reaction catalyzed by alanine aminotransferase. This reaction is the major mechanism of transporting ammonia from nonhepatic tissues to the liver. The liver is the only organ capable of carrying out the urea cycle, the pathway for removal of ammonia waste. Alanine is converted back to pyruvate in the liver and diverted to the gluconeogenesis pathway for the synthesis of glucose. Its function in ammonia transport is

the major reason that alanine is the principal glucogenic amino acid. Aspartate (choice B) and glutamate (choice D) are good sources of TCA cycle intermediates through the action of transaminases and as such are glucogenic amino acids. However, they do not supply major sources of carbon for glucose synthesis. Cysteine (choice C) is oxidized to pyruvate, which makes it glucogenic, but like most glucogenic amino acids, it is not the major source of carbon for glucose synthesis. Serine (choice E) is interconvertible with glycine, or can be oxidized to pyruvate, but like other glucogenic amino acids, the latter reaction does not constitute a major source of carbons for glucose synthesis.

25. **(B)** Lesions involving the left lentriculostriate branches result in damage to upper motor neuron axons coursing through the posterior limb of the internal capsule on the left side. This results in motor deficits involving the contralateral extremities, as well as in the musculature innervated by cranial nerves VII, IX, X, XI, and XII, which have been deprived of their motor cortex input. Damage to the left anterior spinal artery (choice A) produces ipsilateral lower motoneuron signs in the musculature innervated by the damaged levels of the spinal cord. Lesions involving the right lenticulostriate vessels (choice C), the paramedian branches of the basilar bifurcation on the right (choice D), and the right posterior spinal artery (choice E) do not lead to upper motoneuron signs on the right side, or cause the protruded tongue to deviate to the right.

26. **(C)** When present in high concentration, glucose can react nonenzymatically with protein amino groups to form an unstable intermediate, or Schiff base, which subsequently undergoes an internal rearrangement to form a stable glycated protein. The glycation of the amino acids valine and lysine on the β chain of hemoglobin A results in hemoglobin A_{1c} (HbA_{1c}), or glycated hemoglobin. One hypothesis for the pathogenesis of diabetic microvascular disease is that prolonged glucose elevation leads to the glycation of basement

membrane proteins in the same manner. Because red blood cells circulate for an average of 90 to 120 days, assaying HbA_{1c} provides an index of a diabetic patient's glucose control over the preceding 3 to 4 months. Although normal values vary between laboratories, on average nondiabetic subjects have HbA_{1c} levels roughly between 4% and 6%. Fasting levels of insulin and C peptide (choice A) (C peptide is an amino acid component of the insulin precursor proinsulin) are not used in the evaluation of glycemic control. A glucose tolerance test (choice B) is used in the diagnosis of diabetes mellitus by measuring glucose levels during a 2-h period following the ingestion of 75 g of oral glucose. A random serum glucose value (choice D) is of little value in estimating glucose control because it represents only the blood glucose level at any single point in time and is influenced by dietary conditions. A urine ketone body level (to test for ketonuria) (choice E) is obtained in conjunction with urine glucose (to test for glycosuria), serum glucose, and serum ketone levels in the diagnosis of diabetic ketoacidosis. Insufficient insulin results in mobilization of free fatty acids from adipose tissue, which are then oxidized in the liver through the stimulatory effects of glucagon and eventually converted into ketone bodies. Ketone bodies are moderately strong acids and lead to the onset of diabetic ketoacidosis.

27. **(A)** Injuries affecting upper cervical segments (above C3) usually quickly cause death from loss of respiratory muscle function. However, transection of the spinal cord between C8 and T1 only severs neural connections between the brainstem and some of the muscles involved in respiration (e.g., intercostal and abdominal muscles), while sparing connections to the diaphragm (phrenic nerves come off spinal neurons in segments C3-C5 ["three, four, and five keep the diaphragm alive"]). Normal, quiet expiration is passive. However, forced expiration, as in the latter part of vital capacity measurement, requires active participation by expiratory muscles. By definition, functional residual capacity (FRC) is the volume at which the respiratory system stays when all respiratory muscles are inactive. On the other hand, residual volume (RV) is the volume left after maximal expiratory effort (involving intercostal and abdominal muscles). RV is normally about 1 L less than FRC. Because this patient has no expiratory muscle function, there cannot be an RV less than FRC; in this patient, FRC = RV. Additionally, you might expect a vital capacity (choice E) that is at best only about 50% of normal. In this quadriplegic patient there is essentially complete loss of expiratory muscle function, but only modest loss of inspiratory action (choices B and C) because the diaphragm is the major muscle of inspiration. Because inspiration is less compromised than forced expiration in this patient, any increase in tidal volume during exercise (choice D) is contributed by the inspiratory reserve volume.

28. **(B)** The child has celiac disease, a disorder resulting from a hypersensitivity reaction to gluten in the diet. Withdrawal of gluten from the diet is usually curative. Clinically, there is diarrhea, malabsorption, and steatorrhea. Histologically, there is villous atrophy of the small intestinal mucosa. A referral to hospice for supportive care (choice A) is unlikely to be necessary; more than 95% of patients respond to the removal of gluten from their diet. Recalcitrant cases are rarely life threatening and may be successfully treated with various forms of hyperalimentation that bypass the small intestine. Because the disease is usually cured by dietary measures, the use of antineoplastic drugs (choice C), β-interferon therapy (choice D), and surgical resection of the small intestine (choice E) are not appropriate treatment options.

29. **(B)** The ECG shows prolongation of the QT interval, the interval that reflects the ventricular repolarization time (i.e., the duration of the ventricular action potential). Ibutilide is a group III antiarrhythmic drug that prolongs action potential duration and the QT interval by blocking the delayed rectifier potassium channel (I_{Kr}). Flecainide (choice A), a group IC antiarrhythmic drug, prolongs the QRS

duration because it selectively inhibits sodium channels. Lidocaine (choice C) is a highly selective group IB agent that has little effect on the ECG. Propranolol (choice D), a β-blocker, prolongs AV conduction time and PR interval. Verapamil (choice E), a group IV calcium channel blocker, also prolongs PR interval and has little effect on the QT interval.

30. **(A)** Glutamate dehydrogenase utilizes both nicotinamide nucleotide cofactors; NAD⁺ in the direction of nitrogen liberation and NADPH for nitrogen incorporation. The reaction catalyzing the liberation of ammonia and α-ketoglutarate (α-KG) from glutamate is a key anapleurotic process linking amino acid metabolism with TCA cycle activity. This reaction allows glutamate to play an important role in energy metabolism. Glutamate dehydrogenase provides an oxidizable carbon source used for the production of energy as well as a reduced electron carrier, NADH. In the forward reaction, as shown in Figure 8–6, glutamate dehydrogenase is important in converting free ammonia and α-KG to glutamate, forming one of the 20 amino acids required for protein synthesis. As expected for a branch point enzyme with an important link to energy metabolism, glutamate dehydrogenase is regulated by the cell energy charge. ATP (choice B) and GTP (choice E) are positive allosteric effectors of the formation of glutamate, whereas ADP and GDP are positive allosteric effectors of the nitrogen-liberating reaction. Thus, when the level of ATP is high, conversion of glutamate to α-KG and other TCA cycle intermediates is limited; when the cellular energy charge is low, glutamate is converted to ammonia and oxidizable TCA cycle intermediates. Citrate (choice C) and glutamine (choice D) do not allosterically affect glutamate dehydrogenase.

31. **(D)** The abducens nerve is motor to the lateral rectus muscle. Paralysis of this muscle produces medial deviation of the pupil due the unopposed action of the medial rectus muscle. Damage to the oculomotor nerve results in a loss of visual accommodation (choice A) due to interruption of parasympa-

thetic innervation to the sphincter pupillae and ciliary muscles. Dilatation of the pupil (choice B) results from interruption of the parasympathetic innervation to the sphincter pupillae muscle carried by the oculomotor nerve. Lateral deviation of the pupil (choice C) can result from damage to the oculomotor nerve supplying the medial rectus muscle. Lateral deviation of the pupil results from unopposed action of the lateral rectus muscle. Ptosis of the upper lid (choice E) can result from damage to the oculomotor muscle supplying the levator palpebrae superioris muscle or from interruption of the sympathetic innervation to the superior tarsal muscle.

32. **(B)** All typical antipsychotic drugs, such as haloperidol, are dopamine receptor antagonists and increase serum prolactin levels. They are likely to be effective for the positive symptoms, such as hallucinations, delusions, loosening of association, and catatonia. Unlike the atypical antipsychotics (e.g., risperidone, olanzapine), they are not effective in treating the negative symptoms (such as flat affect, paucity of thought) of schizophrenia. For the pseudoparkinsonian side effect of typical antipsychotics, anticholinergic agents such as benztropine may be used. They tend to be sedating.

33. **(A)** The ECG shows atrial fibrillation characterized by an irregularly undulating baseline, absence of P waves, and irregular QRS intervals. Atrial fibrillation is a common arrhythmia that accompanies several forms of chronic heart disease. It probably represents some form of reentry phenomenon in which part of the tissue may be excited at an inappropriately early part of the cardiac cycle. A number of drugs are available to prolong the effective refractory period of selective parts of the heart, and these drugs would be effective in restoring normal atrial contraction. The strength of ventricular contraction is related to the timing of filling, and thus failure of the atria to effectively contract alters ventricular filling. This produces an irregular pulse (choice B). Direct current shock (choice E) is

an effective treatment to return the heart to normal rhythm and reverse atrial fibrillation. However, atrial fibrillation per se is not a life-threatening event, and placing the entire myocardium into a refractory period usually is not the appropriate course of action. Activation of conducting tissue in the atrioventricular node becomes variable in time from cycle to cycle, and thus the QRS complex interval becomes less constant (choice C). Because the atria do not contract, there are no P waves in this ECG recording (choice D).

34. **(B)** A maximum T-helper cell proliferation and induction of cytotoxic T lymphocytes are seen in mixed lymphocyte reactions when disparity occurs at MHC class I and class II loci. Because these cells play primary roles in the rejection of transplanted tissue, the chance of successful transplant between donor and recipient is minimal when the donor and recipient have different MHC class I and II molecules.

35. **(D)** The Henderson–Hasselbalch equation describes the relationship between the dissociation constant for any acid or base and the negative log of the hydrogen ion ($-\log[H^+]$ = pH) concentration. This is defined as:

$$pH = pK_a + \log[A^-]/[HA]$$

From this equation it is clear that the pH of a solution of any acid (for which the equilibrium constant is known) can be calculated knowing the concentration of the acid, HA, and its conjugate base $[A^-]$. At the point of the dissociation where the concentration of the conjugate base $[A^-]$ is equal to that of the acid $[HA]$:

$$pH = pK_a + \log[1]$$

The log of 1 = 0. Thus, at the midpoint of a titration of a weak acid pK_a = pH. In other words, the term pK_a is that pH at which an equivalent distribution of acid and conjugate base (or base and conjugate acid) exists in solution. The term K_a (choice A) is the dissociation constant and reflects the equation:

$[H^+][A^-]/[HA]$. The terms $\log[A^-]$ (choice B) and $[HA]$ (choice C) are parts of the Henderson–Hasselbalch equation and as such by themselves do not define the midpoint of titration of an acid or base.

36. **(D)** Movement of an individual to a higher altitude (with decreased partial pressure of oxygen) requires greater oxygen-carrying capacity of blood and is thus a stimulus for an increased rate of erythrocyte production. This is reflected by an increased percentage of circulating erythrocytes that are newly developed (reticulocytes). Exposure to allergens (choice A), infectious agents (choices B and C), or vaccines (choice E) elicit responses involving distinct populations of leukocytes.

37. **(E)** This patient has developed pernicious anemia (PA), an autoimmune disease that results in vitamin B_{12} deficiency due to the inability of gastric parietal cells to produce intrinsic factor (IF). Her biopsy results are typical of type A chronic gastritis, which occurs at the end stage of the disease. Patients with PA have an increased risk of gastric carcinoma and endoscopic surveillance with biopsy is indicated in all patients with the disease. Three different antibodies have been identified: (1) about 75% of patients have an antibody that blocks the binding of B_{12} to IF (blocking antibody); (2) about 50% of patients have an antibody that binds with the B_{12}–IF complex, thus interfering with the binding of the complex to ileal mucosal receptors (binding antibody); and (3) about 90% of patients have antibodies against gastric parietal cells (sometimes called parietal canalicular antibody). Vitamin B_{12} deficiency results in subacute combined degeneration of the spinal cord, which is caused by demyelination of the posterior and lateral columns. These changes may lead to paresthesias, loss of position and vibration sense, weakness, sensory ataxia, and spastic paraparesis. Peripheral neuropathy is a result of segmental demyelination of nerves. The incidence of PA is substantially increased in patients with other autoimmune diseases, particularly of the thyroid and adrenal glands. Peripheral neuropathy may

occur as a result of alcohol abuse (choice A), but would not explain the biopsy findings. Heavy alcohol ingestion may cause acute gastropathy that would reveal hemorrhage into the lamina propria on biopsy. Chemotherapy (choice B) would be a possible choice for gastric carcinoma; biopsy results would show poorly differentiated cells distended by intracellular mucin (signet ring cells). NSAID use is associated with gastric ulcerations; biopsy would show a necrotic base with acutely inflamed debris and a zone of granulation tissue that does not match the findings here so replacement of NSAID with acetaminophen (choice C) is not appropriate here. Triple antibiotic therapy (choice D) is used to treat *Helicobacter pylori* that is present in nearly all chronic duodenal ulcers and approximately 75% of chronic gastric ulcers.

38. (C) The femoral head shows marked degenerative osteoarthritis. The gradual destruction of articular cartilage can eventually lead to joint compromise through eburnation, osteophyte formation, subchondral cysts, and osteochondral loose body formation. Clinically, these anatomic changes are reflected as joint pain and a restricted range of motion. Figure 8–8 does not display evidence of a benign neoplasm (choice A), coagulopathy (choice B), infection (choice D), or malignant neoplastic process (choice E).

39. (A) Chronic granulomatous disease patients cannot generate hydrogen peroxide metabolically because of their genetic defect in NADPH oxidase. Thus, they are repeatedly infected with catalase positive microorganisms such as staphylococci. In contrast to this, these patients are rarely infected with catalase-negative bacteria such as streptococci (choices B, C, D, and E). This occurs because catalase-negative bacteria accumulate hydrogen peroxide, activating the defective myeloperoxidase–hydrogen-peroxide–halide system of the host neutrophils.

40. (B) Opioids with μ- and κ-agonistic properties cause miosis by an excitatory action on the parasympathetic nerve innervating the pupil. Some tolerance develops, but miosis is seen even in addicts. Intestinal spasm and constipation, rather than hypermotility (choice A), are seen with opioids. Tolerance does not develop to the constipating effect. Opioids do not relax the lower end of the common bile duct (choice C), but rather constrict the sphincter of Oddi, causing a large increase in bile duct pressure. This may produce symptoms of biliary colic. Respiratory rate is depressed by opioids (choice D), but tolerance to this effect is marked. Depression of respiratory drive at the level of the brainstem may lead to respiratory arrest, the most common cause of death in morphine intoxication. Opioids depress rather than stimulate the cough reflex (choice E). Codeine is an effective antitussive agent. The antitussive agent dextromethorphan is chemically related to the opioids, but has no actions on opioid receptors and does not possess analgesic or addictive properties.

41. (A) The bifunctional enzyme phosphofructokinase-2 (PFK-2) contains a kinase and a phosphatase domain. The kinase domain phosphorylates fructose 6-phosphate (F6-P) to yield fructose 2,6-bisphosphate (F2,6-BP), whereas the phosphatase dephosphorylates F2,6-BP yielding F6-P. F2,6-BP is a potent allosteric activator of the rate-limiting enzyme of glycolysis, phosphofructokinase-1 (PFK-1), as well as a potent allosteric inhibitor of the gluconeogenic enzyme fructose-1,6-bisphosphatase. The activity of PFK-2 is regulated by cAMP-dependent protein kinase (PKA)-mediated phosphorylation. When phosphorylated, PFK-2 functions as a phosphatase, and as a kinase when dephosphorylated. The PKA-mediated change in activity of PFK-2 allows the level of F2,6-BP to be regulated by circulating hormones such as glucagon and epinephrine, ultimately controlling the flux through glycolysis. PFK-2 itself is not an allosteric effector (choice B), but is responsible for regulating the levels of F2,6-BP, which is an allosteric effector. As indicated, PFK-2 acts as a phosphatase, not as a kinase, when it itself is phosphorylated. Therefore, when phosphorylated, PFK-2 removes phosphate from its substrate (choice C). The substrate for the kinase activity of PFK-2 is F6-P (choice D). PFK-2 functions as a regulatory enzyme in glycolysis, not the TCA cycle (choice E).

42. **(D)** The muscles of the tongue are innervated by the paired hypoglossal nerves. On protrusion of the tongue, deviation occurs to the side of the damaged nerve and paralyzed muscles. Damage to the left hypoglossal nerve (choice A) results in deviation of the protruded tongue to the left side. Damage to the left lingual nerve (choice B) has no effect on movement of the tongue, but produces a loss of general sensation and taste on the left half of the anterior two-thirds of the tongue. Damage to the right glossopharyngeal nerve (choice C) has no effect on movement of the tongue, but produces a loss of general sensation and taste on the right half of the posterior one-third of the tongue. Damage to the right lingual nerve (choice E) has no effect on movement of the tongue, but produces a loss of general sensation and taste on the right half of the anterior two-thirds of the tongue.

43. **(C)** All cancers may be associated with depression (choices A, B, D, and E). However, some neoplasms, particularly cancer of the tail of the pancreas, are particularly likely to cause, and often present with, clinical depression.

44. **(C)** Glaucoma is characterized by increased intraocular pressure with resultant pressure atrophy of the optic disc and decreased visual activity. Medicinal treatment with papillary constrictors can provide temporary relief. Arcus senilis (choice A) is a ring of fatty material in the outer cornea commonly seen in elderly individuals. The ocular pressures and visual acuity are unaffected by this change. A cataract (choice B) is an opacity of the lens and is not associated with increased intraocular pressure. Pinguecula (choice D) is an actinically induced growth that does not alter intraocular pressure. Retrolental fibroplasia (choice E) is seen in premature infants exposed to high concentrations of oxygen.

45. **(A)** Acute spinal transection causes immediate flaccid paralysis and loss of all sensation and reflex activity below the level of injury. This initial phase is called "spinal shock" and lasts for hours or days. If the spinal cord below the lesion is intact, reflex activity later returns and the flaccid paralysis changes to a spastic paralysis with exaggerated (choice B) or normal (choice D) stretch reflexes. The bladder reflex normalizes only gradually (choice C), eventually resulting in an automatic bladder because central control remains lost. All sensation including sense of vibration (choice E) is absent in parts of the body innervated by spinal cord segments below the lesion.

46. **(E)** Individuals exposed to acute radiation doses of between 0 and 50 cGy do not show any immediate clinical symptoms. However, low-level exposure may increase the likelihood of neoplasia in the future. Exposures between 50 and 200 cGy usually produce acute radiation syndrome (choice A) characterized by fatigue, nausea, and vomiting. Hematopoietic syndrome (choice D) is characterized by leukopenia and thrombocytopenia, in addition to the clinical findings of acute radiation sickness. Exposure dosages are usually between 200 and 600 cGy. The acute mortality rate is between 20% and 50%. Exposures of 600 to 1000 cGy may produce mucosal ulceration, diarrhea, and electrolyte loss as part of the GI syndrome (choice C). Acute mortality rates are between 50% and 100%. The cerebral syndrome (choice B) has a 100% mortality rate and is seen with acute doses above 1000 cGy.

47. **(E)** Fibrinogen is activated by conversion to fibrin monomers through the action of thrombin, which cleaves several peptide bonds in fibrinogen to yield fibrin. The fibrin monomers, thus formed, aggregate to form a clot. Thrombin itself is derived by proteolytic cleavage of its precursor, prothrombin (choice D). Antithrombin III (choice A) is an inhibitor of thrombin activity. It inactivates the enzyme by forming an irreversible complex with it. This inhibition can be enhanced

by the presence of heparin (choice B) and is the basis of the latter's anticoagulant properties. Fibrin clots can be dissolved by the action of plasmin (choice C), a serine protease.

48. **(D)** The best bone marrow donor for this patient is her mother, because the results of the mixed lymphocyte reaction correlate with the degree of dissimilarity of histocompatability (i.e., high counts indicate enhanced stimulation suggesting immunologic unrelatedness of tissue tested). Twins who have identical leukocyte antigens do not stimulate mixed leukocyte reactions, indicating that their tissues are mutually transplantable.

49. **(D)** Deficiencies of vitamin C and vitamin D can produce similar skeletal abnormalities such as those listed. However, a major difference is that vitamin C deficiency is accompanied by hemorrhages, as seen in this child. This also leads to hemarthrosis (bleeding into joints) that makes movement very painful. Vitamin A deficiency (choice A) is associated with night blindness, with or without keratomalacia and papular dermatitis. Vitamin B_1 deficiency (choice B) produces beriberi marked by polyneuropathy, heart failure, and edema (or Wernicke syndrome in chronic alcoholics). Vitamin B_{12} deficiency (choice C) produces megaloblastic anemia and subacute combined degeneration of the spinal cord. Vitamin D deficiency (choice E) produces osteomalacia in adults and rickets in children due to defective mineralization of bone. Vitamin K deficiency (choice F) can result in a bleeding diathesis because it is required for the activity of clotting factors II, VII, IX, and X.

50. **(B)** Tissue plasminogen activator (t-PA) directly catalyzes the proteolytic conversion of plasminogen to plasmin. When used early, the thrombolytics significantly reduce morbidity from myocardial infarction. The early use of t-PA also offers a significant advance for occlusive strokes. The activation of antithrombin III (choice A) is one of the mechanisms of action of regular heparin. Formation of an active complex with plasminogen (choice C) is a property of streptokinase, a

protein produced by β-hemolytic streptococci. Streptokinase has no intrinsic enzymatic activity, but rather forms a stable complex with plasminogen that is enzymatically active in cleaving free plasminogen to plasmin. Inhibition of activated factor X (choice D) is an effect of regular heparin and low-molecular-weight heparins. Proteolytic activation of fibrinogen (choice E) to fibrin is a property of thrombin in the formation of the fibrin mesh leading to clot formation.

51. **(A)** Direct and indirect inguinal hernias can be distinguished by their location in relation to the inferior epigastric vessels. An indirect inguinal hernia is located lateral to the inferior epigastric vessels, whereas a direct inguinal hernia develops medially. Because the pulse of the inferior epigastric artery is felt laterally to the swelling in the groin area, the hernia is a direct inguinal hernia and not an indirect one (choice D). Furthermore, because the swelling is situated superior and medial to the pubic tubercle, it is not a femoral hernia (choice B), which would be located inferior and lateral to the pubic tubercle. Direct inguinal hernias tend to develop in older men with weak abdominal muscles, resulting from a sedentary existence. The chronic cough precipitated the development of the hernia by increasing intra-abdominal pressure. A sliding hiatal hernia (choice C) occurs when the upper part of the stomach and the gastroesophageal junction protrude into the posterior mediastinum. An umbilical hernia (choice E) is a defect in the midline of the anterior abdominal wall; the intestines protrude through the abnormal umbilical opening.

52. **(A)** Dry social kissing is considered to be safe. Unsafe sex and IV injection with a contaminated needle are the major causes of dissemination of HIV, and affected individuals should always prevent blood and semen from entering another person's body. Therefore, choice E is incorrect. Safe sex with a condom, however, need not be avoided. Choice B is incorrect because HIV may cause an encephalopathy with prominent subcortical dementia. Choice C is incorrect because mastur-

bation does not involve body fluids entering another person. Choice D is incorrect because affected individuals should not donate blood, whether or not they are receiving treatment.

53. **(A)** Phosphofructokinase-1 (PFK-1) is the rate-limiting enzyme of glycolysis catalyzing the phosphorylation of fructose 6-phosphate yielding fructose 1,6-bisphosphate. PFK-1 is under tight allosteric control, being maximally active when energy levels are low and inhibited when energy levels are high. When the level of AMP is rising in the cell, it signals a decrease in overall energy charge. AMP is an allosteric activator of PFK-1. In contrast to AMP, ATP is a potent allosteric inhibitor of PFK-1 by binding to a site distinct from that of the ATP substrate site. As the level of ATP declines, there is less allosteric inhibition of PFK-1 and a concomitant increase in allosteric activation by AMP. This allows PFK-1 to "sense" the energy status of the cell and in turn regulate the flux through the glycolytic pathway. Rising NADH levels (choice B) signal that the energy charge of a cell is increasing and would be concomitant with rising ATP levels. PFK-1 is allosterically activated, not inhibited, by fructose 1,6-bisphosphate (choice C). Fructose-1,6-bisphosphatase, a gluconeogenic enzyme, (choice D) has no effect on the activity of PFK-1. ATP is a negative allosteric regulator of PFK-1 activity. PFK-1 does not function in the capacity of substrate level phosphorylation as is characterized by phosphoglycerate kinase and pyruvate kinase (choice E).

54. **(B)** Exercise promotes glucose utilization and increased insulin sensitivity. All the other conditions or hormones listed (choices A, C, D, and E) tend to exacerbate insulin resistance.

55. **(A)** This 30-year-old man has influenza, which is caused by the influenza viruses A, B, or C. These viruses are single-stranded RNA microbes. Their genome is segmented into eight moieties, and is surrounded by an envelope covered with distinct hemagglutinin and neuraminidase spikes. Antigenic changes in these spikes lead to worldwide epidemics. Influenza virus is a circular virus, not a bullet-shaped virus (choice B). The rabies virus is bullet shaped. Influenza virus has hemagglutinating (H) antigen, it has neuraminidase (N) antigen, and it has an envelope; thus, choices C, D, and E are incorrect.

56. **(B)** The human embryo is most susceptible to malformations caused by environmental factors during days 15 to 60 of gestation. This period is referred to as the embryonic or "organogenic period" because most of the major organ systems are organized and begin to grow. Environmental factors acting during the first 2 weeks after fertilization (choice A) usually lead to abnormalities of embryo implantation that result in complete fetal wastage rather than malformations. During the second trimester (choice D), third trimester (choice E), and at delivery (choice C) all of the major organ systems have already formed their requisite component structures and are unlikely to suffer subsequent malformation by environmental agents introduced at these times.

57. **(C)** The most obvious distinctive feature of the simple columnar epithelium that lines the oviduct is that it contains a mixture of two main cell types. The ciliated cells are recognizable by the apical cilia extending from basal bodies that appear as a row of darkly stained bars underlying the cilia. The secretory cells, which have no cilia, have a tapered shape (narrow at the base and broad at the apex), hence the name peg cell. The apical surfaces of peg cells tend to bulge out into the lumen. The epithelial lining of the small intestine (choice D) is also simple columnar, but the most abundant cell type is an absorptive cell that has a brush border composed of tightly packed microvilli. Microvilli can be distinguished from cilia because microvilli have no basal bodies, and they are much thinner and shorter than cilia. Goblet cells are mucus-secreting cells scattered among the absorptive cells of the epithelium. Like the peg cells of the oviduct, these are tapered cells, but the broad apical portion of the cell

is packed with large secretory granules that appear washed out in most histologic preparations. The trachea (choice E) is lined by respiratory epithelium, a ciliated, pseudostratified columnar epithelium. As in the oviduct, ciliated cells are the most abundant cell type, but the oviduct does not have the goblet cells and basal cells that are seen in respiratory epithelium. Like the respiratory epithelium of the trachea, the lining of the epididymal duct (choice A) is a pseudostratified columnar epithelium. However, the columnar cells do not have cilia; rather, the apical specialization is the presence of extraordinarily long microvilli called stereocilia. The oropharynx (choice B) is lined by a stratified squamous epithelium.

58. **(A)** Edrophonium is an ultrashort-acting cholinesterase inhibitor because it binds to cholinesterase via ionic interactions rather than forming a covalent complex as do the other clinically used cholinesterase inhibitors. It is used in the diagnosis of myasthenia gravis but, because it must be used parenterally and its duration of action is only 5 to 15 minutes, it is not useful for chronic treatment of the disease. Metrifonate (choice B) is a prodrug organophosphate inhibitor of cholinesterase. It is used in the treatment of schistosomiasis. Neostigmine (choice C) is a quaternary ammonium reversible anticholinesterase that is used in the treatment of myasthenia gravis. It does not show specificity for nicotinic or muscarinic synapses. Its limited lipid solubility probably contributes to lack of actions at the ganglionic level. Physostigmine (choice D) is a tertiary ammonium reversible anticholinesterase with sufficient penetration of the blood–brain barrier to allow its use in treating atropine intoxication. Pralidoxime (choice E) is an oxime-type reactivator of organophosphate-inhibited cholinesterase. It is used to treat organophosphate intoxication, but must be administered within a few hours of exposure because chemical rearrangement of the organophosphate–cholinesterase complex is rapid and leads to forms not reactivated by pralidoxime.

59. **(B)** The most common site for secondary tuberculosis is the lung apices because this area is more oxygenated and provides a better environment for this aerobic bacterium. The clinical manifestation of the disease is quite variable but typically includes chronic cough with hemoptysis, low-grade fever, night sweats, and weight loss. A single mass lesion (choice A) could indicate, given the rapid clinical progression of this case, a malignant tumor. However, this is less likely given this patient's age. Bilateral hilar lymphadenopathy (choice C) could be due to a number causes including sarcoidosis and various infections and neoplastic processes but given the details of the case, this finding is less likely. Lobar consolidation (choice D) is the classical finding of lobar pneumonia, which would follow a much more acute course than indicated. Patchy diffuse interstitial infiltrates (choice E) are associated with such agents as *Mycoplasma*, various viruses, and *Pneumocystis*. These interstitial processes are not usually productive.

60. **(B)** The diagram shows a right-sided homonymous hemianopsia, a loss of vision in the right optical field of both left and right eyes (nasal part of left eye and lateral part of right eye). The lesion must be in the left optical tract, which carries nerve fibers originating from the lateral retina of the left eye and the nasal retina of the right eye. Note that the lateral visual fields project onto the nasal retinas and the nasal visual fields project onto the lateral retinas. Complete damage to the left optical nerve (choice A) or right optical nerve (choice D) results in total blindness of the left and right eye, respectively. Damage to the optic chiasma (choice C), which is commonly caused by pituitary tumors, results in a bitemporal hemianopsia (loss of the right visual field of the right eye and loss of the left visual field of the left eye). This is because fibers from the nasal portions of the retinas cross over in the chiasm to form the optical tracts. The right optical tract (choice E) carries nerve fibers originating from the lateral retina of the right eye and the nasal retina of the left eye and when damaged would result in a left-sided homonymous hemianopsia.

61. **(C)** Under normal conditions, lactate delivered to the liver is oxidized to pyruvate with the concomitant reduction of NAD+ to NADH. The pyruvate is then transported to the mitochondria for conversion to oxaloacetate (OAA) catalyzed by pyruvate carboxylase. In the presence of mitochondrial phosphoenolpyruvate (PEP) carboxykinase the OAA is converted to PEP. In cells lacking mitochondrial PEP carboxykinase, OAA is transaminated to aspartate for transport to the cytoplasm. In the cytoplasm the aspartate is converted back to OAA. Cytoplasmic OAA is then converted to PEP by the cytoplasmic PEP carboxykinase. When alcohol is consumed, cytoplasmic alcohol dehydrogenase (ADH) catalyzes the following reaction:

$$\text{Ethanol} + \text{NAD}^+ \rightarrow \text{acetaldehyde} + \text{NADH}$$

Ethanol metabolism occurs primarily in the liver and leads to an inhibition of hepatic gluconeogenesis. The large amounts of NADH generated by ADH must be transported to the mitochondria by the malate–aspartate shuttle. The excess cytoplasmic NADH forces the lactate dehydrogenase and cytoplasmic malate dehydrogenase reactions in the direction of lactate and malate production, respectively. The direction of the lactate dehydrogenase reaction inhibits the use of lactate as a gluconeogenic substrate. The direction of the cytoplasmic malate dehydrogenase reaction rapidly converts any cytoplasmic OAA to malate, preventing its conversion to PEP by PEP carboxykinase. The net effect of the oxidation of ethanol on the direction of these two reactions is that ethanol and OAA are converted to acetaldehyde and malate, respectively. Although the increase in cytoplasmic NADH favorably drives the glyceraldehyde 3-phosphate dehydrogenase reaction in the gluconeogenic direction (choice D), the equilibrium shift in lactate dehydrogenase and malate dehydrogenase reduces the concentrations of pyruvate and OAA for use by the gluconeogenic enzyme pyruvate carboxylase and PEP carboxykinase, respectively. Ethanol metabolism does not activate glycolysis (choice A) at any step (choice B), nor

does it signal altered levels of hepatocyte ATP (choice E).

62. **(C)** Degeneration of the substantia nigra is pathognomic for Parkinson disease and results in progressive rigidity and slowness of movement (bradykinesia) and difficulty initiating movements. On examination, passive movement of the limbs is met with constant resistance. Superimposed tremors give it a "cog wheel"-like quality. Athetosis (choice A)—writhing involuntary movements of the proximal extremities—and chorea (choice B)—brief purposeless movements of the distal extremities—are examples of hyperkinesias due to dopaminergic overactivity in the basal ganglia. Hyperkinesia (choice D) is an excess of movement often due to disorders of the basal ganglia. Parkinson disease is characterized by poverty of movement and a mask-like facial expression. Intention tremor (choice E) is characteristic of cerebellar lesions.

63. **(E)** Arrow #3 indicates the trachea, which is filled with air and thus, like the lungs is not radiopaque. The superior vena cava (choice D, arrow #1) is anterior and to the right; the arch of the aorta (arrow #2) forms an elongated structure anteriorly and to the left. The esophagus (choice C) is the rounded structure immediately anterior to the vertebra and posterior to the trachea. The trachea has an elongated appearance at this level because this is the level of the carina (the division of the trachea into right and left bronchi).

64. **(A)** Colestipol and cholestyramine are bile acid–binding resins. By sequestering bile acids in the intestinal lumen, the bile acid–binding resins decrease reabsorption of steroids into the liver. The resulting lower intracellular cholesterol level causes increased expression and activity of hepatic LDL receptors that mediate endocytosis of LDL particles. Bile acid–binding resins produce less lowering of LDL cholesterol levels than the statins because HMG-CoA reductase activity is also increased with both treatments, but this activity is inhibited only by the statins. Dietary therapy (choice B) is antihyperlipidemic because it shunts more cholesterol into bile acids, leaving less cholesterol to be secreted into the blood as lipoproteins. Etretinate (choice C) is not a lipid-lowering agent, but rather is a retinoic acid analog that is used in the treatment of inflammatory psoriasis. Gemfibrozil (choice D) and the other fibric acid derivatives reduce plasma triglyceride levels by decreasing the apoprotein CIII content of VLDL particles; this apoprotein normally acts as an inhibitor of lipoprotein lipase activity. The resulting increased lipoprotein lipase activity allows more rapid catabolism of VLDL particles in skeletal muscle and adipose tissue vascular beds. Gemfibrozil also causes a beneficial increase in HDL cholesterol levels through unknown mechanisms. Niacin (choice E) functions as an antihyperlipidemic agent through inhibition of VLDL secretion by an unknown mechanism with subsequent lowering of VLDL and LDL.

65. **(E)** The biological activity of an antibody molecule centers on its ability to specifically bind antigen. The combining site is located on the amino terminal end of the antibody molecule and is composed of hypervariable segments within the variable regions of both light and heavy chains. Antibody specificity is a function of both the amino acid sequence and its three-dimensional configuration.

66. **(C)** The kidney in Figure 8–12 demonstrates severe hydronephrosis characterized by dilation of the renal pelvis at the expense of the subadjacent renal medulla and cortex. Postrenal obstruction, such as a ureteral stone, is the most likely etiology. Abuse of analgesics (choice A) may be associated with necrosis of the renal papillae. The papillae in the photo are not necrotic. Hypertension (choice B) mainly affects the blood vessels of the renal cortex, sparing the pelvic region of the kidney. Renal cell carcinoma (choice D) displays a yellowish cortical-based tumor, not hydronephrosis. An acute renal infarct (choice E) demonstrates a pale, wedge-shaped area with its base along the renal capsule. A chronic infarct shows either fibrous scarring or cyst formation. The renal pelvis is usually unaffected with renal infarcts.

67. **(C)** The Crypts of Lieberkuhn are important sites of cellular proliferation and fluid and electrolyte secretion. There are no specific sites of iron secretion (choice B). Bile secretion (choice A) occurs across the apical hepatocyte membrane and absorption from the terminal ileum by specific transporters. Dead enterocytes (choice D) slough from the villus tip, not the crypts. Membrane-bound enzymes (choice E) of the enterocytes that make up the surface of the villi are not limited to cells at the crypts.

68. **(C)** Uncal herniation syndrome includes contralateral hemiplegia and ipsilateral oculomotor nerve signs such as paralysis of the ipsilateral medial rectus muscle. Paralysis of the contralateral (not ipsilateral lower, choice B, or contralateral upper, choice A) lower portion of the facial expression muscles may also be present. Typically, ipsilateral hemiplegia (choices D and E) is not seen, although it is possible for the contralateral cerebral peduncle to be compressed against the tentorial notch and if this occurs, then paralysis might also be present in the extremities ipsilateral to the herniated uncus.

69. **(D)** Clotting factors that are unique to the intrinsic pathway include factors VIII, IX, XI, and XII. The activation of factor X (choice E) represents the point of convergence of the intrinsic and extrinsic pathways. Factors required for clotting that are activated subsequent to activation of factor X are all part of the common pathway. Activated factor X proteolytically cleaves prothrombin (choice B) to thrombin, which in turn cleaves fibrinogen (choice A) to fibrin. Factor V (choice C) stimulates the activation of factor X, and fibrin-stabilizing factor (factor XIII) stabilizes the clot by cross-linking fibrin. The defect in hemophilia A is a deficiency in factor VIII, or the antihemophilic factor. This factor acts at the last step of the intrinsic pathway. Factor VIII, which is activated by minute amounts of thrombin, acts in concert with activated factor IX, a proteolytic enzyme, to activate factor X (Figure 8–18).

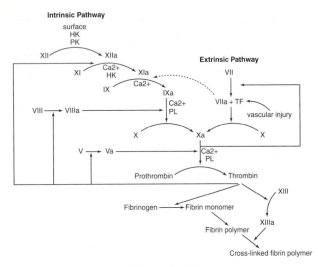

Figure 8–18

70. **(D)** Hypothyroidism is often characterized by confusion, anxiety, and depression combined with fatigue, insomnia, and weight gain (myxedema). A dexamethasone suppression test (choice A) may be positive in major depression as well as in Cushing syndrome, but is of questionable clinical value in this case. Increased serum calcium level (choice C) may be associated with depressive symptoms, but is of questionable value in this case. Psychological tests such as Rorschach and trail-making (choices B and E) are also unlikely to be of much help.

71. **(D)** Psychomotor retardation refers to decreased motoric and speech response, which often occurs in depression. Increased activity (psychomotor agitation) (choice C) may also be seen in depression. Emotional lability may be seen in hysteria and pseudobulbar palsy (choices A and B), but there is no history to support these diagnoses. Restless leg syndrome (choice E) involves motoric activity not connected with depressive syndrome with agitation.

72. **(A)** A patient who has suicidal intentions and agitated depression is a very high-risk patient, and hospitalization is indicated. Choice B would result in her having in her possession amitriptyline, 1500 mg. If she takes it as prescribed, 50 mg/d, it is probably a subtherapeutic dose. However, if all 1500

mg are taken together, the dose would be lethal. All other therapies (choices C, D, and E) may be helpful but may not prevent the patient's suicide.

73. **(E)** Past suicidal attempts increase the risk of successful suicide. Therefore, coupled with agitated depression, the patient's suicidal intent should be taken very seriously. Choices A and D are therefore incorrect. Suicide attempts are common in psychosis (choice C), but there is no evidence of it at present. Antisocial personality (choice B) is not usually associated with suicide attempt.

74. **(A)** Family history of bipolar disorder is most relevant because it may indicate that the patient may be bipolar as well, and one should carefully look for evidence for bipolarity in this patient. Mood stabilizers may be needed if there is an indication that this patient may have bipolar disorder. Family history of all other conditions (choices B, C, D, and E) is important but perhaps not as immediately useful as that of bipolar disorder.

75. **(E)** Valproic acid is a mood stabilizer often used to treat bipolar disorder. Buspirone (choice A) is an antianxiety agent for generalized anxiety disorder. Fluoxetine (choice B), nefazadone (choice C), and tranylcypromine (choice D) are antidepressants that may be useful in treating the depression in bipolar disorder, but not the mania or hypomania.

76. **(B)** Arrow #4 points to the left ventricle. In the chest, the heart points to the left side of the body. For this reason, the right side of the heart always lies anteriorly and the left side lies more posteriorly. The larger chamber on the left side of the heart is then the left ventricle and the smaller chamber, the left atrium (arrow #2, choice A). In this scan, the interventricular wall can be seen as the dark line separating the right ventricle (arrow #3, choice D) from the left ventricle (arrow #4). The right atrium is indicated by arrow #1 (choice C).

77. **(D)** The proteolytic blood enzyme thrombin has a specificity for arginine–glycine bonds in

a manner similar to trypsin. Thrombin is synthesized as prothrombin, which contains γ-carboxyglutamate residues *(gla)* deriving from vitamin K–dependent, posttranslational modification of glutamate. To be activated, prothrombin is proteolytically cleaved by factor Xa (activated factor X) after being anchored to platelet membranes in a calcium–γ-carboxyglutamate-dependent reaction. The γ-carboxyglutamate end of the prothrombin molecule is removed, leaving an active thrombin. Active thrombin then hydrolyzes fibrinogen to fibrin at four arginine–glycine bonds. The A and B fibrinopeptides that are released spontaneously associate to form a clot of insoluble fibrin fibers. Thrombin does not complex with fibrinopeptides in a clot (choice C), and is a monomeric protein (choice A). The requirement for vitamin K is as a cofactor in the γ-carboxylation of glutamates. The *gla* residues are required for proper localization of prothrombin, but are not required when prothrombin is activated by proteolytic cleavage to thrombin, a process that (as indicated) removes the *gla* residue–containing portion of the protein (choices B and E).

78. **(C)** In cardiogenic shock, an agent that increases myocardial contractility without increasing heart rate and peripheral resistance is required. In cardiogenic shock resulting from acute myocardial infarction, it is particularly important to select an agent that does not increase cardiac workload and further extend myocardial damage. Dobutamine, a selective β₁-adrenoceptor agonist, increases myocardial contractility without producing significant increases in heart rate or peripheral resistance. The β₂-selective agonist albuterol (choice A) may produce a modest increase of myocardial contractility, but is not useful in cardiogenic shock. Digoxin (choice B) produces a positive inotropic effect along with a reduction in heart rate, but its onset of action is not rapid enough to treat this medical emergency. Furthermore, it sometimes increases peripheral resistance. Although epinephrine (choice D) can increase myocardial contractility, it also increases heart rate and,

at doses that produce increased contractility, increases peripheral resistance. The result is an increase in the cardiac workload, an undesirable effect in cardiogenic shock. Phenylephrine (choice E) is a nonselective α-agonist that increases peripheral resistance, a very undesirable effect in cardiogenic shock.

79. **(B)** The blood gas data from this patient illustrate chronic respiratory alkalosis with renal compensation. A lowlander at high altitude for 2 weeks is expected to have low P_{O_2} plus low P_{CO_2} because of hypoxia-induced hyperventilation. Renal compensation in the form of bicarbonate excretion reduces plasma bicarbonate and returns pH to a nearly normal value. Either severe chronic lung disease (choice A) or an overdose of heroin (choice E) would have caused respiratory acidosis due to abnormally high arterial P_{CO_2} (not the low P_{CO_2} this subject has). Breathing a low-oxygen gas mixture (choice C) is similar to being at high altitude, but if this is only for a few minutes, there is no time for renal compensation. Acute aspirin overdose (choice D) in adults usually presents first with a respiratory alkalosis, which includes a low P_{CO_2}, but not a low P_{O_2}.

80. **(C)** The subdiaphragmatic parietal peritoneum is innervated by the phrenic nerve (C3, 4, and 5). Irritation of the parietal peritoneum gives rise to referred pain over the shoulder because the supraclavicular nerves (C3 and 4) innervate the skin of this region. None of the other choices innervate the subdiaphragmatic parietal peritoneum. The least splanchnic nerve (choice A) carries preganglionic sympathetic and visceral afferent fibers. The iliohypogastric nerve (choice B) innervates muscles of the anterior abdominal wall and the skin over the lateral gluteal and suprapubic areas. The subcostal nerve (choice D) innervates subcostal and abdominal muscles, and anterior gluteal skin. The vagus nerve (choice E) carries preganglionic parasympathetic and visceral afferent fibers.

81. **(E)** *Helicobacter pylori* is a small, spiral microbe that produces large amounts of urease.

Thus, tests for urease activity have been employed as rapid and useful diagnostic assays. Patients with gastritis caused by *H. pylori* do not show elevation in their IgE levels. *Helicobacter pylori* does not have any unusual carbohydrate utilization patterns that can be used for the diagnosis of gastritis (choice A). Culture of gastric contents on blood agar containing metronidazole and bismuth salts (choice B) results in the inhibition of growth of *H. pylori*, which is susceptible to metronidazole and bismuth salts. Patients with parasitic infections have high IgE levels in their serum (choice C). Gram stains do not provide any reliable information for the diagnosis of gastritis caused by *H. pylori*, because there are many microbes that resemble *H. pylori* (choice D).

82. **(D)** A stenotic mitral valve produces a diastolic murmur with a loud S_1 as the valve closes, followed by a normal S_2 as the aortic valve closes, and then a click or snap as the abnormal valve opens. None of the other choices match these findings. With aortic regurgitation (choice A), there is an early diastolic murmur, the aortic valve closure sound may be diminished or absent, and quite commonly there is a third heart sound. Aortic stenosis (choice B) produces a midsystolic murmur and because systemic pressure is decreased, there is a soft closure of the aortic valve (i.e., a soft S_2). Mitral regurgitation (choice C) produces a pansystolic murmur due to regurgitation of blood from the left ventricle to the left atrium during systole. During diastole, the blood flows back over the valve producing a third heart sound and a diastolic flow murmur. Pulmonic regurgitation (choice E), pulmonic stenosis (choice F), tricuspid regurgitation (choice G), and tricuspid stenosis (choice H) are much less common and do not match the findings described.

83. **(A)** Seemingly normal full-term infants suffering from urea cycle defects usually become lethargic and need stimulation to feed within 24 to 72 h after birth. When presented in the Emergency Department, many are comatose.

One obvious outward clinical sign is a bulging fontanel due to ammonia-induced encephalopathy. If a correct diagnosis of hyperammonemia is not made in a timely manner, these infants die. Elevated levels of various urea cycle intermediates are indicative of a particular defect in the pathway so that high argininosuccinate (choice B) is indicative of argininosuccinase deficiency, high citrulline (choice C) is indicative of argininosuccinate synthetase deficiency, and high orotic acid levels (choice D) are indicative of ornithine transcarbamoylase deficiency. When excess fatty acids are oxidized the acetyl-CoA that cannot be utilized, the TCA cycle is diverted into the production of the ketone bodies, acetoacetate, and β-hydroxybutyrate. If the concentration of ketone bodies is high, such that they are not utilized by nonhepatic tissues, much of the acetoacetate spontaneously decarboxylates to acetone. Much of the acetone is then volatilized in the lungs. The odor of acetone on the breath (choice E) indicates severe ketoacidosis, which occurs in individuals with type I (insulin-dependent) diabetes.

84. **(A)** Filtration pressure (P_{uf}) is calculated from the Starling equation involving four forces:

$$P_{uf} = (P_{GC} - P_{BS}) - (\Pi_{GC} - \Pi_{BS})$$

Normally, the filtrate in Bowman space has such negligible amounts of protein that Π_{BS} is considered to be 0 and is often left out of the Starling equation for glomerular filtration. Choices B, C, and D all give $P_{uf} = 0$ (i.e., glomerular filtration equilibrium). Choice E gives a negative filtration pressure of –5 mm Hg, which favors absorption instead of filtration.

85. **(B)** Koplik spots on the buccal mucosa are characteristic of infection with the measles virus. Microscopic examination of these lesions reveals giant cells containing viral nucleocapsids. Macroscopically, these lesions appear as small, erythematous macules with white centers. Rubella (German measles,

choice C) is an acute febrile disease characterized by fever, maculopapular rash, and respiratory symptoms. It does not produce Koplik spots. Rubella infections during the first trimester of pregnancy lead to congenital malformations. Herpangina (choice A) is caused by coxsackie group A viruses, which are not known to induce Koplik spot formation. Scarlet fever (choice D) is cutaneous rash produced by *S. pyogenes.* This infection does not include Koplik spot formation. Thrush (choice E) is production of white spots due to overgrowth of *Candida albicans* in the oral cavity.

86. **(C)** All of the nondepolarizing neuromuscular blockers (except succinylcholine) can be reversed with acetylcholinesterase inhibitors. Pancuronium is a relatively long-acting nondepolarizing blocker and neostigmine is often used to reverse its action. Atracurium (choice A) breaks down spontaneously as its major mode of elimination. An important breakdown product of atracurium, laudanosine, is a convulsant at high concentrations. It is metabolized rapidly in the plasma by plasma cholinesterase. Mivacurium (choice B) is one of the shortest-acting nondepolarizing blockers. Succinylcholine (choice D) is the shortest-acting neuromuscular blocker. Tubocurarine can cause histaminic reactions (choice E) because it releases histamine from mast cells in some individuals. It has no antihistaminic properties.

87. **(E)** Interactions among antigen-presenting cells, T lymphocytes, and B lymphocytes are necessary for immune responses, and these cellular associations are promoted by the organization of lymph nodes. The deep cortical (paracortical) zone of a lymph node is the T-lymphocyte domain, and it does not develop if the thymus fails in its function of T-lymphocyte production. The presence of germinal centers in the outer cortex indicates that B-lymphocyte responses are under way, precluding a condition of agammaglobulinemia (choice A) or combined immunodeficiency (choice C). An acute bacterial infection (choice B) can lead to enlargement of all zones in lymph nodes. Thrombocytopenia (choice D), a deficiency in platelet numbers, does not change lymph node organization.

88. **(A)** Figure 8–15 depicts a fibroadenoma, a common benign tumor of the female breast. The microscopic features of this tumor include compressed benign ducts, which are surrounded by nonatypical and normally cellular connective tissue. Intraductal carcinoma (choice B) displays a proliferation of atypical epithelial cells within the ducts. Medullary carcinoma (choice C) displays syncytial groups of anaplastic epithelial cells with a peripheral lymphoplasmocytic inflammatory reaction. Paget disease (choice D) is an intraepidermal adenocarcinoma that presents clinically as an ulcerated or scaly lesion of the nipple. In most instances, a palpable mass is not present. Scirrhous carcinoma (choice E) is a common form of breast malignancy characterized by anaplastic epithelial cells in a fibrous reactive stroma.

89. **(C)** Pulmonary arterioles are unique for their ability to constrict under conditions of hypoxia. This results in a local adjustment of perfusion to ventilation. For example, if a bronchiole is obstructed, the lack of O_2 causes contraction of the pulmonary vascular smooth muscle in the corresponding area, shunting blood away from the hypoxic region to better-ventilated regions. Similarly, systemic hypoxia causes an increase in pulmonary artery resistance and increased workload for the right ventricle. Coronary (choice A), GI (choice B), renal (choice D), and skeletal muscle (choice E) arteries all dilate under hypoxic conditions, resulting in enhanced blood flow to their respective organs.

90. **(A)** Aminotransferases are the class of enzymes involved in the interconversion of one amino acid and one α-keto acid into their respective counterparts. Aminotransferases exist for all amino acids except threonine and lysine. The most common compounds involved as a donor/acceptor pair in transamination reactions are glutamate and α-keto-

glutarate (α-KG), which participate in reactions with many different aminotransferases. Serum aminotransferases such as serum glutamate-oxaloacetate-aminotransferase (SGOT; also called aspartate aminotransferase [AST]) and serum glutamate-pyruvate aminotransferase (SGPT; also called alanine transaminase [ALT]) have been used as clinical markers of tissue damage, with increasing serum levels indicating an increased extent of damage. Alanine transaminase has an important function in the delivery of skeletal muscle carbon and nitrogen (in the form of alanine) to the liver. In skeletal muscle, pyruvate is transaminated to alanine, thus affording an additional route of nitrogen transport from muscle to liver. In the liver, alanine transaminase transfers the ammonia to α-KG and regenerates pyruvate. The pyruvate can then be diverted into gluconeogenesis. Dehydrogenases (choice B) are the class of enzymes involved in oxidation-reduction reactions such as the reaction of glycolysis catalyzed by glyceraldehye-3-phosphate dehydrogenase. Hydrolases (choice C) are the class of enzymes that utilize water in the process of hydrolyzing bonds. Nitrogenases (choice D) are bacterial enzymes involved in the fixation of atmospheric nitrogen.

91. **(C)** With the patient seated and the head tilted anteriorly (chin on chest), irrigation of the right ear with warm water produces increased output from the right vestibular sensory apparatus, and this leads to activation of the left lateral rectus and right medial rectus muscles. These two muscles then produce slow (not fast, choices A and B) conjugate horizontal movement of the eyes to the left (not right, choices D and E), followed immediately by rapid conjugate movement to the right.

92. **(D)** Because of changes in sexual behaviors (practice of safe sex), the percentage of gay and bisexual men with HIV has gradually declined in the United States. Choice A is incorrect because more women are now being infected through heterosexual intercourse than IV substance abuse. Choice B is incor-

rect because the number of infected women is growing four times faster than the number of infected men. As for choice C, because there is a decrease in the percentage of infected gay and bisexual men, there is an increase in infected heterosexual men. Choice E is incorrect because the ratio of men to women who are infected with HIV is estimated at 6:1.

93. **(D)** Cirrhosis is often associated with diminished albumen synthesis by the liver; loss of protein oncotic pressure in the plasma results in transudation of fluid into the extravascular space. The loss of circulating blood volume results in marked compensatory secretion of aldosterone. Increased aldosterone results in retention of salt and water by the kidney and massive fluid accumulation may result. The most direct physiologic therapy is to administer an aldosterone antagonist, spironolactone. Spironolactone is a pharmacologic antagonist at the aldosterone receptor. The resulting diuresis is often greater than that achieved with a loop diuretic. Captopril (choice A) is an indirect aldosterone antagonist; it reduces the production of angiotensin II. It is not as effective as spironolactone. Digoxin (choice B) is a useful therapy for some patients with congestive heart failure, but rarely benefits a patient with edema due to cirrhosis. Hydrochlorothiazide (choice C) is a moderately efficacious diuretic that acts in the distal convoluted tubule. It is more efficacious than spironolactone in patients with low aldosterone levels, but considerably less efficacious in patients with cirrhotic edema. Triamterene (choice E) is a potassium-sparing diuretic like spironolactone; unlike spironolactone, it physiologically inhibits aldosterone's effects by blocking sodium channels in the collecting tubules. It is not nearly as effective as spironolactone.

94. **(E)** DiGeorge syndrome is a form of glandular aplasia due to defective embryonic development of the third and fourth pharyngeal pouches, which give rise to the thymus, parathyroid, and thyroid glands. This anomaly results in a depletion of thymic-dependent

areas in lymphoid tissues. A defect in the killing of intracellular bacteria by neutrophils (choice A) occurs in chronic granulomatous disease, but not in DiGeorge syndrome. A depletion of B-dependent areas (choice B) in lymph nodes occurs in Bruton X-linked agammaglobulinemia, not in DiGeorge syndrome. A depletion of lymph node lymphocytes (choice C) in both T- and B-dependent areas occurs in combined immune deficiency disease (SCID), not in DiGeorge syndrome. In DiGeorge syndrome, T-cell production is affected. The number of B-cells that are involved in the production of antibodies, including isohemagglutinins (choice D), is not affected.

95. **(B)** The fine-needle biopsy demonstrates a fairly monomorphic population of small, mitotically active neoplastic lymphocytes with associated starry sky histiocytes. The morphology of the tumor and the clinical history are typical for endemic Burkitt lymphoma. The diagnosis of adenocarcinoma (choice A) is incompatible with the photograph because malignant epithelial elements are not seen. Chronic lymphocytic leukemia-lymphoma (choice C) is distinctly uncommon in children and features mature lymphocytes without a starry sky background. There are no parasitic elements (choice D) evident in the photograph. Salivary gland lymphoepithelioma (choice E) is usually seen in an older age group, contains some remaining epithelial elements, and has larger immunoblastic-type lymphocytes.

96. **(C)** The development of endemic Burkitt lymphoma is strongly linked to prior infection by the Epstein–Barr virus. Aflatoxin (choice A) ingestion increases the risk of hepatocellular carcinoma, not lymphoma. The occurrence of endemic Burkitt lymphoma is not due to a lack of an essential dietary nutrient (choice B). Infections with *W. bancrofti* (choice D) produce an obstructive lymphadenitis called filariasis. This parasitic infection is not related to the development of Burkitt lymphoma. Sjögren syndrome (choice E) is associated with a higher risk of subsequently developing lymphoma,

most often occurring in middle-aged or elderly females. The lymphomas are not of the Burkitt cell type.

97. **(C)** When lactate enters hepatocytes for conversion to glucose, it is oxidized to pyruvate by lactate dehydrogenase. In this direction lactate dehydrogenase reduces NAD^+ to NADH. The NADH thus generated can be used by glyceraldehyde-3-phosphate dehydrogenase in the gluconeogenic direction converting 1,3-bisphosphoglycerate to glyceraldehyde 3-phosphate. During this reduction reaction NADH is oxidized to NAD^+, completing the cycle between the two enzymes of the gluconeogenesis pathway that require nicotinamide nucleotide as a cofactor/substrate. Glucose-6-phosphate dehydrogenase requires $NADP^+$ as a cofactor and does not function in the gluconeogenesis pathway (choice A). The primary direction of the glycerol-3-phosphate dehydrogenase-catalyzed reaction (choice B) is in the transfer of electrons from cytoplasmic NADH to mitochondrial $FADH_2$. The direction of this reaction generates cytoplasmic NAD^+, not NADH. The cytoplasmic malate dehydrogenase reaction (choice D) does function in gluconeogenesis and yields cytoplasmic NADH, but is involved in the process when pyruvate is the direct source of carbon (e.g., from amino acids), not lactate. The phosphoenol pyruvate carboxykinase reaction (choice E) does not yield any reduced electron carriers.

98. **(B)** Peptic ulcerations seen in Zollinger–Ellison syndrome are due to ectopic hypersecretion of gastrin. An islet cell tumor of the pancreas is the most frequent ectopic site. Antibodies to intrinsic factor (choice A) are seen with pernicious anemia and usually cause gastric mucosal atrophy and metaplasia. Gastric mucosal hypertrophy, not atrophy (choice C), is the expected result with an increased secretion of gastrin as is seen with Zollinger–Ellison syndrome. Pressure ulceration from bezoars (choice D) and vascular abnormalities (choice E) are not the etiology of the peptic ulcerations seen with Zollinger–Ellison syndrome.

99. **(A)** The facial veins communicate with the cavernous sinus by way of the inferior ophthalmic veins. The cavernous sinus is located on either side of the sella turcica in the middle cranial fossa. All the other bony sinuses (choices B, C, D, and E) do not have communication with the facial vein.

100. **(A)** In contrast to the other agents listed, acetaminophen, while expressing analgesic and antipyretic activity, is a poor inhibitor of cyclooxygenase and possesses little anti-inflammatory activity. The reasons for this difference are not clear. All of the other agents listed are NSAIDs, effective inhibitors of cyclooxygenase, the enzyme responsible for the initial step in the conversion of arachidonic acid to the prostaglandin mediators of inflammation, fever, and pain perception. Anti-inflammatory activity correlates with the ability to inhibit cyclooxygenase. Aspirin (choice B) is both the prototype and exception to the NSAIDs. It is the exception in that it causes acetylation of cyclooxygenase to produce an irreversible inhibition, whereas the other NSAIDs cause a reversible inhibition. The irreversible inhibition is particularly important for platelet function because platelets, unlike most other cells, are not capable of synthesizing new cyclooxygenase molecules. The result is a loss of ability of the affected platelets to produce thromboxane A_2, a platelet-aggregating agent. This is the basis for the use of low-dose aspirin in prevention of thrombosis and resulting myocardial infarction and occlusive stroke. Indomethacin (choice C) is a potent cyclooxygenase inhibitor, but its use in chronic situations is limited because of the high rate (35% to 50%) of patients experiencing adverse reactions. These include GI pains, ulceration, and severe headache. It is used in the treatment of gout and to produce closure of patent ductus arteriosus. Nabumetone (choice D) is an amine form of NSAID given as a prodrug that is converted to the active acid form in the body. Tolmetin (choice E) is an NSAID in the heteroaryl acetic acid class, used in the treatment of osteoarthritis and rheumatoid arthritis.

REFERENCES

Aidley DJ. *The Physiology of Excitable Cells,* 4th ed. Cambridge, England: Cambridge University Press; 1998.

Berne RM, Levy MN. *Physiology,* 4th ed. St. Louis: Mosby-Year Book; 1998.

Braunwald E, Fauci AS, Kasper DL, et al. *Harrison's Principles of Internal Medicine,* 15th ed. New York: McGraw-Hill; 2001.

Brooks GF, Butel JS, Morse SA. *Jawetz, Melnick, and Adelberg's Medical Microbiology,* 22nd ed. Stamford, CT: Appleton & Lange; 2001.

Chandrasoma P, Taylor CR. *Concise Pathology,* 3rd ed. Stamford, CT: Appleton & Lange; 1998.

Devlin TM. *Textbook of Biochemistry: With Clinical Correlations,* 4th ed. New York: John Wiley & Sons; 1997.

Elkin GD. *Introduction to Clinical Psychiatry.* Stamford, CT: Appleton & Lange; 1998.

Ganong WF. *Review of Medical Physiology,* 20th ed. Stamford, CT: Appleton & Lange; 2001.

Guyton AC, Hall JE. *Textbook of Medical Physiology,* 10th ed. Philadelphia: WB Saunders; 2000.

Hall-Craggs ECB. *Anatomy as a Basis for Clinical Medicine,* 3rd ed. Baltimore: Williams & Wilkins; 1995.

Hardman JG, Limbird LE, Molinoff PB, et al. *Goodman & Gilman's The Pharmacological Basis of Therapeutics,* 9th ed. New York: McGraw-Hill; 1996.

Johnson LR. *Gastrointestinal Physiology,* 5th ed. St. Louis: Mosby-Year Book; 1997.

Kandel ER, Schwartz JH, Jessel TM. *Principles of Neural Science,* 5th ed. Stamford, CT: Appleton & Lange; 2000.

Kaplan HI, Sadock BJ. *Comprehensive Textbook of Psychiatry/VI CD-ROM.* Teton Data Systems, Jackson, Wyoming, Baltimore: Williams & Wilkins; 1998.

Kaplan HI, Sadock BJ. *Kaplan and Sadock's Synopsis of Psychiatry,* 8th ed. Baltimore: Williams & Wilkins; 1998.

Katzung BG. *Basic & Clinical Pharmacology,* 8th ed. Stamford, CT: Appleton & Lange; 2001.

Leigh H, Reiser MF. *The Patient: Biological, Psychological, and Social Dimensions of Medical Practice,* 3rd ed. New York: Plenum Press; 1992.

Levinson WE, Jawetz E. *Medical Microbiology & Immunology: Examination and Board Review,* 6th ed. Stamford, CT: Appleton & Lange; 2000.

Lewis WH, Elvin-Lewis MPF. *Medical Botany.* New York: John Wiley & Sons; 1977.

McArdle WD, Katch FI, Katch VL. *Exercise Physiology: Energy, Nutrition, and Human Performance,* 4th ed. Philadelphia: Lea & Febiger; 1996.

Moore KL. *Clinically Oriented Anatomy,* 3rd ed. Baltimore: Williams & Wilkins; 1992.

Mountcastle VB. *Medical Physiology,* 14th ed. St. Louis: Mosby-Year Book; 1980.

Murray PR, Rosenthal KS, Kobayashi GS, Pfaller MA. *Medical Microbiology,* 3rd ed. St. Louis: Mosby-Year Book; 1998.

Murray RK, Granner DK, Mayes PA, Rodwell VW. *Harper's Biochemistry,* 25th ed. Stamford, CT: Appleton & Lange; 2000.

Roitt I, Brostoff J, Male D. *Immunology,* 5th ed. London, UK: Mosby-Year Book; 1998.

Rose DB, Post T. *Clinical Physiology of Acid-base and Electrolyte Disorders,* 6th ed. New York: McGraw-Hill; 2001.

Rosse C, Gaddum-Rosse P. *Hollinshead's Textbook of Anatomy,* 5th ed. Philadelphia: Lippincott Raven Publishers; 1997.

Rubin F, Farber JL. *Pathology,* 3rd ed. Philadelphia: JB Lippincott; 1999.

Vander AJ. *Renal Physiology,* 5th ed. New York: McGraw-Hill; 1995.

West JB. *Pulmonary Pathophysiology—The Essentials,* 5th ed. Baltimore: Williams & Wilkins; 1998.

Woodburne RT, Burckel WE. *Essentials of Human Anatomy,* 9th ed. New York: Oxford University Press; 1994.

Subspecialty List: Practice Test I

Question Number and Subspecialty

1. Biochemistry
2. Anatomy
3. Pharmacology
4. Pharmacology
5. Behavioral sciences
6. Pathology
7. Biochemistry
8. Microbiology
9. Microbiology
10. Microbiology
11. Physiology
12. Anatomy
13. Behavioral sciences
14. Biochemistry
15. Pharmacology
16. Pathology
17. Physiology
18. Biochemistry
19. Anatomy
20. Physiology
21. Pathology
22. Pharmacology
23. Behavioral sciences
24. Biochemistry
25. Anatomy
26. Pathology
27. Pathology
28. Pathology
29. Pharmacology
30. Biochemistry
31. Anatomy
32. Behavioral sciences
33. Physiology
34. Microbiology
35. Biochemistry
36. Physiology
37. Pathology
38. Pathology
39. Microbiology
40. Pharmacology
41. Biochemistry
42. Anatomy
43. Behavioral sciences
44. Pathology
45. Physiology
46. Pathology
47. Biochemistry
48. Microbiology
49. Pathology
50. Pharmacology
51. Anatomy
52. Behavioral sciences
53. Biochemistry
54. Physiology
55. Microbiology
56. Pathology
57. Anatomy
58. Pharmacology
59. Pathology
60. Anatomy
61. Biochemistry
62. Physiology
63. Anatomy
64. Pharmacology
65. Microbiology
66. Pathology
67. Physiology
68. Anatomy
69. Biochemistry
70. Behavioral sciences
71. Behavioral sciences
72. Behavioral sciences
73. Behavioral sciences
74. Behavioral sciences

75. Behavioral sciences
76. Anatomy
77. Biochemistry
78. Pharmacology
79. Physiology
80. Anatomy
81. Microbiology
82. Pathology
83. Biochemistry
84. Physiology
85. Microbiology
86. Pharmacology
87. Anatomy

88. Pathology
89. Physiology
90. Biochemistry
91. Anatomy
92. Behavioral sciences
93. Pharmacology
94. Microbiology
95. Pathology
96. Pathology
97. Biochemistry
98. Pathology
99. Anatomy
100. Pharmacology

CHAPTER 9

Practice Test II
Questions

DIRECTIONS: (Questions 1 through 100): Each of the numbered items or incomplete statements in this section is followed by answers or by completions of the statement. Select the ONE lettered answer or completion that is BEST in each case.

1. A research assistant is involved in the production of anthrax vaccine. He must destroy all vegetative cells and spores of *Bacillus anthracis* that have contaminated the glassware he used. This can best be accomplished by

    (A) autoclaving
    (B) boiling
    (C) use of anionic detergents
    (D) use of ethyl alcohol
    (E) use of oxidizing agents

2. Benign prostatic hypertrophy can be treated in several ways, including

    (A) α_1-adrenergic receptor agonist
    (B) androgens
    (C) estrogens
    (D) 5-α-reductase inhibitors
    (E) surgical section of the detrusor muscle

3. On physical examination a 17-year-old man is noted to have only minimal secondary sexual development, gynecomastia, and an eunuchoid tall habitus. Of the following, the syndrome that best describes these findings is

    (A) Down
    (B) Edwards
    (C) Klinefelter
    (D) multi-X
    (E) Turner

4. Symptoms of von Gierke disease include massive enlargement of the liver, severe hypoglycemia, ketosis, hyperlipemia, and hyperuricemia. Biopsy of the tissues of an affected person shows that the liver has a specific deficiency of the enzyme

    (A) glucokinase
    (B) glucose-6-phosphatase
    (C) α-1,4-glucosidase
    (D) hexokinase
    (E) phosphofructokinase-1

5. Figure 9–1 shows a cardiac pacemaker potential (bold line = normal). Which of the curves best represents the effect of sympathetic stimulation on the pacemaker potential?

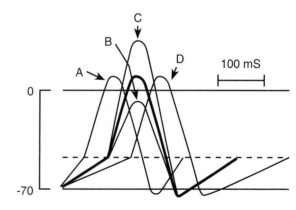

Figure 9–1

    (A) Curve A
    (B) Curve B
    (C) Curve C
    (D) Curve D
    (E) Sympathetic stimulation does not alter the pacemaker potential

6. An indication for HIV testing is

   (A) homosexuality
   (B) induction into the military
   (C) medical students
   (D) patients who request testing
   (E) psychiatric hospitalization

7. Neuronal cell bodies innervating the intrinsic muscles of the larynx may be found in the

   (A) dorsal motor nucleus of the vagus
   (B) hypoglossal nucleus
   (C) inferior (nodose) ganglion of the vagus nerve
   (D) nucleus ambiguous
   (E) superior (jugular) ganglion of the vagus nerve

8. Methimazole is useful in the treatment of

   (A) diabetes
   (B) hyperthyroidism
   (C) hypoparathyroidism
   (D) infertility due to anovulatory cycles
   (E) osteoporosis

9. In a positive viral hemagglutination inhibition test, hemagglutination is inhibited by which of the following substances in the serum?

   (A) Antiviral antibody
   (B) Hemolysin
   (C) Latex agglutinins
   (D) Rh antibody
   (E) Virus

10. An important dimension of the liver's impact on physiology and disease is due to its protein synthetic capacity. Blood-borne proteins synthesized in the liver include

    (A) fibrinogen
    (B) growth hormone (GH)
    (C) insulin
    (D) renin
    (E) von Willibrand factor

11. Figure 9–2 demonstrates Michaelis–Menton kinetics of

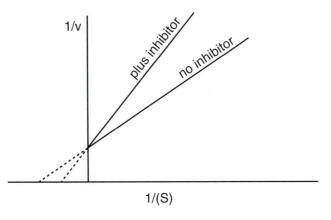

Figure 9–2

   (A) a competitively inhibited enzyme
   (B) a noncompetitively inhibited enzyme
   (C) an allosteric enzyme with and without effector
   (D) an irreversibly inhibited enzyme
   (E) an uncompetetively inhibited enzyme

12. Effects of glucocorticoids on intermediary metabolism include

    (A) decreased glucose production by the liver
    (B) decreased protein breakdown
    (C) diminished serum free fatty acid levels
    (D) increased lipolysis in the periphery with redistribution of fat stores
    (E) increased peripheral protein synthesis

13. A serious adverse effect that may occur with a single dose of one aspirin tablet is

    (A) bronchoconstriction
    (B) cardiac arrhythmia
    (C) hemolytic anemia
    (D) hepatotoxicity
    (E) nephrotoxicity

14. In an influenza virus complement-fixation procedure, the indicator system consists of complement, sheep RBCs, plus

(A) antibody to influenza virus

(B) antibody to sheep RBCs

(C) ^{51}Cr-labeled sheep RBCs

(D) fluorescent-tagged virus

(E) neuraminidase

15. A 67-year-old man has a primary, well-differentiated adenocarcinoma of the sigmoid colon that invades into, but not through, the muscularis propria. Eleven lymph nodes in the sigmoid resection specimen are examined pathologically and two are found to contain metastatic carcinoma. During surgery there is no evidence of distant metastases to the liver. How would you stage this cancer?

(A) T1 N0 M0

(B) T2 N0 M1

(C) T2 N1 M0

(D) T3 N0 M1

(E) T4 N0 M1

16. A 40-year-old man with brittle diabetes mellitus notes high fasting blood glucose in the morning. When he increases his bed time insulin dose, his morning blood glucose is even higher. He also reported nightmares and vivid dreams. You recommend that he

(A) cut his bed time insulin dose

(B) decrease in his food intake, especially at night

(C) further increase in his bed time insulin dose

(D) modify his life style to eliminate sources of stress

(E) switch from insulin to oral hypoglycemic agents

17. A 36-year-old avid hiker has a 4-week history of migratory arthritis and malaise. Her serum contains IgM and IgG antibodies against *Borrelia burgdorferi*. The likely diagnosis is

(A) achondroplasia

(B) Lyme disease

(C) ochronosis

(D) osteoarthritis

(E) rheumatoid arthritis

18. The appearance of high levels of phenylpyruvate and phenyllactate in the urine is indicative of which disorder?

(A) Alcaptonuria

(B) Hartnup disease

(C) Hepatorenal tyrosinemia

(D) Maple syrup urine disease

(E) Phenylketonuria

19. The microscopic manifestation of highly condensed, transcriptionally inactive DNA is

(A) euchromatin

(B) heterochromatin

(C) nuclear pore

(D) nucleolus

(E) rough endoplasmic reticulum (rER)

20. Which of the following drugs has been shown effective in both epilepsy and bipolar disorder?

(A) Amitriptylline

(B) Clonazepam

(C) Haloperidol

(D) Lithium

(E) Valproic acid

21. A graft-versus-host reaction may occur

(A) because the graft has histocompatibility antigens not found in the recipient

(B) because the graft is contaminated with gram-negative microorganisms

(C) only when tumor tissues are grafted

(D) when a histocompatible graft is irradiated before engraftment

(E) when immunocompetent lymphoid cells are present in the graft and the recipient is immunosuppressed

Questions 22 and 23

A 28-year-old man has a long history of intermittent bloody diarrhea.

22. The colon is surgically removed and displayed in Figure 9–3. The most likely diagnosis is

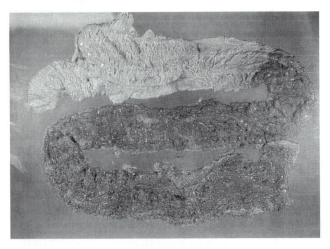

Figure 9–3

(A) amebic colitis
(B) collagenous colitis
(C) gangrenous colitis
(D) pseudomembranous colitis
(E) ulcerative colitis

23. The rationale for a colonic surgical resection relates to an increased risk of developing

(A) amyloidosis
(B) carcinoma
(C) liver abscess
(D) melanoma
(E) stricture

24. Endocrine–metabolic changes characteristic of renal failure include

(A) diminished progression of atherosclerosis
(B) hypotension
(C) increased insulin requirements in patients with diabetes mellitus
(D) polycythemia
(E) secondary hyperparathyroidism

25. The Philadelphia chromosome is the result of a translocation between chromosomes 9 and 22 leading to the generation of a chimeric tyrosine kinase gene, BCR-ABL. This chromosomal abnormality is associated with

(A) Burkitt lymphoma
(B) Chronic myeloid leukemia
(C) Fanconi anemia
(D) Li–Fraumeni syndrome
(E) von Hippel–Lindau syndrome

26. A resident is about to perform a needle biopsy of the liver. She has marked the location for entry of the needle at the midaxillary line. To not penetrate the costodiaphragmatic recess, she asks the patient to breathe out forcefully and then to hold her breath before insertion of the needle. The resident remembered that, in the midaxillary line, the lower border of the pleura crosses the

(A) fourth rib
(B) sixth rib
(C) eighth rib
(D) tenth rib
(E) twelfth rib

27. Propranolol is beneficial in the treatment of angina because it

(A) dilates capacitance vessels
(B) increases coronary blood flow
(C) increases oxygen delivery
(D) inhibits renin release
(E) reduces oxygen demand

28. A 30-year-old patient with cystic fibrosis has fever and is coughing sputum, which when grown on nutrient agar produces gram-negative, motile rods that elaborate a blue-green color. This microorganism most likely is

(A) *Legionella pneumophila*
(B) *Mycoplasma pneumoniae*
(C) *Pseudomonas aeruginosa*
(D) *Staphylococcus aureus*
(E) *Staphylococcus epidemidis*

29. The term "personality" may best be defined as a person's

    (A) characteristic means of relating with reality
    (B) characteristic patterns of thought, behavior, and feelings
    (C) defensive armamentarium
    (D) ego
    (E) ego and superego combined

30. A 17-year-old man is admitted with a gunshot wound to his left temporal cortex. Damage to Wernicke area of the cerebral cortex is associated with

    (A) dyslexia
    (B) impaired comprehension of speech
    (C) impaired recognition of visual forms
    (D) impaired vocalization
    (E) loss of short-term memory

31. Rh$_o$-specific immune globulin (RhoGAM) therapeutic preparations are correctly described as composed of

    (A) anti-allergen antibodies
    (B) anti-inflammatory agents
    (C) antilymphocyte antibodies
    (D) blocking antibodies
    (E) enhancing antibodies

32. Which glycosaminoglycan is a major component of mast cells lining the blood vessels?

    (A) Chondroitin sulfate
    (B) Dermatan sulfate
    (C) Heparin
    (D) Hyaluronate
    (E) Keratan sulfate

33. A 56-year-old man suffers from prostatic cancer. Treatment requires surgical removal of the prostate along with the seminal vesicles, ejaculatory ducts, and terminal portions of the vas deferens. However, the surgeon attempts to preserve the nerves and blood vessels to the penis to increase the patient's chance for retention of sexual function. The nerves fibers to the prostate in this region derive directly from the

    (A) celiac plexus
    (B) inferior hypogastric plexus
    (C) inferior mesenteric plexus
    (D) superior hypogastric plexus
    (E) superior mesenteric plexus

34. In a patient suffering from severe anaphylactic shock, the drug of choice for restoring circulation and relieving angioedema is

    (A) dopamine
    (B) epinephrine
    (C) isoproterenol
    (D) norepinephrine
    (E) phenylephrine

35. A 66-year-old woman initially develops some subtle changes in memory, judgment, and behavior. However, this is followed by a very severe and rapidly progressive dementia that is accompanied by startle myoclonus. She dies 8 months after the first onset of her symptoms. Her disease is most likely the result of a (an)

    (A) acquired or inherited prion
    (B) hereditary lysosomal storage disease
    (C) increased neurofibrillary tangles
    (D) protozoan infection
    (E) repeated exposure to a chemical toxin

36. A medical student has been immunized with hepatitis B virus (HBV) recombinant vaccine. The curve in Figure 9–4 represents the production of protective antibodies to the viral component present in the recombinant vaccine. This viral component most likely is

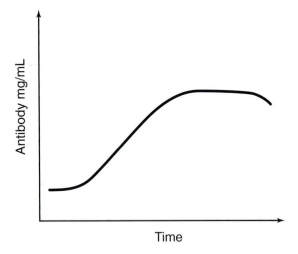

Figure 9–4

(A) nucleocapsid proteins of HBV
(B) RNA genome of HBV
(C) viral core antigen (HBcAg)
(D) viral e antigen (HBeAg)
(E) viral surface antigen (HBsAg)

37. The central processes of muscle (spindle) afferents from the upper extremity terminate within the

(A) contralateral cuneate nucleus
(B) dorsal horn from C3 to C5
(C) ipsilateral lateral (accessory) cuneate nucleus
(D) ipsilateral nucleus gracilis
(E) nucleus dorsalis from C5 to T1

38. E.W. is a 67-year-old woman who follows a vegetarian diet. She complains of weakness and a "pins and needles" sensations throughout her body. The woman's daughter confides that her mother has undergone a personality change with periods of irritability and confusion. Examination of a blood sample shows the presence of macrocytic anemia.

This patient will probably require administration of

(A) ferrous sulfate
(B) folic acid
(C) intrinsic factor
(D) thiamine
(E) vitamin B_{12}

39. Two reactions of the urea cycle that occur within the mitochondria are shown in Figure 9–5 (depicted by the enclosure). The enzyme denoted by the letter B catalyzes the condensation of ornithine with carbamoyl phosphate. A defect in this enzyme leads to

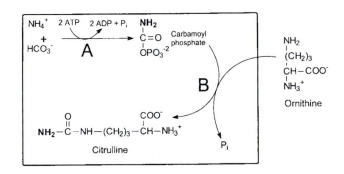

Figure 9–5

(A) argininosuccinic aciduria
(B) citrullinemia
(C) hyperargininemia
(D) type I hyperammonemia
(E) type II hyperammonemia

40. The photomicrograph in Figure 9–6 displays the organism that may cause

(A) aspergillosis
(B) phycomycosis
(C) tinea barbae
(D) tinea corporis
(E) tinea pedis

41. Some clinical improvement has been noted in a limited number of patients with Alzheimer disease with the chronic use of

(A) atracurium
(B) atropine

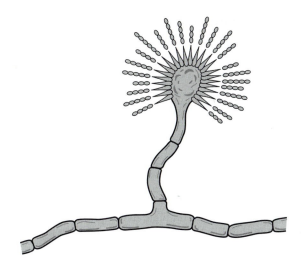

Figure 9–6

(C) cimetidine

(D) ipratropium

(E) tacrine

42. A patient is suffering from eruptions and multiple draining sinuses with copious suppuration. The lesions are located in the cervicofacial region. Microscopic examination of material taken from the lesions reveals small sulfur granules. This patient is most likely suffering from

   (A) actinomycosis
   (B) amebiasis
   (C) candidiasis
   (D) histoplasmosis
   (E) mucormycosis

43. You are attending a patient with a long-standing history of angina pectoris. Left coronary blood flow normally is greatest

   (A) at the peak aortic systolic
   (B) in early diastole
   (C) in early systole
   (D) near the end of diastole
   (E) near the end of systole

44. Which statement concerning the processing of precise tactile localization on the face is correct?

   (A) Pain sensation from the upper (maxillary) teeth is carried in the contralateral spinal trigeminal tract.
   (B) Signals from the right side of the face reach the ipsilateral chief sensory nucleus.
   (C) Signals from the right side of the face reach the ipsilateral spinal trigeminal nucleus.
   (D) The ventral posterior medial nucleus of the thalamus receives information from the ipsilateral side of the face.
   (E) The ventral trigeminothalamic tract terminates in the chief sensory trigeminal nucleus.

45. A 35-year-old apparently healthy African-American man undergoes a medical examination while applying for purchasing life insurance. He is not anemic. His hemoglobin electrophoresis is reported as: HbA, 62%; HbS, 35%; HbF, 1%; HbA_2, 1%; no variant C, D, G, or H bands detected. The most likely diagnosis is

   (A) sickle cell disease
   (B) sickle thalassemia minor
   (C) sickle trait
   (D) thalassemia major
   (E) thalassemia minor

46. The purpose of the Cori cycle is to shift the metabolic burden from

   (A) brain to liver
   (B) cytoplasm to mitochondria
   (C) liver to brain
   (D) liver to muscle
   (E) muscle to liver

47. Ondansetron is effective in reducing chemotherapy-induced vomiting by acting on

   (A) acetylcholine muscarinic receptors
   (B) DOPA receptors
   (C) glucocorticoid receptors
   (D) histamine H_1 receptors
   (E) 5-HT_3–gated ion channels

48. A banker has been told by his physician that the rash on his arm is due to delayed-type hypersensitivity. If this is actually the case, which one of the following statements is accurate?

   (A) Delayed-type hypersensitivity can be transferred passively to volunteers by sensitized lymphocytes.
   (B) Delayed-type hypersensitivity is suppressed by antihistaminic drugs.
   (C) This type of allergy does not cause tissue damage.
   (D) This type of allergy is due to IgE absorbed on mast cells.
   (E) This type of allergy occurs usually after inhalation of grass pollens.

49. The adverse effects of severe alkalemia include

   (A) arteriolar dilatation
   (B) hyperkalemia
   (C) hypoventilation
   (D) increased cerebral blood flow
   (E) increased ionized calcium concentration

50. Which of the following drugs acts by inhibiting viral reverse transcriptase?

   (A) Acyclovir
   (B) Amantadine
   (C) Didanosine
   (D) Ribavirin
   (E) Saquinavir

51. For hormones to carry out their actions, there is a requirement that receptor–ligand interactions activate pathways of intracellular signal transduction, of which pathways mediated by cAMP and phosphatidylinositol are major examples. Which of the following examples are known to be mediated by cAMP?

   (A) Amylase secretion in response to acetylcholine
   (B) Histamine release from mast cells in response to antigen
   (C) Glycogen breakdown in response to vasopressin

   (D) Serotonin and PDGF secretion by platelets in response to thrombin
   (E) Triglyceride breakdown in fat cells in response to epinephrine

52. A 47-year-old man has radiographic evidence of a pulmonary abnormality. A photomicrograph of his sputum is shown in Figure 9–7. What is the likely pulmonary disorder?

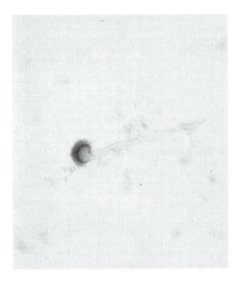

Figure 9–7

   (A) Asbestosis
   (B) Aspergillosis
   (C) Blastomycosis
   (D) Histoplasmosis
   (E) Tuberculosis

53. A housewife has warts caused by the human papillomavirus (HPV). The infectious HPV are most likely to be found

   (A) in terminally differentiated squamous cells
   (B) in the basal layer of warts
   (C) in the surface cell layer of warts
   (D) only in transformed cancer cells
   (E) throughout the warts

54. Imaging studies conducted in the emergency room indicate that a young accident victim has a skull fracture involving the posterior cranial fossa. A fracture involving the posterior cranial fossa is most likely to injure

(A) cranial nerve VIII as it enters the internal acoustic meatus

(B) the abducens nerve in the cavernous sinus

(C) the mandibular division of the trigeminal nerve

(D) the temporal lobe of the cerebral hemisphere

(E) the temporomandibular joint

55. You received the patient's consent for a bone marrow biopsy for possible multiple myeloma yesterday. Today, when you are preparing for the biopsy, the patient asks you why he needs the biopsy. This may be an example of

(A) dementia

(B) denial

(C) depression

(D) malingering

(E) repression

56. The pathway of creatine phosphate synthesis is shown in Figure 9–8. Which amino acid is required in this pathway as indicated by the letter A?

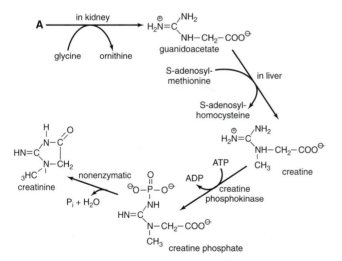

Figure 9–8

(A) Arginine

(B) Asparagine

(C) Aspartate

(D) Glutamate

(E) Glutamine

57. A 3-month-old baby has been immunized with the poliomyelitis vaccine. Biochemical analysis of the baby's serum 6 days after immunization indicates the presence of the immunoglobulin shown in Figure 9–9. This immunoglobulin is

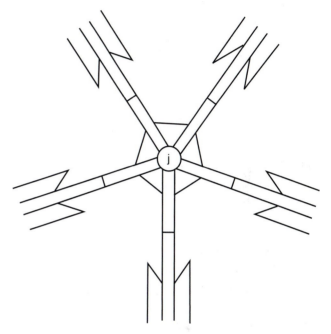

Figure 9–9

(A) IgA

(B) IgE

(C) IgD

(D) IgM

(E) IgG

58. During a recent visit to an infertility special-
ist, a 35-year-old woman reports an inability
to get pregnant over the past 2 years. During
this time she also reports having irregular
menses, menorrhagia, occasional suprapubic
pain and dysuria, and occasional dyspareunia and painful defecation. A diagnostic laparoscopy reveals thickened adnexa, abdominal adhesions, two hemorrhagic cysts on the
right ovary, and one ruptured hemorrhagic
cyst on the left ovary. Microscopically, fibrotic
patches of tissue found on the rectum and
urinary tract reveal hemosiderin-laden glandular and stromal tissue. These collective
findings most likely suggest a diagnosis of

   (A) endometriosis
   (B) luteal phase dysfunction
   (C) ovarian carcinoma
   (D) pelvic inflammatory disease
   (E) polycystic ovary disease

59. A 23-year-old student has been infected with
HIV. Which of the following is the most frequent early clinical manifestation of HIV infection?

   (A) Cytomegalic inclusion disease
   (B) Dermatologic disease
   (C) *Mycobacterium avium-intracellulare* dis-
       seminated disease
   (D) Non-Hodgkin lymphoma
   (E) Toxoplasmosis encephalitis

60. A 24-year-old nullipara primigravida comes
in for her routine obstetric checkup at 18
weeks gestation. Her serum human chorionic
gonadotropin (hCG) is 8 U/mL (normal at 18
weeks gestation, 20 U/mL). Which of the following is a possible cause of her abnormally
low hCG levels?

   (A) Choriocarcinoma
   (B) Hydatidiform mole
   (C) Threatened abortion
   (D) Trisomy 21
   (E) Twin pregnancy

61. A 46-year-old woman had rheumatic fever as
a child and now presents with heart failure.

On examining her heart, you will most likely
find an abnormality in the

   (A) coronary arteries
   (B) epicardium
   (C) mitral valve
   (D) pulmonary valve
   (E) right ventricle

62. Occlusion of branches of the posterior spinal
artery that irrigate the dorsomedial portion
of the left side of the caudal medulla might
result in damage to a pathway conveying somatosensory signals. If this is the case, which
of the following symptoms might be observed?

   (A) Hemiplegia involving the right side
   (B) Hyperactive reflexes in the left upper ex-
       tremity
   (C) Loss of pain and temperature sensation
       in the left upper extremity
   (D) Loss of position sense in the left upper
       extremity
   (E) Loss of vibratory sensation in the right
       upper extremity

63. Which of the following statements best describes the mechanism of action of glipizide?

   (A) Binds to the peroxisome proliferator-
       activated receptor-γ (PPAR-γ) in
       peripheral tissues
   (B) Closes potassium channels in pancreatic
       B cells
   (C) Directly stimulates glucose uptake by
       skeletal muscle
   (D) Euglycemic actions, including reduced
       glucagon secretion and reduced hepatic
       gluconeogenesis
   (E) Inhibits α-glucosidase in the intestine

Questions 64 and 65

A 45-year-old African-American woman complains
of gradually increasing fatigue. On physical examination she is noted to have obesity, hypertension, a
buffalo hump deformity of her back, moon facies,
abdominal striae, and muscle weakness. Radiographic imaging studies identify an abnormality of
her right adrenal gland.

64. The right adrenal gland is surgically resected. The intact specimen weighed 24 g. A hemisection of the gland is displayed in Figure 9–10. What is the diagnosis?

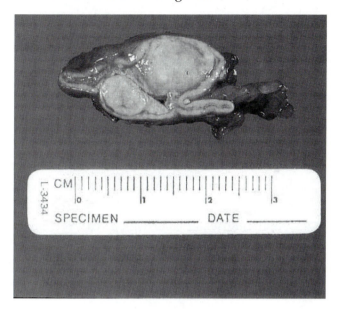

Figure 9–10

  (A) Adrenal cortical adenoma
  (B) Krukenberg tumor
  (C) Multifocal infarction
  (D) Neuroblastoma
  (E) Pheochromocytoma

65. Tests on this patient's serum are likely to reveal an elevation of

  (A) CA-125
  (B) carcinoembryonic antigen
  (C) cortisol
  (D) neuron-specific enolase
  (E) norepinephrine

66. Glutathione (GSH) functions in red blood cells to directly reduce oxidizing agents such as hydrogen peroxide. When oxidized, a disulfide bond forms between 2 molecules of GSH and the compound is designated GSSG. For GSSG to be reduced to 2 moles of GSH requires

  (A) NADH produced during fatty acid oxidation
  (B) NADH produced during glycolysis

  (C) NADH produced from the TCA cycle
  (D) NADPH produced during fatty acid synthesis
  (E) NADPH produced from the pentose phosphate pathway

67. A physician wishes to isolate *Mycoplasma pneumoniae* from a clinical specimen. This can most likely be accomplished by incorporating into the culture medium

  (A) doxycycline
  (B) erythromycin
  (C) minocycline
  (D) oxytetracycline
  (E) penicillin

68. A 78-year-old man has mild congestive heart failure. Which of the following agents is most likely to increase myocardial contractility without producing a concomitant increase in heart rate?

  (A) Captopril
  (B) Digoxin
  (C) Furosemide
  (D) Metoprolol
  (E) Nitroprusside

69. A 22-year-old white man is found dead at home. Urine obtained at autopsy contains benzoylecgonine. What conclusion can be drawn from this result?

  (A) A chromosomal abnormality was present.
  (B) A congenital deformity of the lower limb is likely.
  (C) Death was due to status asthmaticus.
  (D) The decedent had recently used cocaine.
  (E) The decedent was taking chemotherapy for cancer.

Questions 70 through 74

A patient with a history of unexplained polydipsia is admitted for evaluation of possible diabetes insipidus. After several hours of fluid deprivation, the following measurements are made:

Plasma osmolarity: 300 mosm/L
Urine osmolarity: 150 mosm/L
Urine solute output: 900 mosm/d

70. The rate of urine production in this patient is

    (A) 1.5 L/d
    (B) 2.0 L/d
    (C) 3.0 L/d
    (D) 6.0 L/d
    (E) unable to be calculated unless plasma volume is also known

71. Solute clearance in this patient is

    (A) 1.5 L/d
    (B) 2.0 L/d
    (C) 3.0 L/d
    (D) 6.0 L/d
    (E) unable to be calculated unless plasma volume is also known

72. Free water clearance in this patient is

    (A) −3.0 L/d
    (B) −1.5 L/d
    (C) +1.5 L/d
    (D) +3.0 L/d
    (E) unable to be calculated unless insulin clearance is also known

73. Because this patient's urine concentration is less than expected after water deprivation, additional tests are performed. Figure 9–11 shows several relationships between urine flow and urine solute excretion. Which of these relationships supports a diagnosis of diabetes insipidus in this patient?

    (A) Line A
    (B) Line B
    (C) Line C
    (D) Line D
    (E) Line E

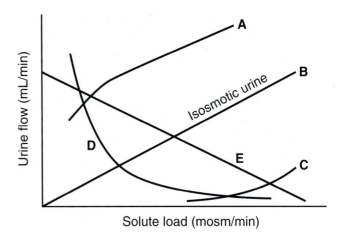

Figure 9–11

74. Following water deprivation, vasopressin is injected intravenously into the patient (arrow in Figure 9–12) and urine osmolarity is monitored. Based on the graph in Figure 9–12, the patient most likely has

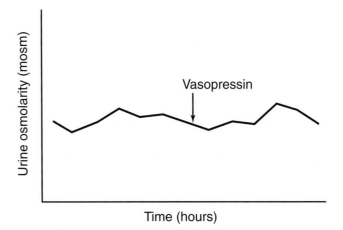

Figure 9–12

    (A) central diabetes insipidus
    (B) diabetes mellitus
    (C) no abnormality
    (D) psychogenic polydipsia
    (E) renal diabetes insipidus

75. A test is available for a fairly common disease (prevalence = 10%). The sensitivity is 90% and the specificity is 90%. You order the test for one of your patients and a positive result is reported. What is the probability (to the near-

est whole number) of this result being a true positive rather than a false positive; that is, what is the predictive value positive?

(A) 1%
(B) 10%
(C) 50%
(D) 90%
(E) 100%

Questions 76 through 82

An 18-year-old student is brought to the hospital because she had not come out of her room for 3 days, missing school. She would eat only when a tray was brought in.

76. If the patient is observed in her room folding and unfolding her bed sheet hundreds of times, this is probably an example of

(A) bipolar disorder
(B) obsessive-compulsive behavior
(C) panic behavior
(D) schizophrenia
(E) undoing

77. Upon further examination, you find that it is frustrating to listen to the patient; she keeps elaborating on topics and then goes on to related topics that seem peripheral to your question for protracted periods. This phenomenon is called

(A) autistic thinking
(B) circumstantiality
(C) folie à deux
(D) loose association
(E) thought blocking

78. While you are trying to understand her, she suddenly looks at an IV pole in front of the next bed, and tries to hide from it. She probably has

(A) ambivalence
(B) delusion
(C) hallucination
(D) illusion
(E) negativism

79. All of a sudden, she stands up and starts pacing rapidly. She keeps on saying, "I have to get out of here." This is an example of

(A) agitation
(B) catalepsy
(C) cataplexy
(D) catatonia
(E) hebephrenia

80. A useful immediate treatment for the condition described in question 79 is

(A) hypnosis
(B) psychoanalysis
(C) reassurance
(D) restraints
(E) sertraline

81. Further history reveals that the patient has been socially withdrawn since menarche at age 13, and has been preoccupied with the thought that her blood is impure. There seems to be no history of substance abuse. Family history reveals that her maternal grandmother died in a state hospital. The most likely diagnosis for this patient is

(A) bipolar disorder type I
(B) delusional disorder
(C) folie à deux
(D) psychosis secondary to a general medical condition
(E) schizophrenia

82. For this patient, an effective drug to treat many of her symptoms is

(A) benztropine
(B) chlordiazepoxide
(C) lithium chloride
(D) fluoxetine
(E) risperidone

83. A 79-year-old man complains of flank pain and red-colored urine. Radiographic studies indicate an increased size of his left kidney. The kidney is surgically resected and displayed in Figure 9–13. The cause of the kidney enlargement is most likely

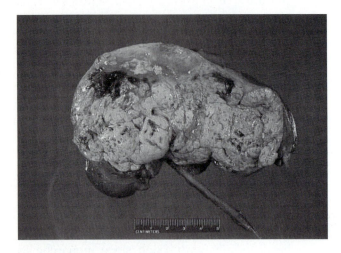

Figure 9–13

(A) abnormality of ureter or bladder
(B) congenital abnormality
(C) infectious process
(D) neoplastic process
(E) stone formation

84. A 45-year-old woman suffers from a para-esophageal hiatus hernia. Radiographic examination reveals that the portion of her stomach involved in the hernia is the

(A) body
(B) cardia
(C) fundus
(D) pyloric antrum
(E) pylorus

85. Staphylococcal enterotoxin

(A) blocks release of acetylcholine
(B) disrupts the cytoplasmic membrane
(C) disrupts the stratum granulosum in the epidermis
(D) is produced by over 90% of the strains of *S. epidermidis*
(E) resists boiling for 10 minutes

86. In some parts of the world, chronic arsenic poisoning may arise from ingestion of ground water supplies contaminated with arsenic. The best current treatment for chronic arsenic poisoning is

(A) calcium disodium edetate
(B) deferoxamine
(C) dimercaprol
(D) folic acid
(E) thiosulfate

87. A 3-year-old girl who has not been immunized against the usual childhood viral diseases has fever, runny nose, conjunctivitis, rash, a hacking cough, and a red-based, blue-white centered lesion in her mouth. The virus responsible for this girl's symptoms most likely is

(A) adenovirus
(B) corona virus
(C) hantavirus
(D) measles virus
(E) orthomyxovirus

88. A 12-year-old boy complains of a painful, enlarging mass on his left fourth rib. By x-ray, this lesion is seen to be well defined, circumscribed, and radiolucent with a ground glass appearance. Microscopically, it is found to be composed of a benign, fibroblastic proliferation in which there are random, curvilinear spicules of woven bone. The lesion is most likely a (an)

(A) chondroma
(B) fibrous dysplasia
(C) giant cell tumor
(D) osteoblastoma
(E) osteoid osteoma

89. During development, neural crest cells give rise to the

(A) microglia
(B) motoneurons in the spinal cord
(C) oligodendroglia
(D) protoplasmic astroglia
(E) sympathetic ganglion cells

90. A 68-year-old woman has a dislocated right hip joint due to a fall. The attending physician is concerned because the patient has loss of sensation below the knee, except for a narrow area along the medial side of the lower portion of the leg and medial border of the foot. Although she has weak flexion of the knee, her hamstring muscles and all muscles below the knee are paralyzed. Her right foot is in the plantar flexed position (foot drop). The nerve involved in this injury is the

(A) common peroneal (fibular) nerve
(B) femoral nerve
(C) obturator nerve
(D) sciatic nerve
(E) tibial nerve

91. A sewer worker arrives at the Emergency Room with intense headache, stiff neck, hepatitis, and nephritis. Examination of centrifuged urine by dark-field microscopy reveals many small spirochetes with thin, tightly coiled turns and hooks at both ends. The most likely diagnosis is

(A) legionellosis
(B) leptospirosis
(C) pinta
(D) relapsing fever
(E) yaws

92. Which of the following structures is directly associated with the vestibular system?

(A) External cuneate nucleus
(B) Scarpa's ganglion
(C) Stria vascularis
(D) Tunnel of Corti
(E) Zone of Lissauer

93. A 27-year-old man who is known to be allergic to penicillin is inadvertently given an injection of the antibiotic and within minutes develops upper respiratory obstruction followed by hypotension and shock. This hypersensitivity reaction is classified as type

(A) I
(B) II
(C) III
(D) IV

94. High plasma levels of the lipoprotein particle identified as lipoprotein(a) [Lp(a)] have been shown to be a primary risk factor for coronary heart disease and stroke. Lp(a) is a unique lipoprotein assembled from LDL and a single glycoprotein called apolipoprotein(a) or apo(a). Apo(a) is associated with LDL via a disulfide linkage to which other apolipoprotein?

(A) ApoA-I
(B) ApoB-48
(C) ApoB-100
(D) ApoC-II
(E) ApoE

95. An eruption of shingles over the cutaneous distribution of the ophthalmic nerve (herpes zoster ophthalmicus) is a common and often painful affliction. Your patient has involvement over the dorsum of the nose extending to the tip. Which of the following cutaneous branches of the ophthalmic nerve is involved?

(A) External nasal nerve
(B) Lacrimal nerve
(C) Supraorbital nerve
(D) Supratrochlear nerve
(E) Zygomaticotemporal nerve

96. The health benefits of regular exercise are well recognized and it is important to understand the cardiovascular changes normally occurring during exercise. With different levels of aerobic exercise under steady-state conditions,

(A) arterial diastolic blood pressure decreases substantially
(B) blood perfusion of the skin decreases
(C) blood pressure in the pulmonary artery approaches that of the systemic arteries
(D) cardiac output is almost linearly related to oxygen uptake
(E) stroke volume is linearly related to oxygen uptake up to maximal oxygen consumption

97. N-acetylcysteine is the preferred antidote for overdosage with which drug?

    (A) Acetaminophen
    (B) Diazepam
    (C) Ferrous sulfate
    (D) Morphine
    (E) Pentobarbital

98. A 43-year-old man has a routine chest x-ray and a subpleural parenchymal "coin" lesion measuring 2×2 cm is observed. The lesion is excised and sectioned and is shown in the photomicrograph in Figure 9–14. The best diagnosis is

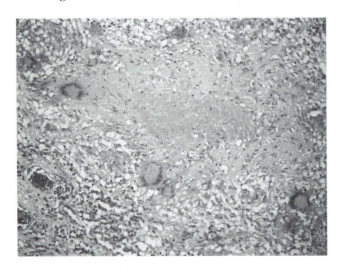

Figure 9–14. (See also Color Insert.)

    (A) abscess
    (B) carcinoma
    (C) granuloma
    (D) infarct
    (E) thrombus

99. B-cell receptors play a significant role in the development of immune responses. Which of the following statements about B-cell antigen-specific receptors is correct?

    (A) It appears that different receptor isotypes do not have different functions on the same cell.
    (B) Surface immunoglobulin is dimeric and contains only two heavy chains.

    (C) Surface immunoglobulin synthesized by a B-cell clone does not serve as an antigen receptor for that clone.
    (D) The mature B cell has IgE on its surface.
    (E) The surface immunoglobulin of the immature B cells is IgM.

100. A 12-month-old girl exhibits severe developmental delay with associated macrocephaly, dysmorphic facies, hypotonia, and hepatosplenomegaly. Clouding of the corneas is not evident. A pebbly, ivory-colored lesion is present over the infant's back. The activity of iduronate sulfatase in the plasma is not detectable. These symptoms are indicative of which mucopolysaccharidosis?

    (A) Hunter
    (B) Hurler
    (C) Maroteaux–Lamy
    (D) Morquio B
    (E) Sanfilippo A

Answers and Explanations

1. **(A)** *Bacillus anthracis* is a gram-positive, spore-forming microbe. Autoclaving is the best option for killing both the vegetative cells and spores of *B. anthracis*.

2. **(D)** The pathophysiology of benign prostatic hypertrophy involves a role for both prostatic smooth muscle and epithelial cells. Smooth muscle proliferation and hypertrophy constricts the urethra, as does epithelial cell proliferation under the influence of dihydrotestosterone (DHT). α_1-Adrenergic receptor blockers (choice A) often reverse smooth muscle hypertrophy and contraction (e.g., terazosin). Therapy with anti-androgens (choice B) blocks epithelial hypertrophy and proliferation. Finasteride, a specific inhibitor of the 5-α-reductase enzyme that converts testosterone to DHT, is often an effective treatment, decreasing prostate volume by 20%. Thus, therapy with either androgens, estrogens (choice C), or with an α_1-adrenergic agonist exaccerbates rather than treats the problem. Finally, surgical resection of the detrussor muscle (choice E) causes side effects including lack of control over urination, without any clear benefit.

3. **(C)** Klinefelter syndrome has a 47,XXY karyotype, testicular atrophy, eunuchoid tall habitus, gynecomastia, and a female distribution of hair. Down syndrome (choice A) is characterized by trisomy 21, congenital cardiac defects, epicanthic folds, mental retardation, dysplastic ears, and an increased risk of developing leukemia. Edwards syndrome (choice B) is a trisomy of chromosome 18. Individuals with Edwards syndrome may display mental retardation, micrognathia, rocker bottom feet, and prominent occiput. Patients with multi-X syndrome (choice D) are usually phenotypically normal females. Turner syndrome (choice E) has a 45,X karyotype, webbing of the neck, amenorrhea, streak gonads, short stature, and cardiac defects.

4. **(B)** Of the enzymes listed, only glucokinase and glucose-6-phosphatase are found in the liver and not in most other tissues. Hexokinase (choice D) is the glucose phosphorylating enzyme of nonhepatic tissues. A deficiency in glucokinase, which is the hepatic-specific glucose phosphorylating isozyme (choice A), leads to increased blood sugar levels and hyperglycemia, not hypoglycemia. This occurs because of the liver's decreased ability to phosphorylate free glucose. In contrast, a defect in glucose-6-phosphatase causes the symptoms observed in von Gierke disease. This endoplasmic reticulum enzyme catalyzes the dephosphorylation of glucose-6-phosphate, allowing glucose to be released into the blood when levels are low. A lesion at this point results in massive storage of glycogen in the liver. A deficiency in phosphofructokinase-1 (choice E) also results in a glycogen storage disease, called Tarui disease, and it is restricted to muscle and erythrocyte involvement. It leads to exercise-induced cramping and hemolytic anemia. A deficiency in lysosomal α-1,4-glucosidase (choice C), also called lysosomal acid α-glucosidase or acid maltase, results in the glycogen storage disease termed Pompe disease. This disorder leads to glycogen accumulation in most tissues, but the effects are

most pronounced in skeletal and cardiac muscle. Affected individuals die at an early age due to massive cardiomegaly.

5. **(A)** Sympathetic stimulation releases the neurotransmitter norepinephrine at the nerve terminals. Norepinephrine acts by increasing membrane permeability to Na$^+$ and Ca^{2+} ions, resulting in an increased slope of the diastolic depolarization. Therefore, membrane potential reaches the threshold for self-excitation (broken line) earlier, increasing the heart rate. The amplitude of the action potential (curves B and C) is little affected by sympathetic stimulation. Curve D represents the effect of parasympathetic stimulation.

6. **(D)** Not all patients admit to the presence of risk factors, but may request testing. Other indications include being a member of a high-risk group, patients with symptoms of AIDS, women belonging to a high-risk group planning pregnancy, and blood, semen, or organ donors. Homosexuality (choice A) per se without having had sexual contact with a possibly infected person is not an indication, nor is being in the military (choice B), medical school (choice C), or a psychiatric hospital (choice E).

7. **(D)** Neurons of the nucleus ambiguous give rise to the branchial efferent fibers of the cranial portion of the accessory nerve. The cranial portion of the accessory nerve joins the vagus nerve outside of the skull, to be distributed to the intrinsic muscles of the larynx. The dorsal motor nucleus of the vagus (choice A) provides visceral efferent fibers to the thoracic and abdominal viscera. The hypoglossal nucleus (choice B) innervates intrinsic and extrinsic muscles of the tongue. The inferior (nodose) ganglion of the vagus nerve (choice C) gives rise to visceral afferent fibers from the pharynx, larynx, trachea, esophagus, and viscera of the thorax and abdomen. The superior (jugular) ganglion (choice E) sends out somatic afferent fibers to the external auditory meatus, part of the ear lobe, and the dura of the posterior cranial fossa.

8. **(B)** Methimazole acts within the thyroid gland to inhibit the peroxidase responsible for the incorporation of iodine into thyroglobulin and the coupling of iodotyrosyl residues to form the iodothyronines. It is used to treat hyperthyroidism prior to surgery or radioiodine ablation, or in anticipation of remission of the hyperthyroid state. Diabetes (choice B) is treated with insulin and in the noninsulin-dependent form, with oral agents. Hypoparathyroidism (choice C) arises from the lack of parathyroid hormone and is characterized by hypocalcemia with muscle spasms and paresthesias in the extremities. It is treated with calcium and vitamin D. Infertility due to anovulatory cycles (choice D) may result from a variety of abnormalities. It is most often treated with hormonal stimulation of the pituitary, using drugs such as clomiphene. This partial estrogen agonist reduces estrogen feedback suppression of pituitary luteinizing hormone (LH) and follicle-stimulating hormone (FSH), and the increased levels of these hormones may result in restoration of ovulation. Osteoporosis (choice E) most commonly results from loss of estrogenic protection of bone in postmenopausal women. In women without contraindications, estrogen replacement therapy, with or without progestin replacement, is effective in restoring protection. Raloxifene, a selective estrogen receptor modulator, is an estrogen agonist in bone that has antagonist effects in breast tissue, so this drug is more suitable for women with a high risk of breast cancer. Bisphosphonates such as alendronate are effective in preventing further bone loss and appear to also increase bone density to some degree.

9. **(A)** In a positive viral hemagglutination test, the virus is the hemagglutinating particle. Antibody specific to the viral hemagglutinin blocks this activity and inhibits hemagglutination. The assay is similar to a neutralization test, with the erythrocyte taking the place of a susceptible nucleated host cell. Latex agglutinins are antibodies that agglutinate antigens that have been bound on the surface of latex spheres. Hemolysin is a mole-

cule that lyses red blood cells. *Staphylococci, streptococci,* and other bacteria produce various types of hemolysins (choice B). Viral hemagglutination takes places between red blood cells and viruses (choice C). Rh antibody is directed toward the D antigen found on red blood cells (choice D). Certain viruses such as influenza, measles, mumps, and parainfluenza viruses produce hemagglutinins that agglutinate red blood cells, but these viruses promote hemagglutination, they do not inhibit it (choice E).

10. **(A)** Fibrinogen is one of the remarkable array of proteins of diverse function that are made in the liver. Renin (choice D) is made by cells of the juxtaglomerular apparatus in the kidney; however, its action is to cleave circulating angiotensinogen, which is made by the liver. Growth hormone (choice B) is made by cells in the anterior pituitary gland. However, much of GH action is mediated by insulin-like growth factor-1 (IGF-1), a protein secreted from the liver in response to stimulation by GH. Insulin (choice C) is made in cells of the endocrine pancreas and acts on the liver, but is not produced there. von Willibrand factor (choice E) is made by endothelial cells.

11. **(A)** The double-reciprocal Lineweaver–Burk plot shown in Figure 9–2 illustrates a competitively inhibited enzyme. In competitive inhibition, the intercept on the y axis, which is equal to I/V_{max}, does not change. This points out that at significantly high substrate concentration, the inhibition can be overcome. In noncompetitive inhibition (choice B), the V_{max}, and hence the y-axis intercept, does change. Noncompetitive inhibition cannot be overcome by increasing the substrate concentration. Allosteric enzymes (choice C) do not obey Michaelis–Menten kinetics and cannot be plotted as straight lines on double-reciprocal curves. Irreversibly (choice D) and uncompetitively (choice E) inhibited enzymes cannot be treated by Michaelis–Menten kinetics.

12. **(D)** Patients with glucocorticoid excess have fat redistribution due to the differential effect on the periphery versus central distribution. This is a good example of the nuances that account for why there are so many different "counterregulatory" hormones that oppose insulin action—they each oppose insulin in different ways and to different degrees. This is also a good corrollary to the notion that central fat generates more insulin resistance than peripheral fat. All the other options (choices A, B, C, and E) are opposite to what is seen with high-dose glucocorticoids.

13. **(A)** Some individuals exhibit an intolerance to aspirin even at low doses. This is manifested by a range of symptoms from rhinitis to acute bronchoconstriction, angioedema, and shock. The reaction does not appear to be of immunologic origin. The suggestion has been made that the condition arises from inhibition of cyclooxygenase and shunting of arachidonic acid into the 5-lipoxygenase pathway. For reasons that are not understood, aspirin intolerance is associated with the presence of nasal polyps. Cardiac arrhythmias (choice B) are not associated with the use of aspirin. Hemolytic anemia (choice C) does not occur with aspirin, but mild hemolysis may occur in individuals with a deficiency of erythrocytic glucose-6-phosphate dehydrogenase activity. Hepatotoxicity (choice D) is rarely associated with chronic aspirin therapy and usually occurs with plasma concentrations maintained at 150 µg/mL or greater. Elevation of liver enzyme activity in the plasma is the usual sign of hepatotoxicity. Nephrotoxicity (choice E) is rarely seen with aspirin used alone, but may occur with chronic high-dose therapy and more so with newer NSAIDs.

14. **(B)** Complement-fixation procedures are performed in two stages. The test system consists of antigen and antibody (one of which is unknown) plus complement. The indicator system consists of sheep erythrocytes and hemolysin (an antisheep-RBC serum), which sensitizes the cells to the lytic action of complement. If complement is fixed in the test system, it is effectively bound (or consumed) in the antigen–antibody complexes there and

is not free to participate in the lysis of the sensitized erythrocytes present in the indicator system. In an influenza virus complement-fixation test, the indicator system consists of complement, unlabeled sheep RBCs, and antibody to sheep RBCs (choice C). The indicator system does not need antibody to influenza virus (choice A), fluorescent-tagged virus (choice D), or neuraminidase (choice E).

15. **(C)** Each organ site has specific rules by which to stage the extent of tumor involvement. The colon invasion of the tumor into, but not through, the muscularis propria is T2. The presence of pericolic lymph nodes with metastatic carcinoma is N1. The absence of distal non-nodal metastases, such as in the liver, is M0. T1 N0 M0 (choice A) is incorrect because the tumor is T2 and the nodal status is N1. The M status is correct as M0. T2 N0 M1 (choice B) is incorrect because the nodal status is N1 and distant metastatic status is M0. The tumor is correct as T2. T3 N0 M1 (choice D) has all three items coded incorrectly. T4 N0 M1 (choice E) also has all three items coded incorrectly.

16. **(A)** "Brittle" is a term used to describe patients whose blood glucose swings wildly from too high to too low despite standard approaches to blood glucose control. Patients often relate the scenario described, and are puzzled at the "paradoxical" increase in blood glucose despite an increase in the amount of insulin injected. Unbeknownst to them, the problem is that they were already taking too much insulin. It was dropping their blood glucose to levels that stimulated secretion of counterregulatory hormones, including glucagon and epinephrine, which in turn raises blood glucose. This is what the patient observes in the morning, termed the Somogyi phenomenon. The tip-off here is the patient's noting nightmares and vivid dreams, both signs of nocturnal hypoglycemia. Decreasing his night time food intake (choice B), a further increase in his bed time insulin dose (choice C), and a modification of his life style (choice D) would only worsen the nocturnal hypoglycemia. Switch-

ing to an oral hypoglycemic drug (choice E) is unlikely to address the current problem.

17. **(B)** Lyme disease is due to a systemic infection by the spirochete *B. burgdorferi*. Infections are usually transmitted to humans through a tick bite. Campers, hikers, and outdoor enthusiasts are at risk, particularly in the northeastern United States. A transient rash followed by migratory arthritis is the typical clinical course. Antibiotics are curative. Achondroplasia (choice A) is an autosomal dominant genetic disorder characterized by dwarfism and arthritis. Antibodies directed against *Borrelia* species are not a feature of osteoarthritis. Ochronosis (choice C) is an autosomal recessive disorder characterized by early arthritis, pigmented cartilage, and excess homogentisic acid in the urine. Osteoarthritis (choice D) is uncommon in a person only 36 years old. Rheumatoid arthritis (choice E) should demonstrate an elevated serum rheumatoid factor, not antibodies against *B. burgdorferi*.

18. **(E)** Normal catabolism of phenylalanine involves hydroxylation to tyrosine catalyzed by phenylalanine hydroxylase. Mutations in the phenylalanine hydroxylase gene lead to deficiencies in the enzyme and manifest as phenylketonuria (PKU). Patients suffering from PKU have elevated levels of phenylalanine in their blood as well as the transamination product, phenylpyruvate. Phenylpyruvate is converted to phenyllactate and phenylacetate by reduction and oxidation, respectively; all three byproducts are excreted in the urine. The standard test for PKU is for elevated phenylalanine in the blood of newborns. Alcaptonuria (choice A) results from a defect in homogentisate oxidase, which is involved in tyrosine catabolism. The urine of afflicted individuals darkens upon exposure to air due to the presence of homogentisic acid. Hartnup disease (choice B) results from a defect in intestinal and renal transport of neutral amino acids with general neutral aminoaciduria. Hepatorenal tyrosinemia (choice C) is a form of tyrosinemia, all forms of which lead to elevated levels of tyrosine, or

its various metabolites, in the blood. Maple syrup urine disease (choice D) results from a defect in α-keto acid decarboxylase and leads to elevated levels of the branched-chain amino acids, leucine, isoleucine, and valine, in the blood and urine.

19. **(B)** Heterochromatin is a highly condensed form of chromatin in which the DNA is inaccessible to transcription. In light microscopy, heterochromatin stains intensely with basic stains, and the amount and distribution pattern of heterochromatin in the nucleus is a useful feature in identifying both normal and abnormal cells in tissue sections. Euchromatin (choice A) stains less intensely than heterochromatin because the chromatin is in a more dispersed form, and consequently the DNA is accessible to transcription. Cells that are active in either protein synthesis or division tend to have large nuclei containing mostly euchromatin. Nuclear pores (choice C) provide a regulated portal for movement of material between the nucleus and the cytoplasm. The nucleolus (choice D) is the site of ribosomal RNA production. The rER (choice E) is the site of translation and initial posttranslational modification of proteins destined for export, sequestration within vesicles such as lysosomes, or incorporation into membranes. Those mRNAs coding for such proteins contain a sequence of bases at the 5′ end that codes for a signal sequence of mostly hydrophobic amino acids. This leads to docking of the ribosome–mRNA complex on the membrane of the endoplasmic reticulum. As the newly synthesized protein is inserted into the lumen of the rER, the signal sequence is enzymatically removed by the signal peptidase.

20. **(E)** Valproic acid has unusual versatility. It is effective in both absence and partial (tonic–clonic) seizures and in the management of bipolar disorder. Its mechanism in each of these conditions is poorly understood. Amitriptylline (choice A) is a first-generation antidepressant that may cause seizures. Clonazepam (choice B) is a useful drug for generalized seizures of the absence type, but is sedating at effective doses. It is not used in bipolar disorder. Haloperidol (choice C) is a very effective antipsychotic, but is rarely used in bipolar disorder unless mania is not controlled by lithium. It is of no value in epilepsy. Lithium (choice D) is the usual drug of choice in bipolar disorder (valproic acid and carbamazepine are also used), but is of no value in epilepsy.

21. **(E)** The graft-versus-host reaction occurs when immunocompetent lymphoid cells are transferred to a histoincompatible recipient who is unable to reject them. The donor cells then mount an immune response against the foreign histocompatibility antigens of the recipient and attempt to reject them. This usually occurs in bone marrow transplantation performed as a therapeutic modality in patients with certain leukemias or other blood diseases, such as aplastic anemia. Contamination of the graft with gram-negative bacteria (choice B) is not known to be the key factor for the graft-versus-host reaction. Graft-versus-host reactions can occur with any type of tissue grafting be that of neoplastic or non-neoplastic origin (choice C). A graft-versus-host reaction does not occur because the graft has histocompatibility antigens not found in the recipient, but because the reaction occurs when immunocompetent lymphoid cells are transferred to a histoincompatible recipient who is unable to reject the immunocompetent lymphoid cells (choice A). For the reasons stated, a graft-versus-host reaction does not occur when a histocompatible graft is irradiated before engraftment (choice D).

22. **(E)** The colon segment in Figure 9–3 demonstrates ulcerative colitis. The disease is limited to the colon and preferentially involves in continuity the rectum, sigmoid, and descending colon. The affected colon demonstrates a red, granular mucosa with occasional pseudopolyp formation. Deep fissures, skip lesions with alternating areas of diseased and normal colon, and strictures do not typically occur. Amebic colitis (choice A) is usually limited to the right colon and displays multiple, scattered, separate ulcerations. In collagenous

colitis (choice B), the colon appears grossly normal. Gangrenous colitis (choice C) has an acute clinical course. Grossly, the colon demonstrates a transmural area of blackened, thinned tissue. Pseudomembranous colitis (choice D) is usually an acute colitis occurring after antibiotic therapy. White, custard-like debris that partially coats the mucosal surface is the characteristic gross observation of pseudomembranous colitis.

23. **(B)** Chronic ulcerative colitis carries an increased risk for developing adenocarcinoma. Most patients are followed by annual endoscopies with histologic evaluation of random colonic biopsies. The presence of high-grade dysplasia usually is an indication for prophylactic pancolonic resection. Amyloidosis (choice A) does not occur with increased frequency in ulcerative colitis. A liver abscess (choice C) is a known complication of amebic colitis. There is no increased risk to develop melanoma (choice D) with ulcerative colitis. It is not observed with ulcerative colitis. Strictures (choice E) are not a typical feature of ulcerative colitis. Most strictures are focal lesions capable of being treated by a local resection rather than a pancolectomy.

24. **(E)** Vitamin D is a steroid hormone that plays a crucial role in calcium homeostasis. It has to be activated in a two-step process involving first the liver, then the kidney. In renal failure, the kidney's ability to generate active vitamin D (1,25-dihydrocholecalciferol) is impaired or lost. Thus, serum calcium falls, serving as a stimulus to parathyroid hormone secretion, which in turn stimulates bone resorption. The latter response elevates serum phosphate that is not cleared by the kidney due to renal failure and therefore serves to bind calcium and lower the ionized calcium that triggers further PTH secretion, and so on. All of the other options are the opposite of what is generally observed in renal failure. Increased oxidative products not cleared by the kidneys results in accelerated atherosclerosis (choice A). Volume overload in renal failure tends to give hypertension, not hypotension (choice B). Insulin clearance

occurs largely by the kidney; thus, an important tip-off of progression of renal failure is unexplained diminution in a patient's insulin requirements (choice C). Loss of erythropoietin results in anemia, not polycythemia (choice D).

25. **(B)** Chronic myeloid leukemia is characterized as a pluripotent stem cell disease of the hematopoietic system that results from a consistent chromosomal translocation. This translocation is known as the Philadelphia chromosome and results from a translocation between chromosomes 9 and 22. The translocation occurs within the protooncogenic tyrosine kinase gene, c-abl on chromosome 9 and the bcr locus on chromosome 22 (t9:22). The ABL gene was first identified as the transforming protein of Abelson murine leukemia virus. Therefore, the term c-abl differentiates the cellular version from the viral version (v-abl). The bcr (*b*reakpoint *c*luster *r*egion) locus is so named because it was a region on chromosome 22 identified in numerous chromosomal breakpoints. The result of the Philadelphia translocation is a fusion protein, bcr-abl, that has uncontrolled tyrosine kinase activity leading to the ability to transform cells. Burkitt lymphoma (choice A) results with high frequency due to a chromosomal translocation between chromosomes 8 and 14 (t8:14). The translocation occurs within the protooncogene MYC on chromosome 8 and the immunoglobulin heavy chain locus on chromosome 14. The result of the translocation is the placement of the strong immunoglobulin gene enhancer element near the MYC gene leading to uncontrolled MYC expression. Fanconi anemia (choice C) is caused by chromosomal instability and frequent breakage leading to a predisposition to acute myelogenous leukemia. Li–Fraumeni syndrome (LFS) (choice D) is a rare inherited form of cancer that involves breast and colon carcinomas, soft tissue sarcomas, osteosarcomas, brain tumors, leukemia, and adrenocortical carcinomas. These tumors develop at an early age in LFS patients. The p53 tumor suppressor gene is responsible for LFS. Mutant forms of p53 are found in approximately 50%

of all tumors. The normal p53 protein functions as a transcription factor that can induce either cell cycle arrest or apoptosis (programmed cell death) in response to DNA damage. von Hippel–Lindau (VHL) syndrome (choice E) is an inherited form of renal carcinoma caused by mutations in a tumor suppressor gene identified as the VHL gene.

26. **(D)** The lower border of the pleura crosses the tenth rib at the midaxillary line. It crosses the eighth rib (choice C) at the midclavicular line and the twelfth rib (choice E) at the sides of the vertebral column. The lower border of the lungs cross the sixth rib (choice B) at the midclavicular line, the eighth rib at the midaxillary line, and the tenth rib at the sides of the vertebral column. The space between the lower borders of the lungs and the pleura forms the costodiaphragmatic recess. Rib 4 (choice A) is superior to the nipple and thus to the lower border of the pleura.

27. **(E)** The β-blocker propranolol, by blocking cardiac $β_1$-adrenoceptors, prevents the sympathetic nervous system from increasing heart rate and contractility in response to exertion. This prevents the normal increase in cardiac workload and reduces myocardial oxygen demand. This effect is prophylactic. Propranolol does not dilate capacitance vessels (choice A). In contrast, the nitrovasodilators such as nitroglycerin dilate capacitance vessels, an effect that reduces cardiac preload. This effect reduces the workload and results in a decrease in myocardial oxygen demand, thus terminating an anginal attack. There is no net change in coronary blood flow (choice B) with propranolol. Propranolol does not increase oxygen delivery (choice C). Propranolol does inhibit the release of renin (choice D) from the juxtaglomerular apparatus. This effect may be important in its antihypertensive actions, but does not contribute to the prevention of anginal attacks.

28. **(C)** *Pseudomonas* infections often occur in patients suffering from cystic fibrosis or burns. These infections are most frequently caused by *P. aeruginosa*, which produces a characteristic blue-green pigment. *Legionella pneumophila* (choice A) and *M. pneumoniae* (choice B) do not produce pigments. *Staphylococcus aureus* (choice D) and *S. epidemidis* (choice E) produce yellow and white pigments, respectively.

29. **(B)** Although all the other items (choices A, C, D, and E) are components of personality, patterns of thought, behavior, and feelings combined are the most comprehensive.

30. **(B)** Wernicke area, located at the posterior end of the superior temporal gyrus, is believed to play an important role in the understanding of language, either written or spoken. Patients with lesions in this area have a form of fluid aphasia in which the ability to vocalize is not impaired, but the subject matter of speech is not intelligible. Moreover, the ability to understand either speech or writing is impaired. This is in contrast to lesions of Broca area, in which understanding is preserved, but the ability to vocalize speech is impaired (choice D). Deficits in the processing of visual information (choice C), dyslexia (choice A), or disorders of short-term memory (choice E) may each result from cerebral lesions, but are not specifically associated with Wernicke area.

31. **(D)** Erythroblastosis fetalis can occur when an Rh_o-positive child is being carried by an Rh_o-negative mother. If the mother makes antibodies against the $Rh_o(D)$ antigen, these may cross the placenta and destroy fetal erythrocytes. The induction of this immune response can be blocked if an antibody specific for the Rh_o antigen is injected into the mother at the time of her first exposure to the fetal RBCs, which usually occurs at parturition. Rh_o immune globulin (RhoGAM) is a human γ-globulin preparation rich in antibodies specific for the Rh_o antigen. It is used to prevent the sensitization of the mother, which then protects a subsequent antigenically incompatible fetus from this disease. Anti-allergen antibodies (choice A), anti-inflammatory agents (choice B), antilymphocyte antibodies (choice C), and enhancing antibodies (choice E) are

not the components of Rh$_0$-specific immunoglobulin (RhoGAM).

32. **(C)** Heparin is an important glycosaminoglycan (GAG) involved in the regulation of the clotting cascade. Abundant levels of heparin are found in granules of mast cells lining the blood vessels. In response to injury, mast cells release the contents of their granules. Release of heparin inhibits the clotting cascade by complexing with and activating antithrombin III, which in turn inhibits the serine proteases of the clotting cascade. It is this function of the naturally occurring GAG heparin that has been exploited in the use of injected synthetic heparin for anticoagulation therapies. Chondroitin sulfates (choice A) predominate in cartilage and are also found in bone and heart valves. Dermatan sulfates (choice B) are found in skin, heart valves, and vessels. Hyaluronate (choice D) predominates in synovial fluid and vitreous humor. Keratan sulfates (choice E) are found in cornea and bone, and in aggregates with chondroitin sulfates in cartilage.

33. **(B)** The inferior hypogastric plexus lies lateral to the posterior part of the urinary bladder, prostate, seminal vesicle, and rectum. It thus supplies sympathetic and parasympathetic nerve fibers to the prostate gland. The celiac (choice A), superior (choice E), and inferior (choice C) mesenteric plexuses supply mainly digestive and urinary organs. The superior hypogastric plexus (choice D) sends right and left hypogastric nerves into the pelvis to contribute to the formation of the inferior hypogastric plexus.

34. **(B)** Epinephrine is the drug of choice in the treatment of anaphylaxis because it provides a pressor response through α_1-adrenoceptor actions, cardiac stimulation through β_1-adrenoceptor actions, and bronchodilation and prevention of mast cell release of histamine and leukotrienes through actions on β_2-adrenoceptors. The actions of dopamine (choice A) on the cardiovascular system are complex; dopamine exerts effects on renal, mesenteric, and myocardial vascular D$_1$ re-

ceptors (vasodilation), cardiac β_1-receptors (positive inotropic effect), and vascular α_1-receptors (vasoconstriction), depending on the dopamine concentration. Dopamine also causes release of norepinephrine from sympathetic nerve terminals, but it does not inhibit mast cell release of mediators of shock. Dopamine is useful in hypovolemic and cardiogenic shock in maintaining renal perfusion. Isoproterenol (choice C) inhibits mast cell release of mediators and provides cardiac stimulation, but does not provide needed pressor activity. Norepinephrine (choice D) provides pressor activity to treat shock, but does not inhibit mast cell release of mediators of shock and does not dilate the bronchi. Phenylephrine (choice E), like norepinephrine, provides pressor activity, but not the cardiac stimulation or inhibition of mast cell function.

35. **(A)** Creutzfeldt–Jakob disease is caused by a prion that may either be inherited or acquired during life. Prions are composed of protein only and behave like a slow viral infection. Human prion disease has recently become more prominent with the outbreak of mad cow disease in England due to human consumption of beef tainted with prions. Creutzfeldt–Jakob disease is not known to be inherited as a lysosomal storage disease (choice B) or to be caused by protozoan infections (choice D). Increased neurofibrillary tangles (choice C) are seen with Alzheimer disease, not Creutzfeldt–Jakob disease. Repeated exposure to chemical toxins (choice E) can cause dementia. Alcohol is a common example. However, the histology of chemical dementia usually differs in character and distribution from the cortical spongiform changes seen in Creutzfeldt–Jakob disease.

36. **(E)** The envelope of HBV contains an antigen known as HbsAg. This antigen is of germane importance because production of antibodies against HBsAg indicate immunity against HBV, which resulted either from infection or vaccination with HVsAg. Treatment of HBV with nonionic detergent removes the envelope and produces the viral core, which con-

tains the HVcAg. Neither the nucleocapsid proteins of HBV (choice A) nor the RNA genome of HBV (choice B) are protective. Antibodies to HVcAg are not protective (choice C). Treatment of the viral core with strong detergents result in the release of a soluble core antigen called HVeAg. Production of antibody against HVeAg (choice D) signals active disease, during which period the patient is infectious.

37. **(C)** Afferents from muscle spindles in the upper extremity terminate in the lateral cuneate nucleus of the medulla after entering the spinal cord in dorsal roots from C5 to T1. Upper limb muscle spindle afferents do not terminate in the dorsal horn from C3 to C5 (choice B), the nucleus dorsalis (choice E) at any level where this nucleus is present, or in the ipsilateral nucleus gracilis (choice D), which is reserved for lower extremity sensory input. Some muscle spindle afferents from the upper limb may reach the ipsilateral, but not the contralateral (choice A), nucleus cuneatus.

38. **(E)** The description of symptoms suggests B_{12} deficiency. Definitive diagnosis requires the measurement of plasma vitamin B_{12} levels. Plant sources of food lack vitamin B_{12}. Macrocytic megaloblastic anemia arises from derangements in DNA metabolism and is a symptom of both vitamin B_{12} and folate deficiency. Diagnosis of the underlying cause of the anemia must precede the treatment because folate administration (choice B) corrects the anemia but allows neurologic damage associated with B_{12} deficiency to progress. Neurologic problems and even psychotic states may result from demyelination that takes place with B_{12} deficiency. Ferrous sulfate (choice A) is the agent of choice for treating simple iron deficiency anemia. Iron deficiency results in a microcytic, hypochromic anemia. Intrinsic factor (choice C) is a secreted glycoprotein involved in intestinal absorption of vitamin B_{12}. The absence of intrinsic factor leads to B_{12} deficiency. Alcoholism is the most common cause of thiamine deficiency (choice D) in the United States.

The deficiency may lead to neurologic problems and Wernicke syndrome, sometimes manifested as a global confusion. This condition is treated with thiamine. Anemia is not a feature of thiamine deficiency.

39. **(E)** The enzyme designated by the letter B is ornithine transcarbamoylase (OTC). Deficiencies in OTC result in type II hyperammonemia, the most commonly occurring urea cycle defect. Symptoms include hyperammonemia, elevated serum glutamine, and orotic aciduria. Argininosuccinic aciduria (choice A) results from deficiencies in argininosuccinate lyase (argininosuccinase), the enzyme that catalyzes the hydrolysis of argininosuccinate to fumarate and arginine. Citrullinemia (choice B) results from deficiencies in argininosuccinate synthetase, the enzyme that catalyzes the condensation of asparate and citrulline forming argininosuccinate. Hyperargininemia (choice C) results from deficiencies in arginase, the enzyme that catalyzes hydrolysis of arginine to urea and ornithine. Type I hyperammonemia (choice D) results from deficiencies in carbamoyl phosphate synthetase I (the enzyme depicted by the letter A in Figure 9–5), which catalyzes the ATP-dependent condensation of ammonium ion and bicarbonate ion forming carbamoyl phosphate.

40. **(A)** The position of the conidiospores in strings arising from the columella is characteristic of the genus *Aspergillus*. The organism in Figure 9–6 is septate (note the divisions, or cross-walls) in the hypha. This observation rules out any of the phycomycetes (choice B), because these organisms are cyanoacytic. The dermatophytes that are the causative agents of the tinea infections (choices C, D, and E) usually have single conidiospores and are characterized by their macroconidial forms.

41. **(E)** Studies of autopsy samples from Alzheimer disease patients indicate a loss of cholinergic neurons such as those in the nucleus basalis of Maynert. Following the model of enhancing dopamine to treat the loss of dopaminergic neurons in Parkinson disease, anticholinesterase treatment has been used

to treat patients with Alzheimer disease. Tacrine is an aminoacridine inhibitor of cholinesterase. Use of tacrine appears to slightly slow the decline in cognitive function, but does not arrest the underlying neurodegenerative process. Reversible hepatotoxicity is an important adverse effect. Atracurium (choice A) is a competitive antagonist at the nicotinic receptor of the neuromuscular junction. Because of the drug's high polarity, it does not gain access to the CNS and exerts no action there. Although its use has not been reported in the treatment of Alzheimer disease, the muscarinic antagonist atropine (choice B) would exacerbate the loss of cognitive function. The H_2-blocker cimetidine (choice C) has no effect in Alzheimer disease. Ipratropium (choice D) is a muscarinic antagonist used in treatment of asthmatic bronchoconstriction. It does not enter the CNS and would not have beneficial effects in Alzheimer disease if it did.

42. **(A)** Cervicofacial actinomycosis (lumpy jaw) is an endogenous infection usually preceded by a tooth extraction or some other traumatic injury to the mouth. The lesion commonly drains to the cheek or submandibular area. The presence of sulfur granules is of great diagnostic importance. These are actually small (approximately 1 mm in diameter) colonies of the organism in a calcium phosphate matrix. They consist of a central filamentous mass of branching bacilli surrounded by radially oriented, club-shaped structures. Amebiasis (choice B), candidiasis (choice C), histoplasmosis (choice D), and mucormycosis (choice E) are caused by a protozoan and fungi that do not produce sulfur granules.

43. **(B)** When cardiac muscle contracts, it squeezes blood vessels that course through it, and this extravascular compression has a significant effect on coronary blood flow. In early systole, there is an actual reversal of blood flow, and although coronary blood flow increases during systole, it is not until the ventricle relaxes that maximal left coronary artery blood flows are obtained. Peak flows are obtained in early diastole, when the ventricle is relaxed and aortic pressure has not declined to its diastolic level. During systole (choices A, C, and E), ventricular muscle contraction impedes coronary blood flow. During late diastole (choice D), coronary blood flow decreases because of the lower aortic blood pressure compared to early diastole.

44. **(B)** Precise tactile discriminative sensations from the right side of the face (including the teeth) travel via the ipsilateral trigeminal nerve to the ipsilateral principal (chief) sensory trigeminal nucleus (not the spinal trigeminal nucleus, choice C). Sensation from the maxillary teeth is carried to the chief sensory nucleus in the ipsilateral (not contralateral, choice A) spinal trigeminal tract. Somatosensory information from the face travels across the midline via the contralateral ventral trigeminothalamic tract to eventually reach the contralateral (not ipsilateral, choice D) ventral posteromedial thalamic nucleus. The ventral trigeminothalamic tract originates (not terminates, choice E) in the contralateral chief sensory and spinal trigeminal nuclei.

45. **(C)** Individuals with sickle trait are healthy and not anemic. Hemoglobin electrophoresis demonstrates a minor proportion of hemoglobin S and a major proportion of hemoglobin A. Fetal hemoglobin and A_2 hemoglobin are usually normal. Sickle trait confers the benefit of protecting erythrocytes from some forms of malarial infection. About 9% of blacks in the United States have sickle trait. In sickle cell disease (choice A), almost all hemoglobin is hemoglobin S. No hemoglobin A is detected and patients have a clinical history of severe anemia. Sickle thalassemia minor (choice B) presents as a chronic microcytic anemia with a major hemoglobin S component and an elevated hemoglobin A_2. Thalassemia major (choice D) and thalassemia minor (choice E) do not demonstrate hemoglobin S on electrophoresis.

46. **(E)** During anaerobic glycolysis, that period of time when glycolysis is proceeding at a high rate, the oxidation of NADH occurs

through the reduction of an organic substrate. Erythrocytes and skeletal muscle (under conditions of exertion) derive all of their ATP needs through anaerobic glycolysis. The large quantity of NADH produced is oxidized by reducing pyruvate to lactate. This reaction is carried out by lactate dehydrogenase (LDH). The lactate produced during anaerobic glycolysis diffuses from the tissues and is transported to highly aerobic tissues such as liver. The lactate is then oxidized to pyruvate in these cells by LDH and the pyruvate is further oxidized in the TCA cycle. If the energy level is high in liver cells, the carbons of pyruvate are diverted back to glucose via the gluconeogenesis pathway. The cycle of glucose oxidation to lactate in skeletal muscle with the delivery of the lactate to liver for its conversion to glucose, which can then be delivered to skeletal muscle for oxidation, is referred to as the Cori cycle. The metabolism of lactate by liver effectively shifts this metabolic burden from muscle to liver. None of the other choices (A, B, C, and D) refers to the process of the Cori cycle.

47. **(E)** Ondansetron is a very effective antiemetic in chemotherapy-induced and postsurgical vomiting. Muscarinic acetylcholine receptors (choice A) do not appear to be involved in chemotherapy-induced emesis, although scopolamine is effective in preventing vomiting due to motion sickness. DOPA receptors (choice B) are not recognized, but dopamine receptors are involved in the action of the dopamine antagonist metoclopramide, another drug used to control chemotherapy-induced emesis. Glucocorticoid receptors (choice C) are important for the action of dexamethasone, another useful drug for chemotherapy-induced vomiting. Histamine H_1 receptors (choice D) are blocked by diphenhydramine, a drug that is useful in both chemotherapy- and motion sickness-induced vomiting.

48. **(A)** Unlike other types of hypersensitivity (types I through III), which are associated with antibodies, histamine, and antigen–antibody complexes, delayed-type hypersensitivity reactions are initiated by antigen-specific T cells. Delayed-type hypersensitivity can be transferred in vivo with sensitized T cells alone. Immediate-type allergy (choice B), but not delayed-type, is suppressed by antihistaminic drugs. Anaphylaxis and allergic rhinitis (type I hypersensitivity) is due to IgE absorbed on mast cells. IgE is not involved in delayed-type (type IV) hypersensitivity (choice D). The destruction of lung tissue seen in tuberculosis, histoplasmosis, and blastomycosis is believed to be associated with delayed-type hypersensitivity. Therefore, this allergy causes tissue damage (choice C). Inhalation of grass pollens, molds, house dust, and dandruff are the usual allergens that induce type I or immediate hypersensitivity, not delayed-type allergy (choice E).

49. **(C)** Alkalemia is the presence of lower than normal levels of H^+ ions in blood. Because ventilation and elimination of CO_2 is a major and rapid mechanism of blood pH adjustment, severe alkalemia results in hypoventilation to elevate P_{CO_2} to buffer blood pH toward the normal range. The other options (choices A, B, D, and E) are all opposite of what is observed in alkalemia.

50. **(C)** All of the drugs listed are antiviral agents. Didanosine is a nucleoside that acts on HIV by inhibiting reverse transcriptase. Acyclovir (choice A) is an antiherpes agent that blocks DNA transcriptase. Amantadine (choice B) is an anti-influenza agent that interferes in a poorly understood manner with viral absorption and uncoating in the host cell. Ribavirin (choice D) is useful in respiratory syncitial virus infections and probably acts on viral RNA synthesis. Saquinavir (choice E) is an anti-HIV drug that blocks viral protease.

51. **(E)** The ability of epinephrine to signal breakdown of triglyceride to free fatty acids and glycerol is mediated by cAMP (see Figure 9–15). Epinephrine binds to receptors of the β-adrenergic class on the surface of adipose cells that, in turn, triggers the activation of adenylate cylcase. Adenylate cyclase con-

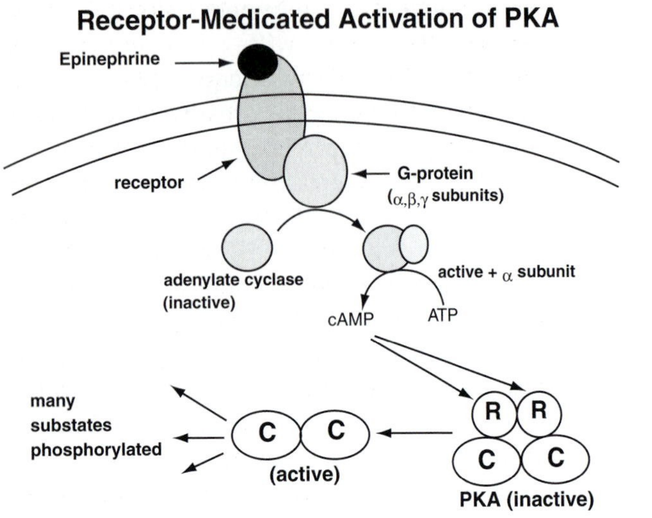

Receptor-Medicated Activation of PKA

Figure 9–15

verts ATP to cAMP. When cAMP is formed, it binds to the regulatory subunits of cAMP-dependent protein kinase (PKA), resulting in release and activation of the catalytic subunits. In the context of fat release from adipose tissue triglycerides, PKA phosphorylates and activates hormone-sensitive lipase. Hormone-sensitive lipase then hydrolyzes fatty acids from stored triglycerides. The free fatty acids and the glycerol backbone can be released to the blood and then taken up by various tissues, such as the liver. Choices A, B, C, and D represent hormones that function to regulate pathways of phosphatidylinositol signaling.

52. **(B)** The photomicrograph displays the distinctive fruiting head structure diagnostic for *Aspergillus* species. Pulmonary infections by these organisms may include allergic bronchopulmonary aspergillosis, cavity-occupying aspergilloma, or invasive aspergillosis. Asbestosis (choice A) displays iron-encrusted, baton-shaped asbestos bodies. Fungal bodies are not seen. Blastomycosis (choice C) is diagnosed if large, encapsulated budding yeasts are evident. Histoplasmosis (choice D) demonstrates small, yeast-shaped organisms or multinucleate giant cells. Microscopic examination of sputum from individuals with tuberculosis (choice E) may reveal multinucleate giant cells.

53. **(A)** Warts caused by papillomaviruses are nonmalignant tumors of squamous cells. Thus, infectious papillomaviruses are most likely to be found in terminally differentiated squamous cells, and not in the basal cells (choice B), in the surface layer of warts (choice C), only transformed cancer cells (choice D), or throughout the wart (choice E).

54. **(A)** The internal acoustic meatus is a feature of the posterior cranial fossa. It transmits cranial nerves VII and VIII. The abducens nerve in the cavernous sinus (choice B) lies in the middle cranial fossa along the body of the sphenoid bone. The mandibular division of the trigeminal nerve (choice C) exits the middle cranial fossa through the foramen ovale. The temporal lobe of the cerebral hemisphere (choice D) occupies the middle cranial fossa. The temporomandibular joint (choice E) is the joint between the head of the mandible and the mandibular fossa of the squamous part of the temporal bone. The mandibular fossa is related superiorly to the middle cranial fossa.

55. **(E)** Repression is the psychological defense mechanism that relegates unpleasant memories into the unconscious. Denial (choice B) blocks perception and therefore unpleasant facts never become processed as memory. The patient gave consent yesterday, indicating that the reason for the biopsy was understood then. The other options (choices A, C, and D) are obviously inappropriate.

56. **(A)** Creatine and the energy reserve form phosphocreatine are present in skeletal muscle, brain, and blood. Creatine synthesis begins in the kidney from arginine and glycine. The products of the first reaction are ornithine and guanidoacetate. Guanidoacetate is transported to the liver where it is converted to creatine by methylation from S-adenosylmethionine. Phosphorylation of creatine is carried out by creatine kinase (CK). CK plays an important role in the reversible transfer of phosphate from ATP to creatine when energy levels are high, and then from creatine to ADP when energy levels fall and

demand for energy is high. Creatine can spontaneously cyclize to creatinine. Creatinine clearance by any given individual is amazingly constant from day to day and is proportional to muscle mass. None of the other amino acid choices (B, C, D, and E) are involved in creatine synthesis.

57. **(D)** Of the five immunoglobulin classes, only IgM has a pentameric configuration displayed in Figure 9–9. IgM is the first immunoglobulin to appear in the serum upon initial exposure of an antigen to the immune system. Peak levels of IgM occur about 1 week after initial exposure to the sensitizing antigen. IgA (choice A) may be encountered as either a monomer or dimer, but not as a pentamer. IgE (choice B), IgD (choice C), and IgG (choice E) only exhibit a monomer configuration.

58. **(A)** Endometriosis is the presence of endometrial tissue in a site other than the lining of the endometrial cavity. It most commonly occurs in the ovaries, wall of a fallopian tube, parametrial soft tissue, and serosa of the intestine but can also occur at many other locations. This condition may be asymptomatic but is an important cause of infertility, dysmenorrhea, and pelvic pain. Repeated episodes of hemorrhage result in fibrosis, which can lead to peritoneal adhesions or intestinal obstruction. Involvement of the fallopian tubes can block the lumen and lead to infertility and an increased risk of ectopic pregnancy. Luteal phase dysfunction (choice B) is also a cause of infertility. Even though ovulation may occur, insufficient progesterone is produced to prepare the endometrial lining for implantation. This is not associated with the other findings of the case described. Ovarian carcinoma (choice C) may be divided into three main types: primary epithelial tumors, germ cell tumors, and sex cord–stromal tumors. Most of these tumors remain clinically silent until quite advanced; although the prognosis varies depending on the type and stage of the tumor, it is generally not good. The presentation of the case does not match that of ovarian carcinoma.

Pelvic inflammatory disease (choice D) is a common disorder in women in which there is infection of the fallopian tubes and ovaries as well as surrounding tissues. The most common causative agent is *Neisseria gonorrhoeae*, but several other organisms including *Chlamydia* have been implicated. Pelvic inflammatory disease is a cause of dyspareunia and sterility (as well as many other conditions), but the case does not indicate an infectious process and the hemorrhagic cysts are classic for endometriosis. Polycystic ovary disease (choice E) is characterized by bilaterally enlarged ovaries, numerous cystic follicles, and absence of corpora lutea (indicating failure of ovulation). In the presence of amenorrhea, this is referred to as the Stein–Leventhal syndrome. These patients have persistent anovulation, obesity, and hirsutism. This is one of the more common causes of infertility, but the other aspects of the case are not explained by polycystic ovary disease.

59. **(B)** The most frequent, early clinical manifestation of HIV infection is the development of a maculopapular rash on the trunk. Fever, generalized lymphadenopathy, lethargy, and sore throat also occur 2 to 4 weeks following infection. This is the acute phase of HIV infection. In the middle stage of HIV infection, which lasts for years, the patient is asymptomatic. Cytomegalic inclusion disease (choice A), disseminated *Mycobacterium avium-intracellulare* infections (choice C), non-Hodgkin lymphoma (choice D), or toxoplasmosis encephalitis (choice E) have all been associated with the late stage of HIV infection.

60. **(C)** Human chorionic gonadotropin is a glycoprotein similar in structure and function to LH from the anterior pituitary gland. hCG is produced by the syncytial trophoblast and prevents involution of the corpus luteum during pregnancy. Measurement at 16 to 18 weeks is recommended for all pregnant women as part of the triple screen. Ectopic pregnancy and trisomy 18 are associated with low serum hCG levels. Low levels of hCG also frequently indicate a threatened abortion. Choriocarcinoma (choice A), hyda-

tidiform mole (choice B), trisomy 21 (choice D), and twin pregnancy (choice E) are all associated with elevated levels of plasma hCG.

61. **(C)** Fibrosis is the major pathologic feature seen with chronic rheumatic heart disease. The mitral valve is almost always involved in this fibrotic process. Valvular stenosis is the usual late clinical sequela. The coronary arteries (choice A) are rarely affected by fibrotic, chronic rheumatic heart disease. The epicardium (choice B) may sustain some degree of adhesive pericarditis with chronic rheumatic heart disease, but it is seen far less frequently than mitral valve fibrosis. The pulmonary valve (choice D) is also less likely to be deranged than are the mitral or aortic valves. The right ventricle (choice E) is infrequently involved by endocardial fibrosis with chronic rheumatic heart disease.

62. **(D)** The vascular infarct in this case affects the left dorsal columns and dorsal column nuclei resulting in a loss of position sense in the left upper and lower extremities, but no involvement of dorsal column modalities on the right side (choice E). Damage to the dorsal medulla does not involve the pyramidal tract, and thus no hemiplegia (choice A) is expected. Pain and temperature sensibility (choice C) are unaffected, and there are no hyperactive reflexes in the left upper extremity (choice B).

63. **(B)** Glipizide is a second-generation sulfonylurea oral hypoglycemic drug. Like glyburide and glimepiride, it is extremely potent but otherwise similar to the older sulfonylureas such as tolbutamide. Its mechanism of action is to increase insulin release from B cells by closing K^+ channels and depolarizing pancreatic cells. The thiazolidinediones (e.g., rosiglitazone, pioglitazone) reduce peripheral insulin resistance by binding to nuclear PPAR-γ receptors (choice A). Direct stimulation of glucose uptake (choice C) has only been proven for insulin. The mechanism of action of the biguanides (e.g., metformin) is still not understood, but suggestions include those listed for choice D as well as increased glu-

cose removal from the blood and reduced glucose absorption from the intestine. Intestinal α-glucosidase inhibitors in current use (choice E) include acarbose and miglitol. By reducing the breakdown of starch and disaccharides in the intestine, they reduce postprandial hyperglycemia.

64. **(A)** The adrenal gland contains a cortical adenoma. Grossly, these neoplasms appear as well-demarcated, round to oval, yellowish, solitary nodules arising within the adrenal cortex. The surrounding non-neoplastic cortex is thinned and atrophic. The underlying medulla is normal. The associated clinical findings suggest Cushing syndrome due to excessive secretion of cortisol by the adenoma. Krukenberg tumor (choice B) is an enlarged ovary due to metastatic carcinoma. Adrenal infarcts (choice C) may be associated with certain bacterial infections and shock. The gland appears diffusely hemorrhagic and necrotic, without the formation of a discrete tumor nodule. Neuroblastoma (choice D) is an adrenal tumor of infancy. The typical gross appearance is a large, tan hemorrhagic mass. Hypercortisolemia is not seen. A pheochromocytoma (choice E) appears as a hemorrhagic, red-tan medullary tumor. Clinically, there may be signs of excessive norepinephrine secretion.

65. **(C)** The clinical and gross anatomic findings suggest a diagnosis of Cushing syndrome due to a functioning adrenal cortical adenoma. Cortisol is the most likely analyte to be elevated. Elevations of CA-125 (choice A) can be seen with serous carcinomas of the ovary. Carcinoembryonic antigen (choice B) is usually elevated with carcinomas of the breast, lung, or GI tract. Neuron-specific enolase (choice D) may be elevated with neuroblastoma. Norepinephrine (choice E) may be elevated episodically with pheochromocytomas.

66. **(E)** Oxidized glutathione (GSSG) is reduced through the action of glutathione reductase. The activity of glutathione reductase is dependent upon the oxidized cofactor NADPH. NADPH is derived during the two oxidative

reactions of the pentose phosphate pathway, glucose-6-phosphate dehydrogenase and 6-phosphogluconate dehydrogenase. Because NADPH is required in the glutathione reductase reaction and not NADH, choices A, B, and C are incorrect. NADPH is required for fatty acid synthesis (choice D), but is not produced during this process.

67. **(E)** *Mycoplasma pneumoniae* is a microorganism that lacks cell wall, and therefore is resistant to penicillin, which inhibits cell wall synthesis. Thus, incorporation of penicillin into a culture medium used for the isolation of *M. pneumoniae* has no effect on its growth but prevents the growth other organisms. Doxycycline (choice A), erythromycin (choice B), minocycline (choice C), and oxytetracycline (choice D) are effective antibiotics for the treatment of mycoplasmal infections.

68. **(B)** All of the drugs listed can be used in congestive heart failure. The cardiac glycosides such as digoxin inhibit Na^+/K^+-ATPase at the plasma membrane. Inhibition of the sodium pump causes an elevation of intracellular sodium ion concentration and a resultant decrease in sodium–calcium exchange. The increased intracellular calcium concentration produces the therapeutic increase in cardiac contractility needed in congestive heart failure. The cardiac glycosides decrease heart rate by enhancing baroreceptor sensitivity and producing a reflex withdrawal of the elevated sympathetic tone associated with heart failure. Captopril (choice A) has no direct effect on contractility or heart rate but reduces sympathetic tone and may indirectly reduce heart rate. It is a first-line agent in chronic failure because of its combination of antiangiotensin, antisympathetic, and anti-remodeling actions. Furosemide (choice C) is a first-line agent in acute failure, especially if pulmonary edema is present. It is one of the most efficacious diuretics available and in addition reduces pulmonary vascular pressure. Metoprolol (choice D) is a β-blocker that has been shown to reduce morbidity and mortality in chronic failure. It should not be initiated in acute failure because of its negative inotropic action. Nitroprusside (choice E) is an extremely efficacious vasodilator that is particularly useful in severe acute failure with elevated preload and afterload. It must be used parenterally by IV infusion.

69. **(D)** Benzoylecgonine is the urinary metabolite of cocaine. It is detectable in urine for about 24 h after the last episode of cocaine use. There is no evidence of a chromosomal abnormality (choice A) or a congenital deformity (choice B) from the given history. Status asthmaticus (choice C) is an occasional cause of sudden death in young males. Autopsy findings of bronchial mucous plugs and distended lungs are the usual correlates. If the decedent was taking chemotherapy for cancer (choice E), either residual neoplasm or chemotherapeutic metabolites should have been noted at necropsy.

70. **(D)** Remember that concentration equals amount of substance divided by volume. Therefore,

$$\begin{aligned} \text{urine volume} &= \text{urine solute output}/ \\ &\quad \text{urine osmolarity} \\ &= 900 \text{ mosm/day}/150 \\ &\quad \text{mosm/L} \\ &= 6.0 \text{ L/day} \end{aligned}$$

Plasma volume (choice E) is not required for this calculation.

71. **(C)** Clearance is the amount of plasma contained the solute excreted. Because, in this patient, the urine solute concentration is half the plasma concentration, the amount of plasma concentration (the amount of plasma contained this solute) must be half the urine volume per day. Alternatively, you can calculate clearance from the usual equation:

$$\begin{aligned} \text{Clearance} &= \text{urine flow} \bullet [\text{urine} \\ &\quad \text{concentration}]/[\text{plasma} \\ &\quad \text{concentration}] \\ &= 6.0 \text{ L/d} \bullet 150 \\ &\quad \text{mosm/L}/300 \text{ mosm/L} \\ &= 3.0 \text{ L/d} \end{aligned}$$

Plasma volume (choice E) is not required for this calculation. Clearance is the fraction of plasma volume that contained the excreted amount of solutes (per day or minute).

72. **(D)** Free water clearance (C_{H_2O}) is the gain or loss of water by excretion of concentrated or diluted urine. In dilute urine it equals the amount of water lost that did not contribute to excretion of solutes. In other words

$$C_{H_2O} = \text{urine flow} - \text{solute clearance}$$
$$= 6.0 \text{ L/d} - 3.0 \text{ L/d}$$
$$= +3.0 \text{ L/d}$$

Choices A and B: Negative values indicate water conservation, and positive values indicate water loss. If the urine were more concentrated than the plasma, free water clearance would be < 0 (antidiuresis). Calculation of free water clearance requires knowledge of solute clearance, but not knowledge of inulin clearance (choice E).

73. **(A)** Generally speaking, urine flow increases with solute load (amount of solutes excreted). Patients with diabetes insipidus are unable to concentrate their urine and require a larger urine volume to excrete the solute load. Therefore, relationship A supports a diagnosis of diabetes insipidus. Line B indicates excretion of urine that is isosmotic to plasma. Line C indicates urine production in the presence of maximal vasopressin effect. Lines D and E are false, because urine flow increases with solute load.

74. **(E)** Vasopressin generally increases urine concentration and results in antidiuresis. Patients with renal diabetes insipidus have defective vasopressin receptors and IV injection of vasopressin fails to increase urine osmolarity. These patients already have a high level of circulating vasopressin. In central diabetes (choice A), the posterior pituitary gland fails to produce adequate amounts of vasopressin. However, the kidneys respond normally (i.e., concentrating the urine) when vasopressin is injected. Patients with diabetes mellitus (choice B) often are in a state of osmotic di-

uresis because of the high plasma and urine glucose concentration. Vasopressin increases urine osmolarity in these patients. Therefore, water deprivation tests should not be performed in patients with diabetes mellitus because of severe risk of hyperosmolar coma. Because the patient's kidneys do not respond to vasopressin, choice C must be false. Patients with psychogenic polydipsia (choice D) should have concentrated urine following water deprivation.

75. **(C)** In a population of 100,000, 10,000 will have the disease and 90,000 will be disease free (the prevalence of the disease equals 10%). The sensitivity is 90%, which indicates that in a population of people with the disease, 90% will have a positive test result (true positives) and 10% will have a negative test result (false negatives). The specificity also equals 90%, which indicates that in a population of people without the disease, 90% will have a negative test result (true negatives) and 10% will have a positive test result (false positives). Thus, looking at the positive test results, there were 9,000 true positives (90% of the 10,000 people with the disease) and 9,000 false positives (10% of the 90,000 people without the disease). Therefore the chances of the test result being a true positive are (true positives)/(true positives + false positives) = (9,000)/(9,000 + 9,000) = 50%. Mathematically, 1% (choice A), 10% (choice B), 90% (choice D), and 100% (choice E) can be eliminated.

76. **(B)** In obsessive-compulsive behavior, the patient recognizes the irrationality of the compulsion but not engaging in it causes extreme anxiety. Bipolar disorder (choice A) and schizophrenia (chioce D) are possible diagnoses in which some obsessive-compulsive behavior may or may not occur. In panic states (chioce C), the patient experiences extreme anxiety but does not engage in repetitive behavior. Undoing (choice E) may be a component of compulsive behavior when the meaning of the behavior is elucidated.

77. **(B)** Circumstantiality is an inability to get to the point without laborious elaborations.

Autistic thinking (choice A) is a more generic term denoting psychotic thinking. Folie à deux (choice C) is delusion shared by two people. Loose association (choice D) is characterized by loosening of the associative (thought process) linkages. Thought blocking (choice E) is sudden absence of thought.

78. **(D)** An illusion is a misperception of sensory stimulus, as in this case she seems to perceive the IV pole as a threatening object. Hallucination (choice C), on the other hand, is perception without apparent sensory stimulus. Ambivalence (choice A) is having strong opposing feelings at the same time, a delusion (choice B) is a belief not based on reality, and negativism (choice E) is persistent negative response.

79. **(A)** Agitation refers to a state of anxiety and increased activity as manifested by pacing in this case. Catalepsy (choice B) refers to waxy flexibility seen in catatonia. Cataplexy (choice C) is sudden loss of muscle tone. Catatonia (choice D) is characterized by rigid muscle tone, immobility, and mutism. Hebephrenia (choice E) is a disorganized type of schizophrenia.

80. **(C)** For acute agitation, reassurance is helpful, followed by an antianxiety agent if necessary. Restraints (choice D) increase agitation and are not indicated in the absence of any dangerous behavior. Sertraline (choice E) is an antidepressant and is unlikely to have an immediate effect. The other choices are inappropriate because they require preparation (choice A) or lengthy treatment (choice B).

81. **(E)** The patient has loosening of association, catatonic rigidity, and delusions, making schizophrenia the most likely diagnosis. The onset of symptoms in her teens supports this diagnosis. Bipolar disorder (choice A) is not impossible, but there is no evidence of mania or severe depression. There is no evidence of a general medical condition (choice D) that may cause psychosis, and she has more symptoms of schizophrenia than just a delusion (choice B). Folie á deux (choice C) involves two people.

82. **(E)** An atypical antipsychotic drug such as risperidone is likely to be effective for the hallucinations, delusions, loosening of association, and catatonia. Unlike typical antipsychotics such as haloperidol, the atypical antipsychotics also tend to treat the negative symptoms of schizophrenia, and have fewer extrapyramidal side effects. Benztropine (choice A), an anticholinergic, may be useful if she develops neuroleptic-induced pseudoparkinsonism. Chlordiazepoxide (choice B), a benzodiazepine, is usually ineffective as a primary drug for psychosis. Lithium chloride (choice C) is useful for manic symptoms. Fluoxetine (choice D) is an antidepressant.

83. **(D)** The kidney contains a large renal cell carcinoma. These malignant tumors are more frequent in the elderly, and may first become apparent as flank pain or hematuria. Grossly, there is a large, solitary cortical mass whose surface displays a variegated red, yellow, and tan coloration. Necrosis is usually evident. The tumor may erode through the renal capsule or into the renal vein. There is no evidence of postrenal process (choice A), congenital anomaly (choice B), an infectious process (choice C), or calculi (choice E) in Figure 9–13.

84. **(C)** In a paraesophageal hiatus hernia, part of the fundus contained within a peritoneal pouch extends through the esophageal hiatus of the diaphragm. The hernia is normally located anterior to the esophagus. All the other portions of the stomach—body (choice A), cardia (choice B), pyloric antrum (choice D), and pylorus (choice E)—remain in their normal position.

85. **(E)** The enterotoxins are considered to be quite heat resistant; after boiling crude solutions for 30 minutes, some toxicity remains. They are also resistant to proteolytic enzymes such as trypsin, chymotrypsin, rennin, and papain. Approximately 30% of strains of *S. aureus* isolated from patients produce enterotoxins. Synthesis of enterotoxins by *S. epidermidis* is doubtful. Six antigenically distinct types of enterotoxins—A, B, C, C2, D, and

E—are produced by *S. aureus*. Enterotoxin A has been most frequently implicated in food intoxication in the United States (choice D). Botulinum toxin is responsible for the blockage of the release of acetylcholine at the neuromuscular junction (choice A). Disruption of the cytoplasmic membrane (choice B) is due to the action of the various hemolysins elaborated by *S. aureus*. Disruption of the stratum granulosum (choice C) in the epidermis is due to the action of exfoliative toxins, which are produced by some strains of *S. aureus*. The exfoliative toxins A and B are responsible for the development of the staphylococcal scalded skin syndrome.

86. **(C)** Arsenic exists naturally in both inorganic and organic forms. Arsenate can substitute for phosphate in oxidative phosphorylation to form an unstable ATP analog that spontaneously hydrolyzes, thus essentially uncoupling oxidative phosphorylation. The trivalent forms readily react with sulfhydryl compounds including enzymes and lipoic acid. Pyruvate dehydrogenase is particularly sensitive to this inhibition. Arsenic poisoning is treated with chelation therapy using dimercaprol, succimer (2,3-dimercaptosuccinic acid), or penicillamine. Calcium disodium edetate (choice A) binds any available divalent or trivalent metal that has a greater affinity for EDTA than calcium. In lead poisoning, for example, the calcium ion in calcium disodium edetate is readily displaced by lead, forming a lead chelate that is excreted in the urine. Deferoxamine (choice B) is an iron-chelating agent used in the treatment of toxicity from iron. This may arise from ingestion of iron supplements (as with children swallowing adult preparations), or diseases such as thalassemia. Folic acid (choice D) is a necessary dietary constituent that functions in synthesis of purines and pyrimidines. Thiosulfate (choice E) is used to treat cyanide toxicity. The mitochondrial enzyme rhodanese combines cyanide and thiosulfate to form thiocyanate, which is excreted by the kidney.

87. **(D)** The infection caused by measles virus is characterized by hacking cough, fever, runny nose, conjunctivitis, rash, and the presence of the red-based, blue-white centered oral lesions known as Koplik spots. Adenovirus (choice A), coronavirus (choice B), and orthomyxovirus (choice E) produce influenza-like infections without rash or Koplik spots. Hantavirus (choice C) is the etiologic agent of Korian hemorrhagic fever. This disease causes petechial hemorrhages, renal failure, fever, and shock, but it does not produce Koplik spots.

88. **(B)** Fibrous dysplasia of bone is a benign lesion that may involve a single bone (monostotic, 70% of cases) or multiple bones (polyostotic). A single lesion may be clinically silent and come to attention incidentally, may cause pain, or may result in a pathologic fracture. Polyostotic disease is more likely to produce progressive disease with more severe complications including bone deformities. The lesions are readily recognized by their radiologic and microscopic appearance as described. Chondroma (choice A) is a common benign neoplasm most frequently found in the diaphysis with the bones of the hands and feet being most commonly involved. Microscopically, hyaline cartilage is seen. Giant cell tumor (choice C) is another fairly common benign neoplasm, but it usually arises in the epiphysis. Microscopically, it is composed of fibroblast-like spindle cells with numerous osteoclast-like giant cells. Osteoblastoma (choice D) is an uncommon, benign lesion that is more often found in the vertebrae but can occur anywhere in the skeleton. It has a similar microscopic appearance to an osteoid osteoma (see below) but is larger (> 2 cm) and produces a dull rather than sharp pain that is not relieved by aspirin. Osteoid osteoma (choice E) is a small, painful bone lesion that is more often found in men under 25 years of age. The associated sharp pain is unusually severe for a small lesion but is readily relieved by aspirin. Microscopically, it is found to be well circumscribed by a rim of reactive bone in the center of which is a mass of thin, irregular trabeculae.

89. **(E)** All neurons within the peripheral nervous system, including sympathetic ganglion

cells, arise from neural crest cells. Microglia (choice A) are derived from mesenchymal cells, which invade the nervous system during development. Motoneurons in the spinal cord (choice B) arise from the neuroepithelium of the neural tube and so do the oligodendroglia (choice C) and protoplasmic astroglia (choice D).

90. **(D)** The neurologic signs point to an injury of the sciatic nerve. The sciatic nerve supplies the hamstring muscles and, by its tibial and common peroneal (fibular) divisions, all muscles below the knee. Sensory innervation below the knee is also mediated by the tibial and common peroneal nerves, except for a narrow area along the lower leg and medial border of the foot. This area is innervated by the saphenous nerve, a branch of the femoral nerve (choice B). The patient still has weak flexion of the knee because of the action of the sartorius and gracilis muscle. These latter muscles are innervated by the femoral and obturator nerves, respectively. Isolated injury of the common peroneal (fibular) nerve (choice A) or tibial nerve (choice E) is not sufficient to give rise to all the neurologic signs described. The femoral (choice B) and obturator (choice C) nerves innervate muscles of the anterior and medial aspect of the thighs, which are functional in this patient.

91. **(B)** The clinical features of leptospirosis (Weil disease) include intense headache, stiff neck, hepatitis, and nephritis. This disease is caused by *Leptospira interrogans,* a spirochete. The germ has tightly coiled spirals with hooks at its ends that serve to differentiate it from spirochetes belonging to genera *Treponema* and *Borrelia.* Legionellosis (choice A) is caused by *Legionella pneumophila,* which is a gram-negative rod. This organism causes an influenza-like illness that can progress to severe pneumonia, mental confusion, diarrhea, proteinuria, and microscopic hematuria. Pinta (choice C) is caused by *Treponema carateum,* a spirochete similar to *T. pertenue* and *T. pallidum.* Pinta is another nonvenereal disease characterized by hyperpigmentation of the skin. Relapsing fever (choice D) is caused

by *B. recurrentis.* This spirochete is twice as big as *L. interrogans,* has large spirals, and lacks hooks at its ends. Relapsing fever begins with a high fever of 100 to 102°C, headache, muscle spasms, and splenomegaly. It has a characteristic spiking curve, which is due to emergence of various antigenic variants. Yaws (choice E) is characterized by the development of cauliflower-like lesions. It is caused by *Treponema pertenue.* This spirochete has acute spiral curves and pointed ends. It is a nonvenereal disease that is transmitted by direct contact with infected persons.

92. **(B)** Scarpa's ganglion contains the cell bodies of the primary afferent neurons whose peripheral processes form synaptic contact with hair cells of the vestibular sensory end organs. The stria vascularis (choice C) and tunnel of Corti (choice D) are parts of the auditory system. The external cuneate nucleus (choice A) and zone of Lissauer (choice E) are parts of the somatosensory system.

93. **(A)** Type I hypersensitivity, or anaphylaxis, is an IgE-mediated reaction to a previously sensitizing antigen. Mast cells and basophils orchestrate this process through the release of preformed substances such as histamine, heparin, and chemotactic factors. Type II hypersensitivity (choice B) occurs as an antigen–antibody reaction on the surface of the host cell. A hemolytic transfusion reaction is an example of this type of immune injury. Type III hypersensitivity (choice C) uses circulating antigen–antibody complexes such as Arthus reaction or serum sickness to produce immune injury. Type IV hypersensitivity (choice D) is a cell-mediated delayed reaction that usually involves a granulomatous inflammatory response.

94. **(C)** Apo(a) is a large glycoprotein with a striking degree of homology to the clotting factor plasminogen, in that apo(a) contains numerous kringle IV domains. There are more than 30 size alleles of apo(a) due to differing numbers of kringle IV domains, which in turn yield more than 500 potential different phenotypes of the protein. The apo(a) protein is

disulfide bonded to apoB-100 of LDLs, generating a lipoprotein particle identified as Lp(a). The size of apo(a) allows it to occupy the exterior surface of the resultant Lp(a) particle, exposing its kringle IV domains to the vasculature. The presence of the plasminogen-like kringle domains in apo(a) suggests that it interferes with the normal process of thrombosis at the endothelial cell surface by inducing a prothrombotic state, and evidence indicates that this does indeed occur. This leads to the deposition of fibrin clots and atherosclerotic plaque formation. ApoA-I (choice A) is a major component of HDLs necessary for the activation of lecithin-cholesterol acyltransferase (LCAT) and is not associated with apo(a). ApoB-48 (choice B) is exclusively associated with chylomicrons and therefore is not found in association with apo(a). ApoC-II (choice D) is required in chylomicrons, VLDLs, LDL, and IDLs for the activation of endothelial cell-associated lipoprotein lipase, but is not linked to apo(a). ApoE (choice E) is necessary for chylomicron remnant and LDL interaction with the hepatic LDL receptor and is not associated with apo(a).

95. **(A)** The external nasal nerve is the terminal cutaneous branch of the anterior ethmoidal nerve (from the nasociliary branch of the ophthalmic nerve). It emerges from the inner surface of the nasal bone to be distributed to the skin down the dorsum of the nose. The lacrimal nerve (choice B) is a branch of the ophthalmic nerve that supplies the lacrimal gland and then becomes cutaneous to supply the conjunctiva and skin of the upper eyelid. The supraorbital nerve (choice C) is a cutaneous branch of the frontal nerve (from the ophthalmic nerve) and is distributed to the skin of the forehead, scalp, and upper eyelid. The supratrochlear nerve (choice D) is a cutaneous branch of the frontal nerve (from the ophthalmic nerve) and is distributed to the skin of the lower medial forehead. The zygomaticotemporal nerve (choice E) is a cutaneous branch of the maxillary nerve.

96. **(D)** In dynamic (isotonic) aerobic exercise, workload and body oxygen consumption are directly related (indeed it is often easier to calculate the workload from the oxygen consumption than to measure it directly). Although mean arterial blood pressure and systolic arterial blood pressure rise with increasing levels of dynamic exercise, diastolic blood pressure (choice A) remains virtually constant. With increasing levels of exercise, blood flow to the skin (choice B) decreases at first, but then as heat production from the exercising muscles begins to increase, blood flow to the skin also increases to aid in temperature regulation. Blood pressures in the pulmonary circulation (choice C) are much lower than in the systemic circulation. Even if the cardiac output were to increase fourfold during exercise, there would be only about a doubling of the pulmonary arterial blood pressure (e.g., from 12 to 24 mm Hg), which would be nowhere near systemic arterial pressures. With increased workload (or increased oxygen consumption), there is an almost perfectly linear increase in heart rate, whereas the curve for stroke volume (choice E) increases at first, but then levels off (plateau) at about half maximal workload (or half maximal oxygen consumption). Thus, for strenuous exercise, the increased levels of cardiac output depend almost entirely on increases in heart rate (at essentially a constant stroke volume).

97. **(A)** Acetaminophen is relatively nontoxic in ordinary dosage in individuals with normal hepatic function. In overdose and in individuals with impaired hepatic function, the drug may accumulate enough to overwhelm the normal sulfate and glucuronide conjugation pathways of metabolism. The alternative route of metabolism is a phase I-type P-450–dependent oxidation that produces reactive intermediates that may bind essential macromolecules in the hepatocyte. Hepatic failure and death may result. In patients with normal glutathione stores, these intermediates are scavenged and excreted as glutathione adducts. In the absence of glutathione, another sulfhydryl donor such as acetylcysteine can function as an antidote. Flumazenil is the antidote for benzodiazepine

overdosage (choice B). Deferoxamine is the chelator used for iron overdose (choice C). Naloxone is the preferred antidote for opioid overdose (choice D). No drugs are available that provide adequate antidotal effects for barbiturate overdosage (choice E). However, good symptomatic support, especially of respiration and circulation, reduces mortality from barbiturates to near zero.

98. **(C)** The photomicrograph shows a granuloma with central amorphous caseous necrosis and a number of Langhans giant cells and mononuclear cells in the periphery. This is a classic finding for tuberculosis, but can also be seen with other infectious agents such as *Coccidioides.* An abscess (choice A) would also show a central area of amorphous necrosis, but it would be accompanied by a neutrophilic rather than a mononuclear response. Carcinoma (choice B) is recognized by the presence of pleomorphic cells with invasion into adjacent tissue. Infarct (choice D) is the result of ischemic necrosis and appears as an area of coagulative necrosis in which tissue outlines can still be recognized, but there is no nuclear staining. Thrombus (choice E), by definition, appears within a vessel and, because this is the lung, would most likely be a thromboembolus. The lesion shown is not within a vessel and does not have the appearance of a thrombus (i.e., fibrin, trapped blood cells).

99. **(E)** The surface immunoglobulin of the immature B cell is IgM. The surface immunoglobulin synthesized by a B-cell clone serves as an antigen receptor for that clone (choice C). The surface immunoglobulins are not dimeric; they also contain a kappa or lambda chain (choice B). It is generally believed that different receptor isotypes have been generated to perform diverse functions on the same cells (choice A). Mature B cells have IgD on their surface (choice D) not IgE.

100. **(A)** Although multiorgan involvement, liver and spleen enlargement, and skeletal abnormalities are common to all the mucopolysaccharidotic (MPS) diseases, each encompasses specific and unique features. Each different MPS is caused by defects in different enzymes which allows for specific diagnosis. Hunter syndrome is characterized by progressive multiorgan failure and premature death. Hallmark features include enlargement of the spleen and liver, severe skeletal deformity, and coarse facial features (which are associated with the constellation of defects referred to as dystosis multiplex). Unlike Hurler syndrome, whose symptoms are similar (but more severe), Hunter syndrome does not cause corneal opacities. Hunter syndrome results from a defect in iduronidate sulfatase activity and this activity can be measured in the plasma. Hurler syndrome (choice B) has features similar to Hunter, but with the added symptom of corneal clouding. Hurler syndrome results from a defect in α-L-iduronidase. Maroteaux–Lamy syndrome (choice C) encompasses symptoms similar to Hurler, but with normal mental development. Maroteaux–Lamy syndrome results from a defect in *N*-acetylgalactosamine-4-sulfatase (also called arylsulfatase B). Morquio syndrome (choice D) comprises two related disorders (Morquio A and B), both of which are characterized by short-trunk dwarfism, fine corneal deposits, and a skeletal dysplasia (spondyloepiphyseal) distinct from other MPS. Morquio B results from a defect in β-galactosidase. Sanfilippo syndrome (choice E) comprises four recognized types (A, B, C, and D), all of which result from defects in the degradation of heparan sulfates. Sanfilippo syndromes are characterized by severe central nervous system degeneration with only mild involvement of other organ systems. Symptoms do not appear until 2 to 6 years of age. Sanfilippo A is the result of defects in α-*N*-acetyl-D-glucosaminidase.

REFERENCES

Aidley DJ. *The Physiology of Excitable Cells*, 4th ed. Cambridge, England: Cambridge University Press; 1998.

Berne RM, Levy MN. *Physiology*, 4th ed. St. Louis: Mosby-Year Book; 1998.

Braunwald E, Fauci AS, Kasper DL, et al. *Harrison's Principles of Internal Medicine*, 15th ed. New York: McGraw-Hill; 2001.

Brooks GF, Butel JS, Morse SA. *Jawetz, Melnick, and Adelberg's Medical Microbiology*, 22nd ed. Stamford, CT: Appleton & Lange; 2001.

Chandrasoma P, Taylor CR. *Concise Pathology*, 3rd ed. Stamford, CT: Appleton & Lange; 1998.

Devlin TM. *Textbook of Biochemistry: With Clinical Correlations*, 4th ed. New York: John Wiley & Sons; 1997.

Elkin GD. *Introduction to Clinical Psychiatry*. Stamford, CT: Appleton & Lange; 1998.

Ganong WF. *Review of Medical Physiology*, 20th ed. Stamford, CT: Appleton & Lange; 2001.

Guyton AC, Hall JE. *Textbook of Medical Physiology*, 10th ed. Philadelphia: WB Saunders; 2000.

Hall-Craggs ECB. *Anatomy as a Basis for Clinical Medicine*, 3rd ed. Baltimore: Williams & Wilkins; 1995.

Hardman JG, Limbird LE, Molinoff PB, et al. *Goodman & Gilman's The Pharmacological Basis of Therapeutics*, 9th ed. New York: McGraw-Hill; 1996.

Johnson LR. *Gastrointestinal Physiology*, 5th ed. St. Louis: Mosby-Year Book; 1997.

Kandel ER, Schwartz JH, Jessel TM. *Principles of Neural Science*, 5th ed. Stamford, CT: Appleton & Lange; 2000.

Kaplan HI, Sadock BJ. *Comprehensive Textbook of Psychiatry/VI CD-ROM*. Teton Data Systems, Jackson, Wyoming, Baltimore: Williams & Wilkins; 1998.

Kaplan HI, Sadock BJ. *Kaplan and Sadock's Synopsis of Psychiatry*, 8th ed. Baltimore: Williams & Wilkins; 1998.

Katzung BG. *Basic & Clinical Pharmacology*, 8th ed. Stamford, CT: Appleton & Lange; 2001.

Leigh H, Reiser MF. *The Patient: Biological, Psychological, and Social Dimensions of Medical Practice*, 3rd ed. New York: Plenum Press; 1992.

Levinson WE, Jawetz E. *Medical Microbiology & Immunology: Examination and Board Review*, 6th ed. Stamford, CT: Appleton & Lange; 2000.

Lewis WH, Elvin-Lewis MPF. *Medical Botany*. New York: John Wiley & Sons; 1977.

McArdle WD, Katch FI, Katch VL. *Exercise Physiology: Energy, Nutrition, and Human Performance*, 4th ed. Philadelphia: Lea & Febiger; 1996.

Moore KL. *Clinically Oriented Anatomy*, 3rd ed. Baltimore: Williams & Wilkins; 1992.

Mountcastle VB. *Medical Physiology*, 14th ed. St. Louis: Mosby-Year Book; 1980.

Murray PR, Rosenthal KS, Kobayashi GS, Pfaller MA. *Medical Microbiology*, 3rd ed. St. Louis: Mosby-Year Book; 1998.

Murray RK, Granner DK, Mayes PA, Rodwell VW. *Harper's Biochemistry*, 25th ed. Stamford, CT: Appleton & Lange; 2000.

Roitt I, Brostoff J, Male D. *Immunology*, 5th ed. London, UK: Mosby-Year Book; 1998.

Rose DB, Post T. *Clinical Physiology of Acid-base and Electrolyte Disorders*, 6th ed. New York: McGraw-Hill; 2001.

Rosse C, Gaddum-Rosse P. *Hollinshead's Textbook of Anatomy*, 5th ed. Philadelphia: Lippincott Raven Publishers; 1997.

Rubin F, Farber JL. *Pathology*, 3rd ed. Philadelphia: JB Lippincott; 1999.

Vander AJ. *Renal Physiology*, 5th ed. New York: McGraw-Hill; 1995.

West JB. *Pulmonary Pathophysiology—The Essentials*, 5th ed. Baltimore: Williams & Wilkins; 1998.

Woodburne RT, Burckel WE. *Essentials of Human Anatomy*, 9th ed. New York: Oxford University Press; 1994.

Subspecialty List: Practice Test II

Question Number and Subspecialty

1. Microbiology
2. Physiology
3. Pathology
4. Biochemistry
5. Physiology
6. Behavioral sciences
7. Anatomy
8. Pharmacology
9. Microbiology
10. Physiology
11. Biochemistry
12. Physiology
13. Pharmacology
14. Microbiology
15. Pathology
16. Physiology
17. Pathology
18. Biochemistry
19. Anatomy
20. Pharmacology
21. Microbiology
22. Pathology
23. Pathology
24. Physiology
25. Biochemistry
26. Anatomy
27. Pharmacology
28. Microbiology
29. Behavioral sciences
30. Physiology
31. Microbiology
32. Biochemistry
33. Anatomy
34. Pharmacology
35. Pathology
36. Microbiology
37. Physiology
38. Pharmacology
39. Biochemistry
40. Microbiology
41. Pharmacology
42. Microbiology
43. Physiology
44. Anatomy
45. Pathology
46. Biochemistry
47. Pharmacology
48. Microbiology
49. Physiology
50. Pharmacology
51. Physiology
52. Pathology
53. Microbiology
54. Anatomy
55. Behavioral sciences
56. Biochemistry
57. Microbiology
58. Pathology
59. Microbiology
60. Physiology
61. Pathology
62. Anatomy
63. Pharmacology
64. Pathology
65. Pathology
66. Biochemistry
67. Microbiology
68. Pharmacology
69. Pathology
70. Physiology
71. Physiology
72. Physiology
73. Physiology
74. Physiology

75. Pathology
76. Behavioral sciences
77. Behavioral sciences
78. Behavioral sciences
79. Behavioral sciences
80. Behavioral sciences
81. Behavioral sciences
82. Behavioral sciences
83. Pathology
84. Anatomy
85. Microbiology
86. Pharmacology
87. Microbiology
88. Pathology
89. Anatomy
90. Anatomy
91. Microbiology
92. Anatomy
93. Pathology
94. Biochemistry
95. Anatomy
96. Physiology
97. Pharmacology
98. Pathology
99. Microbiology
100. Biochemistry

CHAPTER 10

Practice Test III
Questions

68

DIRECTIONS: (Questions 1 through 100): Each of the numbered items or incomplete statements in this section is followed by answers or by completions of the statement. Select the ONE lettered answer or completion that is BEST in each case.

Questions 1 and 2

A 67-year-old white woman complains of gradually increasing fatigue. On physical examination she is found to be anemic and has a peripheral neuropathy characterized by loss of position and vibratory sense. Laboratory studies document an anemia, which is found to be macrocytic in character. In addition, her white blood cell count and platelets are both decreased.

1. What pathologic mechanism accounts for these findings?

    (A) A diet deficient in folate
    (B) Autoantibodies against parietal cells or intrinsic factor
    (C) Chronic blood loss
    (D) Diabetes mellitus
    (E) Myelodysplastic sideroblastic anemia

2. If this condition persists, which organ is at most risk for developing carcinoma?

    (A) Central nervous system (CNS)
    (B) Genital tract
    (C) Lung
    (D) Pancreas
    (E) Stomach

3. Symptoms such as resting tremor, akinesia, and bradykinesia are associated with Parkinson disease. Which of the following is currently thought to be related to the primary neural substrate of this disease?

    (A) Degeneration of neurons in the pars compacta of the substantia nigra
    (B) Facilitation of pyramidal tract neurons in the primary motor cortex
    (C) Loss of cholinergic interneurons in the caudate nucleus
    (D) Loss of GABA neurons in the ventrolateral nucleus of the thalamus
    (E) Vascular infarct in the subthalamic nucleus

4. A 62-year-old man develops a temperature of 101°F and bacteremia 7 days following the insertion of a mitral prosthesis. He was also fitted with IV catheters. Following the operation, this patient was treated for 5 days with penicillin, streptomycin, and methicillin. When his temperature rose to 101°F on the 7th postoperative day antibiotic treatment was changed to ampicillin. A blood culture yielded *Escherichia coli* that was sensitive to ampicillin. The most important initial step is to

    (A) avoid disturbing the mitral valve
    (B) continue treatment with ampicillin
    (C) culture the patient's urine
    (D) remove the IV catheters
    (E) treat with gentamycin

5. The dural reflection that separates the occipital lobe of the cerebrum from the cerebellum is the

(A) crista galli
(B) diaphragma sellae
(C) falx cerebelli
(D) falx cerebri
(E) tentorium cerebelli

6. Which enzyme in muscle glycogen metabolism can be activated by calcium?

(A) Glycogen branching enzyme
(B) Glycogen synthase-b
(C) Phosphorylase-a
(D) Phosphorylase-b
(E) Phosphorylase kinase-b

7. Patients who develop a blood clot (thrombophlebitis) are typically treated first with heparin and then with coumadin. A reason for not starting directly with coumadin is that

(A) coumadin also blocks synthesis of anticoagulant proteins S and C
(B) coumadin works immediately while the onset of heparin action is delayed
(C) coumadin's effect to increase hepatic drug metabolizing enzymes takes a few days
(D) heparin is a necessary cofactor for coumadin action
(E) heparin's primary effect is to prolong the partial thromboplastin time, not the prothrombin time, which is affected by coumadin

8. Flumazenil is an effective antidote for overdosage with

(A) buspirone
(B) diazepam
(C) ethanol
(D) morphine
(E) phenobarbital

9. If food poisoning is assumed to be due to enterotoxin produced by *Clostridium perfringens*, final confirmation will rest on

(A) demonstration of spores in suspected food
(B) enterotoxin production in food and neutralization by its antiserum
(C) growth of gram-positive bacilli in thioglycolate broth
(D) the presence of antibodies against *C. perfringens* in the patient's serum
(E) the presence of many gram-positive rods in food

10. Which of the following can be used to treat or prevent both Parkinson disease and influenza type A?

(A) Amantadine
(B) Benzotropine
(C) Bromocriptine
(D) Oseltamivir
(E) Ribavirin

11. Patients who exhibit a prolonged mucocutaneous bleeding time with a normal coagulation time, clot retraction, and platelet count, and have normal levels of the coagulation factor VIII, exhibit a deficiency in which protein involved in hemostasis?

(A) Factor IX
(B) Fibrinogen
(C) Thrombin
(D) Tissue factor (factor III)
(E) von Willebrand factor

12. A 63-year-old man has a 2-month history of back pain. An autopsy specimen of his spine is displayed in Figure 10–1. What abnormal process is evident?

(A) Degeneration
(B) Infection
(C) Ischemia
(D) Neoplasia
(E) Trauma

13. A patient has suffered a severe laceration in the right forearm in a work-related accident in a machine shop. His right hand has no sensory function in the medial part of the

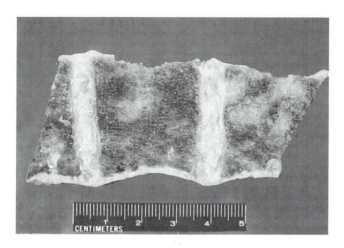

Figure 10–1

palm and the medial one and half digits. When the patient attempts to flex the wrist joint, the hand is drawn to the lateral side. When you ask the patient to make a fist, the patient cannot flex his fourth or fifth digits at the distal interphalangeal joints. These signs are typical of a lesion of the

(A) median nerve
(B) palmar cutaneous branch of the ulnar nerve
(C) radial nerve
(D) superficial branch of the radial nerve
(E) ulnar nerve

14. A 26-year-old man has peptic ulcer caused by *Helicobacter pylori.* Which of the following is the most likely natural habitat of this organism?

(A) Animals
(B) Feces
(C) Food
(D) Human stomach
(E) Water

15. Your patient is being overly controlling and exacting about his care, and complains about "sloppy" treatment. If he turns out to have a newly diagnosed serious medical condition, you should

(A) ask the patient if he would like to hear the bad news
(B) tell the family about the diagnosis, and tell the patient he should discuss it with the family
(C) tell the patient about the diagnosis in great detail
(D) tell the patient about the diagnosis in very general terms, with a cheerful attitude
(E) withhold the information from the patient

16. A woman with insulin-dependent diabetes (IDDM) is late for her tennis match and does not have time to eat breakfast. She injected her usual dose of insulin, normally given 30 minutes before breakfast. The insulin injection coupled with playing tennis will

(A) cause severe hypoglycemia, by stimulating the transport of glucose into skeletal muscles where it will be rapidly oxidized due to the increased level of activity
(B) have little effect because her tissues are utilizing fatty acids under these conditions
(C) increase the uptake of glucose into brain, thereby preventing her from developing hypoglycemic symptoms
(D) inhibit gluconeogenesis in liver by decreasing the concentration of fructose 2,6 bisphosphate
(E) inhibit glycogenolysis in liver by stimulating the conversion of liver glycogen phosphorylase to the phosphorylated and less active form

17. H.D., an HIV-positive man, has developed severe *Candida albicans* septicemia. The treatment of choice is

(A) amphotericin B
(B) clarithromycin
(C) flucytosine
(D) ketoconazole
(E) vancomycin

18. A 27-year-old man has schistosomiasis. Which of the following statements concerning this disease is correct?

    (A) It is caused by a microbe that has a head with hooks and suckers.
    (B) It is not likely to induce high eosinophil counts.
    (C) It is not usually diagnosed by the demonstration of ova in clinical specimens.
    (D) It may cause blockage of the portal venous system. ┿
    (E) Its incidence cannot be significantly reduced by proper disposal of human fecal waste.

19. Which of the following drugs is most likely to be effective in the prevention of recurrent atrial fibrillation in a patient with long-standing severe congestive heart failure (CHF)?

    (A) Adenosine
    (B) Amiodarone
    (C) Digoxin ┿
    (D) Lidocaine
    (E) Propafenone

Questions 20 through 22

A patient with multiple rib fractures following an automobile accident is brought to the Emergency Room.

20. Which of the following arterial blood gas values would you expect in this patient?

	pH	BICARBONATE (mmol/L)	PCO₂ (mm Hg)
(A)	7.25	26	60
(B)	7.35	18	33
(C)	7.35	31	60
(D)	7.50	22	30
(E)	7.45	19	30

21. Which of the following statements about renal handling of bicarbonate (HCO_3^-) in this patient is correct?

    (A) Filtered HCO_3^- enters tubular cells by a HCO_3^-/Cl^- exchange mechanism.

(B) For each HCO_3^- recovered by the renal tubular cells, one H^+ is secreted.
    (C) Most of the filtered HCO_3^- is recovered by the distal tubular cells.
    (D) Most of the HCO_3^- filtered through the glomeruli is lost with the urine.
    (E) This patient's kidneys generate less net HCO_3^- than kidneys from a healthy subject.

22. After several days of chronic acidosis, the main route of renal H^+ excretion in this patient is as

    (A) bicarbonate ✓
    (B) free protons (urine pH < 5)
    (C) nontitratable acid
    (D) phosphoric acid
    (E) uric acid

23. Shown in Figure 10–2 are the sequences that constitute the consensus sequences for eukaryotic mRNA splicing. The nucleotides depicted by Xs are invariant in all introns sequenced (i.e., these sequences appear 100% of the time at the indicated locations). What are the invariant sequences found at the 5′ and 3′ ends, respectively, of all mRNA introns?

Splicing Consensus Sequences

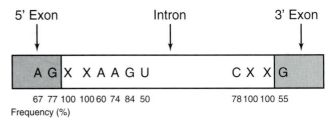

Figure 10–2

    (A) AT and GT
    (B) CT and TA
    (C) GC and AG
    (D) GG and AA
    (E) GT and AG ┿

24. Acquired immune deficiency syndrome (AIDS) is caused by a virus that

    (A) destroys CD4⁺ T lymphocytes ┿
    (B) has a double-stranded genome

(C) is a member of the adenovirus group

(D) lacks a viral envelope

(E) lacks reverse transcriptase

Questions 25 and 26

"Alternating hemiplegia" is the result of damage to descending corticospinal fibers in combination with a cranial nerve. Typically, hemiplegia is present contralateral to the lesion side, and cranial nerve signs are observed ipsilateral to the lesion. Three varieties have been described and they include superior, middle, and inferior alternating hemiplegia. The following two questions pertain to the clinical entity known as inferior alternating hemiplegia.

25. The cranial nerve involvement associated with inferior alternating hemiplegia affects which of the following muscles or muscle groups?

(A) Extraocular muscles

(B) Laryngeal musculature

(C) Muscles of facial expression

(D) Muscles of mastication

(E) Tongue musculature

26. The alternating hemiplegias are typically the result of vascular infarcts. The vessel(s) most commonly involved in inferior alternating hemiplegia is (are) the

(A) lenticulostriate arteries

(B) penetrating branches of anterior spinal artery

(C) posterior inferior cerebellar artery

(D) thalamoperforating vessels

(E) vertebral artery

Questions 27 and 28

Shortly after birth a neonate is diagnosed with a meconium ileus. Laboratory tests indicate an abnormally high content of sodium chloride in the infant's sweat. Genetic testing confirms an abnormality of chromosome 7.

27. What disorder does the child have?

(A) Alkaptonuria

(B) Cystic fibrosis

(C) Hemophilia A

(D) Phenylketonuria

(E) Wilson disease

28. Damage to which organ system accounts for most deaths with this disorder?

(A) Brain

(B) Intestine

(C) Liver

(D) Lung

(E) Pancreas

29. As a medical examiner, you are investigating a suspected homicide. The victim gives the appearance of having been poisoned with strychnine. You wish to confirm the presence of the poison in the victim. If a steady-state concentration of strychnine had been present in the systemic circulation and equilibration between the systemic circulation and tissue compartments had been achieved before death, which of these fluid compartments would have the largest total fluid:blood concentration ratio for the weak base strychnine (pKa = 6)?

(A) Cerebrospinal fluid at pH 7.35

(B) Jejunum and ileum contents at pH 7.6

(C) Stomach contents at pH 2.0

(D) Synovial fluid at pH 7.3

(E) Urine in bladder at pH 6.0

30. A 24-year-old man has a long history of an obsessive personality disorder. Which pain-control technique may be most efficacious for this patient?

(A) As-needed pain medication (prn medication)

(B) General anesthesia

(C) Hypnosis

(D) Patient-controlled analgesia (PCA)

(E) Placebo

31. A 21-year-old student has been informed by his physician that he is suffering from allergic rhinitis. Which of the following statements concerning his allergy is correct?

    (A) Administration of sodium cromolyn increases the release of histamine.
    (B) His allergic antigen–antibody reactions do not neutralize the toxicity of the antigen.
    (C) His immunologic responses are highly unspecific.
    (D) His type of allergy does not lead to IgE production.
    (E) The mast cells in his circulation do not possess any immunoglobulin on their surface.

32. Muscles arising from the second pharyngeal arch mesoderm include the

    (A) masseter
    (B) mylohyoid
    (C) stapedius
    (D) stylopharyngeus
    (E) superior pharyngeal constrictor

33. The current drug of choice for treatment of combined intestinal and hepatic amebic (E. histolytica) infections is

    (A) dehydroemetine
    (B) diloxanide
    (C) mefloquine
    (D) metronidazole
    (E) paromomycin

34. A 2-day-old boy delivered by normal labor (with no known prenatal risk factors) has become lethargic and requires stimulation for feeding. When vomiting and hyperventilation ensue, routine laboratory results show BUN < 1 mg/dL. The infant quickly lapses into a coma and is placed on a ventilator. Bulging of the fontanel suggested an intracranial hemorrhage, but a CT scan revealed only cerebral edema. Within several hours, the infant dies. Death is ascribed to sepsis; however, a postmortem analysis of the plasma samples taken at admission show dramatically elevated serum ammonia and citrulline levels—100 times normal. The enzyme deficiency found to be associated with these severe neonatal symptoms is

    (A) argininosuccinate synthetase
    (B) carbamoylphosphate synthetase I
    (C) 3-hydroxy-3-methylglutaryl-CoA lyase
    (D) medium-chain acyl-CoA dehydrogenase
    (E) pyruvate carboxylase

35. A 45-year-old woman is admitted with a chief complaint of cold, painful legs. She is found to have a blood pressure of 140/90, heart rate 60, and no arterial pulses in her legs. A history of severe migraine headache is elicited and the fact that she consumed 10 tablets of ergotamine over a 2-day period preceding the onset of symptoms. Which of the following drugs is most likely to prevent gangrene in this patient's lower extremities?

    (A) Histamine
    (B) Hydralazine
    (C) Minoxidil
    (D) Nitroprusside
    (E) Phentolamine

36. A patient with advanced HIV disease is receiving highly active anti-retroviral therapy (HAART). This treatment most likely is a regimen consisting of

    (A) acyclovir, zidovudine, and indinavir
    (B) acyclovir, zidovudine, and lamivudine
    (C) ganciclovir, indinavir, and zidovudine
    (D) indinavir, zidovudine, and lamivudine
    (E) zidovudine, laviduvine and ganciclovir

37. The structure indicated by arrow #2 in Figure 10–3 is the

    (A) cerebral aqueduct of Sylvius
    (B) cerebral peduncle
    (C) red nucleus
    (D) superior colliculus
    (E) vermis of the cerebellum

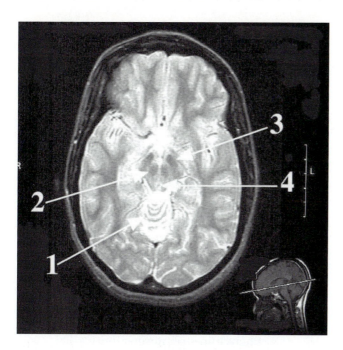

Figure 10–3

38. The structure identified in Question 37 (Figure 10–3 arrow #2) is part of the

    (A) diencephalon
    (B) mesencephalon
    (C) metencephalon
    (D) myelencephalon
    (E) telencephalon

39. When exposed to air, the urine of persons with alkaptonuria turns dark. Late in the course of the disease patients exhibit increased pigmentation of the connective tissues and develop a form of arthritis. Alkaptonuria results from a defect in

    (A) homogentisate oxidase
    (B) α-keto acid dehydrogenase
    (C) phenylalanine hydroxylase
    (D) tryptophan oxygenase
    (E) tyrosine transaminase

40. The plateau phase of the cardiac myocyte action potential is most closely associated with which of the following phases of the ECG?

    (A) P wave
    (B) QRS complex

    (C) QT interval
    (D) ST segment
    (E) T wave

41. A 46-year-old woman complains of abdominal pain in the right upper quadrant after eating fatty foods. A photograph of her opened gallbladder is displayed in Figure 10–4. What abnormal process is evident?

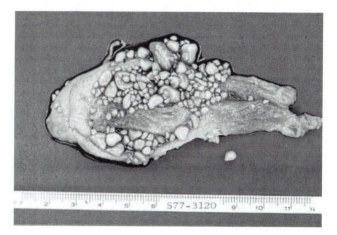

Figure 10–4

    (A) Congenital malformation
    (B) Infection
    (C) Neoplasia
    (D) Stone formation
    (E) Thrombosis

42. Which of the following is useful in the treatment of generalized anxiety disorder with the lowest incidence of sedation?

    (A) Alprazolam
    (B) Amitriptyline
    (C) Buspirone
    (D) Clozapine
    (E) Methylphenidate

43. A 17-year-old boy with influenza has a hemagglutination inhibition titer of 1:400. Which of the following statements is correct?

    (A) A 400-fold dilution of his serum will have no effect in a hemagglutination inhibition assay.
    (B) A 400-fold dilution of his serum will prevent agglutination of red blood cells.
    (C) Each red blood cell can bind 400 viral particles.
    (D) There are 400 hemagglutinins on each red blood cell.
    (E) There are 400 viral particles per milliliter of serum.

44. Following a tonsillectomy, your patient reports numbness on the back of the tongue and a reduced awareness of taste. After examination, you confirm a loss of general sensation and taste from the posterior third of the tongue. You suspect injury to the

    (A) facial nerve
    (B) glossopharyngeal nerve
    (C) hypoglossal nerve
    (D) lingual nerve
    (E) vagus nerve

45. The severe neural toxicity associated with hyperammonemia is due to

    (A) ammonia incorporation into α-ketoglutarate, forming glutamate, leads to a consequent reduction in TCA cycle activity and energy production in the brain
    (B) ammonia incorporation into α-ketoglutarate limits the transfer of ammonia to glutamate from glutamine leading to glutamate poisoning
    (C) ammonium ions alter the pH of neurons, which leads to their depolarization
    (D) ammonium ions alter the pH of neurons, which leads to their hyperpolarization
    (E) ammonia is incorporated into γ-aminobutyrate (GABA), which prevents GABA from carrying out its neurotransmitter function

46. A 34-year-old woman has an ovarian tumor surgically excised. Pathologic examination shows that the tumor is derived from ovarian germ cells. Which neoplasm is compatible with this observation?

    (A) Brenner tumor
    (B) Endometrioid adenocarcinoma
    (C) Mature cystic teratoma
    (D) Mucinous cystadenoma
    (E) Serous papillary carcinoma

47. Which of the following correctly matches an antiepileptic agent with its primary toxicity?

    (A) Carbamazepine—trigeminal neuralgia
    (B) Ethosuximide—gingival hyperplasia
    (C) Lamotrigine—visual field defects
    (D) Phenytoin—photosensitivity
    (E) Valproic acid—hepatotoxicity

48. A 12-year-old boy without diabetes exhibited extensive eruptive xanthomas, hepatosplenomegaly, and milky plasma. The milky plasma was due to a massive accumulation of chylomicrons and triglycerides. Upon switching to a fat-free diet, the lipemia and all other symptoms disappeared. A deficiency in which apolipoprotein would account for the observed symptoms of hyperlipoproteinemia?

    (A) ApoA-I
    (B) ApoB-100
    (C) ApoC-II
    (D) ApoD
    (E) ApoE

49. A 5-month-old baby has a constant, nonproductive cough, wheezing, and a temperature of 100°F. Radiographs and laboratory tests indicate that the baby has viral bronchiolitis. Which one of the following viruses is most likely to cause this illness?

    (A) Adenovirus
    (B) Influenza virus
    (C) Parainfluenza serotype 3 virus
    (D) Respiratory syncytial virus
    (E) Rotavirus

50. Figure 10–5 represents five left ventricular pressure-volume loops, each labeled by a letter (A through E). Loop D shows the normal pressure-volume loop of a healthy adult at rest. Which curve represents a patient with mitral stenosis?

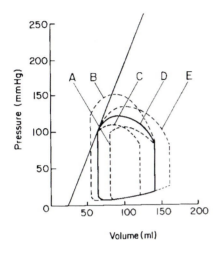

Figure 10–5

(A) A

(B) B

(C) C

(D) D

(E) E

51. Anastomoses between which of the following vessels could potentially provide collateral circulation to the brain in the event of a blockage of the internal carotid artery?

(A) Angular artery and dorsal nasal artery

(B) Lingual artery and facial artery

(C) Superficial temporal artery and middle meningeal artery

(D) Superficial temporal artery and occipital artery

(E) Superior thyroid artery and inferior thyroid artery

52. A young man, who had been active in sports as a youth, experiences leg muscle pain, weakness, cramping and stiffness following even slight exercise. He finds that if he rests during his exercising he gets a "second wind." However, he is particularly alarmed by the occasional appearance of burgundy-colored urine after his attempts at running sprints. On a visit to his physician, it is found that his blood lactate levels fall during a treadmill test instead of the expected increase. Biopsy from his quadriceps muscle finds a deficiency in phosphorylase activity. These clinical findings are indicative of which glycogen storage disease?

(A) Anderson

(B) Hers

(C) McArdle

(D) Tarui

(E) von Gierke

53. The sensory (somatosensory) decussation occurs at the level of the

(A) medulla

(B) midbrain

(C) pons

(D) posterior limb of internal capsule

(E) thalamus

54. A 27-week-old male fetus is delivered prematurely and subsequently dies of respiratory distress syndrome. What pathologic process most likely lead to his demise?

(A) Congenital pulmonary malformation

(B) Inadequate conjugation of bilirubin

(C) Inadequate humoral immunity

(D) Inadequate pulmonary surfactant

(E) In utero viral infection

Questions 55 through 57

A 47-year-old man is brought to the clinic for evaluation of a movement disorder.

55. If the patient is observed to have a resting tremor, an important part of history taking is

(A) family history of seizure disorder

(B) history of alcoholism

(C) history of exposure to von Economo disease

(D) history of treatment with an antipsychotic drug

(E) history of treatment with an anxiolytic drug

56. In addition to the resting tremor, the patient shows slow, rhythmic movements of the lips. A useful test to perform would be

(A) the Babinski test

(B) the Hoover test

(C) to ask the patient to close his eyes and smile

(D) to ask the patient to open his mouth, then protrude his tongue

(E) to ask the patient to run

57. If the patient also exhibits choreiform movements of the arms and legs, the most likely diagnosis is

(A) Creutzfeldt–Jakob disease

(B) multiple sclerosis

(C) Sydenham chorea

(D) tardive dyskinesia

(E) vascular dementia

58. The graph shown in Figure 10–6 shows a viral multiplication curve. Which of the following statements is correct?

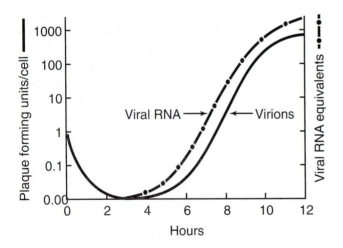

Figure 10–6

(A) During the time period of 0 to 6 hours the virus retains its infectivity.

(B) The time from 0 to 6 hours represents the eclipse period.

(C) The time from 6 to 8 hours represents the appearance of immature virus.

(D) The time from 6 to 8 hours represents the uncoating of the viral particle.

(E) The viral growth curve is similar to bacterial growth curve.

59. The primary mechanism for resistance to saquinavir in the treatment of HIV is

(A) deletion of thymidine kinase

(B) deletion of thymidylate synthase

(C) mutations in the sequence of reverse transcriptase

(D) mutations in the sequence of viral DNA polymerase

(E) mutations in the sequence of viral protease

60. A 50-year-old white woman complains of a lump in her thyroid gland. Fine-needle aspiration of this lump is reported as medullary carcinoma. A test of her serum would most likely reveal an increased level of

(A) α-fetoprotein

(B) CA 125

(C) CA 15–3

(D) calcitonin

(E) human chorionic gonadotropin

61. Hemoglobin is nonenzymatically glycosylated as glucose enters erythrocytes. Because erythrocytes routinely die and are replaced, the level of glycosylated hemoglobin is a good measure of glucose levels in the blood, a measure of the length of time glucose levels were elevated. Glycosylated hemoglobin is designated as

(A) HbA_{1c}

(B) HbA_2

(C) HbC

(D) HbE

(E) HbS

62. Osteopetrosis is an inherited disease characterized by defective osteoclasts that lack the ruffled border characteristic of this cell type. An expected consequence of osteoclast inactivity is

(A) abnormal deposits of calcium in arterial walls and the kidneys

(B) elevation in blood Ca^{2+} levels

(C) enlarged marrow spaces

(D) low concentration of circulating parathyroid hormone

(E) overgrowth and thickening of bones

63. A drug with a half-life of 2 hours is administered by continuous IV infusion. How long will it take for the drug to reach 94% of its final steady-state level?

(A) 2 h

(B) 4 h

(C) 8 h

(D) 16 h

(E) 48 h

64. A postoperative patient with a febrile episode is carefully monitored. Temperatures measured are rectal and given in degrees Centigrade in Figure 10–7. At which point or period does the patient begin to behave as if in a hot environment (sweats and complains of "burning up")?

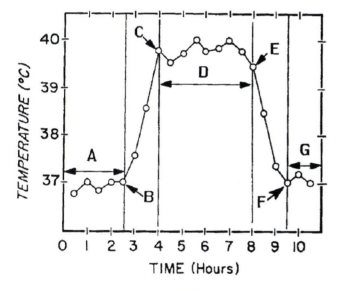

Figure 10–7

(A) Period A

(B) Period D

(C) Period G

(D) Point B

(E) Point C

(F) Point E

(G) Point F

65. Adenosine deaminase (ADA) deficiency is associated with severe combined immunodeficiency. The immune dysfunction occurs because the enzyme deficiency

(A) causes lysis of T and B lymphocytes due to their extreme sensitivity to the increased levels of inosine, which accompany the enzyme deficiency

(B) leads to an inability of immune cells to salvage ATP from inosine, resulting in their death from lack of energy production

(C) leads to elevations in dATP levels, which inhibits ribonucleotide reductase, thereby limiting production of deoxyribonucleotides for DNA synthesis in T and B lymphocytes

(D) leads to elevations in uric acid, which is toxic to T and B lymphocytes

(E) prevents the generation of inosine required for the rapid salvage of thymidine nucleotides needed for DNA replication in T and B lymphocytes

66. A 66-year-old woman is found at autopsy to have shrunken kidneys with granular irregular cortex, combined with the microscopic appearance of a greatly reduced number of nephrons, diffuse glomerular sclerosis, and interstitial fibrosis as well as the presence of IgG, IgA, and C3 under immunofluorescence. Based on these findings the most likely diagnosis is

(A) chronic glomerulonephritis

(B) diabetic nephropathy

(C) lupus nephritis

(D) renal amyloidosis

(E) Wegener granulomatosis

67. You are undertaking a surgical dissection of the posterior triangle of the neck to remove a small tumor mass. Which of the following structures is at risk in the posterior triangle?

(A) Accessory nerve

(B) Superior thyroid artery

(C) Thoracic duct

(D) Vertebral artery

(E) Vagus nerve

68. A 50-year-old woman appears to be infected with a fungus that causes cutaneous mycosis. Which of the following tests is likely to be of little value for the diagnosis of this fungus?

   (A) Agglutination assays
   (B) Cultivation on Sabouraud medium at pH 5.5
   (C) Examination of the fungal colonies
   (D) Growth on Sabouraud agar plates at a temperature of 25°C
   (E) Microscopic examination of skin scrapings, hair, and nails

69. An internist tells the psychiatric consultant that she is having difficulty with a patient. The patient is very upset about the "sloppiness" of the hospital personnel. He insists on having all medicine administered exactly at the scheduled minute, on the dot. He complains if his medicine is only 5 minutes late. The patient most likely has traits of

   (A) antisocial personality
   (B) borderline personality
   (C) depressive personality
   (D) narcissistic personality
   (E) obsessive personality

70. Which enzyme catalyzes the following reaction?
   $$Fe^{2+} + O_2 + 4H^+ \rightarrow 2H_2O + Fe^{3+}$$

   (A) Catalase
   (B) Cytochrome oxidase
   (C) Ferrochetalase
   (D) Peroxidase
   (E) Superoxide dismutase

71. A 55-year-old woman with lobular carcinoma of the breast underwent radical mastectomy and chemotherapy 4 years ago. Two out of 14 axillary lymph nodes at the time were positive for malignant cells. She now presents with bone metastases, and during her lab workup a peptide with PTH-like activity is found in her plasma. The physiologic effect of this substance is to

   (A) decrease metabolism of vitamin D to the 1,25-OH form
   (B) decrease renal phosphate excretion

   (C) decrease serum calcitonin levels
   (D) decrease serum calcium
   (E) stimulate bone resorption

72. The graph in Figure 10–8 shows the blood pressure responses to an IV infusion of epinephrine followed by infusion of drug X. The top of the bars indicate the systolic pressure, the bottom the diastolic pressure, and the filled circles the mean pressure. Heart rate increased from 70 to 105 per minute during the infusion of drug X. Identify drug X.

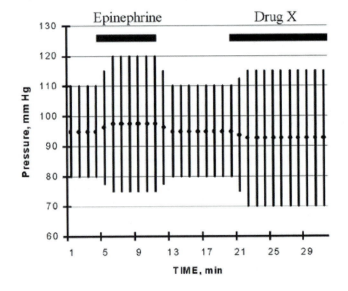

Figure 10–8

   (A) Amphetamine
   (B) Atropine
   (C) Isoproterenol
   (D) Norepinephrine
   (E) Phenylephrine

73. A 52-year-old woman presents to the Emergency Room with new-onset hematemesis. Her only other complaints are progressive pruritis and intermittent nausea. She is otherwise healthy with no history of medical conditions. History is also negative for alcohol, tobacco, and other drug use. Findings on a liver biopsy revealed a micronodular appearance without regenerative nodules. Other findings include periportal fibrosis, scant lymphocytic white blood cell infiltration, and

destruction of bile ducts. The most likely diagnosis is

(A) cholangiocarcinoma

(B) cholangitis

(C) cholestasis

(D) chronic hepatitis A

(E) primary biliary cirrhosis

74. A loss of gastric parietal cells (oxyntic cells) as a result of atrophic gastritis would most likely result in a deficiency in

(A) absorption of vitamin B_{12}

(B) neutralization of chyme by bicarbonate

(C) pepsinogen secretion

(D) secretion of gastrin

(E) the mucus coating of the gastric lining

75. A 10-year-old girl exhibits the following symptoms: marked hepatomegaly, variceal bleeding, chronic bilateral pulmonary infiltrates, chronic liver disease, hepatic encephalopathy, and only 5% of normal sphingomyelinase activity in peripheral blood leukocytes. What is the most likely diagnosis?

(A) Fabry disease

(B) Gaucher disease

(C) Krabbe disease

(D) Niemann–Pick type B disease

(E) Tay–Sachs disease

76. Which of the following statements regarding systemic hemodynamics is correct?

(A) The compliance of the venous circulation is less than that of the arterial circulation.

(B) The greatest cross-sectional area is within the small veins.

(C) The greatest drop in pressure occurs in the arterioles rather than in the large arteries.

(D) The greatest percentage of blood volume is in the capillaries.

(E) The velocity of blood flow is highest in the capillaries.

77. This agent is used in combination therapy for Hodgkin lymphoma. Its most serious toxicity is peripheral neuropathy.

(A) Bleomycin

(B) Cisplatin

(C) Doxorubicin

(D) Mechlorethamine

(E) Vincristine

78. A 65-year-old man is admitted to a neurosurgical unit due to rapidly worsening dementia. Radiology studies reveal multiple lesions in the cerebral cortex. A stereotactic biopsy of one of the lesions is obtained. A touch imprint cytology of the biopsy is shown in Figure 10–9. What is the nature of this man's cerebral lesions?

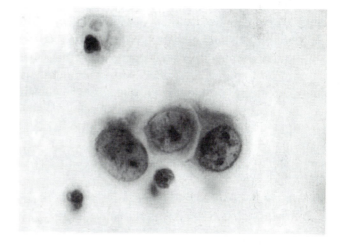

Figure 10–9

(A) Chronic demyelinating disorder

(B) Deficient in an essential nutrient

(C) Malignant neoplasm

(D) Parasitic infection

(E) Viral infection

79. Following clindamycin therapy, a farmer developed severe pseudomembranous enterocolitis. This disease most likely was caused by

(A) *Clostridium difficile*

(B) echovirus

(C) *Entamoeba histolytica*

(D) *Escherichia coli* (enterotoxigenic)

(E) *Salmonella enteritidis*

80. Which of the following is a predictable adverse effect of treatment with haloperidol?

    (A) Diarrhea
    (B) Excessive salivation
    (C) Hyperprolactinemia
    (D) Nausea and vomiting
    (E) Tourette syndrome

81. During surgical removal of the thyroid gland, injury to the external laryngeal nerve may result due to its close proximity to the

    (A) inferior thyroid artery
    (B) recurrent laryngeal nerve
    (C) second and third rings of the trachea
    (D) superior thyroid artery
    (E) thyroid ima artery

82. Tumors of the adrenal medulla that are actively producing catecholamines are called pheochromocytomas. Patients with these tumors experience sudden, periodic increases in catecholamine blood levels. During such an episode, patients may experience

    (A) cardiac ischemia
    (B) decreased blood glucose
    (C) decreased blood pressure
    (D) decreased heart rate
    (E) decreased sweat secretion

83. Which of the following correctly matches an immunosuppressive agent with its mechanism of action?

    (A) Azathioprine—negative regulation of T-cell expression of lymphokines
    (B) Cyclophosphamide—inhibition of antigen presentation
    (C) Cyclosporine—prevention of clonal expansion of T and B lymphocytes
    (D) Prednisone—inhibition of IMP dehydrogenase
    (E) Tacrolimus—inhibition of activation of T-cell transcription factors for cytokine expression

84. A 72-year-old man with a known history of chronic essential hypertension dies unattended at home. The medical examiner determines the cause of death to be a hypertensive intracerebral hemorrhage. The most likely site of the hemorrhage is

    (A) basal ganglia or thalamus
    (B) cerebellum
    (C) frontal lobe
    (D) occipital lobe
    (E) pons

85. Which of the following viruses produces a rash and has an RNA genome?

    (A) Herpesvirus
    (B) Measles virus
    (C) Molluscum contagiosum virus
    (D) Papovavirus
    (E) Variola virus

86. Cushing syndrome results from chronic glucocorticoid therapy. The symptoms of Cushing syndrome are similar to those of Cushing disease, which is caused by pituitary tumors that secrete excess amounts of which hormone?

    (A) Adrenocorticotropic hormone (ACTH)
    (B) Follicle-stimulating hormone (FSH)
    (C) Growth hormone (GH)
    (D) Prolactin (PRL)
    (E) Thyroid-stimulating hormone (TSH)

87. A lung autopsy specimen with an abnormality of the vasculature is depicted in Figure 10–10. What is the most likely associated clinical finding?

    (A) Chronic idiopathic thrombocytopenic purpura
    (B) Disseminated intravascular coagulation
    (C) Hemoptysis due to aneurysmal rupture
    (D) Hemoptysis due to tumor eroding into blood vessel
    (E) Sudden death due to occlusive embolus

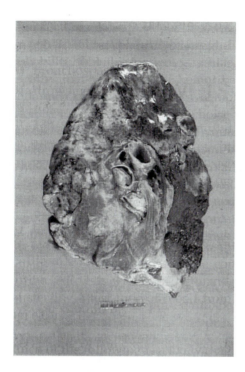

Figure 10–10

88. The fractional excretion of sodium (FeNa) compares the ratio of urine sodium × plasma creatinine to plasma sodium and urine creatinine. Based on your understanding of renal physiology, what would you expect its value to be in pre-renal azotemia?

    (A) < 1
    (B) 0
    (C) 1
    (D) > 1
    (E) > 10

89. Which of these drugs is used in treatment of gouty arthritis to increase the urinary excretion of uric acid?

    (A) Allopurinol
    (B) Colchicine
    (C) Indomethacin
    (D) Piroxicam
    (E) Probenecid

90. Puromycin inhibits translation by

    (A) catalyzing ADP-ribosylation and inactivation of eEF-2
    (B) inhibiting eukaryotic peptidyltransferase
    (C) inhibiting prokaryotic aminoacyl-tRNA binding to the ribosome small subunit
    (D) inhibiting prokaryotic peptidyltransferase
    (E) resembling an aminoacyl-tRNA and interfering with peptide transfer resulting in premature termination in both prokaryotes and eukaryotes

91. The EEG during a petit mal epileptic attack is characterized by

    (A) generalized, high-voltage spikes
    (B) irregular spikes limited to the temporal lobes
    (C) no consistent EEG abnormalities
    (D) 3-per-second "spikes and domes"
    (E) REM-onset sleep

92. A 32-year-old man has a 4-month history of glomerulonephritis and recurrent pulmonary hemorrhage. His serum contains an antibody directed against basement membrane. He most likely suffers from

    (A) fibrosing alveolitis
    (B) Goodpasture syndrome
    (C) Kartagener syndrome
    (D) systemic lupus erythematosus
    (E) Wegener granulomatosis

93. Slow but progressive pulmonary edema, alveolitis, and irreversible fibrosis is characteristic of intoxication by

    (A) dichlorophenyltrichloroethane (DDT)
    (B) dioxin
    (C) paraquat
    (D) polychlorinated biphenyls (PCBs)
    (E) rotenone

94. The use of antibiotics in the treatment of disorders in urea cycle function has as its basis of utility the fact that they

    (A) acidify the intestinal tract leading to ionization of ammonia, which can then be excreted in the feces

    (B) complex intestinal ammonia leading to their excretion

    (C) lead to a reduction of intestinal ammonia-producing bacteria

    (D) promote the conjugation of ammonia with glutamate aiding excretion

    (E) promote the conjugation of ammonia with glycine aiding excretion

95. The graph in Figure 10–11 shows the response of retinal photoreceptors as a function of light wavelength. Which of the following statements is correct?

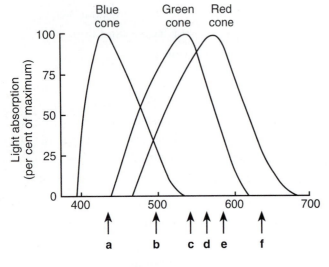

Figure 10–11

    (A) A green sensation is elicited by maximally stimulating the green cone (arrow c).

    (B) A red sensation is elicited by maximally stimulating the red cone (arrow e).

    (C) A yellow sensation is elicited by about equal stimulation of the green cone and red cone (arrow d).

    (D) Color is a subjective sensation and cannot be measured objectively.

    (E) There are four receptor types in the retina corresponding to the primary colors (red, green, blue, and yellow).

96. J.M. is a 14-year-old boy with severe and worsening asthma that has been responsible for three hospitalizations in the last 18 months. He has been using an albuterol inhaler, two puffs 4 times daily. He is referred for consultation on modification of his therapy. Which of the following regimens is most likely to reduce the incidence and severity of his attacks?

    (A) Aminophylline twice daily and albuterol 4 times daily

    (B) Beclomethasone twice daily and albuterol for acute attacks

    (C) Prednisone once daily and salmeterol for acute attacks

    (D) Terbutaline 4 times daily and salmeterol during acute attacks

    (E) Zafirlukast twice daily and prednisone once daily

97. A 59-year-old man has pneumonia caused by *Streptococcus pneumoniae*. The virulence of this microbe is associated with the presence of

    (A) cell wall teichoic acid

    (B) M protein

    (C) peptidoglycan

    (D) pneumolysin

    (E) polysaccharide capsule

98. A component of mitochondrial electron transport that can act as either a one- or two-electron carrier is

    (A) coenzyme Q

    (B) cytochrome c

    (C) NADH

    (D) nonheme iron

99. A 66-year-old man developed intermittent dysphagia a few months ago. This is now constant and accompanied by pain and some weight loss. X-rays of the esophagus with barium swallow show structural and filling defects, and reduced peristalsis. A biopsy is taken and is shown in Figure 10–12. The best diagnosis is

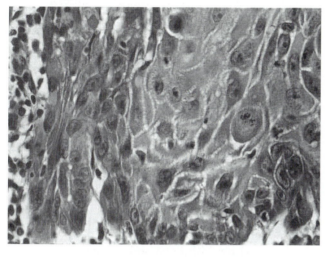

Figure 10–12. (See also Color Insert.)

(A) adenocarcinoma of the esophagus
(B) Barrett esophagus
(C) *Candida* esophagitis
(D) fibrous stricture of the esophagus
(E) squamous cell carcinoma of the esophagus

100. In cases of acute cyanide poisoning, cyanide binds to the Fe^{3+} of a cytochrome. Which statement best describes this cytochrome?

(A) It binds carbon monoxide.
(B) It directly oxidizes cytochrome b.
(C) It directly reduces cytochrome c_1.
(D) It is found in complex I of the respiratory chain.
(E) It is found in complex II of the respiratory chain.

Answers and Explanations

1. **(B)** The clinical and laboratory findings suggest a diagnosis of pernicious anemia. Almost all cases are due to autoantibodies against parietal cells or intrinsic factor. These autoantibodies disrupt the normal absorption of vitamin B_{12}. The inability to absorb vitamin B_{12} leads to a macrocytic pancytopenia and peripheral neuropathy. A diet deficient in folate (choice A) can cause a macrocytic anemia. In folate deficiency, there are no concomitant neuropathic findings. Chronic blood loss (choice C) usually results in microcytic hypochromic anemia due to iron deficiency. Anemia and peripheral neuropathy commonly occur with diabetes mellitus (choice D). However, the anemia is normocytic and the neuropathy is sensory. Myelodysplastic sideroblastic anemia (choice E) may present hematologically with a macrocytic pancytopenia. A peripheral neuropathy is not seen.

2. **(E)** There is an increased risk to develop adenocarcinoma of the stomach with pernicious anemia. Before developing carcinoma, the stomach mucosa usually displays metaplastic or dysplastic changes for a variable time period. Carcinomas of the CNS (choice A), genital tract (choice B), lung (choice C), and pancreas (choice D) are not statistically increased in patients with pernicious anemia.

3. **(A)** Degeneration of dopaminergic neurons of the substantia nigra pars compacta is thought to be the primary defect in Parkinson disease. Loss of GABA neurons in the VL thalamus (choice D) and facilitation of pyramidal tract neurons (choice B) might be secondary or indirect factors in this disease. Vascular lesions involving the subthalamic nucleus (choice E) lead to the condition known as hemiballism. Huntington disease might involve loss of cholinergic interneurons in the caudate nucleus and putamen (choice C).

4. **(D)** It is not possible to determine if the bacteremia was caused by *E. coli*, an IV catheter infection, or endocarditis. A reculture of blood after the IV catheters have been removed could be of value in determining between these possibilities. Bacteremia induced by infected IV catheters is not uncommon. The infection is usually localized and removal of the catheter, which tends to be infected with *S. aureus*, suppresses bacteremia. When bacteremia persists following the removal of catheters, there is either infection in the vein or some other location. At any rate, in the absence of knowledge concerning antibiotic sensitivity of the etiologic agent of bacteremia, blind antibiotic treatment is of little, if any, value.

5. **(E)** The tentorium cerebelli is a tent-like partition that covers the posterior cranial fossa and the cerebellum, and supports the occipital lobes of the cerebral hemispheres. The crista galli (choice A) is the superior project of the ethmoid bone that gives attachment to the falx cerebri. It is not a dural reflection. The diaphragma sellae (choice B) is a horizontal projection of dura that forms the roof of the hypophyseal fossa. The falx cerebelli (choice C) is a small, sickle-shaped projection between the cerebellar hemispheres that attaches above to the tentorium cerebelli and below to the internal occipital crest of the occipital bone. The falx cerebri (choice D) is a

sickle-shaped, midline fold that extends into the median fissure between the cerebral hemispheres attaching anteriorly to the crista galli and the frontal crest and posteriorly to the tentorium cerebelli.

6. **(E)** Phosphorylase kinase-b is the less active form of the enzyme. The activity of the enzyme is significantly increased in response to phosphorylation by cAMP-dependent protein kinase (PKA). Phosphorylase kinase is a complex that includes a subunit of calmodulin. Calmodulin is a calcium binding protein that, upon binding calcium, changes conformation and in turn alters the conformation of its associated enzyme(s). The calmodulin-induced conformational changes in phosphorylase kinase increases its activity in the absence of phosphorylation. None of the other glycogen metabolizing enzymes (choices A, B, C, and D) are affected by calcium ions.

7. **(A)** Coumadin functions as an anticoagulant by blocking the vitamin K–dependent modification (γ-carboxylation of glutamate residues) of certain clotting factors. Blocking this modification renders them inactive. However, the half-life of factors already synthesized means that coumadin does not achieve therapeutic effectiveness for up to several days. The vitamin K–dependent factors synthesized by the liver include not only procoagulants such as factors II, VII, IX and X, but also proteins S and C, both of which are natural anticoagulants. By blocking their synthesis before complete elimination of the procoagulants, treatment with coumadin alone could actually create a transiently procoagulant state that would worsen the problem it was intended to treat. Heparin is a proteoglycan that works by accelerating the action of antithrombin, a coagulation factor inhibitor that binds and inactivates most activated clotting factors (except factor VII). Thus, treatment with heparin, generally given IV, quickly produces an anticoagulated state (contrary to choice B). Once orally administered coumadin has reached full therapeutic effect, heparin therapy can be discontinued and patients can be discharged from

the hospital. Contrary to (choice D), heparin is not necessary for coumadin's actions. Choices C and E are true but not relevant to the question.

8. **(B)** Flumazenil is a pharmacologic antagonist for benzodiazepines such as chlordiazepoxide and diazepam but not other classes of sedative–hypnotics. Buspirone (choice A) is a nonsedating anxiolytic drug, but is not in the benzodiazepine class. Toxicity from overdosage is low and no antidote has been developed. Ethanol (choice C), another sedative–hypnotic drug, has no pharmacologic antagonists. It is sometimes used as an antidote in methanol and ethylene glycol intoxication because it is the favored substrate for aldehyde dehydrogenase and can prevent this enzyme from oxidizing the other alcohols to their more toxic metabolites. Overdosage with morphine (choice D), an opioid analgesic, is effectively reversed with naloxone. Phenobarbital (choice E), one of the prototype barbiturate sedative–hypnotics, has no direct antidote. Intoxication is treated symptomatically and by hemoperfusion.

9. **(B)** In bacterial food poisoning caused by *C. perfringens,* final confirmation rests on toxin production by *C. perfringens* and its neutralization by specific antiserum. Demonstration of the presence of spores (choice A) or large gram-positive rods (choice E) in the suspected food is not very helpful for the identification of *C. perfringens* because of confusion with other clostridia or of large bacilli in thioglycolate broth (choice C) that will not allow classification of the various anaerobic large gram-positive rods. Demonstration of spores in food indicates that a spore-forming organism contaminates the food, but it does not prove that *C. perfringens* caused the food poisoning. Demonstration of antibodies against *C. perfringens* (choice D) in the patient's serum indicates exposure of the patient to *C. perfringens,* but does not prove that *C. perfringens* caused the food poisoning.

10. **(A)** Amantadine is an unusual drug with activity against the influenza virus and the abil-

ity to reduce the symptoms of Parkinson disease. Its mechanism of action in influenza appears to involve inhibition of viral entry into or uncoating inside host cells. The mechanism in Parkinson disease involves increased dopamine release from neurons in the extrapyramidal system. Benztropine (choice B) is a muscarinic antagonist that enters the CNS readily and is useful in Parkinson disease. It has no efficacy in influenza. Bromocriptine (choice C) is a D_2-receptor agonist that is useful in Parkinson disease and amenorrhea/galactorrhea syndrome. It has no antiviral effects. Oseltamivir (choice D) is a new, orally active anti-influenza drug that inhibits neuraminidase, an enzyme essential for replication of both influenza A and B. Ribavirin (choice E) is a guanosine analog that is useful against influenza, respiratory syncytial virus, HIV, and some other viruses, but it has no role in the treatment of Parkinson disease.

11. **(E)** von Willebrand disease (vWD) is the most common bleeding disorder that occurs in man. It is caused by a deficiency in the protein (von Willebrand factor [vWF]) named after Erik von Willebrand who described the bleeding disorder in 1926, which also bears his name. vWF is a complex multimeric glycoprotein found in plasma, platelet α granules, and subendothelial connective tissue. vWF binds to specific receptors on the surface of platelets (identified as GPIb/IX) and in the collagen of subendothelial connective tissue to form a bridge between the platelet and areas of vascular damage. vWF also binds to and stabilizes coagulation factor VIII, an interaction that is necessary to increase the survival of factor VIII in the circulation. Loss of vWF leads to defective platelet adhesion and activation in response to tissue injury. In contrast to classical hemophilia, where bleeding occurs primarily in the joints and deep tissues, bleeding associated with vWD is primarily mucocutaneous. Loss of factor IX (choice A) is associated with hemophilia B. Loss of fibrinogen (choice B) and thrombin (choice C) has dramatic effects on coagulation time. Loss of tissue factor (choice

D) affects the extrinsic clotting cascade, which is the pathway of clotting initiated in response to loss of vascular integrity from an injury such as a cut.

12. **(D)** The spine demonstrates several discrete white abnormal nodules of metastatic carcinoma within the cancellous bone compartment. The nodules are white because the tumor is a prostatic carcinoma, which invokes an osteoblastic response. Most lytic bony metastases are red and soft on gross inspection. Degeneration (choice A) is common in the spine. Grossly, there is either collapse of the intervertebral disk or vertebral body. In Figure 10–1, the disk space and vertebral height both appear normal. Infection (choice B) in the spine is usually due to either hematogenous spread in septicemia or from the outside as with a postoperative wound infection. Osteomyelitis usually demonstrates pus formation on gross examination. Ischemic changes (choice C) are rare in the spine. Those that do occur are thromboembolic in nature and heal without significant anomaly. The joint space and bony confines show no evidence of trauma (choice E).

13. **(E)** The signs displayed by this patient are characteristic of a lesion of the ulnar nerve in the forearm. Loss of sensory function in the medial part of the palm and the medial one and half digits indicate lesioning of the palmar cutaneous and the dorsal cutaneous branches of the ulnar nerve. The lateral drawing of the hand in flexion of the wrist shows that adduction of the hand is impaired, resulting from loss of ulnar innervation to the flexor carpi ulnaris muscle. Finally, the inability to flex the fourth and fifth digits at the interphalangeal joints suggests paralysis of the medial half of the flexor digitorum profundus muscle, which is normally innervated by the ulnar nerve. The median nerve (choice A) is not lesioned because it normally innervates the lateral part of the palm and the lateral three and a half digits. The palmar cutaneous branch of the ulnar nerve (choice B) is not injured by itself because the extensive neurologic signs point to an injury of the ulnar

nerve at a point more proximal than this branch. A lesion of the radial nerve (choice C) results in the inability to extend the hand (wrist drop); this patient displays impairments with flexion. The superficial branch of the radial nerve (choice D) provides sensory innervation to the lateral side of the dorsum of the hand and the sensory loss in this patient does not correspond to this territory.

14. **(D)** The natural habitat of *H. pylori* is the human stomach. Attempts to isolate *H. pylori* from animals (choice A), feces (choice B), food (choice C), or water (choice E) generally have not been successful.

15. **(C)** Exacting, orderly, controlling personalities gain a sense of control and mastery by having exact information. Detailed explanation about the diagnosis, although initially upsetting, may enhance the collaboration between the patient and the physician, and lead to more effective management plans. Choice A sounds patronizing and choice B tends to increase the patient's level of distrust for the physician and the hospital, in addition to being patronizing. With choice D, the patient's idea that the hospital and physician are incompetent and sloppy is likely to increase. Choice E also results in a mistrustful patient.

16. **(A)** The immediate effect of insulin injection is to stimulate the uptake of glucose from the blood by the tissues. This occurs in response to insulin-mediated movement of glucose transporter protein complexes (GLUTs) to the plasma membrane. In patients with IDDM, insulin injection must be accompanied by food intake to prevent a severe drop in blood glucose levels leading to shock and coma. A patient who has injected insulin without eating and then proceeds to exercise further, and rapidly, exacerbates the hypoglycemia because of the increased consumption of glucose by the exercising muscle. Although skeletal muscle prefers to utilize fatty acids for energy (choice B), insulin injection still leads to increased uptake and oxidation of glucose by skeletal muscle and other tissues, thereby leading to hypoglycemia in the absence of food intake. The brain does not respond to insulin action with an increase in glucose uptake (choice C), because this important organ is freely permeable to glucose. However, because other tissues are induced to take up glucose in response to the insulin (coupled with the absence of food intake), hypoglycemia results, leaving reduced glucose for the brain with ensuing unconsciousness. A decreased concentration of fructose 2,6-bisphosphate (choice D) leads to an increase in gluconeogenesis, not a decrease. This is because fructose 2,6-bisphosphate is a negative allosteric regulator of the activity of the gluconeogenic enzyme, frusctose-1,6-bisphosphatase. Insulin does not lead to an increase in phosphorylated glycogen phosphorylase (choice E). When phosphorylated, glycogen phosphorylase is much more active than when nonphosphorylated, leading to an increased rate of glycogenolysis, not a reduced rate.

17. **(A)** *Candida albicans* is a fungus that often resides in the human pharynx and perineal area without causing clinical disease. Under certain conditions, especially immunosuppression, it can become invasive and cause local or even severe systemic disease. In severe septicemia, amphotericin B is the drug of choice for this (and many other) fungi. Clarithromycin (choice B) is a macrolide related to erythromycin that blocks protein synthesis in bacteria but not in fungi. It is effective against many gram-positive cocci, *Chlamydia*, and *Mycobacterium avium complex*. Flucytosine (choice C) is an antifungal prodrug that is converted in the fungus to 5-fluorouracil, which inhibits thymidylate synthase. It is not effective alone but is sometimes used as an adjunct to amphotericin in systemic *C. albicans* infections. Ketoconazole (choice D) is the prototype azole antifungal agent. It is often used topically in pharyngeal and vaginal candidiasis, but is too toxic for systemic use. Vancomycin (choice E) is a drug of choice for methicillin-resistant staphylococcal and other difficult gram-positive infections. It is not effective in fungal infections.

18. **(D)** The larvae of *Schistosoma mansoni* penetrate the human skin and then are transported by veins into the arterial circulation. The schistosomes that enter the superior mesenteric artery are introduced into the portal circulation where they can cause blockage of the portal venous system. Head suckers and hooks are the cytologic features of *Taenia solium* and *T. saginata* not *S. mansoni* (choice A). Control of schistosomiasis is directed toward proper disposal of human waste (choice E). Human waste may contain ova of *S. mansoni*. The ova hatch into miracidia and infect snails. An individual is infected when the free-swimming larvae of *S. mansoni* penetrate the skin. Schistosomiasis produces eosinophilia (choice B), and this symptom is taken into consideration in the diagnosis of this disease. Schistosomiasis can be diagnosed by the demonstration of ova of *S. mansoni* that has a characteristic lateral spine (choice C).

19. **(B)** Amiodarone is a broad-spectrum antiarrhythmic agent with unequaled efficacy and multiple toxicities. The molecular mechanisms for its antiarrhythmic actions are unclear but it blocks sodium, potassium I_{Kr}, and calcium channels as well as β-adrenoreceptors. It is very heavily used in refractory arrhythmias of all types, but especially in those associated with advanced heart failure. The most serious adverse effect of amiodarone is pulmonary fibrosis, but it also causes photodermatitis and thyroid dysfunction. The naturally occurring nucleoside adenosine (choice A) activates cardiac adenosine receptors that open a hyperpolarizing K^+ channel. It is very short acting and is used almost exclusively in the treatment of acute AV-nodal reentrant arrhythmias. Digoxin (choice C) is a cardiac glycoside that has been traditionally used in atrial fibrillation, but has much lower efficacy than amiodarone. Its major benefit is control of ventricular rate, because it prolongs AV refractory period and reduces the number of atrial impulses transmitted into the ventricles. Lidocaine (choice D) is a group IB antiarrhythmic that is of no value in atrial arrhythmias except those caused by digitalis over-

dose. It is most useful in the treatment of ventricular arrhythmias occurring immediately after myocardial infarction. Propafenone (choice E) is a group IC antiarrhythmic drug with some efficacy in both atrial and ventricular arrhythmias. Like other group IC agents, it is prone to causing new arrhythmias. It is not nearly as efficacious as amiodarone.

20. **(A)** Patients with multiple rib fractures or flail chest are likely to develop respiratory acidosis due to the pain and insufficient rib cage movements. In the acute phase, immediate tissue buffering elevates plasma bicarbonate only slightly, by about 1 mmol/L for each increase of 10 mm Hg in P_{CO_2}. Any increase in plasma bicarbonate beyond this expected value is due to renal compensation. Choice B is typical for a metabolic acidosis; the decrease in pH stimulates respiration and P_{CO_2} is lowered. Typically, each 1 mmol/L decrement in plasma bicarbonate results in a decrease of P_{CO_2} of about 1.2 mm Hg. Choice C represents a respiratory acidosis with renal compensation. Bicarbonate reabsorption in the kidneys is increased due to enhanced excretion of acid. Over a period of several days, plasma bicarbonate rises up to 3.5 mmol/L for each increase of 10 mm Hg in P_{CO_2}. Choice D represents an acute respiratory alkalosis. In acute hypocapnia, plasma bicarbonate falls approximately 2 mmol/L for each decrease in 10 mm Hg in P_{CO_2}. Choice E is typical for a compensated respiratory alkalosis, with a 4 to 5 mmol/L fall in plasma bicarbonate for each decrease of 10 mm Hg in P_{CO_2}.

21. **(B)** Kidneys regulate plasma pH by regulating the concentration of HCO_3^-. Almost all of the filtered HCO_3^- must be reabsorbed and this is accomplished by secretion of $H_2CO_3^-$ derived H^+. The secreted H^+ combines with HCO_3^- in the urine and the resulting H_2CO_3 is "lost." However, in the process of generating each H^+ within the tubular epithelium cells, one HCO_3^- is also produced. As a result, for each H^+ secreted, one HCO_3^- is "recovered" by the kidneys. More than 99.9% of the filtered HCO_3^- (choice D) is recovered by this

mechanism occurring predominantly in the proximal, not the distal tubules (choice C). The HCO_3^-/Cl^- exchange mechanism (choice A) is important in red blood cells, but not in renal tubular cells. Tubular fluid HCO_3^- combines with H^+ to form H_2CO_3, which then dissociates into H_2O and CO_2. The CO_2 diffuses passively through cell membranes and does not require active transport mechanisms. Because this patient is in respiratory acidosis, his kidneys generate more, not less, HCO_3^- than kidneys from a healthy subject (choice E). This renal compensation happens by excess H^+ secretion of the tubular cells, resulting in net generation of HCO_3^-.

22. **(C)** Body metabolism produces about 80 mEq of nonvolatile (i.e., not CO_2) acid per day. The majority of net H^+ excreted by the kidneys is bound to nontitratable acid (i.e., NH_4^+, pK > 7.4) and various titratable acids (i.e., buffers with pK < 7.4). Under normal conditions, about 50% of H^+ eliminated by the kidneys is in the form of NH_4^+. Under conditions of chronic acidosis, this amount can increase more than 10-fold, making the ammonia buffer quantitatively the most important route of renal H^+ excretion. For each bicarbonate (choice A) secreted, one H^+ has been reabsorbed by the kidneys, and net H^+ excretion equals NH_4^+ excretion plus urinary titratable acids minus bicarbonate excretion. Less than 0.1 mEq is excreted as free H^+ (choice B) because urine contains only up to $10^{-4.5}$ Eq/L = 0.03 mEq/L H^+ at pH = 4.5. Phosphoric acid (choice D) and uric acid (choice E) are the main titratable acids and together account for the remaining 50% of the total H^+ excreted.

23. **(E)** Sequencing of thousands of eukaryotic cDNAs and their corresponding genes has led to the identification of sequences that are required for accurate and efficient splicing of introns from precursor mRNAs. Sequences at the 5' and 3' ends of every intron analyzed show characteristic invariance. These sequences are GT at the 5' end and AG at the 3' end of each intron. Alteration in these sequences leads to aberrant or nonfunctional

splicing. No other combination of dinucleotides (choices A, B, C, and D) can substitute for the invariant sequences of the intron boundaries.

24. **(A)** HIV multiplies in CD4 lymphocytes, and this multiplication leads to severe lymphopenia due to the lysis of CD4+ lymphocytes. HIV is a member of the retrovirus group (choice C) that contains a single-stranded RNA genome (choice B) and reverse transcriptase (RNA-dependent DNA polymerase) (choice E) that synthesizes DNA from its RNA genome upon infection of host cells. HIV also has an envelope (choices D).

25. **(E)** Inferior alternating hemiplegia involves cranial nerve XII, which innervates the intrinsic musculature of the tongue. Superior and middle alternating hemiplegia involve extraocular musculature (choice A) innervated by cranial nerves III and VI, respectively. The muscles of mastication (choice D) and facial expression (choice C), as well as the laryngeal musculature (choice B), are not involved in alternating hemiplegia syndromes.

26. **(B)** Branches of the anterior spinal artery supply the medullary pyramid and the laterally adjacent fibers of the hypoglossal nerve. The lenticulostriate (choice A), and thalamoperforating vessels (choice D) and the vertebral artery (choice E) are not associated with alternating hemiplegia syndrome. The posterior inferior cerebellar artery (PICA, choice C) is associated with lateral medullary (Wallenberg) syndrome.

27. **(B)** Meconium ileus is a very common early clinical expression of cystic fibrosis. Increased sweat sodium chloride level confirms the diagnosis. About 70% of children with cystic fibrosis have a deletional abnormality of chromosome 7. Pancreatic insufficiency, recurrent pulmonary infections, and biliary obstruction may complicate the disorder. Alkaptonuria (choice A) is an autosomal recessive disease that causes abnormal pigmentation and degeneration of cartilage. Hemophilia A (choice C) is an X-linked hereditary disease caused

by a relative lack of coagulation factors VIII or IX. Phenylketonuria (choice D) is due to a hereditary lack of the enzyme phenylalanine hydroxylase. Mental retardation is the major clinical finding. Wilson disease (choice E) is an autosomal recessive disorder of copper accumulation that principally affects the liver and brain.

28. **(D)** The abnormal pulmonary mucus seen with cystic fibrosis leads to recurrent pulmonary infections. Eventually the lung becomes fibrotic and the majority of deaths are due to a failure of these organs. The major abnormality in cystic fibrosis is the production of abnormal mucus. Because the brain (choice A) does not synthesize mucus, it is not affected by this disorder. Only a fraction of cystic fibrosis deaths are due to abnormalities of the intestine (choice B). Those rare deaths occur in the neonatal period because of intestinal perforation secondary to undiagnosed meconium ileus. The liver (choice C) is minimally affected by cystic fibrosis. Hepatic failure is not a feature of the disorder. The exocrine pancreas (choice E) usually fails sometime during the disease. However, excellent oral medicines are available to replace most of the missing pancreatic agents.

29. **(C)** Strychnine is a weak base with a pKa value of 6.0. The unprotonated form (or the "free base") is uncharged and is the permeant species that crosses biological membranes. At equilibrium, the concentration of the permeant species is the same on both sides of the membrane, but the total amount (base + protonated form) present in each compartment depends on the pH of the compartment. For a weak base, the total amount is the highest in the most acidic compartment. This is because lower pH values cause protonation of the base to the protonated form that then becomes trapped in the compartment; the charged protonated base cannot cross the membrane. The lower the pH value for the compartment, the greater the total amount present. Stomach contents at pH 2.0 have the lowest pH value. The value for the total amount at any pH may be calculated using the Henderson–Hasselbalch equation [pH = pKa + log (unprotonated form/protonated form)].

30. **(D)** Because being in control is important to this orderly, controlling personality, PCA is especially effective for this type of patient (it is effective in almost all types of patients). A prn schedule (choice A) tends to be troublesome; the patient may become dissatisfied with the lag time between request and delivery. General anesthesia (choice B) may be seen by the patient as loss of control, as would hypnosis (choice C). Use of a placebo (choice E) with this type of patient is likely to be discovered, increasing his level of suspicion.

31. **(B)** In contrast to a classical antigen–antibody reaction, allergic reactions do not result in the neutralization of toxicity or antigen. For example, in type I hypersensitivity IgE binds to the surface of mast cells. Upon subsequent contact with the specific antigen to which an individual has been sensitized, mast cells release histamine and other vasoactive substances. This leads to anaphylaxis, urticaria, or other type I hypersensitivity reactions. In type I hypersensitivity, IgE binds to the surface of mast cells. Thus, IgE is produced in type I allergy such as allergic rhinitis (choice D). Administration of sodium cromolyn prevents release of histamine (choice A) from mast cells, and it is used to treat type I allergy. Type I allergy begins with the formation of IgE, which then binds on the mast cells. Therefore, mast cells in circulation have IgE on their surface (choice E). The reaction of IgE with its allergen is highly specific (choice C).

32. **(C)** The stapedius, posterior digastric, and stylohyoid muscles and the muscles of facial expression arise from the mesoderm of the second pharyngeal arch, and all are innervated by the facial nerve. The muscles of mastication, including the masseter muscle (choice A), the anterior belly of the digastric, the mylohyoid (choice B), the tensor tympani, and the tensor veli palatini muscles are all

derived from the mesoderm of the first pharyngeal arch, and all are innervated by the trigeminal nerve. The stylopharyngeus muscle (choice D) is derived from the mesoderm of the third pharyngeal arch and is innervated by the nerve of the third arch, the glossopharyngeal nerve. The superior pharyngeal constrictor muscle (choice E) is derived from the mesoderm of the fourth pharyngeal arch and is innervated by the nerve of the fourth to sixth arches, the vagus nerve.

33. **(D)** Metronidazole is one of the most effective antiamebic agents for tissue infection and has the lowest toxicity. The mechanism of action appears to involve production of toxic redox metabolites within the parasite. Dehydroemetine (choice A) and emetine are efficacious in tissue amebic infections, but are much more toxic than metronidazole. They cause cardiac toxicity and should only be given in the hospital setting with ECG monitoring. Diloxanide (choice B) is the drug of choice for asymptomatic intestinal infections but is not useful for tissue infections. Mefloquine (choice C) is the drug of choice for prevention of malaria in travelers to countries where chloroquine-resistant malaria predominates. It has no efficacy in amebic infection. Paromomycin (choice E) is an effective intestinal amebicide, but it is not absorbed, so it has no efficacy against tissue infection.

34. **(A)** The clinical presentation of patients with defects in several enzymes of urea synthesis are virtually identical. These enzymes are carbamoyl phosphate synthetase I (CPS-I), ornithine transcarbamoylase (OTC), argininosuccinate synthetase (AS), and argininosuccinase. The hallmark of these urea cycle enzyme defects is a normal birth with no known prenatal risk factors. Within 24 to 72 hours after birth, the infant becomes lethargic and requires stimulation for feeding. Additional symptoms develop within hours, including vomiting, increased lethargy, hypothermia, and hyperventilation. The hyperventilation is often misdiagnosed as pulmonary disease. Sepsis is often suspected. Routine blood work indicates a reduced

BUN. Lack of proper intervention leads to coma and death. Correct analysis of hyperammonemia is paramount to proper treatment because it indicated a urea cycle defect when presenting in the newborn. Analysis of plasma amino acids can aid in the differentiation of which enzyme is defective. Elevated citrulline (to 100 times normal levels) results from a deficiency in argininosuccinate synthetase. Several other inborn errors in metabolism are associated with neonatal hyperammonemia, such as carbamoylphosphate synthetase I (choice B), medium-chain acyl-CoA dehydrogenase (MCAD) deficiency (choice D), 3-hydroxy-3-methylglutaryl CoA (HMG-CoA) lyase deficiency (choice C), and pyruvate carboxylase (choice E) deficiency. Careful clinical assessment accompanying appropriate laboratory studies (e.g., plasma pyruvate and lactate levels, and urinalysis) can distinguish among these disorders. In MCAD deficiency, fatty acid oxidation and gluconeogenesis are impaired, whereas they would not be in an infant with a urea cycle defect. HMG-CoA lyase deficiency is associated with an increase in 3-hydroxy-3-methylglutaric, 3-methylglutaconic, and 3-hydroxyisovaleric acids in the urine.

35. **(D)** Ergot alkaloids cause very long-lasting and marked vasoconstriction that can lead to ischemia, pain, and even gangrene. Both α-adrenoreceptors and 5-HT receptors may be involved. No direct pharmacologic antagonists are available. Prevention of ischemic tissue damage is essential and requires a very efficacious vasodilator such as nitroprusside. The other drugs listed (choices A, B, C, and E) are all vasodilators but are not powerful enough to reverse the effect of an ergotamine overdose. Because of the risk of ischemia from overdosage, patients are instructed to take no more than six tablets for any one migraine episode and no more than 10 tablets in 1 week.

36. **(D)** Currently, HAART for advanced HIV disease follows a regimen consisting of the nucleoside inhibitors zidovudine and lamivudine, combined with a protease inhibitor such as indinavir. Gancyclovir and acyclovir

are nucleotide analogues of guanosine and acycloguanosine, respectively, that are used for the treatment of herpetic infections (choices A, B, C, and E).

37. **(C)** The insert at the bottom right indicates that this axial scan is taken at the level of the midbrain. Arrow #2 points to the red nucleus. The cerebral peduncle (choice B) is indicated by arrow #3. Arrow #4 points to the cerebral aqueduct of Sylvius (choice A) and the superior colliculi (choice D) located posteriorly. Arrow #1 points to the vermis of the cerebellum (choice E).

38. **(B)** The structure indicated by arrow #2 is the red nucleus, a midbrain structure derived from the mesencephalon. The thalamus, hypothalamus and epithalamus arise from the diencephalon (choice A). The metencephalon (choice C) eventually forms the pons and the cerebellum. The myelencephalon (choice D) gives rise to the medulla oblongata. The telencephalon (choice E) gives rise to the cerebral hemispheres.

39. **(A)** Alkaptonuria results from a defect in the enzyme homogentisate oxidase, which is required for the catabolism of tyrosine. Increased homogentisic acid is found in the urine and when exposed to the air it oxidizes to a brownish-black color. Deficiencies in α-keto acid dehydrogenase (choice B) lead to maple syrup urine disease (branched-chain ketonuria), characterized by the burnt sugar odor of the urine of affected individuals. A deficiency in phenylalanine hydroxylase (choice C), an enzyme required for the conversion of phenylalanine to tyrosine, is associated with phenylketonuria (PKU). No deficiencies in tryptophan oxygenase (choice D) are known. Tyrosine transaminase (choice E) deficiency leads to type II tyrosinemia (Richner–Hanhart syndrome), which results in elevated plasma tyrosine levels, eye and skin lesions, and moderate mental retardation.

40. **(D)** The sustained depolarization of the plateau phase is represented by the ST interval (which is not normally associated with any voltage deflection). The depolarization observed in the P wave (choice A) signals the onset of atrial contraction, and the QRS complex (choice B) is associated with the initiation of ventricular contraction. The QT interval (choice C) is composed of not only the plateau phase, but also the rapid upstroke (phase 0) and partial repolarization (phase 1) of the cardiac action potential. The T wave (choice E) is associated with the onset of ventricular repolarization.

41. **(D)** The gallbladder contains numerous stones. Gallstone formation is frequently seen in middle-aged, overweight females. Elevated biliary cholesterol may be conducive to stone formation. Potential complications of gallstones include obstructive jaundice, acute cholecystitis, and perforation. The gallbladder does not display a congenital malformation (choice A). Although infection (choice B) may be a later complication of cholelithiasis, there is no evidence of infection in Figure 10–4. There is no evidence of a neoplastic process (choice C) in the opened gallbladder. The gallbladder does not show any evidence of a thrombotic process (choice E).

42. **(C)** Buspirone is an atypical sedative–hypnotic with no hypnotic or anticonvulsant action and practically no sedative effect. Its mechanism of action does not involve the GABA system (unlike typical sedative hypnotics). Its efficacy as an anxiolytic may involve partial agonist action at 5-HT$_{1A}$ receptors. Alprazolam (choice A) is a benzodiazepine with modest but significant sedative actions. It is particularly useful in panic disorder. Amitriptyline (choice B) is a first-generation tricyclic antidepressant. It is not an anxiolytic. Clozapine (choice D) is an atypical antipsychotic agent that is notable for its lack of extrapyramidal toxicity and its selectivity for D$_4$ rather than D$_2$ dopamine receptors. Methylphenidate (choice E) is an amphetamine analog that is used in attention deficit hyperkinetic disorder.

43. **(B)** A hemagglutination inhibition titer of 400 means that when a patient's serum is diluted

400-fold, it will prevent agglutination of the assay red blood cells.

44. **(B)** The glossopharyngeal nerve conducts the general sensation (GVA) and taste (SVA) from the posterior one-third of the tongue. The facial nerve (choice A) has no general sensory distribution to the mucosa of the tongue, but does provide taste fibers to the anterior two-thirds of the tongue via the chorda tympani and lingual nerve. The hypoglossal nerve (choice C) provides motor innervation to the muscles of the tongue. It has no sensory component. The lingual nerve (choice D) provides general sensation to the anterior two-thirds of the tongue and distributes to the same area taste fibers that communicate from the facial nerve to the lingual nerve via the chorda tympani. The vagus nerve (choice E) has no sensory distribution to the mucosa of the tongue, but does provide taste fibers over the epiglottis.

45. **(A)** Marked brain damage is seen in cases of failure to make urea via the urea cycle or to eliminate urea through the kidneys. The result of either of these events is a buildup of circulating levels of ammonium ion. Aside from its effect on blood pH, ammonia readily traverses the blood–brain barrier and in the brain is converted to glutamate via glutamate dehydrogenase, depleting the brain of α-ketoglutarate. As the α-ketoglutarate is depleted, oxaloacetate falls correspondingly, and ultimately TCA cycle activity comes to a halt. In the absence of aerobic oxidative phosphorylation and TCA cycle activity, irreparable cell damage and neural cell death ensue. In addition, the increased glutamate leads to glutamine formation. This depletes glutamate stores, which are needed in neural tissue because glutamate is both a neurotransmitter and a precursor for the synthesis of GABA, another neurotransmitter. Therefore, reductions in brain glutamate affect energy production as well as neurotransmission. None of the other choices (B, C, D, and E) represent reasonable responses of the nervous system to increased ammonia levels.

46. **(C)** Mature cystic teratoma (dermoid cyst) is a benign ovarian tumor that arises from germ cells. It occurs most frequently in young and middle-aged women. A mixture of hair, sebaceous debris, soft tissue, and teeth may be grossly evident. Microscopically, these mixed elements appear mature. Brenner tumor (choice A) is an uncommon, benign ovarian tumor. Transitional epithelial nests within a fibrous stroma characterize this tumor, which is derived from ovarian epithelium. Endometrioid adenocarcinoma (choice B) is an infrequently seen ovarian malignancy arising from ovarian epithelium. Mucinous cystadenoma (choice D) is a benign ovarian neoplasm that originates from epithelial cells, not germ cells. Serous papillary carcinoma (choice E) is the most common type of ovarian malignancy. It arises from ovarian epithelium, not germ cells.

47. **(E)** Valproic acid is associated with a low but significant incidence of hepatic impairment. The cause is unknown, but the incidence is highest in patients under 2 years of age and in those taking multiple medications. Fatalities have resulted. Carbamazepine (choice A) is effective in the treatment of trigeminal neuralgia. Its major toxicities involve diplopia and ataxia in overdose. Ethosuximide (choice B) causes sedation as its primary toxicity. Lamotrigine (choice C) causes a variety of minor adverse effects, but its most serious toxicity is a potentially life-threatening dermatitis. Vigabatrin causes visual field defects that may be irreversible. Phenytoin (choice D) causes diplopia, ataxia, and gingival hyperplasia. It has been associated with fetal abnormalities when taken by pregnant women.

48. **(C)** Apolipoprotein C-II is required to activate the enzyme lipoprotein lipase, which is present on the surfaces of vascular endothelial cells. The function of lipoprotein lipase is to hydrolyze fatty acids from the triglycerides present in chylomicrons and VLDLs. Therefore, a lack of this enzyme results in the inability to remove the dietary fatty acids packaged in chylomicrons. Afflicted individuals exhibit extremely elevated plasma levels

of both chylomicrons and triglycerides. A deficiency in apoC-II is one type of a family of three related inherited disorders that lead to chylomicronemia and triglyceridemia. The other two related disorders are due to a deficiency in lipoprotein lipase and a familial inhibitor of lipoprotein lipase. The restriction to a fat-free diet prevents elevations in plasma chylomicrons and triglycerides. ApoA-I (choice A) is a major protein of HDLs and is required for the activation of lecithin:cholesterol acyltransferase (LCAT). Deficiency in apoA-I results in Tangier disease, which is characterized by a severe deficiency in HDLs in the plasma. This leads to the accumulation of cholesteryl esters in tissues throughout the body. ApoB-100 (choice B) is found associated with VLDLs and LDLs and is required in conjunction with apoE for LDL receptor recognition of LDLs. Abetalipoproteinemia is due to loss of apoB, whereas familial hypobetalipoproteinemia is due to mutant forms of apoB. The former disorder is characterized by the virtual absence of VLDLs and LDLs from the plasma; hepatic and intestinal accumulation of triglycerides; and acanthocytosis (the erythrocytes exhibit a thorny appearance). The latter disorder is characterized by dramatically reduced levels of plasma VLDLs and LDLs. ApoD (choice D) is also called cholesterol ester transfer protein (CETP) and is found associated with HDLs. No identified disorders are associated with apoD. ApoE (choice E) is required for LDL interaction with the LDL receptor. Familial dysbetalipoproteinemia results in persons with a mutant form of apoE (apoE-2). Symptoms include hypercholesterolemia and hypertriglyceridemia.

49. **(D)** Respiratory syncytial virus is the major cause of bronchiolitis and pneumonia in infants less than 1 year old. Adenoviruses (choice A) can cause pneumonia with cough and fever, particularly among children less than 3 years old. Influenza virus (choice B) is not the most common cause of bronchiolitis in infants and is not associated with wheezing. Parainfluenza serotype 3 (choice C) in older individuals has mostly been associated with

tracheobronchitis. Infections with rotaviruses (choice E) are especially common in children 1 to 24 months of age. However, these viruses cause diarrhea, not bronchiolitis.

50. **(C)** Mitral stenosis impedes the filling of the left ventricle, resulting in decreased end-diastolic filling volume. The actual preload on myocardial fibers is the stretch placed on them at the end of diastole just before the beginning of systole. This stretch determines the resting length of the fibers prior to contraction. For practical purposes, the end-diastolic volume is used as a convenient index of preload (the greater the end-diastolic volume, the greater the stretch). The pressure-volume loop with the lowest end-diastolic volume, and therefore the lowest preload, is loop C. Choice A represents a negative inotropic effect (parasympathetic stimulation). Note that the stroke volume is reduced and the end-systolic volume (blood left in ventricle after systole) is increased. The other two curves (choices B and E) have stroke volumes greater than normal, but only one of these shows increased contractility. Which of the two has increased contractility can be determined from the location of the end-systolic pressure-volume point. The end-systolic pressure-volume point for loop E is on the same line as for the normal individual (diagonal line in illustration). In contrast, loop B has an end-systolic pressure-volume point at a higher level (falls on an end-systolic pressure-volume line that begins at about the same intercept with the abscissa, but has a steeper slope than for normal contractility). Thus, loop B represents a pressure-volume loop for increased contractility. Loop E most closely resembles the pressure-volume loop one might expect if the venous return were increased, resulting in a larger filling volume of the ventricle.

51. **(A)** The angular artery, a branch of the facial artery, anastomoses with the dorsal nasal artery, a branch of the ophthalmic artery, providing a potentially significant anastomosis between the external carotid and internal carotid arteries. The lingual and facial arter-

ies (choice B) are both branches of the external carotid artery. The superficial temporal artery is a branch of the external carotid artery and the middle meningeal artery arises from the maxillary artery, a branch of the external carotid (choice C). The superficial temporal artery and the occipital artery (choice D) are both branches of the external carotid artery. The superior thyroid artery is a branch of the external carotid artery and the inferior thyroid artery arises from the thyrocervical trunk, a branch of the subclavian artery (choice E).

52. **(C)** McArdle disease (type V glycogen storage disease) is the result of a deficiency in skeletal muscle glycogen phosphorylase. Clinical symptoms are characterized by exercise-induced muscle cramping and pain, and usually appear in young adulthood. Anderson disease (type IV glycogen storage disease) (choice A) results from a deficiency in the glycogen branching enzyme. Symptoms present within the first few months of life and include hepatosplenomegaly and failure to thrive. Progressive liver damage along with esophageal varices and ascites lead to death by age 5. Hers disease (type VI glycogen storage disease) (choice B) results from a deficiency in liver phosphorylase. Patients progress with a relatively benign course of hepatomegaly and growth retardation. The hepatomegaly improves and disappears as the patient enters puberty. Tarui disease (type VII glycogen storage disease) (choice D) results from a deficiency in skeletal muscle phosphofructokinase. Symptoms are similar to those of McArdle disease. Differential diagnosis of McArdle and Tarui disease requires assay of muscle phosphorylase and phosphofructokinase activities. Von Gierke disease (type I glycogen storage disease) (choice E) results from a deficiency in glucose-6-phosphatase. Symptoms appear soon after birth and are characterized by hypoglycemia, lactic acidosis, hyperlipidemia, and hyperuricemia following a short fast.

53. **(A)** The medial lemniscus, which contains decussated (crossed) ascending somatosensory fibers originating in the dorsal column nuclei, is formed in the caudal medulla just rostral to the levels of the motor (pyramidal) decussation. The somatosensory fibers of the dorsal column–medial lemniscal system that ascend through the midbrain (choice B), pons (choice C), internal capsule (choice D), and thalamus (choice E) cross at medullary levels and are contralateral to their origin at these levels.

54. **(D)** Surfactant serves to reduce surface tension within the alveoli and prevent atelectasis. In premature infants, inadequate surfactant predisposes to the development of respiratory distress syndrome. Congenital pulmonary malformations (choice A) do not affect the secretion of surfactant. Neonates have a reduced capacity to conjugate bilirubin (choice B) that may lead to hyperbilirubinemia or kernicterus. Pulmonary surfactant is not altered. Infants have a reduced humoral immunity capacity (choice C). The production of surfactant is related to gestational age, not immune status. Several in utero viral infections (choice E) may prove deleterious to neonates. However, these infections do not cause a lack of surfactant in premature infants.

55. **(D)** Neuroleptic-induced pseudoparkinsonism, including pill-rolling tremor, should be ruled out because it can be treated effectively with anticholinergic drugs. von Economo encephalitis (choice C), pandemic in 1917 and 1918, often resulted in Parkinsonism, but this patient's age makes it unlikely. The other items (choices A, B, and E) are of importance in history taking, but not as important in this case as a history of taking neuroleptic drugs.

56. **(D)** When tardive dyskinesia is suspected, the Abnormal Involuntary Movement Scale (AIMS) is useful. A part of the test includes asking the patient to open his mouth and observe his tongue (it may have slow movements), and to protrude the tongue (it may show movements, or there may be quick withdrawal of the tongue). All the other tests (choices A, B, C, and E) are unlikely to docu-

ment involuntary movements associated with tardive dyskinesia.

57. **(D)** Choreoathetoid movements coupled with pseudoparkinsonism are diagnostic of tardive dyskinesia associated with neuroleptic use. There is no evidence of dementia (choices A and E). Multiple sclerosis (choice B) is associated with intention tremor and other neurologic signs, and Sydenham chorea (choice C) is predominantly a disease of childhood not associated with athetoid movements.

58. **(B)** The time interval 0 to 6 hours is called the eclipse period. During this period of viral growth cycle, the virus is absorbed to the host cell, enters the host cell, and the viral nucleic acid is separated from its capsid. The time period of 0 to 6 hours is the eclipse period, and represents events that lead to loss, not retention, of viral infectivity (choice A). The time period of 6 to 8 hours represents a portion of the rise period, which marks the appearance of mature virus (choices C and D). The bacterial growth curve (choice E) is a bell-shaped curve composed of the lag phase (in which the cell population is constant), the logarithmic phase of growth (in which the number of cells increase in a geometric fashion [1–2–4–8–16]), the stationary phase (in which the cell population remains constant), and the phase of decline (in which the cells die in an exponential fashion).

59. **(E)** Saquinavir is an HIV protease inhibitor. The current HIV protease inhibitors are not suitable for monotherapy because of the rapid emergence of resistance due to mutations in the HIV protease sequence. Combination therapy using saquinavir with two of the reverse transcriptase inhibitors such as zidovudine, lamivudine, or didanosine is currently effective in greatly lowering viral load or even making patients (apparently) virus free. The nucleosides zidovudine (AZT), didanosine (ddI), lamivudine (3TC), and zalcitabine (ddC) inhibit viral reverse transcriptase. These nucleosides are metabolized to the triphosphate forms that competitively in-

hibit reverse transcriptase. Deletion of thymidine kinase (choice A) is another mechanism for resistance of herpesvirus to acyclovir. Although thymidylate synthase is a target of 5-fluorouracil action, deletion of the enzyme (choice B) is not a mechanism for resistance, because thymidylate synthase is an essential activity. Combinations of agents must be used because resistance arising from mutations in the reverse transcriptase sequence (choice C) frequently arises with monotherapy. Mutations in the sequence of viral DNA polymerase (choice D) are a mechanism of resistance for the antiherpesvirus nucleosides acyclovir, valacyclovir, famciclovir, and ganciclovir. These agents are metabolized to their nucleotide triphosphate forms that competitively inhibit the herpesvirus DNA polymerase. Acyclovir and valacyclovir also cause DNA chain termination.

60. **(D)** Calcitonin is a hormone secreted by the parafollicular C cells of the thyroid gland. Medullary carcinoma arises from malignant transformation of these cells. α-Fetoprotein (choice A) may be elevated in the serum in association with hepatocellular carcinomas and gonadal tumors. CA 125 (choice B) is a tumor-associated glycoprotein frequently expressed by ovarian carcinomas. CA 15–3 (choice C) is a tumor-associated glycoprotein frequently expressed by breast carcinomas. Elevations of human chorionic gonadotropin (choice E) in the serum may be seen in normal pregnancies, gonadal tumors, and choriocarcinomas.

61. **(A)** The anomeric hydroxyl group of glucose derivatizes the amino groups of lysine side chains in hemoglobin as well as the amino terminals of the globin monomers. When glycosylated, hemoglobin can be separated from normal adult hemoglobin (designated HbA) by ion exchange chromatography. To distinguish glycosylated hemoglobin, it is given the designation, HbA_{1c}. Other modifications of adult hemoglobin occur, such as with glucose-6-phosphate and fructose-1,6-bisphosphate, and these modified hemoglobins are given designations with subscripts like those

for glycosylated hemoglobin (e.g., HbA_{1a1} or HbA_{1b}). Normal levels of glycosylated hemoglobin represent about 5% of the total. About 2% to 3% of normal adults contain a version of hemoglobin that is composed of two α chains and two δ chains (instead of two β chains). This hemoglobin is designated HbA_2 (choice B). The other choices designate defective forms of hemoglobin found in various disease states. HbC (choice C) results when a lysine is substituted for glutamate at position 6 of the β chain. HbE (choice D) is the most common hemoglobin variant in man. It results from a substitution of lysine for glutamate at position 26 of the β chain. HbS (choice E) is the form of hemoglobin found in sickle-cell anemia. This hemoglobin results from a substitution of valine for glutamate at position 6 of the β chain.

62. **(E)** The normal function of osteoclasts is removal of bone matrix, a process that is crucial both in regulation of circulating Ca^{2+} concentration and in modeling and remodeling of bones. Congenital failure of osteoclast function results in development of thick, abnormally dense bones. The regulation of calcium concentration in plasma and tissue fluid depends on a dynamic system of hormone-mediated calcium removal and deposition in bone. Abnormal deposition of calcium in sites such as the kidney and vessel walls (choice A) is a consequence of excessive calcium release from bone into circulation. This is a condition associated with inappropriately high activity of osteoclasts as a result of their stimulation by excessive parathyroid hormone. Low levels of circulating calcium stimulates release of parathyroid hormone, which stimulates calcium release from bone by osteoclasts. Osteoclast activity is an important component of the system, and failure of osteoclast function tends to reduce rather than increase (choice B) calcium in circulation. During bone development, osteoclasts are required for replacement of the initial spongy core of the bone by a marrow cavity. Thus, failure of osteoclast function results in reduced, not enlarged (choice C), marrow cavities. The consequences of this include de-

ficient hematopoietic capacity. Individuals with osteopetrosis typically suffer from anemia and increased susceptibility to infections. Failure of osteoclasts to respond and the consequent failure of circulating calcium levels to return to normal would more likely result in increased, rather than decreased, parathyroid hormone levels (choice D).

63. **(C)** During a constant dosing regimen (constant infusion), the kinetics for the approach to the steady-state concentration are controlled by drug clearance and can be predicted from the elimination half-life. The concentration traverses half of the remaining distance to the steady state in each half-life. In this case, after 2 h (one half-life), the concentration is 50% of the steady-state level. After 4 h (two half-lives), the concentration is 75% of steady state. After 8 h (four half-lives), the concentration is approximately 94% of the steady-state level.

64. **(F)** Endogenous and exogenous pyrogens, resulting from the presence of infecting pathogenic microorganisms, raise the hypothalamic set point and thereby cause a rise in body temperature (fever). If the factors originally responsible for the fever are gone (successfully eliminated by the body's immune system), the hypothalamic set point returns to normal. For a while, the body's core temperature is above the now normal set point. This has the same effect as if the individual were too hot. The patient begins sweating and complains of "burning up" because of his hot skin (due to vasodilation). During period A (choice A), the patient is comfortable because his body temperature matches his set point. When the set point is first raised due to pyrogens (at point B, choice D), the body temperature is temporarily below the new, higher set point, just as if the body were too cool. The hypothalamus stimulates the usual responses to produce additional heat (shivering) and to conserve the heat present (skin vasoconstriction and lack of sweating). The patient subjectively feels chilled and seeks to raise his body temperature until he is more comfortable (piles on blankets, sits by the

fire, or gets a heating pad). Once the patient's temperature has risen to match the newer, higher set point (choices B and E), the patient is comfortable and his new, higher temperature is well regulated around the new set point. Similarly, when the patient reaches his normal temperature at the end of the febrile episode (choices C and G), he once again feels comfortable; his body temperature matches his set point.

65. **(C)** Adenosine deaminase is required for the catabolism of adenosine to inosine. In the absence of ADA, deoxyadenosine is phosphorylated to yield levels of dATP that are 50-fold higher than normal. The levels are especially high in lymphocytes, which have abundant amounts of the salvage enzymes, including nucleoside kinases. High concentrations of dATP inhibit ribonucleotide reductase, thereby preventing other dNTPs from being produced. The net effect is to inhibit DNA synthesis. Because lymphocytes must be able to proliferate dramatically in response to antigenic challenge, the inability to synthesize DNA seriously impairs the immune responses, and the disease is usually fatal in infancy unless special protective measures are taken. There is no increase in inosine levels in ADA deficiency (choice A). ADA deficiency does not impair salvage of ATP (choice B). Loss of adenosine catabolism does not lead to increased uric acid production (choice D). Inosine (a purine) cannot be used to salvage thymidine (a pyrimidine) nucleotides for DNA synthesis (choice E).

66. **(A)** Chronic glomerulonephritis is a common finding probably representing the end stage of many diseases involving the glomeruli. Grossly, the kidneys are shrunken with a granular, irregular surface. Microscopically, the number of nephrons is greatly reduced with hyalinization of glomeruli, tubular atrophy, interstitial fibrosis, and IgG, IgA, and C3 in some of the remaining glomeruli. Diabetic nephropathy (choice B) produces few gross changes but microscopically there is capillary basement membrane thickening, diffuse and nodular glomerulosclerosis, and the pathog-

nomonic finding of hyaline thickening of both the afferent and efferent arterioles. The findings in lupus nephritis (choice C) are quite variable, but usually include focal or diffuse proliferative glomerulonephritis with subendothelial deposits, sometimes with areas of necrosis. Diagnostic "wire loop" lesions, due to massive subendothelial deposits, can sometimes be seen. Renal amyloidosis (choice D) is the most common cause of death in patients with amyloidosis. Nephrotic syndrome is common and hyaline deposits of amyloid may be seen in glomeruli, vessels, and the interstitium. When stained by Congo red, the deposits show green birefringence under polarized light. Renal disease in Wegener granulomatosis (choice E) is characterized by proteinuria, hematuria, and rapidly progressive renal failure. Microscopically, the glomeruli show focal segmental proliferative glomerulonephritis and vessels show a necrotizing granulomatous arteritis.

67. **(A)** The accessory nerve emerges from deep in the sternocleidomastoid muscle and passes posteriorly across the posterior triangle to supply the trapezius muscle. The superior thyroid artery (choice B) arises from the external carotid artery in the carotid triangle and descends through the neck in the anterior triangle. The thoracic duct (choice C) enters the root of the neck on the left side under cover of the sternocleidomastoid muscle and empties at the junction of the internal jugular and subclavian veins. The vertebral artery (choice D) arises from the first part of the subclavian artery in the root of the neck and under cover of the sternocleidomastoid muscle. It is not related to the posterior triangle of the neck. The vagus nerve (choice E) descends in the neck within the carotid sheath. Superiorly it lies in the carotid triangle, and inferiorly it lies under cover of the sternocleidomastoid muscle.

68. **(A)** Serologic tests, such as agglutination reactions, are of little if any value for the diagnosis of dermatophytes because they tend to have common antigens and they grow in clumps. Thus, homogeneous fungal cell sus-

pensions are extremely difficult to produce and use in proper agglutination reactions.

69. **(E)** The patient is an exacting, orderly, controlling person who is very conscious of punctuality. The other personalities (choices A, B, C, and D) do not explain his preoccupation with exactness.

70. **(B)** The reaction shown is that catalyzed during the final step of oxidative phosphorylation, which requires cytochrome oxidase (cytochrome aa_3) of complex IV. Catalase (choice A) is responsible for the destruction of hydrogen peroxide to water. Ferrochetalase (choice C) catalyzes the conversion of protoporphyrin IX to iron protoporphyrin IX, the heme prosthetic group of hemoglobin. Peroxidases (choice D) reduce peroxides such as hydrogen peroxide to water using various electron acceptors. Superoxide dismutase (choice E) catalyzes the conversion of superoxide radicals to hydrogen peroxide and O_2.

71. **(E)** PTH-like peptides are most commonly produced by massive squamous lung carcinomas, renal malignancies, and some breast cancers. Parathyroid hormone and PTH-like substances stimulate bone resorption and vitamin D conversion (choice A), thereby elevating serum calcium levels (choice D). Serum calcitonin is consequently expected to rise. A PTH-like effect on the kidneys increases calcium absorption while markedly increasing phosphate excretion (choice B). Calcitonin levels (choice C) are expected to increase secondary to the elevated blood Ca^{2+} concentration. Hypercalcemia due to malignancy is common, often severe, and difficult to treat.

72. **(C)** With the infusion of epinephrine, we observe an increase in systolic pressure indicative of an increase in cardiac stroke volume. Increased stroke volume results from an increase in cardiac contractility, a cardiac β_1-adrenoreceptor action. The decrease in diastolic pressure indicates that peripheral resistance has decreased. Epinephrine acts on β_2-adrenoreceptors in skeletal muscle blood vessels to relax this vascular smooth muscle.

Because skeletal muscle constitutes a large percentage of body mass, total peripheral resistance decreases even though epinephrine also acts on α_1-adrenoreceptors in arterioles throughout the body to produce vasoconstriction. With the infusion of drug X, we observe a larger decrease in diastolic pressure than that seen with epinephrine and a slight decrease in mean pressure. This is consistent with either blockade of vasoconstricting α_1-adrenoreceptors or vasodilation through activation of β_2-adrenoreceptors. The systolic pressure has increased to a lesser extent than that seen with epinephrine, but there is a significant increase in pulse pressure, suggesting increased stroke volume. This is consistent with β_1-adrenoreceptor stimulation. The increase in heart rate from 70 to 105 per minute is also consistent with β_1-adrenoreceptor stimulation. All of the observations are consistent with infusion of an agent such as isoproterenol that possesses β_1- and β_2-adrenoreceptor agonistic properties. Amphetamine (choice A) is an indirect-acting sympathomimetic that releases norepinephrine from sympathetic nerve endings. Its effects therefore mimic norepinephrine, with increased diastolic, mean, and systolic pressures. Atropine (choice B) is a muscarinic antagonist. It has little direct effect on normal blood pressure, but usually increases heart rate when given in large doses. Norepinephrine (choice D) is a potent α_1-, α_2-, and β_1-agonist. Its primary effect is to produce a large increase in total peripheral resistance, thereby raising diastolic pressure. It also stimulates the contractility of the heart, so that stroke volume increases somewhat; it increases systolic pressure more than diastolic. Phenylephrine (choice E) has α_1- and α_2-agonist activity, but practically no β activity. Therefore, it increases diastolic and systolic pressure about equally, with little change in pulse pressure.

73. **(E)** Primary biliary cirrhosis (PBC) is characterized by destruction of the interlobular bile ducts. Despite its name, it is not a true cirrhosis because no nodular regeneration of the liver is seen in the disease. It is thought to be

an autoimmune disorder and is associated with other immunologic diseases such as Sjögren syndrome and systemic sclerosis. The presence of serum antimitochondrial antibodies in titers exceeding 1:160 is diagnostic. More than 90% of cases occur in middle-aged women and four histologic cases of PBC have been identified that are associated with various degrees of mostly lymphatic and plasma cell infiltration: bile duct destruction, followed by abnormal bile duct proliferation and then progressive bile duct destruction; and progressive fibrosis that eventually encloses individual lobules to create an overt micronodular cirrhosis. Epithelial granulomas with Langhans giant cells occur in about 30% of cases. Clinical presentation follows slow progressive biliary obstruction, and pruritis is the most common first symptom. Serum alkaline phosphatase is elevated early on, but jaundice usually occurs 6 to 18 months after onset. Elevated serum triglyceride and cholesterol levels are common, as are subsequent xanthomas. Portal hypertension and liver failure may result 5 to 15 years following onset. Secondary biliary cirrhosis occurs following prolonged bile duct obstruction and is distinguished from PBC most notably by the presence of regenerative nodules late in the disease. Cholangiocarcinomas (choice A) are usually well-differentiated sclerosing adenocarcinomas that secrete mucin, which is frequently present within cells. It is not associated with cirrhosis. Clinical presentation is with a liver mass. Cholangitis (choice B) is a secondary suppurative infection of the intra-extrahepatic ducts typically following an extrahepatic obstructive lesion, usually an impacted bile duct gallstone. Symptoms include high fever, chills, and jaundice. Cholestasis (choice C) is an obstruction of canalicular bile flow. Bile ducts are normal. Clinical presentation is with jaundice. Hepatitis A (choice D) does not cause chronic disease.

74. **(A)** The major products of parietal cells are hydrochloric acid and intrinsic factor. Intrinsic factor is a glycoprotein that combines with vitamin B_{12} to form a complex that is ab-

sorbed by enterocytes of the ileum. Neutralization of the highly acidic chyme (choice B) that passes from the stomach into the jejunum is mainly a function of bicarbonate secretion by the pancreas in response to signaling by the peptide hormone secretin, a product of enteroendocrine cells in the duodenum. Although atrophic gastritis results in decreased pepsin in gastric juice, pepsinogen (choice C) is secreted by chief cells, the other major cell type of fundic glands of the stomach. Acid secretion by parietal cells is stimulated by gastrin (choice D), but these cells do not produce this polypeptide hormone. Gastrin is secreted by enteroendocrine cells of the stomach and duodenum. The protective mucous coat of the gastric lining (choice E) is mainly a product of the cells of the surface epithelium.

75. **(D)** Niemann–Pick disease (NPD) is composed of three types of lipid storage disorders, two of which (types A and B NPD) result from a defect in acid sphingomyelinase. Type A is a disorder that leads to infantile mortality. Type B is variable in phenotype and diagnosed by the presence of hepatosplenomegaly in childhood and progressive pulmonary infiltration. Pathologic characteristics of NPD are the accumulation of histiocytic cells that results from sphingomyelin deposition in cells of the monocyte–macrophage system. Fabry disease (choice A) is an X-linked disorder that results from a deficiency in α-galactosidase A. This leads to the deposition of neutral glycosphingolipids with terminal α-galactosyl moieties in most tissues and fluids. The most affected tissues are heart, kidneys, and eyes. With advancing age, the major symptoms are due to increasing deposition of glycosphingolipid in the cardiovascular system. Indeed, cardiac disease occurs in most hemizygous males. Three types of Gaucher disease (choice B) have been characterized and are caused by defects in lysosomal acid β-glucosidase (glucocerebrosidase). Defects in this enzyme lead to the accumulation of glucosylceramides (glucocerebrosides), which leads primarily to CNS dysfunction, as well as hepatosplenomegaly and skeletal lesions. Krabbe disease (choice C), also called

globoid-cell leukodystrophy, results from a deficiency in galactosylceramidase (galacto-cerebroside-β-galactosidase). This disease progresses rapidly and invariably leads to infantile mortality. Tay–Sachs disease (choice E) results from a defect in hexosaminidase A leading to the accumulation of G_{M2} gangliosides, particularly in neuronal cells. This defect leads to severe mental retardation, progressive weakness, and hypotonia, which prevents normal motor development. Progression of the disease is rapid and death occurs within the second year.

76. **(C)** Resistance to blood flow primarily occurs in arterioles with smooth muscle, and thus this is the site of the largest pressure drop. Compliance (stretchability) of veins is much larger than that of arteries due to their lack of elastic fibers and thinner walls (choice A). Although the capillaries are the smallest vessels, by virtue of their large number and parallel arrangement, their effective cross-sectional area is very large, larger than that of small veins (choice B). Blood volume is greatest not in the capillaries (choice D), but in the small veins, which serve as a blood reservoir by nature of their high compliance (low elasticity). Because velocity is inversely related to cross-sectional area, the velocity in the capillaries is very low (choice E). This large surface area and low velocity promote exchange of substances between blood and tissue.

77. **(E)** Vincristine is a natural product derived from the vinca plant and acts by interfering with microtubule assembly. It is useful in Hodgkin lymphoma. Its primary toxicity is peripheral neuropathy, manifested as numbness, tingling, and pain. A very similar vinca alkaloid, vinblastine, has the same mechanism of action, but causes myelosuppression rather than neuropathies. Bleomycin (choice A) is an antibiotic chemotherapeutic agent that produces single- and double-strand breaks. It is useful in combination therapy of Hodgkin disease because it produces little myelosuppression, but it does produce serious toxicity involving the lung, including life-threatening pulmonary fibrosis. Cisplatin

(choice B) is used alone and in combination to treat a wide variety of carcinomas. Toxicity is expressed as renal damage. Cisplatin is particularly effective in treating testicular and ovarian cancers in combination with other antitumor agents. Cisplatin exerts a renal toxicity that may be prevented by the infusion of saline prior to drug administration. Ototoxicity involving high-frequency hearing loss is a toxicity that is not prevented by hydration. Doxorubicin (choice C) is another natural product used in Hodgkin disease that acts by DNA intercalation. The primary toxicity of doxorubicin is cumulative cardiac damage, so that lifetime dosage of the drug must be limited. Mechlorethamine (choice D) is a synthetic nitrogen mustard compound used in Hodgkin disease that alkylates DNA, especially at the N^7 position of guanine. Its primary toxicity is myelosuppression.

78. **(C)** The touch imprints show a metastatic carcinoma. The cells demonstrate cytologic features of malignancy such as anaplasia, molding, wrinkled nuclear membranes, and hyperchromatism. The finding of large, atypical cohesive epithelial cells in a cerebral biopsy is diagnostic of a malignant process. A chronic demyelinating disorder (choice A) does not contain atypical epithelial cells on touch imprint. The displayed cells are malignant epithelial cells. The lack of an essential nutrient (choice B) is not pertinent to the observed cells. The cells do not show any cytologic features of parasitic infestation (choice D), such as inclusion body formation, eggs, or cysts. The displayed cells do not demonstrate any cytologic features of viral infection (choice E), such as inclusion bodies or multinucleation.

79. **(A)** *Clostridium difficile* is most commonly associated with severe pseudomembranous enterocolitis following antibiotic therapy, and especially treatment with clindamycin and ampicillin. Echovirus (choice B) may cause aseptic meningitis and encephalitis. *Entamoeba histolytica* (choice C) may cause discrete enteric ulcers, and liver abscesses. *Escherichia coli* (choice D) that can form enterotoxin is a

common cause of traveler's diarrhea. *Salmonella enteritis* (choice E) causes vomiting, fever, and profuse diarrhea.

80. **(C)** Prolactin secretion from the anterior pituitary is under negative regulation by dopamine released by the hypothalamus. Blockade of dopamine receptors by the neuroleptic agents increases prolactin secretion. Hyperprolactinemia is associated with galactorrhea, amenorrhea, and infertility in women, and infertility, impotence, and galactorrhea in men. Butyrophenones such as haloperidol possess weak antimuscarinic activity that causes decreased, not increased, salivation (choice B). Similarly, the weak antimuscarinic activity of the butyrophenones may cause constipation rather than diarrhea (choice A). Nausea and vomiting (choice D) are common effects with many drugs, but the neuroleptic agents have antiemetic actions through their dopamine-blocking effects on the chemoreceptor trigger zone. Tourette syndrome (choice E) consists of chronic multiple motor and phonic tics of unknown etiology. The motor tics commonly affect the face and may consist of repetitive blinking or closing of the eyes. The phonic tics may involve explosive grunts, coughs, or coprolalia (involuntary obscenities). Although the cause is unknown, the symptoms are often controlled with haloperidol treatment, suggesting excess dopamine activity in a brain region.

81. **(D)** The superior thyroid artery runs next to the external laryngeal nerve along the lateral aspect of the larynx to supply the superior pole of the thyroid gland. To avoid injury to the external laryngeal nerve during surgical removal of the thyroid gland, the superior thyroid artery is ligated and resected more superiorly to the gland, away from its close proximity to the nerve. The structures in choices A, B, C, and E are not in close proximity to the external laryngeal nerve. The inferior thyroid artery (choice A) supplies the inferior pole of the thyroid gland. The recurrent laryngeal nerve (choice B) supplies internal laryngeal muscles. The second and third rings of the trachea (choice C) lie under the isthmus of the thyroid gland in the midline. The thyroid ima artery (choice E) supplies the anterior surface of the trachea and the isthmus of the thyroid gland.

82. **(A)** Catecholamines produced by the healthy adrenal medulla are epinephrine and, to a lesser extent, norepinephrine. However, many pheochromocytomas produce predominantly norepinephrine, resulting in α-adrenergic effects. Cardiac ischemia results from increased cardiac oxygen demand and coronary artery spasm. Systemic actions of catecholamines include increased glucose levels (choice B), increased blood pressure (choice C), and increased heart rate (choice D) through insulin suppression and enhanced gluconeogenesis. Sweat glands (choice E) are innervated by sympathetic fibers utilizing acetylcholine as the transmitter substance and are not directly stimulated by circulating catecholamines. However, the paroxysmal release of catecholamines precipitates a generalized activation of the sympathetic nervous system, and episodic profuse sweating is common in these patients.

83. **(E)** Tacrolimus, formerly known as FK506, is used in liver transplantation. It acts intracellularly by binding to a cytoplasmic FK506-binding protein, FKBP12, to form a complex that inhibits the calcium-stimulated phosphoprotein phosphatase calcineurin. Calcineurin is involved in translocation and activation of a T-cell transcription factor that is important in the expression of the genes for cytokines including IL-2 and the IL-2 receptor. The result is that tacrolimus prevents T-cell activation. Azathioprine (choice A) is converted to 6-mercaptopurine, which is metabolized to 6-mercaptopurine nucleotides that inhibit purine synthesis and purine salvage pathways. It is also metabolized to 6-thio-GTP, which damages DNA after incorporation thus preventing immune cell proliferation. Cyclophosphamide (choice B) is an antineoplastic alkylating agent that affects both T and B cells, but the primary effect is on suppression of humoral immunity, because the B-cell population is slower to

recover. Cyclosporine (choice C) works in much the same manner as tacrolimus, except that its cytoplasmic binding protein is cyclophilin. Prednisone (choice D) is a glucocorticoid used in immunosuppression. The glucocorticoids inhibit T-cell proliferation and the expression of cytokines. The mechanism listed, inhibition of IMP dehydrogenase, is the mechanism by which mycophenolic acid exerts its immunosuppressive actions.

84. **(A)** About 65% of hypertensive intracerebral hemorrhages occur within the basal ganglia or thalamus. Chronic hypertension predisposes to weakening of arteriole walls with subsequent production of Charcot–Bouchard aneurysms. A rupture of these aneurysms frequently results in fatal intracerebral hemorrhage. The cerebellum (choice B) is the site of hypertensive hemorrhage about 8% of the time. Hypertensive hemorrhages are very rare in the frontal lobe (choice C). Hypertensive hemorrhages are very rare in the occipital lobe (choice D). The pons (choice E) is the site of hypertensive hemorrhage about 15% of the time.

85. **(B)** Measles is a highly contagious childhood disease associated with a maculopapular rash, fever, and respiratory symptoms. Measles virus is an enveloped, single-stranded RNA, linear, nonsegmented, negative-polarity virus. Some types of herpesvirus (type 1, 3, 6) (choice A) and variola (choice E) are associated with production of rash. However, both variola and herpesvirus are double-stranded DNA viruses. Molluscum contagiosum virus (choice C) is an enveloped, double-stranded DNA virus that causes small, pink, papular wart-like, benign skin tumors. Papovaviruses (choice D) are double-stranded DNA viruses that cause lytic and transforming infections, warts, and cervical carcinoma.

86. **(A)** Cushing disease results from pituitary tumors that lead to the excess secretion of ACTH. Symptoms include obesity with central fat distribution, hypertension, glucose in-

tolerance, and gonadal dysfunction (amenorrhea or impotence). Additional clinical findings are moon-shaped facies, hirsutism, poor wound healing, acne, proximal muscle weakness, and superficial fungal infections. Other pituitary adenomas have been identified and some synthesize gonadotropins such as FSH (choice B), but they do not lead to elevated levels of secretion; others do lead to elevated secretion of TSH (choice E). Neither of these pituitary adenoma classes lead to the symptoms of Cushing disease or syndrome. Excess production of PRL (choice D) or GH (choice C) do not result in Cushing disease symptoms.

87. **(E)** Figure 10–10 depicts a large occlusive embolus in the pulmonary artery. Clinically, this finding is associated with sudden death in an individual with a hypercoagulable state or peripheral venous thrombi. Chronic idiopathic thrombocytopenic purpura (choice A) is an unlikely milieu to form thromboemboli due to the paucity of platelets. Likewise, with disseminated intravascular coagulation (choice B) there is a lack of both clotting factors and platelets, making thrombus formation improbable. The figure does not display an aneurysm (choice C) or a neoplasm (choice D).

88. **(A)** An important distinction is when a patient with renal insufficiency has "crossed the line" from pre-renal azotemia, where renal tubules are functioning but are not being adequately perfused, to acute renal failure, where the aforementioned hypoperfused renal tubules actually undergo necrosis. In the former case, a highly sodium avid state is manifest, hence the low FeNa. However, once acute renal failure has supervened, sodium transport ability is lost and choice A would be manifest.

89. **(E)** All of the drugs listed are used in gout. Probenecid is a uricosuric agent. Renal uric acid excretion is determined by the balance between the amount filtered plus that actively secreted and the amount undergoing passive and active reabsorption in the S_2 seg-

ment of the proximal tubule. At low doses, probenecid inhibits active secretion and thus promotes retention of uric acid. At higher (clinical) doses, both active secretion and active reabsorption are inhibited, with the result that excretion is enhanced. The decreased plasma level of uric acid reduces deposition of uric acid crystals or tophi. Allopurinol (choice A) and its metabolite alloxanthine inhibit xanthine oxidase, thus preventing conversion of xanthine and hypoxanthine to uric acid. Colchicine (choice B) is an inhibitor of microtubule function that brings relief in an acute gout attack by inhibiting the motility of granulocytes and reducing the formation of mediators of inflammation of leukocytes. Indomethacin (choice C) is an NSAID that, by inhibiting cyclooxygenase, prevents formation of prostaglandins and eicosanoids involved in the inflammatory process and pain perception in an acute episode of gouty arthritis. Piroxicam (choice D) is another NSAID; it has a long half-life that allows once-a-day dosing. Piroxicam is also used to treat rheumatoid arthritis and osteoarthritis.

90. **(E)** The structure of puromycin resembles that of the 3′ end of tyrosinyl-tRNA. The antibiotic is incorporated into the A-site of the ribosome, which interferes with subsequent peptide transfer leading to the premature termination of translation. Diphtheria toxin catalyzes the poly-ADP ribosylation of the translational elongation factor (eEF-2) (choice A). Cycloheximide inhibits the activity of eukaryotic peptidyltransferase (choice B). Tetracycline inhibits the binding of prokaryotic aminoacyl-tRNAs to the small ribosomal subunit (choice C). Chloramphenicol inhibits prokaryotic peptidyltransferase (choice D).

91. **(D)** Absence seizures (petit mal or "blank spells") are generalized seizures characterized by momentary loss of responsiveness, during which patients are unaware of their surroundings, but do not lose muscle tone. The EEG shows a characteristic "spike and dome" pattern with a frequency of 3 per second during these blank spells. Generalized

high-voltage spikes (choice A) are characteristic of grand mal seizures. Partial seizures of the temporal lobe (choice B) manifest complex automatic behaviorisms or may spread to become secondarily generalized grand mal attacks. REM-onset sleep (choice E) is characteristic of narcolepsy.

92. **(B)** Goodpasture syndrome consists of antibodies against basement membrane material, recurrent pulmonary hemorrhage, and glomerulonephritis. The pathologic changes are due to a type II hypersensitivity reaction along the basement membranes of the lung and kidney. Steroids, plasmapheresis, and immunosuppressive medicines may help in a minority of cases. Fibrosing alveolitis (choice A) is a pulmonary disorder of unknown etiology. Glomerulonephritis and pulmonary hemorrhage are not observed clinically. Kartagener syndrome (choice C) is a hereditary disease of infancy due to a defect in respiratory ciliary action. Systemic lupus erythematosus (choice D) may present with renal insufficiency. Antibodies are directed against nuclear antigens. Wegener granulomatosis (choice E) may present clinically with pulmonary hemorrhages and renal insufficiency. There are antibodies against neutrophil components, not basement membrane material.

93. **(C)** Paraquat is an herbicide that is nontoxic by inhalation or skin exposure, but causes lethal effects when ingested. Initial symptoms include nausea, with vomiting and diarrhea, but these give way to much slower and progressive pulmonary effects that are frequently lethal. There is no antidote for paraquat intoxication, so removal of the toxin from the GI tract as soon as possible after exposure is the best treatment. DDT (choice A) is an insecticide that interferes with sodium channel function. In humans, it causes neurologic abnormalities, including convulsions. Because of its very lipophilic nature, it accumulates in the food chain for predators and causes important reductions in reproductive capacity in these species. Dioxins (choice B) are contaminants of the herbicide 2,4,5-T ("agent orange"). The best-documented effect

of dioxins is chloracne and other dermatologic conditions, but the substance has been suspected of involvement in immunologic and hepatologic abnormalities and neoplastic disease. PCBs (choice D) have a poorly defined toxicity that includes dermatitis, hepatic alterations, and elevated triglycerides. Rotenone (choice E) is another insecticide that causes local irritation in humans, including conjunctivitis, dermatitis, rhinitis, and cough.

94. **(C)** The use of antibiotics in the treatment of urea cycle defects is related to the need to reduce the level of ammonia in the body. Antibiotics kill intestinal bacteria that produce ammonia, thereby reducing the level of ammonium ions that can be absorbed. Antibiotics do not acidify the intestinal tract and thus have no effect on ammonia ionization (choice A). Antibiotics do not complex intestinal ammonia (choice B). Phenylbutyrate and/or sodium butyrate are often administered to aid in ammonia reduction in urea cycle disorders as these compounds react with glutamine, the transamination byproduct of glutamate (choice D) forming phenylacetylglutamine and with glycine (choice E) forming hippurate, respectively. Antibiotics have no role in the conjugation of phenylbutyrate or sodium benzoate with nitrogenous compounds.

95. **(C)** This question is not meant to make you memorize wavelengths of various light colors, but rather to appreciate the complex relationship between objective wavelength of light and subjective color sensation and the active role the CNS plays in our perception of the world. Based on careful observation of our visual sensations and logical deductions, Helmholtz postulated in the 1860s the existence of three light receptors (blue, green, and red). When these were indeed discovered in 1965, it was found that the light absorption maxima were at 440, 535, and 565 nm, corresponding to blue, yellow-green, and orange. Nevertheless, the old names "blue," "green," and "red" were retained for historical purposes. Further processing of color information in the CNS results in opposition of red and green, as well as yellow and blue (i.e., neurons excited by green are inhibited by red, and so on). Any color of the spectrum can be generated by stimulating the three light receptors in ratios characteristic for each color. For example, yellow sensation is due to 1:1 stimulation of red and green receptors. Green sensation (choice A) is due to stimulation of blue, green, and red receptors at a ratio of 1:2:1 (arrow b), and red sensation is due to stimulation of red cones without simultaneous stimulation of green cones (arrow f). Light waves with a frequency equal to the peak response of red receptors (choice B) also stimulate green receptors and thereby elicit a sensation of orange. Color perception (choice D), although subjective, can be measured in an objective way using Ishihara charts or through color mixing. When mixing yellow from green and red light, patients with protanomaly (low levels of red pigment) require higher red levels than normal subjects to elicit a yellow sensation. The number of distinct retinal color receptors (choice E) is three, as postulated by Helmholtz, not four.

96. **(B)** All of the drugs listed are used in asthma but only the combination of beclomethasone and albuterol is rational as described. Beclomethasone is a very effective corticosteroid in preventing attacks, although it is not a bronchodilator. Used by the inhalation route, it has very low corticosteroid toxicity and can be used routinely. Albuterol is a very effective, short-acting, β_2-selective bronchodilator that should be used for acute symptoms, not on a regular 4-times-daily schedule. Aminophylline (choice A) is a long-acting bronchodilator that is rarely used except for control of nocturnal asthma. Prednisone (choice C) is a long-acting corticosteroid used orally for asthma that cannot be controlled with inhaled steroids. It should not be used unless inhaled steroids are inadequate. Terbutaline (choice D) and salmeterol are both β_2-selective adrenoreceptor agonists, but their roles are reversed in this answer. Terbutaline is short-acting and should only be used to control acute symptoms. Salmeterol is long acting (up

to 12 h) and should not be used for acute attacks. Zafirlukast (choice E) is an antagonist at the cysteinyl leukotriene LTC_4, LTD_4, and LTE_4 receptors. It provides significant relief from asthmatic symptoms with chronic use. This drug, like prednisone, is not a bronchodilator and is ineffective in acute episodes. Choice E provides no protection in case of an acute episode.

97. **(E)** The importance of the capsule in the virulence of the pneumococcus is apparent from the observations that only encapsulated strains are virulent, and vaccine efficacy is type specific (the organisms are divided into more than 80 types on the basis of antigenic differences in the capsular carbohydrate composition). Cell wall teichoic acids (choice A) and peptidoglycan (choice C) are found in pneumococci, and are not involved in the pathogenesis of pneumonia. M protein (choice B) is a potent antiphagocytic cell wall component of group A streptococci, not pneumococci. Pneumolysin (choice D) is a cytolytic enzyme for pneumococci, not human cells, and plays no important documented role in the pathogenesis of pneumonia.

98. **(B)** Coenzyme Q (also called ubiquinone) along with the flavins (FAD and FMN) can undergo either one- or two-electron transfer reactions. Cytochrome c (choice A) and the various nonheme irons (choice D) of the electron transport chain each participate in obligatory two-electron transfer reactions. Normal oxidation of NADH (choice C) is always a two-electron reaction, with the transfer of two hydride ions to a flavin.

99. **(E)** The cells in this photomicrograph are pleomorphic and invasive indicating their malignant character. Additionally, there are many intercellular bridges ("prickles") joining the cells indicating their squamous origin. Therefore, this is a squamous cell carcinoma. The presentation described is fairly typical for squamous cell carcinoma of the esophagus. Its development is closely associated with the risk factors of smoking and alcoholism. Adenocarcinoma of the esophagus (choice A) arises in the lower esophagus in a background of Barrett esophagus and is, of course, composed of malignant glandular cells, not the squamous cells seen here. Barrett esophagus (choice B) demonstrates metaplastic glandular epithelium. *Candida* esophagitis (choice C) is recognized by the presence of yeast and pseudohyphae. Fibrous stricture (choice D) can be caused, for example, by severe chronic reflux from ingestion of corrosives and produces fibrosis. Lye ingestion is associated with a 1000-fold increase in risk for squamous cell carcinoma.

100. **(A)** Cyanide binds to the iron of cytochrome oxidase (cytochrome aa_3). This is the same target as that of carbon monoxide. Cytochrome b (choice B) is oxidized when it in turn reduces cytochrome c_1 (choice C). Cytochrome oxidase is found in complex IV of the oxidative–phosphorylation pathway, not complex I (choice D) or complex II (choice E).

REFERENCES

Aidley DJ. *The Physiology of Excitable Cells*, 4th ed. Cambridge, England: Cambridge University Press; 1998.

Berne RM, Levy MN. *Physiology*, 4th ed. St. Louis: Mosby-Year Book; 1998.

Braunwald E, Fauci AS, Kasper DL, et al. *Harrison's Principles of Internal Medicine*, 15th ed. New York: McGraw-Hill; 2001.

Brooks GF, Butel JS, Morse SA. *Jawetz, Melnick, and Adelberg's Medical Microbiology*, 22nd ed. Stamford, CT: Appleton & Lange; 2001.

Chandrasoma P, Taylor CR. *Concise Pathology*, 3rd ed. Stamford, CT: Appleton & Lange; 1998.

Devlin TM. *Textbook of Biochemistry: With Clinical Correlations*, 4th ed. New York: John Wiley & Sons; 1997.

Elkin GD. *Introduction to Clinical Psychiatry*. Stamford, CT: Appleton & Lange; 1998.

Ganong WF. *Review of Medical Physiology*, 20th ed. Stamford, CT: Appleton & Lange; 2001.

Guyton AC, Hall JE. *Textbook of Medical Physiology*, 10th ed. Philadelphia: WB Saunders; 2000.

Hall-Craggs ECB. *Anatomy as a Basis for Clinical Medicine*, 3rd ed. Baltimore: Williams & Wilkins; 1995.

Hardman JG, Limbird LE, Molinoff PB, et al. *Goodman & Gilman's The Pharmacological Basis of Therapeutics*, 9th ed. New York: McGraw-Hill; 1996.

Johnson LR. *Gastrointestinal Physiology*, 5th ed. St. Louis: Mosby-Year Book; 1997.

Kandel ER, Schwartz JH, Jessel TM. *Principles of Neural Science*, 5th ed. Stamford, CT: Appleton & Lange; 2000.

Kaplan HI, Sadock BJ. *Comprehensive Textbook of Psychiatry/VI CD-ROM*. Teton Data Systems, Jackson, Wyoming, Baltimore: Williams & Wilkins; 1998.

Kaplan HI, Sadock BJ. *Kaplan and Sadock's Synopsis of Psychiatry*, 8th ed. Baltimore: Williams & Wilkins; 1998.

Katzung BG. *Basic & Clinical Pharmacology*, 8th ed. Stamford, CT: Appleton & Lange; 2001.

Leigh H, Reiser MF. *The Patient: Biological, Psychological, and Social Dimensions of Medical Practice*, 3rd ed. New York: Plenum Press; 1992.

Levinson WE, Jawetz E. *Medical Microbiology & Immunology: Examination and Board Review*, 6th ed. Stamford, CT: Appleton & Lange; 2000.

Lewis WH, Elvin-Lewis MPF. *Medical Botany*. New York: John Wiley & Sons; 1977.

McArdle WD, Katch FI, Katch VL. *Exercise Physiology: Energy, Nutrition, and Human Performance*, 4th ed. Philadelphia: Lea & Febiger; 1996.

Moore KL. *Clinically Oriented Anatomy*, 3rd ed. Baltimore: Williams & Wilkins; 1992.

Mountcastle VB. *Medical Physiology*, 14th ed. St. Louis: Mosby-Year Book; 1980.

Murray PR, Rosenthal KS, Kobayashi GS, Pfaller MA. *Medical Microbiology*, 3rd ed. St. Louis: Mosby-Year Book; 1998.

Murray RK, Granner DK, Mayes PA, Rodwell VW. *Harper's Biochemistry*, 25th ed. Stamford, CT: Appleton & Lange; 2000.

Roitt I, Brostoff J, Male D. *Immunology*, 5th ed. London, UK: Mosby-Year Book; 1998.

Rose DB, Post T. *Clinical Physiology of Acid-base and Electrolyte Disorders*, 6th ed. New York: McGraw-Hill; 2001.

Rosse C, Gaddum-Rosse P. *Hollinshead's Textbook of Anatomy*, 5th ed. Philadelphia: Lippincott Raven Publishers; 1997.

Rubin F, Farber JL. *Pathology*, 3rd ed. Philadelphia: JB Lippincott; 1999.

Vander AJ. *Renal Physiology*, 5th ed. New York: McGraw-Hill; 1995.

West JB. *Pulmonary Pathophysiology—The Essentials*, 5th ed. Baltimore: Williams & Wilkins; 1998.

Woodburne RT, Burckel WE. *Essentials of Human Anatomy*, 9th ed. New York: Oxford University Press; 1994.

Subspecialty List: Practice Test III

Question Number and Subspecialty

1. Pathology
2. Pathology
3. Anatomy
4. Microbiology
5. Anatomy
6. Biochemistry
7. Physiology
8. Pharmacology
9. Microbiology
10. Pharmacology
11. Biochemistry
12. Pathology
13. Anatomy
14. Microbiology
15. Behavioral sciences
16. Biochemistry
17. Pharmacology
18. Microbiology
19. Pharmacology
20. Physiology
21. Physiology
22. Physiology
23. Biochemistry
24. Microbiology
25. Anatomy
26. Anatomy
27. Pathology
28. Pathology
29. Pharmacology
30. Behavioral sciences
31. Microbiology
32. Anatomy
33. Pharmacology
34. Biochemistry
35. Pharmacology
36. Microbiology
37. Anatomy
38. Anatomy
39. Biochemistry
40. Physiology
41. Pathology
42. Pharmacology
43. Microbiology
44. Anatomy
45. Biochemistry
46. Pathology
47. Pharmacology
48. Biochemistry
49. Microbiology
50. Physiology
51. Anatomy
52. Biochemistry
53. Anatomy
54. Pathology
55. Behavioral sciences
56. Behavioral sciences
57. Behavioral sciences
58. Microbiology
59. Pharmacology
60. Pathology
61. Biochemistry
62. Anatomy
63. Pharmacology
64. Physiology
65. Biochemistry
66. Pathology
67. Anatomy
68. Microbiology
69. Behavioral sciences
70. Biochemistry
71. Physiology
72. Pharmacology
73. Pathology
74. Anatomy

Path – 16   Anat – 15

Neuro – 14

Bioh – 18 A

Physiol – 13

Pharma – 18

Behar – 6

75. Biochemistry
76. Physiology
77. Pharmacology
78. Pathology
79. Microbiology
80. Pharmacology
81. Anatomy
82. Physiology
83. Pharmacology
84. Pathology
85. Microbiology
86. Biochemistry
87. Pathology

88. Physiology
89. Pharmacology
90. Biochemistry
91. Physiology
92. Pathology
93. Pharmacology
94. Biochemistry
95. Physiology
96. Pharmacology
97. Microbiology
98. Biochemistry
99. Pathology
100. Biochemistry